HEALTH ASSESSMENT
for NURSING PRACTICE

Dr. Thompson has 25 years of experience in the field of nursing, and has been teaching and performing health assessment for 20 of those years. In the late 1970s Dr. Thompson coordinated one of the first nurse practitioner programs in the country at Ohio State University. In that capacity, she, along with other nursing and physician colleagues, defined health assessment that was appropriate and comprehensive for advanced nursing practice. Out of that experience Dr. Thompson co-authored Mosby's nursing health assessment text, Clinical Manual for Health Assessment. The four editions of the text matured along with the field of nursing as health assessment evolved into a core component of both basic and advanced nursing practice. Over the past 20 years, Dr. Thompson has taught hundreds of undergraduate and graduate nursing students the principles and techniques of health assessment. This new text is a synthesis of all that she has learned about health assessment and about teaching health assessment, as well as how to handle the problems and pitfalls that she knows students will experience in learning health assessment.

Dr. Wilson, a family nurse practitioner with a PhD in education, has 28 years of teaching experience, including 20 years of teaching health assessment. She has also taught adult and critical care nursing didactic courses. She has cared for adult clients in a variety of settings from critical care to rehabilitation. Dr. Wilson has supervised undergraduate and graduate students in the care of clients in hospital and clinical settings. In addition to her teaching and administrative duties at Texas Christian University, she currently works as a family nurse practitioner in the office of a family practice physician.

HEALTH ASSESSMENT *for* NURSING PRACTICE

June M. Thompson, RN, DrPH
New Mexico Department of Health,
Division of Epidemiology, Planning and Evaluation,
Santa Fe, New Mexico;
Clinical Nursing Affiliations,
University of New Mexico
  Health Sciences Center Hospital,
Albuquerque, New Mexico

Susan F. Wilson, RN, PhD, FNP
Associate Professor,
Harris College of Nursing,
Texas Christian University,
Fort Worth, Texas;
Family Nurse Practitioner,
Medical Center at Riverside,
Grand Prairie, Texas

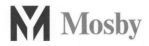

St. Louis Baltimore Boston Carlsbad Chicago Naples New York Philadelphia Portland
London Madrid Mexico City Singapore Sydney Tokyo Toronto Wiesbaden

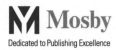
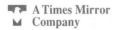

A Times Mirror
Company

Publisher: *Nancy L. Coon*
Senior Editor: *Sally Schrefer*
Developmental Editor: *Gail Brower*
Project Manager: *Dana Peick*
Production Editor: *Cindy Deichmann*
Designer: *Amy Buxton*
Manufacturing Manager: *Betty Richmond*
Cover Photographs: *Bill Leslie*
Cover Design: *Amy Buxton & Bill Leslie*

Printed in the United States of America
Composition by TSI Graphics
Printing/binding by Von Hoffman Press

Mosby-Year Book, Inc.
11830 Westline Industrial Drive
St. Louis, Missouri 63146

International Standard Book Number 0-8151-8774-2

96 97 98 99 00 / 9 8 7 6 5 4 3 2 1

Contributors

Susan R. Carlson, RNC, MSN, CCRN
Nursing Instructor,
Harris College of Nursing,
Texas Christian University,
Fort Worth, Texas

Linda Cox Curry, RN, BSN, MN, PhD
Associate Professor,
Harris College of Nursing,
Texas Christian University,
Fort Worth, Texas

Frances C. Gaskin, RN, PhD
President and Chief Executive Officer,
Frances Christian Gaskin, Inc.,
Albany, New York;
Former Director and Professor of Nursing,
Hostos Community College of the City University
    of New York,
New York, New York

Melanie Gillingham, MS, RD
Clinical Dietitian,
Department of Nutrition and
    Foodservice,
St. Francis Hospital,
Tulsa, Oklahoma

Rae Langford, RN, MS, EdD
Private Practice,
Rehabilitation Nurse Consultant,
Houston, Texas

Elizabeth Petit de Mange, RN, MSN, PhD(c)
Instructor of Nursing,
College of Allied Health/Nursing,
Thomas Jefferson University,
Philadelphia, Pennsylvania

Joy Graham Stone, RN, MN, CS
Administrator,
Summit Home Health Service,
Fort Worth, Texas

Katherine S. Vance, RD, LD, CNSD
Clinical Dietician,
Department of Nutrition and
    Foodservice,
St. Francis Hospital,
Tulsa, Oklahoma

Kerstin West-Wilson, RNC, MS
Clinical Research Coordinator,
Eastern Oklahoma Perinatal Center,
St. Francis Hospital,
Tulsa, Oklahoma

Earl Goldberg, MSN, RN, CS
Associate Professor of Nursing,
Bucks County Community College,
Newtown, Pennsylvania

Barbara C. Martin, RNC, EdD
Assistant Professor,
Nursing Department,
Southern Illinois University at Edwardsville,
Edwardsville, Illinois

La Vone M. Sopher, MSN, ARNP, FNP
Associate Professor,
Department of Nursing Education,
Morningside College,
Sioux City, Iowa

Darla R. Ura, RN, MA
Assistant Professor,
Nell Hodgson Woodruff School of Nursing,
Emory University,
Atlanta, Georgia

Thomas Worms
Assistant Professor,
Department of Nursing,
Truman College,
Chicago, Illinois

Johanna Yurkow, MSN, RN, CS
Director of Clinical Services,
CARE Program,
University of Pennsylvania School of Nursing,
Philadelphia, Pennsylvania

To my mother, Lillian M. Danner
I share the words of Kahlil Gibran,
"You may forget the one with whom you laughed,
but never the one with whom you have wept."
JMT

To Sara Borden, Skip, and Megan
for their continued love, patience, and support
&'to all the exceptional teachers, colleagues, and
students who have taught me through the years.
SFW

If a teacher is indeed wise, he does not bid you enter the house of his wisdom, but rather leads you to the threshold of your own mind.

Kahlil Gibran
The Prophet

So, following this teaching, we have written this text of *Health Assessment for Nursing Practice.* In doing so, we have presented a vast amount of information. It includes growth and development, how to use specific pieces of equipment, how to assess clients of various racial and cultural groups across the lifespan, how to assess clients with special needs, how to promote health and reduce the risk of illness or injury, and how to synthesize information using nursing diagnoses.

UNDERLYING PRINCIPLES

This text is based on the assumption that every client is an interactive, complex being who is more than a collection of his or her parts. Each client's health status depends on the interaction of physiologic, sociocultural, psychologic, and spiritual factors. No person is in this world alone. As living persons we all interact with our environment through what we eat, what kind of activity and work we participate in, where we live, our friends, our family, how we care for our bodies and our health, and when and how we seek health care consultation.

As nurses and health care professionals we are challenged with several responsibilities. First, we are challenged to be knowledgeable and skilled. Second, we are challenged to be objective, nonjudgmental, and to use our knowledge and skill wisely to gather and synthesize an enormous amount of information about the client and the family. And finally, we are challenged to assist clients to mobilize their own resources to optimize their own level of health. This textbook is a *toolbox of information and techniques.* You are challenged to use the threshold of your own mind and potential to use this information to meet these three challenges of responsibility.

ORGANIZATION OF THE BOOK

The textbook is organized into 23 chapters, ranging from overview information to very specific procedures and techniques. Consider each chapter as a different type of tool in the tool box. Collectively, they provide all that you will need to do the work of performing a comprehensive health assessment.

Chapter 1 tells you in a nutshell why you need to learn health assessment.

Chapter 2 presents information on developmental stages that is useful when assessing the client's health status.

Chapter 3 summarizes racial and cultural information that you may find helpful when working with clients and families who are of a culture other than your own.

Chapter 4 guides you through the necessary steps of collecting a comprehensive health history.

Chapter 5 presents detailed information about the equipment that you will need to perform a physical examination.

Chapter 6 teaches you the techniques you will need to know when performing a physical examination.

Chapter 7 provides information on how to perform a systematic nutritional assessment for all ages.

Chapters 8 through 22 provide in-depth history questions with rationales and physical examination techniques with normal and abnormal findings for each body system, along with additional essential content.

Chapter 23 provides the guidelines for putting all of the body system assessments together into one comprehensive examination. It is the integrated finished product, the threshold. A special section on documentation is included.

SPECIAL FEATURES

The 15 chapters that make up the detailed body system assessment chapters have all been developed exactly the same. This provides continuity across chapters and makes information easy to retrieve. Each chapter highlights case examples, nursing diagnoses, specific age variations, ethnic and cultural considerations, health promotion, and a section for clients with special health care needs.

Throughout these chapters are special boxes of information. Some of the boxes include racial or cultural variations. Others include nuggets of information that may assist with an examination procedure or provide factual information that should be factored into the examination.

The following map shows how each clinical chapter is laid out.

■ Anatomy and Physiology ■

The presentation starts with a discussion of the anatomy and physiology of the particular body system and the normal functioning for adults. Following is a discussion about specific variations for infants, children, adolescents, older adults, and pregnant women.

■ History ■

This section presents specific questions that allow you to determine the client's problems, questions, and concerns, as well as to discover their risks for certain health problems. A two-column format is used, with the question on the left and the rationale for asking the question on the right. Following the history questions for the adult are the history sections for specific age groups: infants, children, adolescents, older adults, and, if applicable, pregnant women.

■ Examination Procedures and Findings ■

This section begins with boxed information about the general approach you should consider for the examination of the specific body system, as well as the equipment you will need. The section then sequentially presents the techniques of performing the physical examination, telling you what to do, how to do it, and what you should expect to find. Photographs are provided to enhance your learning. The left-hand column details the techniques of the examination and the normal findings; the right-hand column presents abnormal findings you may encounter. Following this section for examination of adults are sections for all other groups of clients in the lifespan, as well as clients with special situations or cultural diversity.

■ Age-Related Variations ■

This section includes special approaches to clients related to their specific age group and also presents examination findings that are different for that age group.

■ Clients with Situational Variations ■

This unique section includes information about clients with special health problems or situations. The most obvious group is pregnant women, who have time-limited special variations. Examples of other clients who have been included in this section are those with paralysis, individuals with HIV or AIDS, blind or hearing-impaired clients, and clients who have had a mastectomy. In each case, information is presented about unique approaches to use when working with these clients, as well as variations of the examination findings.

■ Ethnic and Cultural Variations ■

This section builds on the information in Chapter 3. Information is presented about the unique approaches that should be considered when examining clients of various racial and cultural groups, as well as variations in examination findings that may be noted for each specific body system or region.

■ Examination Summary ■

This boxed information provides a summary outline of the *order* in which the examination should be performed and *what* to assess for the designated body system.

■ Common Problems ■

This section is an extension of the abnormal findings column in the examination procedures section. Presented is more detailed information about many of the common problems or conditions that are associated with the body system. Numerous illustrations and photographs are provided as examples.

■ Sample Documentation and Nursing Diagnosis ■

In each clinical chapter, two sample cases are presented. These cases provide a client's history (subjective data) and physical examination (objective data) findings and nursing diagnoses that may be derived from the data. The cases demonstrate the type of information that should be collected, serve as excellent examples of proper documentation, and illustrate how appropriate nursing diagnoses are determined.

■ Health Promotion ■

Because many health care problems can be prevented, this section provides recommendations for teaching health promotion to clients. The health history and physical assessment are opportune times for client teaching.

■ Study Questions ■

No text would be worth its weight in gold if it did not present a mechanism for the student to critically evaluate his or her own understanding of the information presented. At the end of every chapter are questions that should challenge your critical thinking and synthesis of the information presented. Whereas many of these questions may be used to evaluate your own understanding of the information in the chapter, they may also be very effectively used in a study or discussion group.

We have presented the information; now you the student are invited and challenged to take this information and use it to your fullest and most creative potential.

June M. Thompson
Susan F. Wilson

Ancillary Package

INSTRUCTOR'S RESOURCE KIT

The Instructor's Resource Kit includes student learning objectives, lecture outlines, learning activities, a test bank of more than 550 multiple choice questions, answers to study questions in the textbook, laboratory checklists, physical examination video summaries, and physical examination interactive videodisc summaries.

TRANSPARENCY ACETATES

Full-color transparency acetates of key illustrations enhance lectures.

AUDIOTAPE OF HEART & LUNG SOUNDS

An audiotape of heart and lung sounds is packaged free with each copy of the text so students can learn normal and common abnormal heart and lung sounds.

MOSBY'S PHYSICAL EXAMINATION VIDEO SERIES

Innovative, thorough, and expertly produced, Mosby's Physical Examination Video Series brings the physical examination process to life. Twenty-four individual videotapes, including *Putting It All Together,* provide a comprehensive visual package for learning how to perform a complete and effective physical examination.

MOSBY'S PHYSICAL EXAMINATION INTERACTIVE VIDEODISC SERIES

This innovative videodisc series provides students with an opportunity to practice "hands-on" physical examination techniques in a simulated setting. Each program contains a technique lab where the learner can review and practice a variety of techniques for physical examination of the body system presented. The second section of the program then presents case studies where the student can evaluate findings from a physical examination. Learners may view the case studies in case study mode (examination with questions), preview mode (view the total examination without interruption), or mentor mode (view the examination with evaluation by an expert) at the end of the case study.

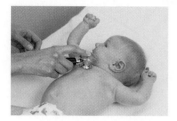

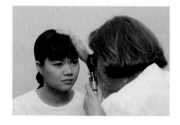

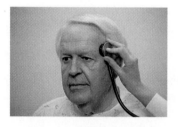

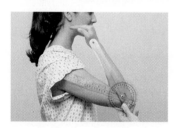

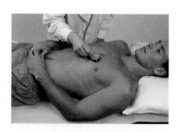

1 Why Learn Health Assessment? *1*

2 Developmental Assessment Through the Life Span, *7*

3 Ethnic and Cultural Considerations, *27*

4 Interviewing to Obtain a Health History, *39*

5 Equipment for Physical Assessment, *61*

6 Techniques of Physical Assessment, *73*

7 Nutritional Assessment, *93*

8 Skin, Hair, and Nails, *115*

9 Lymphatic System, *165*

10 Head and Neck, *185*

11 Nose, Paranasal Sinuses, Mouth, and Oropharynx, *213*

12 Ears and Auditory System, *247*

Contents

13 Eyes and Visual System, *277*

14 Lungs and Respiratory System, *317*

15 Heart and Peripheral Vascular System, *359*

16 Breasts and Axillae, *401*

17 Abdomen and Gastrointestinal System, *437*

18 Female Genitalia and Reproductive System, *481*

19 Male Genitalia, *531*

20 Anus, Rectum, and Prostate, *559*

21 Musculoskeletal System, *683*

22 Neurologic System and Mental Status, *637*

23 Head-to-Toe Examination and Documentation, *685*

APPENDICES

A Sample documentation (adult and child), *701*

B American Nurses Association (ANA) Screening Guidelines, *708*

C Alphabetical List of North American Nursing Diagnosis Association (NANDA) Diagnoses, *712*

D Conversion Tables, *717*

E Conversion Factors to International System of Units (SI Units), *718*

F Abbreviations, *720*

GLOSSARY, *723*

HEALTH ASSESSMENT
for
NURSING PRACTICE

CHAPTER 1

Why Learn Health Assessment?

You are sitting at the clinic desk and a woman with mussed hair and a distressed look on her face tells you that she needs to see someone. You ask her what she needs and she starts to cry softly. She quickly goes on to tell you that she has a headache that won't go away, that she can't keep going on like this, that she can't eat or sleep, and that she hurts all over. As you take a careful look at her, you note that she has bruises on the side of her face and that her lower lip is swollen and split open. You sit back in your chair and the wheels of your mind turn. What do you think? What should you do?*

Every time you interact with a client, a family, or the parents of a young child, you will perform some type of assessment. The nursing process as endorsed by the American Nurses Association (ANA, 1991) includes the steps of *assessment, diagnosis, outcome identification, planning, implementation,* and *evaluation* (see box at right). The first, and foundational, step is assessment. *Assessment* is defined by the ANA as "a systematic, dynamic process by which the nurse, through interaction with the client, significant others, and health care providers, collects and analyzes data about the client." Note that there are two steps in the assessment process. The first involves the collection of data (see box on p. 2), and the second involves the interpretation or analysis of the data. These two components of the assessment process are used differently by nurses in different settings and with different levels of expertise and experience.

Now consider the case presented above. What do you do with the information the client tells you (symptoms) and the physical observations you see (signs) (see box on p. 2)?

- If the nurse is new to the profession and has not had much experience, he or she may collect initial data and "go get help" for the client from someone with more experience.

*Thanks to Vicki Flynn, SN from Madison, Connecticut, for the idea of this case presentation. She believes that every nurse should be alert to the subtle signs and symptoms of domestic violence. We couldn't agree more, and think this example shows the subtle way that a client may present with a significant problem. Thanks, Vicki.

The Nursing Process

Assessment
A systematic, dynamic process by which the nurse, through interaction with the client, significant others, and health care providers, collects and analyzes data about the client.

Diagnosis
A clinical judgment about the client's response to actual or potential health conditions or needs based on an analysis of the data collected.

Outcome Identification
Accomplished by establishing measurable, expected, client-focused goals to meet the client's needs or improve his or her health condition.

Planning
Creating a plan of care that is a comprehensive outline of care to be delivered to attain the outcomes.

Implementation
May include activities or interventions needed to attain the outcome. The client, significant other, or health care provider may be designated to implement the intervention within the plan of care.

Evaluation
The process of determining both the client's progress toward the attainment of expected outcomes and the effectiveness of nursing care.

Modified from American Nurses Association: Standards of clinical nursing practice, *Washington, DC, 1991, The Association.*

- More experienced nurses may interact with the client and collect more information about each of the client's signs and symptoms, and may then determine what clinic and what type of health care provider may best assist the client to ensure correct and timely care.
- The very experienced nurse may reach into his or her past experience, question the client further about the possibility of domestic abuse, determine appropriate referrals,

---

Types of Health Assessment Data

Subjective Data

Those things told to the nurse by clients when asked to describe their current state of health, their previous illnesses and surgeries, and their family history. If the subjective data are acquired from a family member instead of from the client himself or herself, it is referred to as a secondary source of data. Subjective data may also be referred to as the *history*.

Objective Data

Data collected from a variety of data sources. During a physical examination, data are obtained using the techniques of inspection, palpation, percussion, and auscultation. Additional data include measurements of the client's height, weight, pulse, blood pressure, temperature, and respiratory rate. Other sources of objective data include urine, blood, other body excretions, x-rays, and imaging.

Signs and Symptoms

Symptoms

Data that the client or family tell the nurse. They include subjective information about the problem or situation. Examples are pain or itching.

Signs

Data that are observed, felt, heard, or measured by the nurse. They include the objective information or findings collected by the examiner about a problem or situation. Examples of signs are fever, rash, enlarged lymph nodes, or muscle weakness.

---

and ensure that the client receives appropriate immediate care, as well as appropriate follow-up and community referrals.

■ If the nurse is a nurse practitioner or clinical nurse specialist responsible for case management, he or she may perform both in-depth subjective (the history) and objective (the physical examination) data collection, determine appropriate interventions, and actually manage the client's total care both during this and future clinic visits, as well as make and possibly coordinate the appropriate community referrals.

While all the nurses just listed performed some type of assessment, each handled the situation slightly differently based on his or her knowledge and experience. The client provided the same initial signs and symptoms to each nurse. Each nurse, however, collected and analyzed the data slightly differently.

The reason that it is important for you to learn health assessment is that professional nurses have a responsibility to (1) systematically collect objective and subjective information *(assessment)* about the client; (2) make a clinical judgment *(diagnosis)* about the actual or potential health condition or needs of the client; (3) identify the desired outcomes *(outcome identification)* with goals to meet the client's needs or improve the client's health condition; (4) create a comprehensive plan of care *(planning)* to attain the desired outcomes; (5) implement the plan of action *(implementation);* and finally, (6) evaluate the interventions *(evaluation)* to determine the client's progress toward or attainment of the goals (ANA, 1991). These steps of the nursing process are the steps of professional nursing. The first step, *assessment,* is the foundation of all other steps. Without the ability to systematically collect and synthesize information, the entire nursing process is weakened. So whether you are dealing with a client like the one described, dealing with a client in the intensive care unit (ICU) who has a sudden onset of shortness of breath and pink frothy sputum, or whether you are performing a "well" evaluation or "check-up" of a 50-year-old

American Indian man, the first and foundational step of your interaction is always *assessment*. How well you are able to perform this step, and the data patterns identified and inferences made, will determine your abilities as a professional nurse.

WHAT HEALTH ASSESSMENT TELLS US

Health assessment provides a systematic method of collecting all types of data that identify the client's strengths, weaknesses, physiologic status, knowledge, motivation, support systems, and coping ability that may influence the client's health either positively or negatively. The nurse collects information and compares the client's state of health to the ideal state of health for the individual, taking into account the client's age, gender, culture, and physical, psychologic, and socioeconomic status. The weaknesses, problems, or deficits found should guide the plan for assisting the client to maximize his or her health potential. For example, if a 42-year-old Hispanic man is admitted to the hospital for pneumonia and the nurse notices his cholesterol is 260, the nurse should follow the therapeutic medical plan for the pneumonia in addition to developing a nursing plan based on a comprehensive assessment of the client's disease state and his response to the medical treatment. When the time is appropriate and the client is receptive, the nurse teaches the importance of lowering cholesterol and ways to accomplish this through diet and exercise.

WHAT HEALTH ASSESSMENT IS PERFORMED WHERE?

Let's be realistic about where and to what extent health assessment is performed. Many times the student is led to believe that every client in every situation needs a full and complete health assessment performed. Don't believe this; it's unrealistic. What is true is that the nurse must always have within his or her repertoire the complete profile of health assessment questions and examination techniques, so that when the situation presents itself to actually conduct an assessment, the possibilities of data collection suit themselves to the situation. The point of this discussion will become obvious when you reach Chapter 4 of this text, "Interviewing to Obtain a Health History." For pages upon pages you will be taught the spectrum of history questions that may be asked. It is not intended that you ask every client you care for every question on every page. What is important is that you know and learn all of these questions so that when the situation presents itself you will know what to ask, how to ask it, and what the client's response means. Certainly clinical judgment is needed to ensure that the complete complement of questions is asked for any given situation. For example, if you are performing a complete comprehensive health assessment with a client for the first time in a well-client setting, you will want to collect comprehensive subjective and objective information. On the other hand, if you are working in an episodic care clinic or emergency department and the client presents with burns on her hand and chest, that is not the time to conduct a comprehensive assessment. It is important, however, to conduct a focused assessment ensuring comprehensive data collection about all subjective and objective elements that may have direct or indirect impact on the management of the client's burn and potential risk for future injury. For example, it would be important to inquire about last tetanus injection, chronic medical conditions, current medications being taken, and so forth. In addition, if you assess the client to be at risk or in need of further health assessment evaluation, it is very important that the client be referred to a more appropriate site at a later date so that a comprehensive assessment may be made.

health beliefs, and activities to maintain health, as well as his or her health problems and lack of resources for maintaining health.

Now consider the woman who presented at the clinic desk in the beginning of this chapter. This women—let's call her Stacy—has more than mussed hair, a distressed face, headache, facial bruises, a split lip, and general body aching. Stacy is a woman with a physical, psychologic, emotional, spiritual, and socioenvironmental history. Different nurses with different knowledge and skills may interact with Stacy differently. It will not be until some health care professional takes the time to systematically collect comprehensive *health assessment* information about all aspects of Stacy's presenting situation, as well as her motivation for seeking care, that the next steps, beginning with *nursing diagnosis* (see box on pp. 4-5), may be taken.

You are now challenged to diligently study this health assessment text to learn how and when to collect and use both subjective and objective data so that you can be the best nurse possible. Someday you may be the client walking up to the clinic desk and sharing a very difficult problem with the nurse behind the desk. If you are the client, then what you need is for that nurse to be prepared and to collect accurate and comprehensive health assessment data about you, to make accurate clinical judgments about your situation, and to develop an intervention to assist you or to provide care that will improve your actual or potential health status. If the nurse is able to do this, then you will have been well served. An accurate and comprehensive health assessment is indeed one of the important cornerstones of the art and science of professional nursing.

WHAT DO YOU DO WITH ALL THESE DATA?

Subjective and objective data collected from the client and inferences made from data collection are used to initiate a nursing process. This is usually done by documenting the information for use by other health care providers. Complete, accurate, and descriptive documentation of health assessment improves the effectiveness of the entire health care team. Documenting these data also prevents the client from having to provide the same information to another health care provider. The written record serves as a legal document and permanent record of the client's health status at the time of the nurse-client interaction. Thus it serves as a baseline for evaluation of subsequent changes and decisions related to care. Using an outline of data to collect and taking brief notes during the encounter will facilitate the documentation and increase its accuracy. Recorded data must be written concisely, without bias or opinion by the nurse.

The outcome of a health assessment entails a portrait of the client with his or her strengths, abilities, support systems,

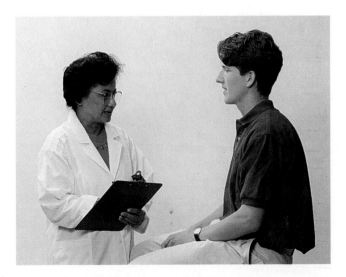

The written record serves as a legal document and permanent record of the client's health status at the time of the nurse-client interaction.

Alphabetic List of NANDA Diagnoses, 1995-1996

Activity intolerance
Activity intolerance, risk for
Adaptive capacity, decreased: intracranial
Adjustment, impaired
Airway clearance, ineffective
Anxiety
Aspiration, risk for
Body image disturbance
Body temperature, altered, risk for
Bowel incontinence
Breastfeeding, effective
Breastfeeding, ineffective
Breastfeeding, interrupted
Breathing pattern, ineffective
Cardiac output, decreased
Caregiver role strain
Caregiver role strain, risk for
Communication, impaired verbal
Community coping, potential for enhanced
Community coping, ineffective
Confusion, acute
Confusion, chronic
Constipation
Constipation, colonic
Constipation, perceived
Coping, defensive
Coping, family: potential for growth
Coping, ineffective family: compromised
Coping, ineffective family: disabling
Coping, ineffective individual
Decisional conflict (specify)
Denial, ineffective
Diarrhea
Disuse syndrome, risk for
Diversional activity deficit
Dysreflexia
Energy field disturbance
Environmental interpretation syndrome, impaired
Family processes, altered: alcoholism
Family processes, altered
Fatigue
Fear
Fluid volume deficit
Fluid volume deficit (2)
Fluid volume deficit, risk for
Fluid volume excess
Gas exchange, impaired
Grieving, anticipatory
Grieving, dysfunctional
Growth and development, altered
Health maintenance, altered
Health-seeking behaviors (specify)
Home maintenance management, impaired
Hopelessness
Hyperthermia
Hypothermia
Incontinence, functional
Incontinence, reflex
Incontinence, stress
Incontinence, total
Incontinence, urge
Infant behavior, disorganized

Infant behavior, disorganized: risk for
Infant behavior, organized: potential for enhanced
Infant feeding pattern, ineffective
Infection, risk for
Injury, perioperative positioning: risk for
Injury, risk for
Knowledge deficit (specify)
Loneliness, risk for
Management of therapeutic regimen, community: ineffective
Management of therapeutic regimen, families: ineffective
Management of therapeutic regimen, individuals: effective
Management of therapeutic regimen, individuals: ineffective
Memory, impaired
Mobility, impaired physical
Noncompliance (specify)
Nutrition, altered: less than body requirements
Nutrition, altered: more than body requirements
Nutrition, altered: risk for more than body requirements
Oral mucous membrane, altered
Pain
Pain, chronic
Parent/Infant/Child attachment, altered, risk for
Parental role conflict
Parenting, altered
Parenting, altered, risk for
Peripheral neurovascular dysfunction, risk for
Personal identity disturbance
Poisoning, risk for
Post-trauma syndrome
Rape-trauma syndrome
Rape-trauma syndrome: compound reaction
Rape-trauma syndrome: silent reaction
Relocation stress syndrome
Role performance, altered
Self-care deficit, bathing/hygiene
Self-care deficit, dressing/grooming
Self-care deficit, feeding
Self-care deficit, toileting
Self-esteem disturbance
Self-esteem, chronic low
Self-esteem, situational low
Self-mutilation, risk for
Sensory/perceptual alterations (specify) (visual, auditory, kinesthetic, gustatory, tactile, olfactory)
Sexual dysfunction
Sexuality patterns, altered
Skin integrity, impaired
Skin integrity, impaired, risk for
Sleep pattern disturbance
Social interaction, impaired
Social isolation
Spiritual distress (distress of the human spirit)
Spiritual well-being, potential for enhanced
Suffocation, risk for
Swallowing, impaired
Thermoregulation, ineffective
Thought processes, altered

Alphabetic List of NANDA Diagnoses, 1995-1996—*cont'd*	
Tissue integrity, impaired Tissue perfusion, altered (specify type)(renal, cerebral, cardiopulmonary, gastrointestinal, peripheral) Trauma, risk for Unilateral neglect	Urinary elimination, altered Urinary retention Ventilation, inability to sustain spontaneous Ventilatory weaning process, dysfunctional Violence, risk for: self-directed or directed at others

From NANDA: Proceedings of the eleventh national conference of the North American Nursing Diagnosis Association, *1994, The Association.*

??????? STUDY QUESTIONS ???????

1. Why is health assessment an important tool in nursing?
2. Identify and describe the steps in the nursing process.
3. Distinguish between subjective and objective data. Give two examples of each.
4. Differentiate a sign from a symptom. Identify each of the following as a sign or a symptom: headache, fever, nausea, vomiting, fatigue, muscle weakness.
5. Describe when you might choose to do a complete profile of health assessment questions and examination techniques. Cite a situation where a complete assessment is not appropriate.

6. What are three purposes of the written medical record?
7. In the case study about Stacy, list three additional concerns that you may identify.
8. Do any of the nursing diagnoses on the NANDA list seem to apply to Stacy?
9. What do the outcomes of a health assessment portray about the client?
10. What is the value of studying health assessment?

Developmental Assessment Through the Life Span

A comprehensive approach to nursing practice includes the assessment of physical, psychosocial, and cognitive aspects of development. Since all three aspects influence health, they must be considered when the nurse interacts with clients.

This chapter is organized by chronological age divisions that correlate with developmental periods. Each division discusses all three aspects of assessment and describes some assessment tools applicable to that age group. Behavioral and psychosocial development for each age division is summarized using Duvall's developmental tasks. During the first six years, however, physical growth and development are so dramatic that additional data are used to describe motor development, social-adaptive behaviors, and language development.

- *Motor development* is made up of two components, gross and fine motor behavior. *Gross motor* behavior refers to postural reactions such as head balance, sitting, standing, creeping, and walking. *Fine motor* behavior refers to the use of hands and fingers in the prehensile approach to grasping and manipulating an object.
- *Social-adaptive behavior* refers to the interactions of the infant or child with other persons, as well as the ability to organize stimuli, to perceive relationships between objects, to dissect a whole into its component parts, to reintegrate these parts in a meaningful fashion, and to solve practical problems. Examples are smiling at other persons and learning to feed self crackers.
- *Language behavior* is used broadly to include visible and audible forms of communication, whether facial expression, gesture, postural movements, or vocalizations (words, phrases, or sentences). Language also includes the comprehension of communication by others.

THEORIES OF DEVELOPMENT

Theories of development help nurses to describe and predict growth and development through the life span. Two widely used theories of psychosocial and cognitive development are described briefly. These theories were developed by Erik Erikson and Jean Piaget.

PERSONALITY DEVELOPMENT: ERIKSON'S THEORY

Erik Erikson (1902-1993) believed that the ego was the primary seat of personality functioning (Erikson, 1950, 1980). He viewed social and cultural influences as the driving forces that create inner conflicts accompanying psychosocial maturation and growth. His theory, a psychodynamic theory of development, defines eight specific developmental stages, by chronological age, in which the resolution of polar conflicts leads to personality development (see box on p. 8). The successful outcome of each stage results in specific lasting effects. For example, in the first stage, during infancy, the conflict is trust versus mistrust. When the infant develops trusting relationships with others, usually the mother, then the lasting outcome tends to be ambition, enthusiasm, and motivation. By contrast, when trust is not developed, that person tends to develop apathy and indifference. Accomplishing each successive task provides the foundation for a healthy self-identity. Each stage depends on the previous stage and must be successfully accomplished for the person to successfully complete the next. Other people and environmental factors influence a person's accomplishment of these tasks; however, the motivation to achieve a healthy identity arises from within each person. While each conflict is described at a particular developmental stage, all the conflicts exist in each person to some extent throughout life. Even though the conflict may be resolved at one time in a person's life, it may recur in similar circumstances (Erikson, 1993).

COGNITIVE DEVELOPMENT: PIAGET'S THEORY

Jean Piaget (1896-1980) described stages of cognitive development from birth to about 15 years of age. Cognition is defined as how the person perceives and processes information about the world. He believed the child's main goal was to master the environment to establish equilibrium between self and environment.

Piaget believed the child's scheme, or view of the world, developed from simple reflex behavior to complex logical and abstract thought. To fully develop cognition, the child needs a

---

Erikson's Eight Stages of Human Development

STAGE (APPROXIMATE)	PSYCHOSOCIAL STAGES	LASTING OUTCOMES
1. Infancy	Basic trust versus basic mistrust	Drive and hope
2. Toddlerhood	Autonomy versus shame and doubt	Self-control and will power
3. Preschool	Initiative versus guilt	Direction and purpose
4. Middle childhood (school age)	Industry versus inferiority	Method and competence
5. Adolescence	Identity versus role confusion	Devotion and fidelity
6. Young adulthood	Intimacy versus isolation	Affiliation and love
7. Middle adulthood	Generativity versus stagnation	Production and care
8. Older adulthood	Ego integrity versus despair	Renunciation and wisdom

Modified from Erikson EH: Childhood and society, *New York, 1993, WW Norton.*

Piaget's Levels of Cognitive Development

STAGE	AGE	CHARACTERISTICS
Sensorimotor	0-2 years	Thought dominated by physical manipulation of objects and events
Preoperational	2-7 years	Functions symbolically using language as major tool
Concrete operations	7-11 years	Mental reasoning processes assume logical approaches to solving concrete problems
Formal operations	11-15 years	True logical thought and manipulation of abstract concepts emerge

Modified from Schuster C, Ashburn S: The process of human development: a holistic lifespan approach, *Boston, 1992, Lippincott.*

---

functioning neurologic system and sufficient environmental stimuli. There are four distinct, sequential stages found (see box above). Each stage represents a qualitative change of thinking and behaving. All children move through the stages in sequential order, but not necessarily at the same age (Piaget and Inhelder, 1969).

ADULT INTELLIGENCE

Though Piaget's work represents the most complete work in cognitive development, it does not progress through adulthood. Horn (1976, 1980, 1982, 1985) and Cattell (1963,1971) describe two types of adult intelligence. *Fluid intelligence* is characterized by abstracting, associated memory, inductive reasoning, understanding relationships between concepts, speed of information processing, and problem solving. This type of intelligence is dependent on central nervous system function and declines with age and physiologic change. *Crystallized intelligence* is characterized by verbal comprehension, concept formation, and word relationships. It is dependent on life experiences and education and remains stable or increases with maturity.

Commons, Richards, and Kuhn (1982) identified two higher-order stages beyond Piaget's formal operations. The first of these stages is *systematic operations,* which involve creating theories or systems of operation and building on previously developed concepts. *Metasystematic operations* involve the ability to compare and contrast between systems and conceptual frameworks.

Shaie (1978, 1989, 1990) proposed four stages of cognitive development of the individual. Stage 1, in childhood and early adolescence, is characterized by knowledge acquisition. Stage 2, in teenage and early adulthood years, is characterized by applying previously learned knowledge. Stage 3, in middle adulthood, is divided into two phases. In the responsible phase, the adults apply skills to complex, real-life problems. In the executive phase, inductive reasoning and complex problem solving are applied to one's social system. Stage 4, in late adulthood, is called the reintegrative stage, in which one's attention is focused on selected aspects of the environment that remain meaningful or gain new meaning and on seeking an understanding of the purpose of life.

INFANTS

Infancy refers to the first year of life. The rapid growth and development that occur during this first twelve months are evident from the data given in Table 2-1, which lists changes in the infant by *month*, whereas subsequent tables document changes by intervals of six months to one year. During this time extensive neurologic and physical development occurs in addition to the acquisition of psychosocial skills.

PHYSICAL GROWTH

Height, weight, and head circumference are measured to assess infant growth. Growth proceeds from head to toe (cephalocaudal) as evidenced by the infant's development of head control before sitting and mastering sitting before standing. Healthy newborns weigh between 5 lb 8 oz and 8 lb 13 oz (2500 and 4000 g). The newborn period is the first 28 days of life. Commonly, newborns lose 10% of their birth weight in the first week, but regain it in 10 to 14 days. In general, they double their birth weight by 6 months of age and triple it by 12 months of age. The infant grows 1 inch (2.5 cm) monthly for the first 6 months, followed by 0.5 inch (1.25 cm) a month from age 6 months to 12 months. Expected head circumference for term newborns averages from 13 to 14 inches (33 to 35 cm) and increases 0.5 inch (1.5 cm) monthly for the first 6 months. By 6 months teeth begin to erupt, with a total of 6 to 8 teeth by the end of the first year.

BEHAVIORAL DEVELOPMENT

A summary of the expected developmental milestones is found in Table 2-1. Piaget identifies the sensorimotor development as the primary task of infancy (Flavell, 1963; Piaget and Inhelder, 1969). Infants utilize their sensorimotor abilities to master motor milestones and to launch relationships with others. Not only can infants advance from crawling to walking and eating some foods, but they also have the ability to win the hearts and attention of others with an intentional smile and showing preference for familiar caregivers. Bonding takes place with caregivers; at about 1 month different cries can be identified as being related to different needs, expressive language progresses to the first word, and receptive language is developed enough to understand and briefly respond to simple disciplinary commands.

The developmental tasks of infancy according to Duvall (1977; Duvall and Miller, 1985) are combined with those of toddlerhood in the box below.

Assessment tools for the infant focus on physical growth and psychosocial development, as well as determining the mother's and father's interactions with the infant. Selected tools are listed in Table 2-4 on p. 21.

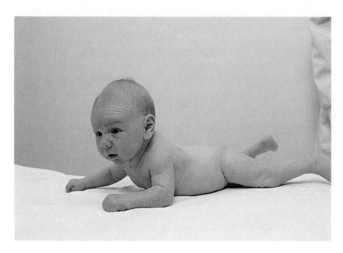

At 4 months infant actively lifts head and looks about.

Developmental Tasks of Infants and Toddlers

Achieving physiologic equilibrium following birth
- Learning to take food satisfactorily
- Learning the know-how and the where-when of elimination
- Learning to manage one's body effectively

Learning to adjust to other people
- Responding to others' expectations
- Recognizing parental authority and controls
- Learning the do's and the don'ts of the immediate world
- Reacting positively to both familiar and strange persons

Learning to love and be loved
- Responding affectionately to others through cuddling, smiling, loving
- Meeting emotional needs through widening spheres and varieties of contacts
- Beginning to give self spontaneously and trustingly to others

Developing systems of communication
- Learning patterns of recognition and responses
- Establishing nonverbal, preverbal, and verbal communication systems
- Acquiring basic concepts such as yes/no
- Mastering basic language fundamentals

Learning to express and to control feelings
- Healthy management of feelings of fear and anxiety
- Developing a sense of trust and confidence with the world
- Handling feelings of frustration, disappointment, and anger appropriately for age
- Moderating demanding attitudes

Laying foundations for self-awareness
- Seeing oneself as a separate entity
- Exploring the rights and the privileges of being an individual
- Finding personal fulfillment with and without others

Data from Duvall, 1977; Duvall and Miller, 1985.

TABLE 2-1	Expected Development of Infants

AGE	FINE MOTOR	GROSS MOTOR	SOCIAL/ADAPTIVE	LANGUAGE
1 month	Follows with eyes to midline Hands predominantly closed Strong grasp reflex	Turns head to side Keeps knees tucked under abdomen When pulled to sitting position, has gross head lag and rounded, swayed back	Regards face	Responds to bell Cries in response to displeasure Makes sounds during feeding
2 months	Follows objects well; may not follow past midline Hands frequently open	Holds head in same plane as rest of body Can raise head and maintain position; looks downward	Smiles responsively	Vocalizes (not crying) Cries become differentiated Coos
3 months	Follows past midline When in supine position puts hands together; will hold hands in front of face Pulls at blanket and clothes	Raises head to 45° angle Maintains posture Looks around with head May turn from prone to side position When pulled into sitting position, shows only slight head lag	Shows interest in surroundings	Laughs Coos, babbles, chuckles
4 months	Grasps rattle Plays with hands together Inspects hands Carries objects to mouth	Actively lifts head up and looks around Will roll from prone to supine position When pulled to sitting position, no longer has head lag When held in standing position, attempts to maintain some weight support	Becomes bored when left alone Begins to show memory	Squeals Vocalizations change with mood
5 months	Can reach and pick up object May play with toes	Able to push up from prone position and maintain weight on forearms Rolls from prone to supine and back to prone Maintains straight back when in sitting position	Smiles spontaneously Playful, with rapid mood changes Distinguishes family	Uses vowel-like cooing sounds with consonantal sounds (e.g., *ah-goo*)
6 months	Will hold spoon or rattle Will drop object and reach for second offered object Holds bottle	Begins to raise abdomen off table Sits, but posture still shaky May sit with legs apart; holds arms straight as prop between legs	Recognizes parents Holds out arms to be picked up	Begins to imitate sounds Uses one-syllable sounds (e.g., *ma, mu, da, di*)

TABLE 2-1	Expected Development of Infants—*cont'd*			
AGE	**FINE MOTOR**	**GROSS MOTOR**	**SOCIAL/ADAPTIVE**	**LANGUAGE**
		Supports almost full weight when pulled to standing position		
7 months	Can transfer object from one hand to other Grasps objects in each hand Bangs cube on table	Sits alone; still uses hands for support When held in standing position, bounces Puts feet to mouth	Fearful of strangers Plays peek-a-boo Keeps lips closed when dislikes food	Says four distinct vowel sounds "Talks" when others are talking
8 months	Beginning thumb-finger grasping Releases object at will Grasps for toys out of reach	Sits securely without support Bears weight on legs when supported May stand holding on	Responds to word "no" Dislikes diaper changes	Makes consonant sounds *t, d, w* Uses two syllables such as *dada,* but does not ascribe meaning to them
9 months	Continued development of thumb-finger grasp May bang objects together Use of dominant hand evident	Steady sitting; can lean forward and still maintain position Begins creeping (abdomen off floor) Can stand holding onto established object when placed in that position	Seems interested in pleasing parent Show fears of going to bed and being left alone	Responds to simple commands Comprehends *no-no*
10 months	Practices picking up small objects Points with one finger Will offer toys to people but unable to let go of objects	Can pull self into sitting position; unable to let self down again Stands while holding on to furniture	Inhibits behavior in response to command *no-no* Repeats actions that attract attention Plays interactive games such as pat-a-cake Cries when scolded	Says *da da, ma ma* with meaning Comprehends *bye-bye*
11 months	Holds crayon to mark on paper Drops object deliberately for it to be picked up	Moves about room holding onto objects Preparing to walk independently; wide-base stance Stands securely holding on with one hand	Experiences satisfaction when task is accomplished Reacts to restrictions with frustration Rolls a ball to another upon request	Imitates speech sounds
12 months (1 year)	May hold cup and spoon and feed self fairly well with practice Can offer toys and release them Releases cube in cup	Able to twist and turn and maintain posture Able to sit from standing position May stand alone, at least momentarily	Shows emotions of jealousy, affection, anger, fear May develop habit of "security blanket" or favorite toy	*Da da* or *ma ma* specific Recognizes objects by name Imitates animal sounds Understands simple verbal commands (e.g., "Give it to me")

CHILDREN

TODDLERHOOD

Toddlerhood is the period of growth and development from 12 to 36 months. During this period the child's locomotion is increasing, and the child becomes more independent in moving about. This increased motor autonomy places children at risk, since they possess minimal knowledge or cognitive skills regarding dangerous situations. They have a strong quest for exploration and mastery of the surrounding world and environment. Parents seeking to foster their children's exploratory and inquiring spirit, along with the mastery of motor skills, often feel extremely overwhelmed and exhausted at the end of the day. This exhaustion, coupled with the toddler's low tolerance for frustration, has led to this stage being labeled the "terrible twos."

Physical growth. A slower but steady growth in height and weight occurs during toddlerhood. By 24 months, chest circumference exceeds head circumference. Children are half their adult height by age 2. By 30 months the birth weight is tripled. The usual appearance of a toddler is pot belly, sway back, and short legs. The toddler may be ready for daytime control of bowel and bladder function by age 24 months. Teeth continue to erupt, with 20 teeth expected by 30 months.

Behavioral development. Developmental tasks of infancy and toddlerhood summarized by Duvall (1977; Duvall and Miller, 1985) are listed in the box on p. 9. A summary of the expected development milestones, including fine and gross motor, social, and language behaviors, are found in Table 2-2. Ideally children leave this period less dependent, with the beginnings of autonomy in feeding themselves, in walking, and in communication.

The tool used most frequently by nurses to assess development is the Denver II, used for children age 1 month to 6 years. This tool replaced the original Denver Developmental Screening Test (DDST) and the revised DDST in 1994. The Denver II differs from the DDST by having an increased number of language items, two articulation items, a new age scale, a new category of item interpretation to identify milder delays, a behavior rating scale, and new training materials. The Denver II form is shown in Fig. 2-1. Other tools for this age group provide data about the social, motor, and language development of toddlers.

PRESCHOOLER

The preschooler ranges in age from 3 to 5 years. As the child's locomotion and language mature, he or she moves away from the protective yet confining care of parental figures. Children begin to understand concepts and meanings in a more "real" sense, and begin increased forms of independent play and decision making.

Physical growth. Weight and height increase at a slower rate than during infancy. Typical preschoolers grow 2 to 2.75 inches (5 to 7 cm) a year. By age 4, birth length has doubled, and weight increases by 3 to 5 pounds (1.5 to 2.3 kg). Appearance changes as the long bones grow more than the trunk, and they lose their baby fat and their pot belly. By age 5, children begin to lose deciduous teeth, and first permanent teeth erupt.

Behavioral development. During the preschool years children become more autonomous, communicate easily, become toilet-trained, have an active imagination, demonstrate basic social skills, can delay gratification, use more acceptable outlets to express frustration, and expand their environment beyond home.

The developmental tasks for preschoolers as described by Duvall are listed in the box on p. 16. A summary of the expected development including fine and gross motor, social, and language behaviors of preschoolers is found in Table 2-3 on p. 16.

Assessment tools. Assessment tools focus on readiness for school and social assessment (see Table 2-4 on p. 21).

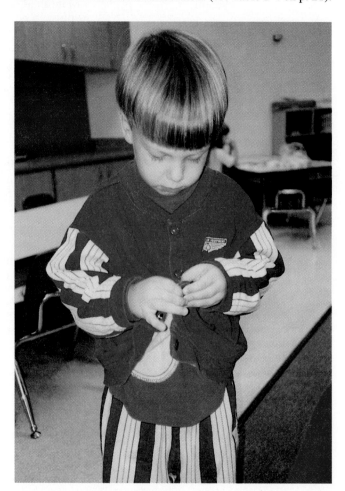

Preschooler develops the ability to help dress self.

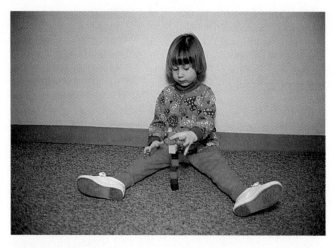

Child building block tower demonstrates fine motor skills.

TABLE 2-2	Expected Development of Toddlers			
AGE	**FINE MOTOR**	**GROSS MOTOR**	**SOCIAL/ADAPTIVE**	**LANGUAGE**
15 months	Can put raisins into bottle Will take off shoes and pull toys Builds tower of 2 cubes Scribbles spontaneously Uses cup well, but rotates spoon	Walks alone well Able to seat self in chair Creeps up stairs Cannot throw ball without falling	Tolerates some separation from parents Begins to imitate parents' activities (e.g., sweeping, mowing lawn)	Says 10 or more words "Asks" for objects by pointing Uses *no* even when agreeing with request
18 months	Builds tower of 3 to 4 cubes Turns pages in book 2 or 3 at a time Manages spoon without rotating	May walk up and down stairs holding hand May show running ability	Imitates housework Temper tantrums may be more evident Has beginning awareness of ownership (e.g., *my toy)*	Says 10 or more words Points to 2 or 3 body parts
24 months (2 years)	Able to turn doorknob Able to take off shoes and socks Able to build 7- to 8-block tower Dumps raisins from bottle following demonstration Turns pages in book one at a time	May walk up stairs by self, two feet on each step Able to walk backward Able to kick ball	Parallel play demonstrated Pulls people to show them something Increased independence from mother	Has vocabulary of 300 words Uses 2- or 3-word phrases Uses pronouns *I, you* Uses first name Refers to self by name
30 months (2½ years)	Able to build 8-block tower Scribbling techniques continue Feeding self with increased neatness Dumps raisins from bottle spontaneously	Able to jump from object Walking becomes more stable; wide-base gait decreases Throws ball overhanded	Separates easily from mother In play, helps put things away In toileting, only needs help to wipe Begins to notice sex differences	Gives first and last name Uses plurals Refers to self by appropriate pronoun Names one color

SCHOOL-AGE CHILDREN

The beginning of school is a developmental landmark for children. Entering school brings a whole new influential environment into children's lives. Information about concepts, life, and interpersonal relationships expands beyond the confines of the family home. Teacher and peer influences may be noticed in school-age children's reactions and behavior. The school-age period lasts from approximately 6 to 12 years of age.

Physical growth. The growth continues at a slow pace, with about a five-pound weight gain and two-inch height increase per year. Growth rates for boys and girls are similar until the growth spurt starts between the ages of 10 and 12 years. By age 8 or 9 there is increased smoothness and speed in motor control, making the child more agile and graceful. Bone replaces cartilage and continues to ossify. Bones of the face and jaw grow at a faster rate than they have in previous

years. The school-age child is slimmer, with less body fat and a lower center of gravity. Eyes and hands are well coordinated, and muscles are stronger and more developed. These changes in growth facilitate fine motor activities such as drawing, needle work, and playing musical instruments, and gross motor activities such as jumping, biking, and swimming. By age 12 the rest of the teeth (except the wisdom teeth) erupt.

Behavioral development. By the time children enter school, their development of fine and gross motor, social/adaptive, and language skills changes more gradually. The focus of assessment changes to identifying the accomplishment of developmental tasks. Tasks for the school-age child are listed in the box on p. 17.

Assessment tools. Assessment tools for school-age children focus on mental abilities, as well as social and emotional behaviors. Table 2-4 (p. 21) lists selected tools to use with this age group.

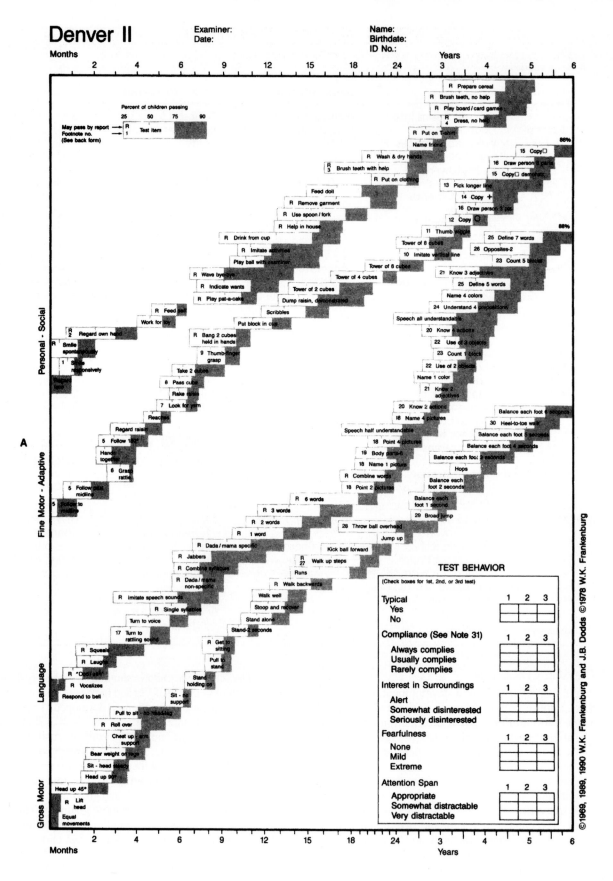

Fig. 2-1 Denver II. *(From Frankenburg, Dodds, 1990.)*

DIRECTIONS FOR ADMINISTRATION

1. Try to get child to smile by smiling, talking or waving. Do not touch him/her.
2. Child must stare at hand several seconds.
3. Parent may help guide toothbrush and put toothpaste on brush.
4. Child does not have to be able to tie shoes or button/zip in the back.
5. Move yarn slowly in an arc from one side to the other, about 8" above child's face.
6. Pass if child grasps rattle when it is touched to the backs or tips of fingers.
7. Pass if child tries to see where yarn went. Yarn should be dropped quickly from sight from tester's hand without arm movement.
8. Child must transfer cube from hand to hand without help of body, mouth, or table.
9. Pass if child picks up raisin with any part of thumb and finger.
10. Line can vary only 30 degrees or less from tester's line.
11. Make a fist with thumb pointing upward and wiggle only the thumb. Pass if child imitates and does not move any fingers other than the thumb.

  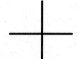 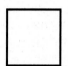

12. Pass any enclosed form. Fail continuous round motions.
13. Which line is longer? (Not bigger.) Turn paper upside down and repeat. (pass 3 of 3 or 5 of 6)
14. Pass any lines crossing near midpoint.
15. Have child copy first. If failed, demonstrate.

When giving items 12, 14, and 15, do not name the forms. Do not demonstrate 12 and 14.

16. When scoring, each pair (2 arms, 2 legs, etc.) counts as one part.
17. Place one cube in cup and shake gently near child's ear, but out of sight. Repeat for other ear.
B
18. Point to picture and have child name it. (No credit is given for sounds only.)
    If less than 4 pictures are named correctly, have child point to picture as each is named by tester.

 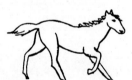 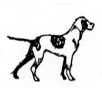 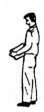

19. Using doll, tell child: Show me the nose, eyes, ears, mouth, hands, feet, tummy, hair. Pass 6 of 8.
20. Using pictures, ask child: Which one flies?... says meow?... talks?... barks?... gallops? Pass 2 of 5, 4 of 5.
21. Ask child: What do you do when you are cold?... tired?... hungry? Pass 2 of 3, 3 of 3.
22. Ask child: What do you do with a cup? What is a chair used for? What is a pencil used for?
    Action words must be included in answers.
23. Pass if child correctly places <u>and</u> says how many blocks are on paper. (1, 5).
24. Tell child: Put block **on** table; **under** table; **in front of** me, **behind** me. Pass 4 of 4.
    (Do not help child by pointing, moving head or eyes.)
25. Ask child: What is a ball?... lake?... desk?... house?... banana?... curtain?... fence?... ceiling? Pass if defined in terms of use, shape, what it is made of, or general category (such as banana is fruit, not just yellow). Pass 5 of 8, 7 of 8.
26. Ask child: If a horse is big, a mouse is __? If fire is hot, ice is __? If the sun shines during the day, the moon shines during the __? Pass 2 of 3.
27. Child may use wall or rail only, not person. May not crawl.
28. Child must throw ball overhand 3 feet to within arm's reach of tester.
29. Child must perform standing broad jump over width of test sheet (8 1/2 inches).
30. Tell child to walk forward, ⟋⟍⟋⟍⟋⟍➤ heel within 1 inch of toe. Tester may demonstrate.
    Child must walk 4 consecutive steps.
31. In the second year, half of normal children are non-compliant.

OBSERVATIONS:

Developmental Tasks of Preschoolers

- Settling into healthy daily routines
    - Enjoying a variety of active play
    - Being more flexible and capable of accepting change
    - Mastering good eating habits
    - Mastering the basics of toilet training
    - Developing physical skills
- Becoming a participating member of the family
    - Assuming responsibility within the family
    - Giving and receiving affection and gifts freely
    - Identifying with the parent of the same sex
    - Developing an ability to share parents with others
    - Recognizing the family's unique ways
- Beginning to master impulses and to conform to expectations of others
    - Outgrowing impulsivity
    - Learning to share, take turns, enjoy companionship
    - Developing sympathy and cooperation
    - Adopting situationally appropriate behavior
- Developing healthy emotional expressions
    - Playing out feelings
    - Delaying gratification
    - Expressing hostility/making up
    - Discriminating between a variety of emotions, feelings

- Learning to communicate effectively with others
    - Developing a vocabulary and speech ability
    - Learning to listen, follow directions, increase attention span
    - Acquiring social skills that allow more comfortable interactions with others
- Developing ability to handle potentially dangerous situations
    - Respecting potential hazards
    - Effectively using caution and safety practices
    - Being able to accept assistance when needed
- Learning to be autonomous with initiative and a conscience of his or her own
    - Becoming increasingly responsible
    - Taking initiative to be involved in situations
    - Internalizing expectations, demands of family/culture
    - Being self-sufficient for stage of development
- Laying foundation for understanding the meaning of life
    - Developing gender awareness
    - Trying to understand the nature of the physical world
    - Accepting religious faith of parents, learning about spirituality

Data from Duvall, 1977; Duvall and Miller, 1985.

TABLE 2-3   Expected Development of Preschoolers

AGE	FINE MOTOR	GROSS MOTOR	SOCIAL/ADAPTIVE	LANGUAGE
36 months (3 years)	Can unbutton front buttons Copies vertical lines within 30° Copies zero Begins to use fork	Walks up stairs, alternating feet on steps Walks down stairs, two feet on each step Pedals tricycle Jumps in place Able to perform broad jump	Dresses self with help with back buttons Pulls on shoes Parallel play Able to share toys	Vocabulary of 900 words Uses complete sentences Constantly asks questions
48 months (4 years)	Able to copy plus sign (+) Picks longer line 3 out of 3 times Uses scissors Can lace shoes	Walks down stairs, alternating feet on steps Able to button large front buttons Able to balance on one foot for approximately 5 seconds Catches ball	Play is associative Imaginary friend is common Boasts and tattles Selfish, impatient, rebellious	Gives first and last name Has 1500-word vocabulary Uses words without knowing meaning Questioning is at a peak
60 months (5 years)	Able to dress self with minimal assistance Able to draw 3-part human figure Draws square (■) following demonstration Colors within lines	Hops on one foot Catches ball bounced to him or her two out of three times Able to demonstrate heel-toe walking Jumps rope	Eager to follow rules Less rebellious Relies on outside authority to control the world	Has 2100-word vocabulary Recognizes 3 colors Asks meanings of words Uses sentences of 6 to 8 words

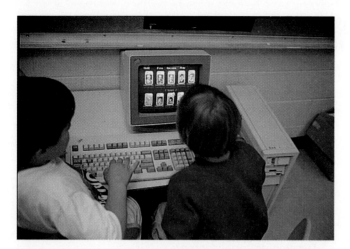

School-age children learn the basic skills required for school.

Developmental Tasks of School-Age Children

■ Learning the basic skills required for school
  Mastering reading and writing
  Developing reflective thinking
  Mastering physical skills

■ Mastering money management
  Obtaining money through socially acceptable ways
  Buying wisely
  Saving
  Delaying gratification
  Understanding role of money and place in life

■ Becoming an active and cooperative member of the family
  Participating in family discussions
  Joining in family decision making
  Being responsible for household chores
  Participating in reciprocal gift giving

■ Extending abilities to relate to others
  Asserting rights
  Developing leadership skills
  Following social mores and customs
  Cooperating in group situations
  Maintaining close friendships

■ Managing feelings and impulses
  Coping with frustrations
  Managing anger appropriately
  Expressing feelings in the right time, place, manner, and to the right person

■ Identifying the sex and gender role
  Differentiating expectations based on gender
  Understanding reproduction and gender-specific physical development
  Managing physical growth spurts
  Conceptualizing life as a mature man or woman

■ Identifying self as worthy individual
  Gaining status and respect
  Growing in self-esteem and self-confidence
  Establishing unique identity

■ Developing conscience and morality
  Determining right from wrong
  Developing moral guided control over behavior
  Learning to live according to identified values

Data from Duvall, 1977; Duvall and Miller, 1985.

ADOLESCENTS

The hallmark of adolescence is puberty, which marks the end of childhood and the onset of adulthood. With hormonal changes, growth spurts, intense sexual impulses, identity crises, and the desire to be loved and to belong, this is a turbulent period. Adolescence occurs from approximately 12 to 13 years of age to 17 to 18 years of age. By the end of this period of growth and development, the individual is physically and psychologically mature. The adolescent reviews the learning, experiences, and values accepted in earlier stages and modifies them into a unique and personalized identity. During this identity clarification process, previously accepted ideas and beliefs may be temporarily or permanently changed. Adolescents may behave in new and different ways, much to the chagrin of their parents, as they "try on" differing roles and values. The adolescent begins testing and evaluating previously accepted notions about life, living, spirituality, relating, and being. The early values of the child often are the accepted values from the parental authority in the family.

The adolescent years bring the young person to a new understanding of self, strong relationships beyond the family, and a new physical image. Advanced intellectual skills allow them to reexamine accepted ideas, which can be a strain within the family, but leads to a stronger sense of self and independence. Developmental tasks for the teen years include those listed in the box on p. 18.

ASSESSMENT TOOLS

Assessment tools for this age group focus on social and emotional behaviors, in addition to identifying and reducing stress. A list of selected tools is found in Table 2-4 on p. 21.

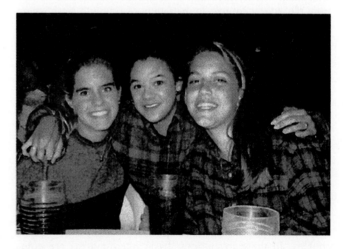

The peer group is a major influence in adolescent development. *(From Wong, 1995.)*

Developmental Tasks of Adolescents

- Accepting physical changes
  - Coming to terms with physical maturation
  - Accepting one's own body
- Achieving a satisfying and socially accepted role
  - Learning masculine/feminine role
  - Realistic understanding of gender role
  - Adopting acceptable practices
- Developing more mature peer relationships
  - Being accepted by peer group
  - Making and keeping friends of both sexes
  - Dating
  - Loving and being loved
  - Adapting to variety of peer associations
  - Developing skills in managing and evaluating peer relationships
- Achieving emotional independence
  - Outgrowing childish parental dependence
  - Developing mature affection for parents
  - Being autonomous
  - Developing mature interdependence

- Getting an education
  - Acquiring basic knowledge and skills
  - Clarifying sex-role attitudes toward work/family roles
- Preparing for marriage and family life
  - Formulating sex-role attitudes
  - Enjoying responsibilities
  - Developing responsible attitudes
  - Distinguishing between infatuation and mature love
  - Developing mutually satisfying personal relationships
- Developing knowledge and skills for civic competence
  - Communicating as a citizen
  - Becoming involved in causes outside oneself
  - Acquiring problem-solving skills
  - Developing social concepts
- Establishing one's identity as a socially responsible person
  - Developing philosophy of life
  - Implementing worthy ideals and standards
  - Assuming social obligations
  - Adopting mature sense of values and ethics
  - Dealing effectively with emotional responses

Data from Duvall, 1977; Duvall and Miller, 1985.

ADULTS

EARLY ADULTHOOD

Young adults (approximately 20 to 35 years of age) are at the height of physical and cognitive capabilities. These individuals have developed an identity and begin to express it through work, recreation, and interpersonal relationships. Adults move away from the dependent role in the family of origin to establishing their own lifestyle. Productivity, self-sufficiency, and intimacy in love relationships are driving tasks for adults, even though adults may shift back and forth in career choices, commitment, and goals as they continually define and redefine a definition of self.

The young adult is ready to enter the adult world and assume a position as a responsible citizen. Achievements are the result of self-direction, with goals changing as a result of reevaluation. Mature relationships with others are important in both the work and home environments. Most young adults choose to marry and start a family. The tasks listed in the box on p. 19 are usually accomplished during this developmental stage.

Assessment tools.   The focus of assessment for young adults is on career choice and mate selection.

Career choice. Many assessment tool inventories have been developed for the young adult contemplating career choices. In these inventories, basic interest areas are compared to occupational themes. The inventory responses will cluster similar interest areas and relate them to an occupation or vocational choice. Stability in interest areas is important to the predictive power of the inventory. If an individual has many, varied interests, then the inventory scores may be less reliable and less valid. Career assessment inventories are commonly used to guide college-bound students, by placement and selection agencies, and for individuals uncertain of a career choice or those planning a career change (Table 2-4).

Mate selection. Along with career choice, mate selection is a primary interest area for individuals in early adulthood.

The field of premarital and couple counseling has rapidly expanded since the 1940s, along with the increasing divorce rate in America. A variety of tools have been used to try to give couples a prediction of potential areas of conflict and mismatching in their relationship. Tools range from diagnostic rating tools, inventories, and checklists to personal or couple interviews, questionnaires, and even games (Table 2-4, p. 21).

MIDDLE ADULTHOOD

Entry into the middle years, between ages 35 and 65, may be met with the feeling that one's best years have passed, especially in light of today's emphasis on youth. There are obvious physical signs of aging, such as wrinkling of the skin, graying or loss of hair, and changes in muscle tone and mass. During this time many decisions have been made concerning career, partner, children, lifestyle, and living arrangements. For persons who have successfully met the developmental tasks of earlier stages, this can be a period of stability, self-understanding, and self-actualization. For others this is the time of the midlife crisis, when they feel life is incomplete. Frustration drives them to search for new directions and goals in life.

During middle age one is adapting to physical changes of aging while reaping the benefits of career success, support of family and friends, and experiences of earlier years. With introspection common to this period, wisdom is nurtured. There is an appreciation that there is more to life than the goals set in one's youth and a desire to be an integral part of one's society. New levels of development emerge as one gains a deeper level of self-understanding and self-comfort.

Most middle-aged adults are an integral part of a family. Changes for the adult affect not only themselves but also members of their family. While many adults experience personal struggles as they progress through this stage, most adults meet normal developmental challenges without a crisis. Despite conflicting research on intellectual changes, the

---

Developmental Tasks of Young Adults

- Establishing one's autonomy as an individual
- Planning a direction for one's life
- Getting an appropriate education
- Working toward a vocation
- Appraising love/sexual feelings
- Becoming involved in love relationships
- Selecting a mate
- Getting engaged
- Being married

Data from Duvall, 1977; Duvall and Miller, 1985.

Developmental Tasks of Middle Adults

- Providing a comfortable and healthful home
- Allocating resources to provide security in later years
- Division of household responsibilities
- Encouragement of both husband/wife role within and beyond the family
- Maintaining emotional and sexual intimacy
- Incorporating all family members into family circle as family enlarges, and caring for extended family
- Participating in activities outside the home
- Developing competencies that maintain family functioning during crises and encourage achievement

Data from Duvall, 1977; Duvall and Miller, 1985.

Developmental Tasks of Older Adults

- Making satisfying living arrangements
- Adjusting to retirement
- Establishing comfortable routines
- Maintaining physical and mental health
- Maintaining love, sex, and marital relations
- Remaining in touch with other family members
- Keeping active
- Finding the meaning in life

Data from Duvall, 1977; Duvall and Miller, 1985.

---

ing positive attitudes about aging and in making society aware of the developmental tasks they experience, as well as the barriers to leading a healthy, happy life in a society that values youth.

Developmental tasks for the aging adult have been summarized in the box above.

Brown (1978) gives recognition to the lengthy time span for this developmental stage and changing life situations. Later adulthood is divided into two stages, the young-old and the old-old. Separate tasks are identified (see box below).

Assessment instruments. As with earlier adult stages, previously discussed tools may be used to assess the adult of later years. However, in the past ten years there has been an increased focus on geriatric assessment and issues more specific to the later years of life. Community resources for the older adult warrant assessment, exploration, and evaluation (Table 2-4, p. 21).

Developmental Tasks of Young-Old and Old-Old

Young-Old (approximately 65-85 years)
- Preparing for and adjusting to retirement
- Adjusting to lower and fixed income of retirement
- Establishing physical living arrangments
- Adjusting to new relationships with adult children and their offspring
- Managing leisure time
- Adjusting to slower physical and intellectual responses
- Dealing with death of parents, spouses, and friends

Old-Old (approximately over 85 years)
- Learning to combine new dependency needs with continued need for independence
- Adapting to living alone
- Accepting and adjusting to possible institutional living
- Establishing affiliation with age group
- Adjusting to increased vulnerability to physical and emotional stress
- Adjusting to loss of physical strength, illness, and approach of one's own death
- Adjusting to losses of spouse, home, and friends

Data from Brown, 1978.

---

middle years are productive years, with energy directed at maintaining a home, relationships, and work. Developmental tasks for this stage include those listed in the box above.

Assessment tools. As the middle-aged adult is concerned with life achievements, many of the assessment tools used in this age group focus on career, home, and personal satisfaction with life (Table 2-4, p. 21).

OLDER ADULTHOOD

The later years, beginning with age 65, are for most adults productive years met with a sense of pleasure and enjoyment. Older adults represent the fastest growing population in the United States, and probably the least understood. They are a very diverse group. Though there are many physical changes that accompany aging, most older adults are active members of society and have independent lifestyles. Chronic health problems are common but usually can be managed. One must deal with various losses during this phase of life. Loss of one's spouse is frequently one of the hardest psychosocial adjustments during this time, other than the adjustment related to retirement. Society is becoming more aware of the presence of ageism and stereotyping against a person due to age. The growing number of older Americans has in itself encouraged society to take steps to better understand the needs and concerns of this stage of development. In addition, older adults are becoming more active in encourag-

FAMILY DEVELOPMENT AND ASSESSMENT

Most individuals in America grow up within the social unit of a family. However, the definition and composition of family structures have changed dramatically over the past several years. Families are no longer traditionally two married heterosexual parents with children who live under one roof. Blended families are composed of stepchildren and children from the current unit. Homosexual couples join as family units, some of which include children. There are single-parent families: some from divorce, some never married, and some formed due to adoption or artificial fertilization. There are also intergenerational families in which multiple generations live together under one roof, or in which grandparents or even great-grandparents raise and care for their grandchildren. Thus defining and understanding the contemporary family is a complex challenge. For our purposes, a family shall be defined as two or more individuals who share bonds of commitment, loyalty, and affection. The family unit typically shares some degree of time, financial and physical resources, and responsibilities for the unit maintenance.

Duvall (1977; Duvall and Miller, 1985) defines the functions and task of the family unit through stages for the traditional family of yesteryear, e.g., the two-parent, married, heterosexual couple with children, in the box at the right.

Nonnuclear or nontraditional families within American culture form a growing population that has been studied by Visher and Visher (1979). They note that in adoptive families the children sustained a primary relationship loss with both biologic parents, but usually the household was composed of an adult heterosexual couple. In foster families, the children also sustained a primary relationship loss with a biologic parent, and the household usually had an adult couple serving as head of household. However, in foster families there may be children as members in more than one household, and the adults in the family may have minimal or even no legal relationship with the foster children.

In stepfamilies, a biologic parent lives elsewhere, and the children commonly are transferred between the homes of two biologic families. Virtually all members of a stepfamily sustain primary relationship loss. The parent and stepparents must repeatedly deal with a part-time relationship with the stepchild if the stepchild is involved with the other biologic parent. The relationship between the adult parents outside of the stepfamily predates the new marriage and the relationship with the stepparent. This can create conflicts and loyalty divisions in parenting strategies and with the child. Children within a stepfamily struggle with being members of more than one household; stepparents cope with parenting a child to whom they are not legally related.

Single-parent families are rising in number due to the increasing divorce rate in America and the decreasing social stigma related to unwed mothers. In single-parent families the child lives with one biologic parent. Both the child and the single parent sustain a loss from the absent biologic parent of the child. There is a great variation in the involvement of the absent parent of the child; some are actively involved with the child, whereas others have minimal to no involvement with the child. Other children may be added to the single-parent family from the same or different biologic parentage. Financial difficulties are the most-noted stressor for single-parent families, as only one adult is present to care for the children, care for the home, and provide for the family.

ASSESSMENT TOOLS

Assessment tools for families focus on structure and function, social environment, interrelationships among members, and identifying and reducing family stress. Selected tools are listed in Table 2-4.

Developmental Tasks of the Family

STAGES	THEMES
Married couple	Without children; establishing satisfying marriage; adjusting to pregnancy; fitting into kin network
Childbearing	Oldest child birth to 30 months; nurturing infants; establishing home
Family with preschoolers	Oldest child 2½ to 6; adapting to needs of children; decreased energy and privacy as parents
Family with school-age children	Oldest child 6 to 13; being part of community of school-age families; encouraging educational achievement of children
Family with teenagers	Oldest child 13 to 20; balancing freedom and responsibility; establish postparental interests
Family launching young adults	First child gone until last child's leaving home; maintain supportive home base
Middle-age parents	Empty nest to retirement; refocus on marriage; maintain kin ties
Aging family members	Retirement to death of both spouses; coping with bereavement; adapting home for aging; adjust to retirement; living alone

SUMMARY

The growth and development of an individual throughout the life cycle is unique. Despite that uniqueness, commonalities form the basis of understanding psychosocial stages of development throughout life. From that knowledge, tools have been designed to assess both the individual and the family structure in which they are nurtured. Objective assessment can be utilized to determine whether an individual is progressing within an acceptable range of development, is at risk for developmental delays, or is experiencing developmental delays. The family can be assessed for style of functioning and success in meeting family tasks. A wide range of assessment instruments is available, with new instruments being developed yearly. Table 2-4 gives a brief summary of the assessment tools discussed in this chapter. The challenge is to identify an appropriate tool for the situation, determine the level of expertise needed for administration and data interpretation, utilize data to most effectively promote psychosocial development, and be knowledgeable of community resources for both professional assessment and implementation of intervention strategies. Results of assessment can be used to maintain family or individual development or to plan active interventions. Early intervention, at its best, can promote optimal development of healthy individuals and families.

TABLE 2-4	Summary of Assessment Instruments		
NAME	**AGE**	**ASSESSMENT FOCUS**	**COMMENTS**
*BNBAS: Brazelton Neonatal Assessment Scale (Brazelton, 1973; 1983)	Newborn	Neurologic deficits	The most widely used neonatal behavioral asseessment scale. Used with all cultural groups. Special training required to administer test. Data from the test may be used to enhance parenting skills and sensitivity to infant behaviors.
National Child Assessment Form (Kaufman and McMurrain, 1992)	0-3 years	Social-emotional, language, cognitive, gross and fine motor	Developmental progression is noted through visual representation. Behavior is considered either consistently present, occasionally present, or not present. Format: checklist.
Assessment Tool for Measuring Maternal Attachment Behaviors (Cropley et al, 1976)	Infancy	Maternal attachment	Used to monitor progression of maternal attachment, evaluate interventions for stimulating and fostering maternal attachment, and identify at-risk situations. Format: checklist.
BSID-II: Bayley Scale of Infant Development (Bayley, 1993)	1-42 months	Mental, psychomotor behavior	Used with children at risk for or suspected risk of developmental delay.
BINS: Bayley Infant Neurodevelopmental Screener (Bayley, 1993)	3-24 months	Mental, psychomotor	Abbreviated form of the BSID II.
Portage Guide to Early Education (1994)	Birth-6 years	Cognitive, motor, self-help, social, communication	A home-teaching program assesses child's development, serves as an educational guide to enhance family functioning, and supports parent in child's development. Translated into 35 languages. Format: checklist.
Lollipop Test (Chew, 1992)	5 years	School readiness—visual perception, numeric ability, color recognition and visual discrimination, spatial recognition	Diagnostic screening tool.
Fathering Assessment Tool (Murphy, 1979)	Not age-specific Infancy-young child	Father-child interactions	Measures father-infant interactions, role gratification, growth potential, and family support. Format: Likert scale.

*Requires training to use

Continued

TABLE 2-4	Summary of Assessment Instruments—*cont'd*		
NAME	**AGE**	**ASSESSMENT FOCUS**	**COMMENTS**
*Denver II (1990)	0-6 years	Personal—social, fine motor–adaptive, language, and motor gross (direct observation)	Used world-wide. Screens for early detection of developmental delays.
Prescreening Developmental Questionnaire (PDQ, RPDQ) (Denver, 1990)	3 months-6 years	Personal—social, fine motor–adaptive, language, and motor gross (completed by parent or during interview)	Abbreviated form of Denver II. Collects data about child from parents. Format: questionnaire.
CABS: Children's Adaptive Behavior Scale Revised (Kicklighter & Richmond, 1983)	5.0-10.11 years	Language and psychosocial	Describes language development, independent functioning, family role performance, economic-vocational activity, and socialization. Used to develop educational plans for handicapped.
Washington Guide to Promoting Development in the Young Child (Powell, 1981)	0-5 years	Feeding, sleep, play, motor, language, toilet training, discipline, dressing	Focuses on social development, requires direct observation; no score calculated; offers objective identification of developmental levels.
Goodenough-Harris Drawing Test (Goodenough, 1926; Harris, 1963)	3-15 years	Mental age, intelligence quotient	Test is composed of two scales: man and woman. Each drawing is scored on 75 specific characteristics.
The Rating-Ranking Scale of Child Behavior	Preschool-adolescence	Social, emotional development	Developed for use by nurse, teachers, as well as diagnosticians
Social Readjustment Rating Scale (Holmes and Rahe Social, 1967)	Adult	Stress	Measures the amount of change an individual has experienced within the last year. Based on the belief that change is stressful.
Change in Life Events Scale for Children (Coddington, 1972)	Preschool-senior high	Stress	Same as Social Readjustment Rating Scale
Overload Index Pace of Life Index (Kemper, Giuffre, and Drabinski, 1986)	Adolescent-adult	Stress from lack of time management and pacing life	Ten- and 15-question indexes to help recognize sources of daily stress and teach health promotion strategies.
VII: Vocational Interest Inventory (Lunneborg, 1981)	Adult	Career interest	
CAI: Career Assessment Inventory (Johansson & Johansson, 1978)	Adult	Career interest	

*Requires training to use

TABLE 2-4	Summary of Assessment Instruments—*cont'd*		

NAME	AGE	ASSESSMENT FOCUS	COMMENTS
Personal Assessment of Intimacy Relationships (Schaefer & Olson, 1981)	Adult	Perception of intimacy and goals for the relationship	Five type of intimacy assessed: emotional, social, sexual, intellectual, and recreational.
*Myers-Briggs Type Indicator (Myers, 1980)	Adult	Personality	Used by pastors, counselors, educators. Used in premarital counseling and coworker/manager interactions. Describes the continuum of complementary vs. opposing personality types in terms of sensing/intuitive, thinking/feeling, perceptive/judging, introvert/extrovert.
Job Descriptive Index (Smith et al, 1969)	Adult	Job satisfaction (tasks)	Determines satisfaction with tasks performed in vocation.
Pay Satisfaction Scale (Cammann et al, 1979)	Adult	Salary/job satisfaction	Determines satisfaction with pay.
Social Rewards Satisfaction Scale (Goldstein & Herson, 1984)	Adult	Job social rewards	Determines satisfaction with workplace social environment.
Intrinsic and Extrinsic Rewards Satisfaction Scale (Goldstein & Herson, 1984)	Adult	Job satisfaction	Determines satisfaction of internal and external rewards of vocation.
Need Satisfaction Questionnaire (Porter, 1961)	Adult	Personal needs in job	Determines how well vocation meets personal needs.
CRICHT: Chrichton Geriatric Rating Scale (Robinson, 1964)	65+	Behavior/functioning	Rates behavior and ability to perform activities of daily living.
SGSS: Stokes/Gordon Stress Scale (1986)	65+	Stress	Similar to Social Readjustment Rating Scale, using belief that change is stressful.
Geriatric Scale of Recent Life Events (Kiyak, Liang, Kahana, 1976)	Older adult	Stress	Similar to Social Readjustment Rating Scale, using belief that change is stressful.
Modes of Adaptation Patterns Scale (Sharma, 1977; Kane, Kane, 1984)	Older adult	Coping skills	Results in four adaptive styles: high activity plus high morale (conformist), high activity plus low morale (ritualist), low activity plus high morale (passive-contented), low activity plus low morale (retreatist).
Sandor Clinical Assessment—Geriatric (SCAG)(Shader, Harmatz, & Salzman, 1974)	Older adult	Behavioral functional	Assesses behavior and ability to perform activities of daily living.

*Requires training to use

Continued

TABLE 2-4   Summary of Assessment Instruments—*cont'd*

NAME	AGE	ASSESSMENT FOCUS	COMMENTS
Calgary Family Assessment (Wright & Leahey, 1984)	Families	Structure, development, function	Developed for use by nurses. Tool is easily modified to fit family being assessed.
FES: Family Environment Scale (Moos & Moos, 1976)	Families	Social environment	Compares real and ideal family social environments. Ten subscales measure relationships, personal growth, system maintenance. Results used as guide for family therapy and education.
Evaluation of Family Functioning Scale (Reidy & Thibaudeau, 1984)	Families	Functioning regarding health	Developed for use by community health nurses. Dimensions evaluated include health/illness, problem solving and coping abilities.
Parenting Satisfaction Scale (Guidubaldi & Cleminshaw, 1994, in Psychological Corporation, 1995)	Adult	Parent-child relationship	Self-report. Format: Likert scale.
FACES: Family Adaptability and Cohesion Evaluation Scales I, II, III (Olson, 1986)	Adult	Family functioning	Families are defined as enmeshed vs. disengaged and structurally rigid vs. chaotically formed.
FILE: Family Inventory of Life Events and Changes (McCubbin & Patterson, 1987)	Family	Stress	FILE and A-FILE are similar to Social Rating Scale for life stressors. Format: questionnaire.
A-FILE: Adolescent-Family Inventory of Life Events and Changes (McCubbin & Patterson, 1987)	Adolescent/Family	Stress	FILE and A-FILE are similar to Social Rating Scale for life stressors. Format: questionnaire.

??????? STUDY QUESTIONS ???????

1. Identify and define the three broad aspects of development.

2. Describe and define the two components of motor development; fine motor development.

3. Define social adaptation. Give examples of social adaptive behavior.

4. Compare and contrast the physical growth of an infant, a toddler, and a preschooler.

5. List and discuss four developmental tasks addressed by infants and/or toddlers.

6. Match the age with the appropriate fine motor skill:

4 months	*Transfers objects hand to hand*
7 months	*Grasps objects*
10 months	*Offers and releases objects*
12 months	*Points with one finger*

7. Match the age with the appropriate gross motor skill:

6 months	*Sits alone*
7 months	*Sits with legs apart*
9 months	*Can pull into a sitting position*
10 months	*Can lean forward while sitting*

8. Match the age with the appropriate language skill:

5 months	*Makes consonant sounds*
6 months	*Uses one-syllable sounds*
7 months	*Makes vowel-like sounds*
8 months	*Uses distinct vowel sounds*

9. Identify two assessment tools that you might use to assess the fine and gross motor skills in infants.

10. Match the age with the appropriate fine motor skill:

15 months	*Dumps raisins spontaneously*
18 months	*Puts raisins in bottle*
24 months	*Builds three-block tower*
30 months	*Can turn knobs*

11. Match the age with the appropriate gross motor skill:

2 years	*Hops on one foot*
3 years	*Balances on one foot*
4 years	*Kicks a ball*
5 years	*Broadjumps*

12. Match the age with the appropriate language skill:

2 years	*Uses 6- to 8-word sentences*
3 years	*Uses pronouns*
4 years	*Makes complete sentences*
5 years	*Has 1500-word vocabulary*

13. List and discuss four developmental tasks addressed by preschoolers.

14. What is the primary focus of assessment tools designed for preschoolers?

15. Compare and contrast the physical growth of school-age children to that of adolescents.

16. What aspect of development is the primary focus of assessment tools for school-age children?

17. List and discuss four developmental tasks addressed by school-age children.

18. How do the developmental tasks of adolescence differ from those of young adulthood? How are the tasks similar?

19. Match the testing need to the appropriate assessment tool:

Educational goals	*Job Expectations Questionnaire*
Career interest	*Occupational Check List II*
Career assessment	*Career Assessment Inventory*
Job satisfaction	*SDS: self-directed search*

20. List two reasons that middle adulthood might be regarded as the best years of life.

21. Identify and discuss four major developmental tasks of the middle adult.

22. Discuss some of the changes that occur as adults reach the age of 50.

23. Identify four developmental tasks of the older adult.

24. Compare and contrast the developmental tasks of the young-old with the old-old.

25. Describe the changes that have taken place in the composition of family structures. Define the term *family unit.*

26. Select and discuss two developmental tasks of the heterosexual nuclear family. Select a nonnuclear family structure. How might these tasks differ in that structure?

CHAPTER 3

Ethnic and Cultural Considerations

As we move into the 21st century, the world is becoming one global village. One of the things that makes the world a wonderful place is our rich cultural diversity. We are indeed a land of many colors, many heritages, and many histories. With this diversity also comes many challenges. As a health care professional, you are challenged with the responsibility to work with and care for individuals who may not have the same skin color, language, health practices, beliefs, and values as your own. When this occurs, the goal is not to force the client and his or her family to comply with your beliefs, values, and health practices, but instead to meet the client where he or she is and to work with his or her belief and value system. The challenge is not when the client is of the same heritage and speaks the same language as the nurse, but it occurs when the cultures and languages are different. Consider the following scenario:

> *You are caring for a 72-year-old Hispanic female, Rosa Martinez, who speaks Spanish as her primary language. Conversing in broken English, she tells you that she has injured her lower back and now has continuing aches and stiffness. She does not want to be at the clinic but is here because her daughter forced her to come. She says that she hasn't seen a physician in years because Maria, her "Cuerandera," takes good care of her. When you inquire whether she has seen Maria for her back, she replies yes, and then goes on to tell you that Maria had given her an herbal formula to take internally and had made herbal poultices to use at home. The client tells you that she believes that these remedies are working and she is not sure why her daughter made her come to the clinic.*

The nurse caring for Mrs. Martinez is potentially challenged by three issues: (1) the language barrier; (2) an alternative health care provider, Maria the Cuerandera, in whom Mrs. Martinez has much confidence; and (3) the use of alternative folk remedies—the herbal formulas and poultices. How the nurse interacts with this client and her family will depend partly on the nurse's own heritage and culture and partly on her knowledge and attitude of other cultures and other cultural health beliefs and practices.

As health care professionals we are each challenged to be as knowledgeable as possible about the health beliefs, practices, and cultural values of cultural and racial groups other than our own. An individual may be from one of the major racial and cultural groups, such as American Indian, African American, Asian, or Hispanic, or one of the sometimes unrecognized cultural groups, such as the homeless, migrant workers, gay men, or lesbians. Each group has special needs, special values, and possibly different beliefs that may affect the type of health care that is sought, needed, and, most important, understood as affecting the client's health.

Improving cultural awareness requires several steps. First, develop a sensitivity to the differences between your own culture and the client's; second, don't stereotype; third, learn the facts; and fourth, develop a template that may be used for cultural assessment of the client and the family.

BECOME CULTURALLY SENSITIVE

The first task you have in caring for clients of races and cultures other than your own is becoming sensitive to the fact that there are differences in health and religious beliefs and practices, values, and family relationships. To begin to become culturally sensitive you must:

1. Recognize that cultural diversity exists.
2. Recognize the uniqueness of and demonstrate respect for individuals and families of cultures other than your own.
3. Respect the unfamiliar.
4. Identify and explore your own cultural beliefs.
5. Recognize that some cultural groups have definitions of health and illness that may differ from your own.
6. Recognize that some cultural groups maintain health and healing practices that may be different from your own.
7. Be willing to modify health care delivery to be more congruent with the client's cultural background.
8. Recognize the cultural diversity and uniqueness of individuals within a recognized cultural group.
9. Recognize and appreciate that each person's cultural values are ingrained and therefore very difficult to change.

Modified from Seidel et al, 1995.

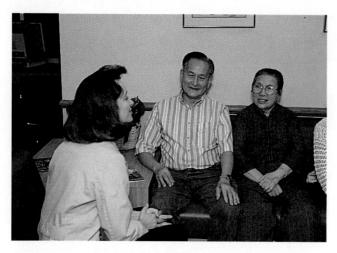

It is important to develop a sensitivity to the differences between your own culture and that of clients from another culture.

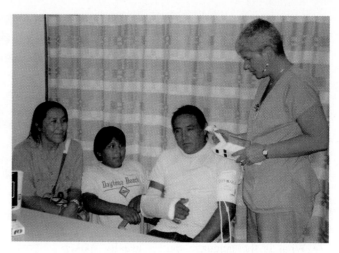

Recognize that some cultural groups maintain health and healing practices that may be different from your own.

DON'T STEREOTYPE

Every individual on this earth is unique. Regardless of skin color, physical features, cultural heritage, or social group, realize each individual's uniqueness. Cultural heritage plays an important part in helping to identify the individual's "roots" and perhaps helps to explain attitudes, beliefs, and health practices, but each major cultural group is made up of unique individuals and families who may have values and attitudes that differ from the cultural norm. Don't assume that because an individual or family is Asian or Pacific Islander that they share all culturally similar beliefs. For example, within the Asian or Pacific Islander race people are Chinese, Filipino, Japanese, Asian Indian, Korean, Vietnamese, Cambodian, Thai, Bangladeshi, Burmese, Indonesian, Malayan, Laotian, Kampuchean, Pakistani, Srilanken, Hawaiian, Samoan, Tongon, Tahitian, Polquan, Fijian, and Northern Mariona Islanders, and each of these groups has a unique heritage and set of beliefs.

Personal beliefs and knowledge about other cultures in the United States have been influenced by stereotyped images and misinformation presented through the media, educational and political institutions, and family beliefs. Some common misbeliefs and stereotyped images include:

- All African Americans have large families
- All African Americans and Hispanics are on welfare
- All welfare recipients are minorities
- The color black connotes evil; the color white connotes goodness and purity
- All Asians excel in math and science
- All American Indians are alcoholics
- All American Indians are supported by the government
- All Hispanics speak Spanish

If you learn nothing else from this text, learn that we are all unique individuals deserving of a unique and personalized assessment of our beliefs, our values, and our culture.

LEARN THE FACTS

In addition to the just-mentioned thesis that every individual is unique and should be respected accordingly, factual information about the four major cultural groups provides background information that gives a backdrop from which the nurse can work (Table 3-1 on p. 30).

DEVELOP A TEMPLATE FOR ASSESSMENT

When assessing the client and family, it is important to include a direct assessment of the client's health beliefs and practices that may be reflective of his or her cultural heritage. Knowing the risks of stereotyping, perform a focused interview that will reflect the client's personal beliefs, values, and attitudes. Assess the following:

WHAT ARE THE CLIENT'S PERSONAL BELIEFS ABOUT HEALTH AND ILLNESS?

- How do you define health and illness?
- Do you believe that you have control over your health?
- Are there particular practices or rituals that you believe will improve your health?
- Do you or have you used any of the alternative healing methods, such as acupuncture, acupressure, ayuveda, healing touch, or herbal products? If so, how effective was the treatment?
- Are there particular practices or rituals that you believe should be used to treat your health problem?
- What are your attitudes toward mental illness? Pain? Handicapping conditions? Chronic disease? Death? Dying?
- Are you the one who makes the health decisions in your family? If not, who is the decision-maker?

WHAT ARE RELIGIOUS INFLUENCES AND SPECIAL RITUALS THAT AFFECT THE CLIENT?

- Is there a religion to which you adhere?
- Is there a significant person to whom you look for guidance and support?
- Are there any special religious practices or beliefs that are likely to feel supportive when you are ill?
- What events, rituals, and ceremonies are considered important within your life cycle, such as birth, baptism, puberty, marriage, and death?

WHAT IS THE CLIENT'S PRIMARY LANGUAGE AND METHOD OF COMMUNICATION?

- What is the language that is usually spoken in your home?
- How well do you speak, read, and write English?
- Are there special rituals of communication in your family? (For example, is there someone special to whom questions should be directed?)

WHAT ARE THE ROLES OF INDIVIDUAL PEOPLE IN THE FAMILY?

- Who makes the decisions in your family?
- What is the composition of your family? How many generations or family members live in your household?
- When the marriage custom is practiced, what is the attitude about separation and divorce?
- What is the role of and attitude toward children in the family?
- When the children are punished, how is it done, and who does it?

- What are the major important events in your family? How are they celebrated?
- Do you or the members of your family have special beliefs and practices surrounding conception, pregnancy, childbirth, lactation, and child-rearing?

DOES THE CLIENT HAVE SPECIAL DIETARY PRACTICES?

- What is the main type of diet eaten in your home?
- Are there special types of foods that are forbidden by your culture, or foods that are a cultural requirement in observance of a rite or ceremony?
- Who in your family is responsible for food preparation?
- Is the food in your culture prepared in any special way?
- Are there specific beliefs or preferences concerning food, such as those believed to cause or cure illness?

Modified from Seidel et al, 1995.

REMEMBER . . .

The most important behaviors in cultural assessment are to be sensitive, ask questions, gather information specific to the individual client, not stereotype, and not assume that just because you took care of a similar client last week that you know exactly how this client feels and what he or she believes.

Regardless of the client's race or cultural heritage, each individual is unique. Before you become involved in the detailed task of a physical assessment, take the time to first get to know the client and his or her family.

TABLE 3-1	Facts About Major Cultural Groups

	AFRICAN AMERICAN	HISPANIC/MEXICAN
Demographic Trends	African Americans make up almost 12% of the U.S. population and are the single largest minority group in the country. African Americans as a group are considered young (over 35% are under age 20), unmarried (61% are not married), urban (81%), and female (53%). Over half of all African-American children are raised in single-parent homes.	Hispanics, including Mexicans, Puerto Ricans, Cubans, and persons from Central and South America, make up 9% of the U.S. population, which makes them the second largest minority. The Hispanic population is young, with one third under the age of 18.
	The proportion of African Americans below the poverty level is 29.5%, compared to 13.1% of all races and 9.8% of white Americans.	The percentage of families below the poverty level is 25.3%, compared to 13.1% for all races and 9.8% for whites.
	The mean household income for African Americans in 1989 was $19,758.	Most Hispanics live in urban areas. The five states with Hispanic populations of more than 10% of the total state population are New Mexico, Texas, California, Arizona, and Colorado.
		The median household income for Hispanic families in 1989 was $24,156.
Education and Employment	The number of African Americans completing both high school and college are fewer than whites—63% and 11.4%, compared to 77.9% and 21.5%, respectively.	The percentage of Hispanics with less than a 9th grade education is 31%. Those with a high school education are 50%, and those with a college education are 9.2%.
	The unemployment rate for African Americans is 13.7%, more than twice that of whites, which is 5.3%. It is estimated that at any one time, more than 40% of African-American teens are looking for work.	The unemployment rate for Hispanic males is 9.8%, compared to 6.4% for all races.
Health Care Utilization	More African Americans than whites have no usual source of health care. As a group, more African Americans than whites have no medical insurance. A greater percentage of African Americans use hospital clinics and emergency departments as their usual source of care than any other single racial group.	A higher percentage of Hispanics than any other minority group do not have health insurance. Because of this, public clinics and emergency departments are often the location of health care.

Data from 1990 U.S. Census; The Office of Disease Prevention and Health Promotion, 1988; Seidel et al, 1995; Indian Health Service, 1994; Wong, 1995.

ASIAN/PACIFIC ISLANDER

Asians and Pacific Islanders make up 3% of the U.S. population and are the fastest-growing minority in this country. According to the 1990 U.S. census, there are 7,273,662 Asians and Pacific Islanders. There are over 20 categories for Asians and Pacific Islanders.

According to 1990 census data, 92% of Asian Americans lived in metropolitan areas, compared to 75% of the general population. The majority of the Asian Americans in the U.S. live in California.

The mean household income for Asian Americans in 1989 was $36,784, compared to $30,056 for all races combined.

Asian Americans as a whole are better educated and better paid than the general U.S. population, although among some groups (e.g., recent refugees from southeast Asia) the reverse is true.

The unemployment rate for Asian Americans is 5.1%, compared to 6.4% for all races.

Asian/Pacific Americans make visits to physicians less frequently than whites. Those Asian Americans over 65 years of age visit the physician half as often as their white counterparts.

Asian/Pacific Americans are more likely to visit pediatricians and obstetricians and less likely to visit surgeons and psychiatrists than whites.

AMERICAN INDIAN/ALASKAN NATIVE

American Indians and Alaskan Natives are a diverse group of people from varied cultural backgrounds. More than 500 tribal groups are recognized by the federal government. The 1990 census reported the number of American Indians/Alaskan Natives to be 1.9 million people, or 0.8% of the entire U.S. population. The American Indian and Alaskan Native population served by the Indian Health Service is young (30% below the age of 15), and is growing at a rate of almost 3% per year. The birth rate is over 1.5 times that of all other races in the U.S.

In general, the Indian population is younger, less educated, and poorer than the rest of the U.S. The 1990 U.S. census reports that the median household income was $19,886, compared to $30,056 per year for U.S.—All Races. The number of Indians living below the poverty level is 32%, compared to less than 13.2% for all U.S. races combined.

Before 1940, 90% of Indians lived on reservations, but by 1980 more than 50% lived in urban areas.

The average family has between four and five members, which makes it the largest family size of any minority or nonminority group. Almost 25% of all American Indian and Alaskan Native households are headed by women.

The proportion of American Indians and Alaskan Natives finishing college is less than half that of all races in the U.S., and the unemployment rate is twice as high as all other combined races.

The unemployment rate for Indian males is 16.2%, compared to 6.4% for all races and 5.3% for whites.

Since 1955, the U.S. Public Health Service through its Indian Health Service (IHS) has been responsible for providing comprehensive health service to American Indians and Alaskan Natives. In 1995 it is estimated that the IHS will provide care for 1.37 million American Indians and Alaskans, or 70% of all Indians. The remainder usually seek care by other private and public health service providers. Care provided by the IHS is provided at no cost to the individual clients.

Although medical care is available at no cost via the IHS hospitals and clinics, many Indians live in remote areas where the availability of physicians is half the national average.

Continued

TABLE 3-1	Facts About Major Cultural Groups—*cont'd*

	AFRICAN AMERICAN	**HISPANIC/MEXICAN**
General Health Status	The life expectancy for both African-American males and females is less than for whites. Infant mortality rates are higher, maternal mortality rates are higher, and African-American males between the ages of 15 and 44 are the highest risk group to be victims of homicide. The lifetime risk of becoming a homicide victim is 1 in 21 for African-American males. When compared to whites, African Americans have slightly different illness patterns: • The prevalence of coronary heart disease and stroke is higher in African-American males and females than white males and females. • The three most common cancers among African-American males are prostate, lung and bronchus, and colorectal. • The three most common cancers among African-American females are breast, colorectal, and lung and bronchus. • Both African-American men and women have a higher prevalence rate and age-adjusted mortality rate for diabetes than their white counterparts. The prevalence of diabetes in African Americans over the age of 65 has been estimated to be twice that of whites. The incidence of teenage pregnancies is almost 3 times higher for African Americans than whites. Over 50% of the first births to African-American women occur before marriage, compared to less than 15% for white women. Compared to white infants, more than twice as many African-American infants are born prematurely. The infant mortality rate for African-American infants is more than twice that for whites. The maternal mortality rate for African-American women is more than 3 times the rate for white women. The percentage of African-American women and men who are overweight is almost double that of white men and women. Cigarette smoking is more prevalent among African Americans than among whites. The prevalence of high blood pressure among African Americans is more than twice that for whites.	Good data about Hispanics are lacking because the national reporting systems often do not list Hispanics as an ethnic group separate from other whites. The prevalence of non–insulin-dependent diabetes is nearly twice that of whites. The group of Hispanics that is most affected is lower socioeconomic group Mexican Americans. Hispanic women are less likely to use any contraceptive than other minority groups. This puts them at higher risk for pregnancy and sexually transmitted diseases, including HIV. Leading causes of mortality for Hispanics are cardiovascular disease (including hypertension), diabetes, cancer, and homicide. Compared to whites and other minority groups, the suicide rate among Hispanics is low.

ASIAN/PACIFIC ISLANDER

The health status of Asian Americans as a group is good. They have a longer life expectancy than whites, and lower death rates from all causes, including heart disease and cancer. The unintentional injury, homicide, and suicide rates are lower than for other groups.

When compared to whites, certain Asian-American groups suffer high rates of illness from specific causes.
- Stomach cancer is higher among Japanese.
- Suicide is higher among elderly Chinese women.
- Southeast Asian refugees have a higher incidence of intestinal parasites, positive tuberculin tests, presence of hepatitis B antigens, and are more anemic than other Asian Americans and whites in general.

The incidence of teenage pregnancies for Asian Americans is lower than for whites. When compared to other racial groups, Asians have the lowest percentage of women having their first child under age 20 and the highest percentage of women having their first child after age 35.

Asian Americans have a lower age-adjusted death rate from homicide than all other racial groups.

AMERICAN INDIAN/ALASKAN NATIVE

Life expectancy for American Indians and Alaskan Natives is 73.2 years, compared to the U.S. expectancy of 75.4 years for all races.

The leading causes of hospitalization at IHS hospitals are obstetric deliveries and complications of puerperium and pregnancy. This is followed in descending order by respiratory system diseases, digestive system diseases, injuries and poisonings, and, finally, circulatory system problems.

Maternal mortality among Indians is 12% higher than in the population in general.

The ten top causes of mortality among Indians, in descending order, are as follows:
- Diseases of the heart (#1 men/#1 women)
- Injury (#2 men/#3 women)
- Malignant neoplasms (#2 women/#3 men)
- Diabetes mellitus (#9 men/#4 women)
- Chronic liver disease and cirrhosis (#5 men/#6 women)
- Cerebrovascular diseases (#8 men/#5 women)
- Pneumonia and influenza (#6 men/#7 women)
- Suicide (#4 in men/not in top 10 for women)
- Homicide and legal intervention (#7 men/not in top 10 for women)
- Chronic obstructive pulmonary disease (#10 men/#8 women)

The more full-blooded the American Indian or Alaskan Native, the more likely it is that the individual will manifest diabetes. The diabetes is almost exclusively the non–insulin-dependent, ketosis-resistant type, with the same manifestations and vascular complications as in non-Indians.

The incidence of teenage pregnancies is almost twice that of white teens but less than that of African Americans.

Indian infants are 3 times more likely to die of meningitides, twice as likely to die of pneumonia and influenza, and 1.8 times more likely to die of sudden infant death syndrome than all other races in the U.S.

Unintentional injuries account for an estimated 21% of all deaths among American Indians and Alaskan Natives. It is further estimated that 75% of all injury deaths are alcohol-related.

Among all Indians discharged from IHS hospitals during 1992, the rate of individuals discharged with a primary alcohol-related diagnosis (alcohol psychosis, alcoholism, or chronic liver disease and cirrhosis) was 37 per 100,000 population. This is compared to 19 per 100,000 population for the general population.

Continued

TABLE 3-1	Facts About Major Cultural Groups—*cont'd*

	AFRICAN AMERICAN	**HISPANIC/MEXICAN**
Health Beliefs	Illness may be classified as *natural* (forces of nature) or *unnatural* (evil influences such as witchcraft, voodoo, hex, or root-work). Some African Americans may believe that serious illness has been sent by God as punishment. Because of this, they may resist health care.	Health beliefs often have a strong religious association. Body balance is a major cause of illness, especially imbalances between *caliente* (hot) and *frio* (cold). Some Hispanics and Mexican Americans believe that good health is the result of "good luck," which is the reward for good behavior. Illness may be prevented by eating the proper foods, working the proper amount of time, wearing religious medals or amulets, and sleeping with relics at home. Illness may be seen as punishment from God for wrongdoing, or from forces of nature and the supernatural.
Health Practices	Self-care and folk remedies are quite prevalent. Many folk therapies may have a religious origin. Because of inadequate health insurance and lack of a regular health care provider, it is common for some African Americans to attempt home remedies first and not seek help until the illness is serious. It is more likely that the individual will seek care from the "Old lady" (a woman in the community with knowledge of herbs or other remedies), a "Spiritualist" (one who received the gift for healing from God), the "Priest" (a most powerful voodoo priest or priestess), or the "Root doctor" (a healer who uses herbs, oils, candies, and ointments).	To deal with severe illness, Hispanics may often make promises, visit shrines, offer medals and candles, and offer prayers.

ASIAN/PACIFIC ISLANDER

Chinese believe that a healthy body is a gift from the parents and should be cared for. Health is a result of the forces that rule the world: *yin* (cold) and *yang* (hot). Illness results when there is an imbalance. *Chi* is innate energy, and the lack of *chi* results in fatigue, poor consitution, and long illness.

Vietnamese also believe in *yin* and *yang*. Health results from harmony and balance with existing universal order, harmony attained by pleasing good spirits and avoiding evil ones. There are many rituals to prevent illness and to prevent the wrath of evil spirits.

Japanese have the religious influence of *shinto,* which is that humans are inherently good and that evil is caused by outside spirits. Illness is caused by contact with polluting agents, such as bad blood, corpses, or skin diseases.

Filipinos believe that God's will and supernatural forces govern the universe. Illness, injuries, and other misfortunes are God's punishment for violations of His will. *Yin* and *yang* balances and imbalances cause health and illness.

Chinese believe that the goal of health care is to restore *yin* and *yang.* Treatments may include acupuncture, acupressure, tai chi, moxibustion (the application of heat to the skin), or medicinal herbs. They are likely to go to a wide variety of folk healers from herbalists, spiritual healers, or temple healers to fortune healers.

Vietnamese will use all possible means before seeking care from outside agencies or health providers. Fortune-tellers determine the event that caused the illness. They may pray at the temple to obtain divine instruction about what to do during an illness. They may use special diets to prevent illness and promote health.

Japanese remove evil and illness by purification. Treatments may include acupuncture, acupressure, massage, and moxibustion along affected meridians. Most Japanese use a combination of Oriental and Western healing methods, including *Kampō* medicine, which is the use of natural herbs. The family is viewed as the party responsible for caring for the ill and disabled.

Filipinos may use amulets as a shield from witchcraft or as a good-luck charm. Religious medals may also be used.

AMERICAN INDIAN/ALASKAN NATIVE

Health is a state of harmony with nature and the universe. Illness indicates that there is disharmony, which may be because of a supernatural force. Violation of a restriction or prohibition is thought to cause illness.

Many American Indians and Alaskan Natives fear witchcraft and may carry objects to protect themselves from witchcraft. Theology and medicine are strongly interwoven.

Many American Indians and Alaskan Natives seek medical care from a medicine person, an altruistic person who must use his or her powers in conjunction with herbs and rituals in a purely positive way to heal the individual. The medicine healer may use negative force powers to act against the sick person's enemies.

One type of medicine healer is the diviner-diagnostician, who may diagnose the problem but who does not have the powers or skills to implement medical treatment. Some medicine healers use herbs and curative but nonsacred medical procedures. Others cure by the power of song and the laying on of hands, with powers obtained from supernatural beings.

Continued

TABLE 3-1   Facts About Major Cultural Groups—*cont'd*

	AFRICAN AMERICAN	**HISPANIC/MEXICAN**
Family Relationships	There is often a strong kinship that bonds family members. The family will come together at a time of crisis. They are less likely to view illness as a burden than other groups. When necessary, there is sex-role sharing among parents.	Family is very important. The family has a strong kinship and may include *compadres* (godparents), who are established by ritual kinship. Older family members and parents are respected. If elders become ill, they are usually cared for at home. Children are highly valued, very desired, and seen as a gift from God. They are usually taken everywhere with the family. Children are taught to obey and to respect the parents. The home often has a shrine area, which contains statues and pictures of saints. The family is usually large and home-centered, which is the core of their existence. The father is the decision-maker and the provider. The wife and children are subordinate.
Communication	African Americans are alert to any evidence of discrimination. Often importance is placed on nonverbal behavior. Because of distrust, there may be "testing" behaviors to assess health care providers before seeking care. The best approach by health care providers is to use a simple, direct, but caring approach.	Most Hispanics are bilingual, speaking both English and Spanish. In some areas of the country, the language may be primarily Spanish. Many Hispanics have a strong preference to speak their native tongue and may show no eagerness to learn or speak English.
Other Comments	There may be a high level of caution and distrust of majority groups. Tradition of humiliation, oppression, and loss of dignity may cause some African Americans to express or demonstrate feelings of social anxiety. If the African American's values are compromised, he or she will most likely retain dignity rather than seek care or follow the advice of a health care provider. The African-American minister is a strong influence in the African-American community and a valued resource to the ill individual.	Hispanics show a high degrees of modesty, which is often a deterrent to seeking medical care. They have a relaxed concept of time and consider being slightly late for an appointment as acceptable. The hospital is often considered as the place to go to die. For many, religion is very important.

ASIAN/PACIFIC ISLANDER	AMERICAN INDIAN/ALASKAN NATIVE
Chinese have strong extended families, and have loyalty to the young and the old. Respect for elders is taught at an early age. The behavior of children is a reflection on the family. Males are valued more highly than females; women are submissive to men in the family.	The family is an extended family, which includes relatives from both sides. Elder members assume the leadership.
Japanese believe that the family provides the anchor. They tend to keep problems within the family. They value self-control and self-sufficiency. The concept of *haji* (shame) imposes strong control. The behavior of the children reflects on the family.	
Vietnamese also believe that the family is the central anchor. Many families are multigenerational, with the elders receiving great respect. Men are the decision-makers, and women are taught to be submissive. Individual needs and interests are subordinate to those of the family. Although children are highly valued, they are expected to respect their parents.	
Chinese believe that the open expression of emotions is unacceptable.	Most American Indians and Alaskan Natives are bilingual, speaking both English and their native tongue. Nonverbal communication and respect are very important.
Japanese may also suppress their emotions. When they do not know what to do or what is wanted of them, they may wait silently for direction.	Making eye contact may be considered invasive during a conversation.
Vietnamese may avoid direct eye contact as a sign of respect. They may hesitate to ask questions because asking questions may be considered impolite.	
Haitians may prefer family/friends to act as translators and confidants. They may smile and nod in agreement when they do not understand. Their quiet and gentle communication style and lack of assertiveness may lead the health care provider to falsely believe that they comprehend even when they do not.	
Chinese respect their bodies and believe that it is best to die with their bodies intact. They may therefore refuse surgery. Older members may believe that the hospital is a place to go to die. Many believe in reincarnation.	Because the hospital is often considered as the place to die, the client may resist hospitalization.
Japanese highly value cleanliness. Time is also valuable and should be used wisely. They may be stoic and not openly show evidence of pain or discomfort.	Great respect is shown to the elders of both the family and the tribe.
Vietnamese value status more than money. There is a high value placed on social harmony.	

??????? STUDY QUESTIONS ???????

1. Identify and discuss at least four things that you can do to increase your personal cultural sensitivity.

2. Identify two stereotypes that you have about those of another culture. Where did those stereotypes come from?

3. What can you do to recognize and correct stereotypes that you will encounter in the health care system?

4. List at least one demographic trend for each major cultural group presented in the chapter that added to your knowledge about that culture.

5. Identify one health statistic for each major cultural group presented in the chapter that differs from the general population. Speculate as to the reason for the difference.

6. Look back at your speculations in the previous question; are they fueled by stereotypes?

7. Identify two health beliefs that you hold. Are they similar to any of the beliefs identified in the chapter?

8. Select one health practice from those described in the chapter. Discuss your selection with someone from that culture. What did you discover?

9. List at least four things that you discovered about possible communication differences that will directly impact how you perform a history and physical examination. Discuss what you will do to make use of that information.

10. Using the template for cultural assessment, do an assessment of yourself and your family. Did you discover anything interesting? Surprising?

11. Do you need to do a cultural assessment on someone who is the same race as yourself? Cite the rationale for your answer.

CHAPTER 4

Interviewing to Obtain a Health History

Therapeutic relationships begin by gathering information about clients—finding out about their current state of health and how it can be maintained or improved. To accomplish this, nurses interview clients to learn about them and the social, economic, and cultural factors that influence their health and their responses to illness.

PURPOSE OF THE HEALTH HISTORY

The purpose of the health history is to obtain subjective data from clients. Together the nurse and the clients use this data base to create a plan to promote health, prevent disease, resolve acute health problems, and minimize limitations related to chronic health problems. Accomplishing this purpose involves both meeting the clients' expectations for health and the nurse's expectations for the health of those clients. Information to be gathered about clients includes how they define health, whether they believe they can attain and maintain health, whether they believe they are responsible for their health, and what health behaviors they practice now and what unhealthy behaviors they are willing to change. The clients' expectations for health are based on their life experiences, the experiences of their families and friends, and the culture in which they live. The nurse has a broader view of health and compares a client's current state of health to a standard needed to attain or maintain optimal health, and then determines how far away the client is from the desired standard.

The American Nurses Association (ANA) Standards of Practice (1991) direct nurses to establish a comprehensive database. Outcome criteria for this standard include (1) obtaining pertinent data using appropriate assessment techniques; (2) involving the client, significant others, and health care providers in data collection, when appropriate; (3) collecting data in a systematic manner; and (4) documenting relevant data in a retrievable form (ANA, 1991, p. 9).

The nursing process is initiated as the nurse begins data collection about the client's history. A variety of factors will have an impact on the outcome of the interviews. These factors include the nurse's personality and behavior, the personality and behavior of the client, how the client is feeling at the time of the interview, the nature of the information being dis-

cussed or problem being confronted, and the physical setting. The nurse's approach must be orderly without being rigid. Random approaches often result in an incomplete data base and incomplete diagnoses and solutions, which reduces the potential of successful outcomes.

PROVIDING A RELAXED SETTING

Introduce yourself to the clients, offer a handshake, and tell them your role in their care. Be sure you know their names and pronounce them correctly. Address clients by their title (for example, Mr., Mrs., Miss, or Ms.) and their surname. Avoid using the first name with clients unless they request it, except when the client is a child. Also avoid substituting the client's role for his or her name, such as referring to the client as "mom" or "grandpa."

When possible, allow clients to remain in street clothes during the interview to obtain the history and then have them change into a gown for the physical examination. You and the client should sit at a distance from each other that provides a comfortable flow of conversation and allows you to establish eye contact. The client's comfort level is related to personal space, that is, the area that surrounds the person's body. How much space clients want from you will vary and is influenced by their cultures and previous experiences in similar situations. Be attentive to how comfortable a client appears and, if you are not sure, ask "Is this a comfortable seating arrangement for you?" When you are learning the interview process, you may want to use an outline to prompt questions and take brief notes during the interview. Both practices are acceptable as long as they do not interfere with your eye contact with the client or with the flow of information.

DECIDING HOW MUCH DATA TO COLLECT

How much data do you collect at one time? Assessment interviews may be comprehensive or focused. The *comprehensive health assessment* provides a complete health history, family history, review of all body systems, psychosocial assessment, and physical examination. This type of assessment may be part

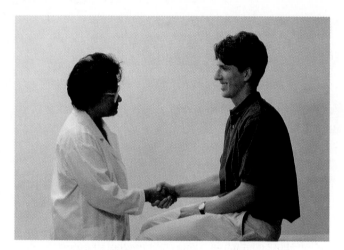

Offer the client a handshake and introduce yourself.

of an admission to a hospital, the first office or home visit, or when the client's reason for seeking care is for relief of generalized symptoms such as weight loss or fatigue. This type of assessment requires more time than usual visits because a comprehensive database is being established. Often clients are given questionnaires to complete about their histories before the interview to reduce the time spent in data collection.

The *focused health assessment* concentrates on episodic health care needs. These needs may be well-child or well-adult visits, screening, or changes that have occurred since the comprehensive health assessment. Well visits include changes in the history since the last visit, a limited physical examination, and education about normal growth and development and health promotion. Screening allows identification of specific risk factors. For example, blood pressure screening provides data on the risk for hypertension. A Mantoux test is given to identify those exposed to tuberculosis. The client may seek help to address a specific topic such as weight reduction, relief from asthma attacks, or an emergency situation.

COMMUNICATING WITH THE CLIENT

From the start there are several points to keep in mind. A stiff, formal demeanor may inhibit the client's ability to communicate, yet being too casual or having a laid-back attitude may fail to instill confidence. Because the client may search for meaning in everything you say, avoid being careless with words. What may seem an innocent comment to you may be vital to the client. Similarly, your face need not be a mask, but avoid the extremes of reaction—startle, surprise, laughter, grimacing—as the client provides information. Your nonverbal demeanor is as important as your words.

The first impression you make starts with the way you appear to the client. The way you are dressed and groomed is important in establishing a positive first impression. Modest dress, clean fingernails, and neat hair are imperative. Avoid extremes in dress and manner so that appearance does not become an obstacle to the client's response.

Interviewing the client with others in the room may present a challenge. Be careful not to assume relationships among the people in the room. For example, when an adult accompanies a child, do not assume the adult is the child's mother; ask "Are you the mother?" Also, when a man and a woman are together, do not assume what their relationship is; ask. Sometimes the relationship will be explained during introductions but, if not, clarify by asking, "What is your relationship?" Trying to interview a mother when her active children are in the room may be disruptive. If the children are too young to wait in the waiting room, find a developmentally appropriate activity for them to do until you complete the interview. When the client speaks a different language, a translator is needed. An objective observer who is the same gender as the client will be a better translator than a family member who may alter the meaning of what is said. The client should respond to the questions if possible. Sometimes the spouse, parent, or another person will answer for the client unless otherwise directed. When this occurs, you must validate with the client that the information is correct. If others persist in answering for the client, you may have to ask the others to allow the client to answer or ask them to wait in another room until the end of the interview.

THE ART OF ASKING QUESTIONS

The art of obtaining information from clients and listening carefully to their responses is an essential competency of nurses. Questions you ask must be clearly spoken and understood by the client. Define words the client may not understand, but do not use so many technical terms that the definitions become confusing. Use the client's terms if possible. Slang words may be used if necessary to describe certain conditions. Comply with the client's level of knowledge and understanding.

Encourage the client to be as specific as possible. For example, if you ask how many glasses of water he drinks each day and he says, "Oh, a few," clarify what he means by asking, "How many is a few? 3? 4? 5?" This approach yields a more specific answer and provides the client's interpretation of "a few."

Ask one question at a time and wait for the reply before asking the next question. If you ask several questions at a time, the client may get confused about which question to answer and you may be uncertain about which question the client is answering. For example, you ask, "Have you had immunizations for tetanus, hepatitis B, and influenza?" If the client answers "yes," you are not sure if he means yes to all three or to one.

If you become confused by something a client says, ask for clarification. The explanation may clear up the confusion, or it may indicate that the client has misinformation or some underlying emotional or thought processing difficulty that impairs understanding.

Be attentive to the feelings that accompany the client's responses to some questions. These responses may signify additional data you need to collect during this interview or a problem that needs to be addressed in the future. For example, if the client reports that her mother died of breast cancer and she seems to have intense feelings, this may indicate a future need for discussing of coping or adjustment method with the client.

Clients may ask you questions during the interview. Answer specific questions using terms that they understand.

Avoid overburdening them with an in-depth answer that, while correct, is far more information than necessary to satisfy them. If a client asks a question you do not feel prepared to answer at the moment or one that is very broad, you can get additional information by asking, "Why do you ask?" This will give you direction in answering the client's specific question. If you do not know the answer to the question, perhaps you can refer the client to a resource for the answer.

TYPES OF QUESTIONS TO ASK

Begin the interview with *open-ended questions,* such as "How have you been feeling?" This broadly stated question encourages a free-flowing, open response. The aim of an open-ended question is to elicit a response that is more than one or two words. Clients will respond to this type of question by describing the onset of signs or symptoms in their own words at their own pace. The open-ended question should, however, focus on the client's health. A question that is too broad, such as "tell me a little about yourself" may be too general to get any useful information. The risk of asking open-ended questions is that clients may be unable to focus on the topic being asked about or may take excessive time to tell their story. In these cases, you will need to focus the interview. Flexibility is needed when using this type of question, however, because the client's associations may be important and you must allow clients freedom to pursue them. You may note topics the client mentions that you want to follow up on later in the interview.

To gain more precise details, you must ask more direct, specific, *closed-ended questions* that require one or two words. For example, you might ask, "Do you become short of breath?" or "Do you frequently get bruises?" Another reason for using this type of question is to give clients options when answering questions, such as "Is the pain in your stomach sharp, dull, or aching?" This type of question is valuable in collecting data, but it must be used in combination with open-ended questions because failure to allow clients to describe their health in their own words may lead to inaccurate conclusions.

Directive questions lead the client to focus on one set of thoughts. This type of question is most often used in reviewing systems or in evaluating functional status. An example would be "Describe the drainage you have had from your nose."

Asking *questions about sensitive issues* can be accomplished by explaining that you have personal or sensitive questions to ask or by describing clients you have interviewed in the past. An example of this type of question is, "I need to know about the drugs you have used that are not prescription or over-the-counter; have you ever used illegal drugs?" An alternative is to say, "Some clients have experimented with illegal drugs; have you ever used illegal drugs?" This method of questioning has been called *permission-giving* because the nurse gives clients permission to report information about a sensitive topic.

TECHNIQUES THAT ENHANCE DATA COLLECTION

The question-answer format is the essential tool used in obtaining a client history. Data collection can be facilitated by using the following techniques.

Active Listening.   Active listening is performed by concentrating on what the client is saying and the subtleties of the message being conveyed. Two behaviors that interfere with active listening are formulating your next question while the client is talking and predicting how clients will answer questions. If you are concentrating on how you are going to word your next question, your attention will be shifted away from the information that client is providing you. When you make assumptions about how the client will respond to questions and plan your next question based on your assumptions, your question may be illogical if your assumption is wrong.

Facilitation.   Facilitation is attained by using phrases to encourage the client to continue talking. These include verbal responses such as "go on," "uh-huh," and "then?" and nonverbal responses such as head nodding and shifting forward in your seat with increased attention.

Clarification.   Clarification is used to obtain more information about conflicting, vague, or ambiguous statements. Examples might be, "What do you mean by 'you almost lost it'?" or "What do you think kept you from returning to work?"

Restatement.   Restatement involves repeating what clients say using different words; it confirms your interpretation of what they said. For example, "Let me make sure I understand what you said. The pain in your stomach occurs before you eat and is relieved by eating. Is that correct?"

Reflection.   Reflection is repeating a phrase or sentence the client just said. This encourages elaboration and indicates you are interested in more information.
Client: "I got out of bed and I just didn't feel right."
Nurse: "You didn't feel right?"
Client: "Uh huh, I was dizzy and had to sit back on the bed before I fell over."

Confrontation.   Confrontation is used when you notice inconsistencies between what the client reports and your observations or other data about the client. For example, "I'm confused here. You say you are staying on your diet and exercising three times a week, yet your weight has increased since your last visit? Can you help me to understand this?" Your tone of voice is important when using confrontation; use a tone that communicates confusion or misunderstanding, rather than one that is accusatory and angry.

Interpretation.   Interpretation is used when you want to share with clients a conclusion you have drawn from data they have given. After hearing your interpretation, clients can either confirm, deny, or revise your interpretation. For example, "Let me share my thoughts about what you just told me; the week you were out of the office you exercised, felt no muscle tension, and had a normal blood pressure. I wonder if your work environment is contributing to your high blood pressure?"

Summary.   Summary condenses and orders data obtained during the interview to help clarify a sequence of events. This is useful when interviewing a client who rambles or does not provide sequential data. Also, summary is useful at the end of the interview to emphasize data that have implications for health promotion, disease prevention, or resolving the client's health problems.

TECHNIQUES THAT DIMINISH DATA COLLECTION

The following communication techniques have been found to interrupt the free flow of the interview, interfere with data collection, and possibly impair the client-nurse relationship. These techniques can be avoided by considering the interview from the client's perspective, such as how you would prefer the flow of the conversation to go and how you would want things explained to you.

Use of Professional Terminology.   Using professional terminology occurs when you use medical terms or abbreviations not commonly known to clients. Some examples include saying "hypertension" instead of "high blood pressure," "dysphagia" rather than "difficulty in swallowing," "CVA" rather than "stroke," or "CA" rather than "cancer." Using these words may be condescending; furthermore, they inhibit the exchange of information and may create a barrier between you and the client.

Expressing Value Judgments.   Including *value judgments* in your questions is always a hindrance. For example, you should ask, "What kind of protection do you use during intercourse?" rather than saying, "You do use protection during intercourse, don't you?" The latter question forces clients to respond in a way that is consistent with your values or causes them to feel guilty or defensive when they must answer to the contrary.

Talking Too Much.   Interviews are about the clients and how to meet their needs. When you monopolize the conversation by talking, you cannot collect sufficient data about the clients' needs.

Interrupting the Client.   Allow clients to finish sentences; do not become impatient and finish their sentences for them. The ending you add to a sentence may not be the ending that the client would have used. Associated with interrupting is *changing the subject* before a client has finished giving information about the last topic discussed. You may feel pressured for time and eager to move on to other topics, but allow clients an opportunity to complete their thoughts.

Being Authoritarian or Paternalistic.   When you use the approach of "I know what is best for you and you should do what I say," you risk alienating the client. Despite what you believe is best for clients, you must always remember that their health is their responsibility. They may choose to follow or ignore your advice and teaching.

Using "Why" Questions.   Using "why" questions may put clients on the defensive. The implication of this question is that they must defend their choices when asked why they did something. Instead of asking, "Why didn't you take all the antibiotic?" you might say, "I noticed you stopped taking the antibiotics before all the pills were gone" and then wait to see if the client offers an explanation. If no explanation is forthcoming, you can follow up with, "I am curious about the reason for not taking all the antibiotic."

MANAGING AWKWARD MOMENTS

Answering Personal Questions.   Questions about you may be asked by clients from time to time. They are curious about you and your life. Often a brief, direct answer will suffice to satisfy the client's curiosity. You may feel comfortable sharing certain experiences that may support clients, such as parenting issues or how you handle stress. Sharing these mutual experiences may enhance the relationship with clients and increase your credibility.

Dealing with Silence.   Silence can be awkward. You may have the urge to break the silence with a comment or question. Remember, however, that clients may need the silence as time to reflect or to gather courage. Some issues can be so painful to discuss that silence is necessary and should be accepted. Silence may provide feedback for you that clients may not be ready to discuss this topic now or that your approach needs to be evaluated. Become comfortable with silence; it can be useful.

Bridging Cultural Diversity.   Cultural diversity has gained awareness among health care providers. Culturally sensitive nursing care refers to the variability in nursing approaches needed to provide culturally appropriate and competent care. To deliver culturally sensitive care, nurses must interact with each individual as a unique person who is a product of past experiences, beliefs, and values that have been learned and passed down from one generation to the next. Remember, however, that all individuals within a specific cultural group will not think and behave in a similar manner. Avoid stereotyping clients just because of their culture. There may be as much diversity within a cultural group as there is across cultural groups. Ask clients about experiences that illustrate what has been of value to them and that characterize their culture. This will increase your knowledge about other cultures and endear you to clients for your interest in them as individuals. (See Chapter 3, "Ethnic and Cultural Considerations.")

Displays of Emotion.   *Crying* is a natural emotion and should be permitted when it occurs. Saying, "Don't cry" is not therapeutic. A more appropriate approach is to provide a tissue and let the client know it is all right to cry by giving a response such as, "Take all the time you need to express your feelings." Postpone further questioning until the client is ready. The crying may indicate a client need that can be addressed at a later time. Compassionate response to a crying client demonstrates caring and may enhance the therapeutic relationship.

Anger of clients may be uncomfortable. The most therapeutic approach is to deal with it directly by first identifying the source of the anger. You may say, "You seem angry; can you tell me the reason for your feelings?" If clients choose to discuss the anger, they hopefully will identify whether the anger is directed at someone else or at you. If clients are angry at someone else, you can discuss with them an ap-

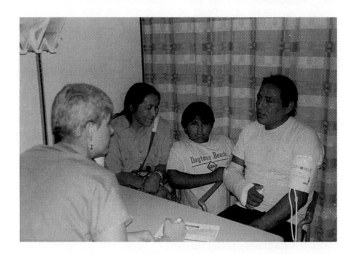

Interact with the client as a unique person and be sensitive to cultural diversities.

proach for discussing the reason for the angry feelings with that person. When clients are angry with you, encourage them to discuss their feelings. Acknowledge the angry feelings and, if appropriate, apologize. You may be able to continue working with these clients after the angry feelings are discussed, but if clients would prefer to interact with another nurse, then you should honor their request. Regardless of the outcome, you have modeled for the clients a healthy, appropriate approach to managing anger.

SCOPE OF THE HEALTH HISTORY

The health history format described in this chapter provides a comprehensive format that may take over an hour to complete. The scope of the history includes the following areas:

- Biographic data
- Reason for seeking care
- Present health status
- Past health history
- Family history
- Review of systems
- Psychosocial status
- Environmental health

BIOGRAPHIC DATA

The biographic data are collected at the first visit and then updated as changes occur. These data begin to form a picture of the client as a unique individual. See the box below for a list of data to be obtained.

REASON FOR SEEKING CARE

The reason for seeking care, also called the chief complaint (CC), is a brief statement of the client's purpose for re-

---

Biographic Data

Name
Address and telephone number
Birth date
Birthplace (important when born in foreign country)
Race—physical features such as skin color, bone structure, or blood group that are genetically determined
Culture—pattern of behavioral responses shaped by values, beliefs, norms, and practices
Religion
Marital status
Family/significant others living in the home
Social security number
Occupation
Contact person
Advanced directive (decisions about end-of-life care)
Durable power of attorney for health care
Source of referral
Usual source of health care
Type of health insurance

---

questing the services of a health care provider. The client's reason for seeking care is recorded in direct quotes. When clients have multiple reasons, list them all and ask clients to indicate the priority of the complaints. Some clients may be uncomfortable giving you the actual reason for seeking care until they feel more comfortable. In this case they may not divulge the true reason they came until the end of the visit.

The client's condition dictates how the examiner will proceed. Urgency dictates expediency. Clients with severe pain, dyspnea, or injury should not be subjected to a prolonged history. Biographic data may be delayed to pursue the health concern, followed by a symptom analysis and selected systems review. This approach enables the examiner to hypothesize quickly and identify the cause of the health concern and to alleviate the signs or symptoms. However, clients with depression may need to be given more time to freely divulge feelings and surrounding circumstances.

PRESENT HEALTH STATUS

The present health/illness status gives clients an opportunity to expand on the reason for seeking care. When the reason is to improve current health status, rather than to relieve illness, the data collected include what clients are doing currently to maintain their health and what they think may be hindering the accomplishment of their health goals. Data included here are as follows:

- Current health promotion activities: diet, exercise, stress management, meditation, yoga, spiritual or religious groups
- Client's perceived level of health
- Current medications
  Herbal preparations
  Type of drug (prescription, over-the-counter, vitamins, illegal)
  Prescribed by whom
  When first prescribed
  Reason for prescription
  Amount of medication and frequency per day
  Effectiveness of medication

In contrast, when clients seek relief from illness, then a *symptom analysis* is completed. A symptom analysis is a systematic way to collect data about the history and status of symptoms and focuses on eight variables: location, quality, quantity, chronology, setting, associated manifestations, alleviating factors, and aggravating factors (see box on Symptom Analysis on p. 44).

PAST HEALTH HISTORY

Past health history is important, since past illnesses may have some effect on the client's current health needs and problems. The following categories of data are included:

- *Allergies:* food, drug, environmental factors, contact substances
- *Childhood illnesses:* measles, mumps, rubella, chicken pox, pertussis, haemophilus influenza, streptococcal throat infection, otitis media. (Ask if there were complications in later years, such as rheumatic fever or glomerulonephritis that can occur after streptococcal throat infection.)

Symptom Analysis

Location—Where are the symptoms?

- Is the location in a specific area? vague and generalized? does symptom radiate?

Quality—Describe the characteristics of the symptom.

- Describe the sensation: stabbing, dull, aching, throbbing, nagging, sharp, squeezing, itching.
- Describe the drainage: color, texture, composition, appearance, and odor.
- Was the onset slow? abrupt? noticeable to others?
- Was the symptom intermittent or continuous?
- How has symptom interrupted your life (e.g., sleeping, eating, working, activities at home or school)?

Quantity—Describe the severity of the symptom.

- Describe the size, extent, number, or amount (e.g., of lesion, rash, blister, discharge).
- Was the symptom so severe that it interrupted your activities?
- On a scale of 1 to 10, with 10 being most severe, how would you rate your symptom?

Chronology—When did the symptom start?

- Ask specific date, time, day of the week.
- How many times a day, week, month did symptom occur?
- How did client feel in between episodes of the symptom?

Setting—Where are you when the symptom occurs?

- Does anyone else with whom you have been in contact have a similar symptom?
- Are there psychologic or physical factors in the environment that may be causing the symptom (e.g., stress or smoke or chemicals)?

Associated manifestations—Do other symptoms occur at the same time?

- What effect does the symptom have on body function? activities? appetite?

Alleviating factors

- What home remedies have you tried?
- What medications have you tried (over-the-counter and prescription)?
- Are there certain body positions that relieve symptom?

Aggravating factors

- Is symptom associated with an activity (e.g., walking, climbing stairs, eating, a body position)?

- *Surgeries:* type, date, outcome
- *Hospitalizations:* illnesses, dates, outcome
- *Accidents or injuries:* fractures, lacerations, loss of consciousness, burns, penetrating wounds
- *Chronic illnesses:* e.g., diabetes, hypertension, heart disease, sickle cell anemia, cancer, seizures, chronic obstructive pulmonary disease, arthritis. Ask how much the illness interferes with daily activities.
- *Immunizations:* tetanus, diphtheria, pertussis; mumps; rubella; poliomyelitis; hepatitis B; influenza, pneumococcus pneumonia, varicella, and, for foreign-born clients, bacillus-Calmette-Guerin (BCG)
- *Last examinations:* physical, dental, vision, hearing, EKG, chest radiograph, skin test for tuberculosis; for women: Papanicolaou (Pap) smear, mammogram
- *Obstetric history:* number of pregnancies (gravidity), number of births (parity), and number of abortions/miscarriages. (For each birth document the course of pregnancy, labor, type of delivery [vaginal or cesarean section], weight of neonate, and postpartum course.)

FAMILY HISTORY

Family history of the client's blood relatives, spouse, and children is obtained to identify any illnesses of a genetic, familial, or environmental nature that might affect the client's current or future health. Trace back at least two generations to maternal and paternal parents and grandparents. Also include siblings, uncles, and aunts. Sometimes health information about significant others, sexual partners, and roommates is relevant to the client's health. Questions about the health of family members should include the following:

- Alzheimer's disease
- Cancer (all types)
- Diabetes mellitus
- Heart disease
- Hypertension
- Seizures
- Emotional problems
- Mental diseases
- Developmental delay
- Alcoholism
- Endocrine diseases (specify)
- Sickle cell anemia
- Kidney disease
- Cerebrovascular accident

Document the absence of the diseases by writing "No history of (disease name)" so that others who read this history will know that you asked the client about the family history of the specific disease. Document the presence of these diseases in a family tree or genogram. Also include the current ages of those who are alive and well (A + W) and cause and age at death of those deceased (Fig. 4-1).

REVIEW OF SYSTEMS

Review of systems (ROS) is conducted to inquire about the past and present health of each of the client's body systems and to ensure no significant data were omitted in the present health status section. In the review of the physical systems, when clients respond positively to a symptom, then a symptom analysis is completed. If the data collection from the present health status section has already provided sufficient data on a body system, you do not need to repeat those questions in this section. For example, if you completed a symptom analysis on "cough" when completing the present health status, you need not repeat questions about cough in the review of systems.

Symptoms are listed in this chapter using medical terms, but a brief definition is included as needed to facilitate your in-

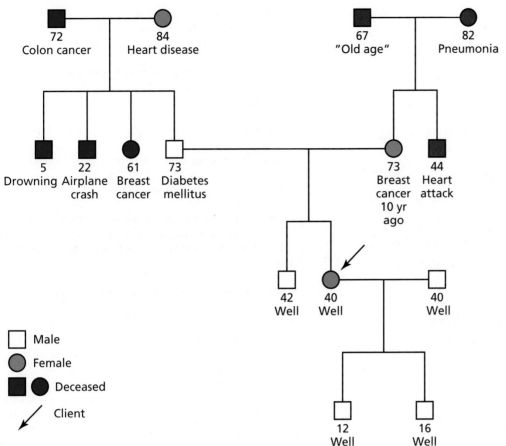

Male
Female
Deceased
Client

Fig. 4-1 Sample genogram identifying grandparents, parents, aunts and uncles, siblings, spouse, and children.

terpretation of the term to the client. For example, if you want to know if the client has dyspnea, you *ask,* "Do you become short of breath?" If the client says "no," you would *document* "denies dyspnea" or "no dyspnea," but if the client says "yes," you would use questions from the symptom analysis and document your findings. Therefore you will need to know the medical terms for documentation and communication with other health care providers, but only terms understood by the client are used during the interview. While some health promotion (HP) data are included in the previous sections titled *present health status* and *past health history,* additional information is collected during the review of systems.

Below is an outline, organized by body region or body system, of the symptoms you ask the client about. In a comprehensive health assessment, you ask most of the questions; but in a focused health assessment, you would only ask about those systems related to the reason for seeking care.

General Health Status
Fatigue, weakness
Sleep patterns
Weight, unexplained loss or gain
Self-rating of overall health status

Integumentary System
Skin
Skin disease, problems, lesions (wounds, sores, ulcers)
Skin growths, tumors, masses
Excessive dryness, sweating, odors
Pigmentation changes or discolorations
Rashes

Pruritus (itching)
Frequent bruising
Texture or temperature change
Scalp itching
HP: Amount of sun exposure, including tanning bed use; use of sun screen; skin self-examination
Hair (refers to all body hair, not just head and pubic area)
Changes in amount, texture, character, distribution
Alopecia (loss of hair)
HP: Use of dyes, permanent waves, or other chemicals
Nails
Changes in texture, color, shape
HP: Type and frequency of nail care

Head
Headache (characteristics, frequency, location and type of pain, duration)
Past significant trauma
Vertigo (dizziness)
Syncope (brief lapse of consciousness)

Eyes
Discharge (describe)
Pruritus
Lacrimation (excessive tearing)
Pain in eyeball
Visual disturbances such as blind spots (floaters), halos around lights, or flashing lights
Swelling around eyes
Redness
Cataracts

History of glaucoma
Unusual sensations or twitching
Vision changes (generalized or vision field)
Use of corrective or prosthetic devices
Diplopia (double vision)
Blurring vision
Photophobia (increased sensitivity to light)
Difficulty reading
Interferences with activities of daily living
HP: Use of protective eyewear

Ears
Pain
Cerumen (wax)
Infection, earache
Discharge (describe)
Hearing changes (describe)
Use of prosthetic devices
Increased sensitivity to environmental noises
Vertigo (dizziness, unable to maintain balance)
Tinnitus (ringing or cracking)
Interference with activities of daily living

Nose, Nasopharynx, and Paranasal Sinuses
Discharge (describe, seasonal occurrence)
Epistaxis (nose bleed)
Sneezing
Obstruction
Sinus pain
Postnasal drip
Change in ability to smell
Snoring
Pain over sinuses

Mouth and Oropharynx
Sore throat (describe)
Tongue or mouth lesion (abscess, sore, ulcer)
Bleeding gums
Voice changes or hoarseness
Use of prosthetic devices (dentures, bridges)
Altered taste
Dysphagia (difficulty swallowing)
Difficulty chewing
HP: Frequency and kind of dental hygiene

Neck
Lymph node enlargement
Swelling or masses
Pain/tenderness
Limitation of movement
Stiffness

Breasts
Pain or tenderness
Swelling
Nipple discharge (describe)
Changes in nipples
Lumps, masses, dimples
Unusual characteristics
HP: Breast self-examination (frequency, method)

Cardiovascular System
Heart
Palpitations
Heart murmur
Hypertension
Chest pain (describe quality, duration)

Dyspnea (shortness of breath)
Orthopnea (person must sit to breathe)
Paroxysmal nocturnal dyspnea (periodic dyspnea during sleep)
HP: Monitor fat in diet; exercise regularly
Peripheral vasculature
Coldness, numbness
Discoloration
Peripheral edema
Varicose veins
Intermittent claudication (leg pain with exercise that ceases with rest)
Paresthesia (abnormal sensations)
Leg color changes
HP: Use of support hose if work involves standing
Avoid crossing legs at the knees
Exercise patterns

Respiratory System
Cold
Cough, nonproductive or productive (describe sputum)
Hemoptysis (coughing up blood)
Dyspnea (short of breath)
Night sweats
Wheezing
Stridor (abnormal, high-pitched, musical sound)
Pain on inspiration or expiration
Smoker; exposure to smoke

Gastrointestinal System
Change in taste
Thirst
Indigestion or pain associated with eating
Pyrosis (burning sensation in esophagus and stomach with sour eructation [belching])
Dyspepsia (heartburn or bloating)
Nausea/vomiting (describe)
Hematemesis (vomiting blood)
Appetite changes
Food intolerance
Abdominal pain (describe)
Jaundice (yellowish color to skin and sclera)
Ascites (abnormal intraperitoneal fluid accumulation)
Bowel habits (frequency)
Flatus
Constipation
Diarrhea
Dyschezia (constipation resulting from habitual neglect in responding to stimulus to defecate)
Changes in stools (color, consistency)
Hemorrhoids (pain, rectal bleeding)
Use of digestive or evacuation aids (what, frequency)
HP: Type of diet; compare diet to food pyramid

Urinary System
Characteristic of urine (color, contents)
Hesitancy
Urinary frequency (in 24-hour period)
Urgency
Change in urinary stream
Nocturia (excessive urination at night)
Dysuria (painful urination)
Flank pain (posterior portion of body between ribs and ileum)

Hematuria
Suprapubic pain
Dribbling or incontinence
Polyuria (excessive excretion of urine)
Oliguria (decreased urination)
Pyuria (white blood cells or pus in urine)
HP: Amount of water drunk daily
  Females—measures to prevent urinary tract infections

Genitalia
General
  Lesions
  Discharges
  Odors
  Pain, burning, pruritus
  Satisfaction with sexual activity
  Sexual preference
  Number of partners
  Method of birth control
  Infertility
  HP: Methods of protection from unwanted pregnancy and sexually transmitted diseases
Men
  Impotence
  Testicular masses/pain
  Prostate problems
  Change in sex drive
  HP: Penis and scrotum self-examination practices
Women
  Menstrual history (date of onset, last menstrual period, length of cycle)
  Amenorrhea (absent menstruation)
  Menorrhagia (excessive menstruation)
  Dysmenorrhea (painful menstruation)
  Metrorrhagia (irregular menstruation)
  Dyspareunia (pain during intercourse)
  Postcoital bleeding (bleeding after intercourse)
  Pelvic pain
  HP: Genitalia self-examination

Musculoskeletal System
Muscles
  Twitching, cramping, pain
  Weakness
Bones and joints
  Joint swelling, pain, redness, stiffness (time of day, duration)
  Joint deformity
  Crepitus (noise with joint movement)
  Limitations in joint range of motion
  Interference with activities of daily living
Back
  Back pain
  Limitations in joint range of motion
  Interference with activities of daily living
  HP: Amount and kind of exercise per week

Central Nervous System
History of central nervous system disease (specify with examples)
Fainting episodes or loss of consciousness
Seizures (characteristics, how treated)

Dysphasia (impairment in speech)
Dysarthria (poorly articulated speech)
Cognitive changes
  Inability to remember (recent vs. dated)
  Disorientation to time, place, person
  Hallucinations
Motor-gait
  Loss of coordinated movements
  Ataxia (balance problems)
  Paralysis (partial vs. complete)
  Paresis
  Tic, tremor, spasm
  Interference with activities of daily living
Sensory
  Paresthesia (abnormal sensations, e.g., "pins and needles," tingling, numbness)
  Anesthesia (absent sensation, location)
  Pain (describe)

Endocrine System
Changes in skin pigmentation or texture
Changes in or abnormal hair distribution
Sudden or unexplained changes in height or weight
Intolerance of heat or cold
Hormone therapy
Presence of secondary sex characteristics
Polydipsia (excessive thirst)
Polyphagia (excessive hunger)
Polyuria (excessive urine output)
Anorexia (decreased appetite)
Weakness

PSYCHOSOCIAL STATUS

Psychologic and sociologic data are important aspects of a health history. The following is an outline of information to be obtained:

General statement of client's feelings about self
  Degree of satisfaction in interpersonal relationships
  Client's position in home relationships
  Most significant relationship
  Community activities
  Work or school relationships
  Family cohesiveness
Activities
  General description of work, leisure, and rest distribution
  Hobbies and methods of relaxation
  Family demands
  Ability to accomplish all that is desired during period (day, week)
Cultural or religious practices
Occupational history
  Jobs held in past
  Current employer
  Education preparation
  Satisfaction with present and past employment
Recent changes or stresses in client's life (e.g., divorce, moving, new job, family illness, new baby, financial stress)
Coping strategies for stressful situations
Changes in personality, behavior, mood
  Feelings of anxiety or nervousness

Feelings of depression (e.g., insomnia, crying, fearfulness, marked irritability or anger)

Use of medications or other techniques during times of anxiety, stress, or depression

Habits

Alcohol/drugs

Type of alcohol/drugs

Frequency per week

Pattern over past 5 years; 1 year

Drinking/drug use companions

Alcohol/drug consumption variances when anxious, stressed, or depressed

Driving or other dangerous activities while under the influence

High-risk groups: sharing/using unsterilized needles and syringes

Smoking

Kind (cigarette, cigar, pipe)

Amount per day

Pattern over 5 years; 1 year

Smoking variances when anxious or stressed

Desire to quit smoking

Exposure to second-hand smoke

Coffee and tea

Amount per day

Pattern over 5 years; 1 year

Consumption variances when anxious or stressed

Physiologic effects

Other

Overeating, sporadic eating, or fasting

Nail biting

"Street drug" use

Financial status

Sources of income

Adequacy of income

Recent changes in resources or expenditures

ENVIRONMENTAL HEALTH

An outline of data to be obtained for the environmental health portion of the history includes the following:

General statement of client's assessment of environmental safety and comfort

Hazards of employment (inhalants, noise, heavy lifting, machinery, psychologic stress)

Hazards in the home (concern about fire, smoke detector, stairs to climb, inadequate heat, open gas heaters, pest control, violent behaviors, loud sound systems including earphones)

Hazards in the neighborhood or community (noise, water and air pollution, heavy traffic on surrounding streets, overcrowding, violence, firearms, sale/use of "street drugs")

Hazards of travel (use of seat belts, motorcycle or bicycle helmets)

Travel outside the United States (when and which countries visited, length of stay)

AGE-RELATED VARIATIONS IN THE HEALTH HISTORY

NEWBORN

The terms *newborn* and *neonate* are used interchangeably and refer to the first 27 days of life. *Infant* is used to describe a baby from 1 to 12 months of age. The gestational age and well-being of the neonate will influence the information needed for the data base; therefore newborns who are at risk should receive additional assessment by neonatal experts.

The purpose of this assessment is to determine the newborn's physical condition and transition from intrauterine to extrauterine life. Maternal history is an important aspect of the total health data base of the newborn, since the mother's behaviors and experiences during pregnancy also may affect the neonate.

Biographic Data.   Biographic data should include the following:

- Name: Mother's name and neonate's name and sex; multiple births may be listed as newborn A or B, etc., until names are given.

- Age: Gestational age, date and time of birth

- Birth weight in pounds and ounces or in grams

- Parent's culture (pattern of behavioral responses shaped by values, beliefs, norms, and practices)

- Socioeconomic factors of family (e.g., parent's employment, on Medicaid)

- Address and telephone number of parents or family

- Siblings and family in home

- Parent's means of transportation for follow-up examinations of newborn

- Description of parent's home and size and type of community

Reason for Seeking Care.   The reason for seeking care is reported by the adult bringing the neonate for care. The visit may be a well-baby or a sick-baby visit. Review with parent or caregiver the schedule for immunizations and well-baby examinations.

Present Health Status.   Ask the adult accompanying the neonate to elaborate on the reason for seeking care. For a sick-baby visit, complete a symptom analysis (see p. 44). For a well-baby visit, the data collected are the same as those listed under the review of systems. Also discuss the physical care of the neonate, including cord care, care after circumcision, use of bulb syringe for suctioning nose secretions, and proper positioning of the neonate for sleep.

Past Health History.   The past health history of the neonate begins with the mother's health status during the pregnancy. This should include the following data:

- Extent of prenatal care

- Complications of pregnancy: bleeding, falls, edema of hands and feet, hypertension, proteinuria, unusual weight gain, infections

- Medications taken, including "street drugs" and tobacco (include dose, duration, and month of gestation when taken)
- Radiographs taken
- Emotional state of mother during pregnancy: crying or depression states
- Planned pregnancy
- Mother's attitude toward neonate
- Father's attitude toward neonate
- Pregnancy history (para, gravida, abortions, miscarriages, time between pregnancies)

Problems that arise during the labor and delivery process also can affect the neonate. The following data should be collected:

Labor and Delivery Process

- Where delivery occurred (hospital, birth center, home)
- Number of weeks of gestation
- Labor—spontaneous or induced, duration, complications
- Type of delivery—vaginal or cesarean section (planned or emergency C-section)
- Type of anesthesia used in delivery
- Presentation of neonate (e.g., vertex, breech)
- Special equipment or procedures required (e.g., forceps)
- Gestational assessment data and neurologic assessment data (APGAR score)
- Medications: Vitamin K, hepatitis B immunization initiated, standard eye care, other medications ordered
- Tests performed (e.g., bilirubin, ABO isoimmunization, phenylketonuria)
- Baby's condition in hospital: oxygen requirements, color, feeding, vigor, cry; duration of baby's stay in hospital and whether infant discharged with mother; prescriptions such as bilirubin phototherapy or antibiotics

Family History.   Family history for the neonate is the same as for the adult, with the addition of congenital anomalies or hereditary disorders in the family.

Review of Systems.   Review of systems for the neonate is the same as for the adult with the following additions:

General Health Status
Nutrition
　Breast or bottle fed, reasons for changes, if any; type of formula used, amount offered and consumed, frequency of feeding and weight gain
Sleep
　Hours of sleep
　HP: Position neonate on side for sleep

Integumentary System
Changes in color of skin or nails
Rashes, petechiae (tiny red spots)
Birthmarks
Healing of cord
HP: Cord care

Eyes
Follows object with eyes
Drainage
Ears
Discharge
Turns toward sounds
Nose, Nasopharynx, and Paranasal Sinuses
Difficulty breathing
Discharge
HP: Use of bulb syringe to suction nose
Mouth and Oropharynx
Strong suck
Respiratory System
Difficulty breathing
Cough, productive or nonproductive
Gastrointestinal System
Amount, type of formula, frequency, method of feeding
Frequency and consistency of stools
Urinary System
Number of diapers used per day
Genitalia
Healing of circumcision
Discharge from vagina
HP: Care after circumcision
Musculoskeletal System
Moving extremities symmetrically
Central Nervous System
Describe cry
Is adult able to console neonate?
Response of touch, noise
Sleep cycle, amount

Psychosocial Status.   Discuss the following with the parent or guardian of the neonate:

- Sibling rivalry, how to deal with it
- Parenting skills
- Stresses of newborn in family, arrangements for infant care, mother's and/or father's plans for return to work

Environmental Health.   Discussion of the neonate's environmental health should include the following:

- Safety: infant seat and seat belts
- Protection from falls
- Appropriate clothing
- Avoiding drafts
- Supporting infant's head
- Absence of smoking in infant's environment

INFANTS

Infancy is the period of life from 1 to 12 months. History for the infant is the same as that for the child.

CHILDREN

Health history for the child is similar to that for the adult, with the additions of prenatal care, growth and development,

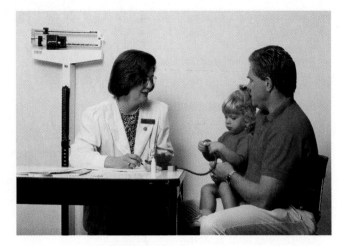

Most data are obtained from the adult accompanying the child.

and behavioral and school status histories. Most data are obtained from the adult accompanying the child but include the child as much as appropriate for his or her age. Also observe the interaction between adult and child during the examination. Depending on the age of the child, it might be helpful to set a time to collect data from the parent without the child's presence. Collecting a complete history is more desirable during a well-child visit rather than when the child is sick. The following format parallels the adult history but includes the significant pediatric data.

Biographic Data.   Biographic data to be gathered for the child include the following:

- Informant: person giving the history (relationship to client)
- Name of child
- Names of children and family members living in the home
- Means of transportation to health care facility, if pertinent
- Description of home, size and type of community

Reason for Seeking Care.   The reason for seeking care portion of the health assessment is the same as for the adult. Data are usually taken from the adult accompanying the child brought for care.

Present Health Status.   The present health status information is also recorded the same as for the adult. If illness is present, record a symptom analysis. If it is a well-child visit, proceed with the data collection about the child's health, growth, and development. (Chapter 2 describes the expected growth and development of children.) Also include information on the following:

- Current medications
  Type (e.g., prescription, over-the-counter, vitamins)
  Prescribed by whom
  Effect of medications
- Allergies (food, drug, environmental factors, contact substances)
- Last examinations (physical, dental, vision, hearing, developmental screening)

- Immunizations: dates administered (see immunization schedule in Chapter 8)

Past Health History.   Health history of mother during pregnancy is the same as for the newborn.

- Birth order
- Neonatal period is the same as described for the newborn
- Illnesses: injuries, hospitalizations, communicable diseases (e.g., colds, earaches, common childhood diseases such as measles, rubella [German measles], chicken pox, mumps, pertussis [whooping cough], diphtheria, scarlet fever, streptococcal infections, tonsillitis, allergic manifestations)

Family History.   Family history should include a maternal gestational history, listing all pregnancies and the health status of living children. For deceased children indicate age, cause of death, and duration of pregnancy if miscarriage.

Other questions about the health of family members are the same as for the adult.

Review of Systems.   The review of systems includes the following additions and variations:

General Health Status
  Fatigue patterns
  Energetic or overactive patterns
  Growth: changes in height and weight appropriate for age
Nutrition
  Breast or bottle fed, reasons for changes, if any; type of formula used, amount offered and consumed, frequency of feeding and weight gain
  Present diet and appetite, age of introduction of solids, age when child achieved three meals a day; present feeding patterns; age weaned from bottle or breast; type of milk and daily intake; food preferences
  Recent weight gain or loss (describe)
  Twenty-four hour recall, including types and amount of food eaten (formula, breast milk, meat, fruits, vegetables, cereals, juices, eggs, milk, sweets, snacks) and frequency
  Does child feed self
  Where does child eat
  Who eats with child
  Parent's perception of child's nutritional status
  Use of vitamin supplements
Integumentary System
  Skin
    Chronic rashes
    Easy bruising, bleeding, or petechiae
  Hair
    Infections, lice
  Nails
    Nail biting
    Hygiene
Eyes
  Crossed eyes
  Complaint of vision changes
  Reading difficulty
  Sits too close to television or video games

Ears

Multiple infections or earaches

Myringotomy tubes in ears

Discharge (describe)

Parent's perception of child's hearing

Mouth and Oropharynx

Dentition: Age of first teeth, loss of deciduous teeth, eruption of first permanent teeth

Sore throat (frequency, describe)

Tonsils present

Mouth sores

Toothaches, caries

Mouth breathing

HP: Tooth brushing and flossing pattern

Breasts

Development of breasts and nipples

Cardiovascular System

Cyanosis (what precipitates it)

Dyspnea (shortness of breath) on exertion

Limitation of activities

Frequent complaints of extremity coldness

Excessive bleeding or easy bruising

Fatigue

Lead exposures

Respiratory System

Snoring

Urinary System

Status of toilet training; plans for; problems

Bed-wetting (associated with emotional upset; family history of bed-wetting)

Use of bubble bath

Genitalia

General

Birth defects

Rashes, irritation

Areas of concern

Female: If menstruating, refer to adult data base for appropriate questions; development of pubic hair

Male: Development of facial and pubic hair, voice changes, emissions, penile/scrotal enlargement

Musculoskeletal System

Gait ability

Curvature of the spine (age when noted)

Generalized aching

Central Nervous System

Birth Injury

Speech

Stuttering

Speech misarticulation

Language delay

Cognitive Changes

Passing out episodes

Staring spells

Learning difficulties

Motor-Gait

Developmental clumsiness

Endocrine System

Precocious or delayed puberty

Psychosocial Status.   The following is an outline of the data collected regarding the child's psychosocial status:

General Status

General statement of child's feelings about self

Parent's observations of child's feelings of self

Development (Following commonly used developmental milestones. Refer to Chapter 2 for comprehensive descriptions.)

Age when able to:

Hold head erect while in sitting position

Roll over from front to back and back to front

Sit alone unsupported

Stand with support and alone

Walk with support and alone

Use words

Talk in sentences

Dress self

Age when toilet trained: approaches to and attitudes regarding toilet training

How sexuality education is handled in the home

Caretakers and Family

Who lives in child's home

Primary care provider for child

Relationships among members of the household

Friends

Child's relationships with friends, classmates, siblings

Age of playmates

Ability to make friends easily

Imaginary friends or animals

Habits

Behavior patterns: nail biting, thumb sucking, pica (habitual ingestion of nonfood substance), rituals ("security" blanket or toy), and unusual movements (head-banging, rocking, overt masturbation, walking on toes)

General description of typical day

Sleep patterns and naps; sound sleeper or fretful; number of hours of sleep per 24 hours; nightmares, night terrors, parent's response

Kinds of play: amount of active and quiet play per 24 hours, television time per 24 hours

Hobbies and methods of relaxation (for older child)

Family

Activities of family as unit

Methods of discipline within family

Effects of discipline

Who disciplines child

Child's reaction to discipline

Parents or providers: type of employment, type of child care provided if both parents work

Availability of emotional support for parents in care of child and opportunity to be away from child

School

Present grade in school or level of nursery care

School performance

Behavior problems

Learning problems; special classes required, if any

Attitude about school

Rate of absenteeism

Ability to Cope with Stress

Child's ability to adapt to new situations

Recent changes or stresses in child's life, (e.g., new baby, financial stress, divorce/separation, move to new home/neighborhood/school)

Behavior patterns child uses to cope with stress

Change in personality, behavior, mood

History of psychiatric care or counseling

Environmental Health.   General statement of parent's assessment of environmental safety and comfort.

Hazards in the home, to include survey of the following:

Toys appropriate for age

Storage of firearms, drugs, toxic chemicals, matches

Stairway protection (e.g., use of gates for toddlers or handrails for older children)

Type of bed (protection device to prevent falls)

Pest control

Open space heaters

Peeling of lead paint in older homes

Injury prevention

Safety belts

Smoke detector in the home

Burn prevention

Medication safety

Hot water heater temperature

Hazards in the neighborhood

Unsafe play area

Stranger safety

Heavily traveled streets

No sidewalks

Water or air pollution

Excessive noise

Isolation or overcrowding from neighbors

Bicycle safety

Other primary prevention measures

Effects of passive smoke

Skin protection from ultraviolet light

ADOLESCENTS

History for an adolescent is similar to that for a child. There are several options to consider when assessing the adolescent. The first is choosing which data base to use, pediatric or adult. Some nurses prefer to use the pediatric data base until the client is 12 to 14 years old and then begin using the adult one, while others modify the pediatric tool and use it throughout adolescence. A second option is whether to assess the adolescent with the parent present. Frequently the history is taken with both present and then the parent is asked to leave so that the adolescent can have time alone with the examiner to discuss health issues privately. Observe the interaction between the adolescent and parent, as well as that with other children in the family who might attend the assessment. A sense of confidentiality should be established so the teenager feels comfortable with the examiner and trusts him or her enough to discuss delicate subjects. In sensitive areas, the nurse should try to approach the teen from a direct but empathetic and nonjudgmental manner. Time should be left at the end of the assessment to summarize the examination and allow time for the adolescent to ask questions. Often adolescents do not reveal what is actually on their minds until the end of the session when the time devoted for the examination is almost gone and they have developed the courage to express concerns. There should be an opportunity at the end of the examination for discussing any risk-taking behaviors such as use of drugs or alcohol, drinking and driving, and sexual practices.

The biographic data, reason for seeking care, present health status, past medical history, and family history for an adolescent are the same as for an adult.

Review of Systems.   ROS for the adolescent is the same as that for the adult with the addition of the following:

Gastrointestinal

Satisfaction with diet and weight

Frequency of binge eating, inducing vomiting, abuse of laxatives, excessive exercise, or prolonged fasting

Genitourinary

Males: age of first night ejaculation

Concern about size of penis

Females: age of onset of menses

Psychosocial Status.   The psychosocial history for adolescents includes those factors listed previously for the adult in addition to specific concerns of this age group. The history is obtained primarily from the adolescent, with or without the parent present. Table 4-1 lists suggested questions to ask the adolescent. The psychosocial history can be summarized using the acronym HEADSS (Home, Education, Activities [including peers], Drugs, Sexuality, Suicide) (Goldenring and Cohen, 1988).

- Home: present family members, intactness of family, relationships between adolescent and other family members or extended family

- Education: grade average, school enjoyment and adjustment, preferred subjects, vocational plans

- Activities: relationships with the same and opposite sex, interests, hobbies, and free-time activities

- Drugs: use of drugs (including alcohol and tobacco) by adolescent, peers, or family members

- Sexuality: knowledge of expected bodily changes during adolescence, dating patterns, sexual activity

- Suicide: feelings of sadness, loneliness, depression, or suicidal thoughts

Environmental Health.   The environmental health history for the adolescent is the same as for the adult.

OLDER ADULTS

There are a variety of definitions, connotations, and meanings for words such as "aging," "aged," "old," and "elderly." The age range from 55 to 74 years has been termed "young-old," while people over 75 are referred to as "old-old." Another differentiation is made between healthy elderly and frail elderly. Often the elderly are described by their functional status, which defines "old" by evaluating the functional performance of clients against standard adult performance (Matteson and McConnell, 1988). The box on p. 54 provides a functional assessment of activities of daily living.

Older adult clients are not different from other adult clients. There is no specific age at which concerns related to

TABLE 4-1	Questions to Ask Adolescents in Obtaining a Psychosocial History

TOPIC	QUESTION
Home	Where do you live and who lives there with you?
Education	What are you good at in school?
	What is hard for you?
	What grades do you get?
Activities	What do you do for fun?
	What things do you do with friends?
	What do you do with your free time?
Drugs	Many teenagers experiment with drugs, alcohol, and cigarettes. Have you or your friends ever tried them? What have you tried? Do any of your family members use drugs, alcohol or cigarettes?
Sexuality	Have you ever had a sexual relationship with anyone?
	Most young people become interested in sexual relationships at your age. Have you had any with boys, girls, or both? Tell me about your sex life.
Suicide	How long does it take you to fall asleep at night?
	How often do you wake up during the night?
	Has there been a change in your appetite or eating pattern? How satisfied are you with your eating patterns? How do you handle your feelings such as anger, sadness, worry, anxiety?

the aging process warrant additional screening questions to complete an accurate data base. The older person may have different concerns and needs due to disability, chronic disease, and changes normal with aging. The older adult client with multiple symptoms, a long history of illness and hospitalizations, and numerous problems at home requires more time for you to adequately analyze the status of each symptom and its interaction with other illnesses. Clients whose speech is impaired from a stroke may need more time to describe their reasons for seeking care.

Reason for Seeking Care. Some older adults have chronic diseases to which they have adapted. Determine if the reason for the visit is related to one of the chronic conditions or is an unrelated problem. Certain problems are not easily identified but, with skilled questioning, they may emerge as the assessment progresses (for instance, depression, weakness, or difficulty caring for self at home).

Older adults may not manifest fever associated with infection to the extent that younger adults do, which is an expected change that comes with aging. Clients may attribute new health problems to "getting old" and therefore not report them as significant.

Patience may be required in identifying priorities of the client's concern, which may be different from the priorities of the nurse.

Present Health Status. Present health status of the older adult should include the following data about current medications:

Type of drug, reason for taking (over-the-counter and prescribed medications)
Prescribed by whom
When first prescribed

Amount of medication per day (compare prescribed with actual doses per day; include over-the-counter drugs also)
How is medication taken
Effectiveness of medication
Side effects of medications
Is there sharing of medications with others
Do visual difficulties affect taking medications
Ability to afford needed medications
Is transportation available to get prescriptions filled

Past Health History. The past health history for an older adult is the same as for the adult. The time span included in the history of course is longer and the client's memory may not be too accurate. Several visits may be required to obtain a comprehensive past health history from an older person.

Family History. Obtaining a family history for an older adult is of questionable value in predicting which diseases the client is at risk for, depending on the age of the client. It does, however, provide data about illnesses and causes of death of relatives.

Review of Systems. The ROS is the same as for the adult.

Psychosocial Status. Obtain data on the following:

General statement of client's feelings about self
Relatives and friends in home or nearby (to meet sexual, affection, support needs)
If client lives alone, to what extent is living alone tolerated? Does client have sufficient and satisfactory access to family and friends? Does client have a pet?
If client lives with family, are relationships satisfactory? Does client participate in family activities and in family decisions? Is there conflict with family members?

Activities of Daily Living (ADL) Assessment

A. Self-care
1. Dressing, undressing, clothing
   a. Keeping clothes in good repair (mending)
   b. Accessing clothes
   c. Getting into and out of underwear (bra, girdle, underpants, pantyhose, stockings, garter belt)
   d. Putting on and removing pants
   e. Getting arms in sleeves
   f. Managing zippers, buttons, snaps (especially in back), ties
   g. Putting on socks, shoes, tying laces
   h. Applying prostheses (e.g., glasses, hearing aids)
2. Grooming and hygiene
   a. Washing, drying, brushing hair
   b. Brushing teeth
   c. Cleaning and putting in dentures
   d. Shaving
   e. Caring for nails (feet and hands)
   f. Applying makeup
   g. Preparing bath water and testing temperature
   h. Getting into and out of tub, shower
   i. Reaching and cleaning all body parts
3. Elimination
   a. Position altered for urination or sitting on toilet
   b. Ability to wipe self
   c. Lowering onto and rising from toilet

B. Mobility
1. Difficulty climbing or descending stairs (Is bedroom/bathroom on upper level? How many stairs/flights to apartment or house?)
2. Sitting up and rising from bed
3. Lowering to or rising from chair
4. Walking (short and long distances); describe necessity for walking
5. Opening doors
6. Reaching items in cupboards
7. Necessity for lifting (and any difficulty)

C. Communication
1. Dialing telephone
2. Reading numbers
3. Hearing over telephone
4. Answering door
5. Immediate access to neighbors, help

D. Eating
1. Access to market
2. Preparing food (opening cans and packages, using stove, reaching dishes, pots, utensils)
3. Handling knife, fork, spoon (cutting meat)
4. Getting food to mouth
5. Chewing, swallowing

E. Housekeeping, laundry, house upkeep
1. Making bed
2. Sweeping, mopping floors
3. Dusting
4. Washing dishes
5. Cleaning tub, bathroom
6. Picking up clutter (to client's satisfaction)
7. Taking out trash, garbage
8. Use of basement (stairs, cleaning)
9. Laundry facilities (in home or near residence, washtub, clothesline)
10. Yard care (garden, bushes, grass)
11. Other home-maintenance concerns (e.g., access to fuse box, storm windows, furnace filters, painting)

F. Medications
1. Large number of prescriptions (may be many)
2. Ability to remember
3. Ability to see labels/directions
4. Medications kept in one area

G. Access to community
1. Busline
2. Walking
3. Driving (self or service from others)
4. Church, dry cleaning, drugstore, bank, health care facility, dentist, other community agencies

H. Other
1. Caring for spouse/relative/companion
2. Financial management (able to write checks, make payments, cash checks)
3. Care of pet(s)

Activities of daily living—Can client independently perform the following:

Dressing, grooming, bathing, preparing meals, grocery shopping, climbing stairs

General description of work, leisure, and rest distribution

Hobbies and methods of relaxation

Family demands

Ability to accomplish all that is desired during period (day/week)

Transportation

Automobile: Does client consider self a safe driver? Is maintaining vehicle a financial burden?

Bus: Easy access? Able to step aboard, does client feel safe when riding bus?

Driving services from others: Availability, convenience

Walking: Problems with distance, carrying packages, fear of traffic

Occupational/volunteer history

Jobs held in past

Current employment

Volunteer and community activities

Satisfaction with present activities

Work/retirement concerns

Reduced/fixed income

Moving/selling home

Role change/time adjustment

Problems in relationship with spouse because of retirement

Recent changes or stresses in client's life (e.g., moving, retirement, illness of self or family member, financial stress, death of friend or family member, new responsibilities)

General statement about client's ability to cope with situation of stress (may also want to get input from spouse, adult child, or close friend)

History of psychiatric care or counseling

Feelings of fear, anxiety, or nervousness

Feelings of depression (e.g., insomnia, crying, fearfulness, marked irritability or anger)

Changes in personality, behavior, mood

Use of medications or other techniques during times of anxiety, stress, or depression

Environmental Health. Data to be obtained should include the following:

General statement of client's assessment of environmental safety and comfort

Hazards of employment (if appropriate): inhalants, noise, heavy lifting, machinery, psychologic stress

Hazards in the home: Concern about fire, stairs to climb, inadequate heat, open gas heaters, pest control, fear of falling

Safety at home for client who has difficulty with activities of daily living:

Gait or balance problems:

Slippery or irregular surfaces (e.g., icy sidewalks, small rugs, risers on stair not fastened down)

Obstructions or clutter on stairs, extension cords

Steep, dark stairs (e.g., cellar)

Stairs without handrails

Inadequate space for maneuvering walker, wheelchair

Slippery bathtub

Decreased vision requires adequate lighting in dark hallway and on stairs, use of a night light

Decreased sensitivity to pain and heat requires caution when using heating pads or hot water bottles, and with hot bath water

Hazards in the neighborhood: Noise, water and air pollution, heavy traffic on surrounding streets, overcrowding, isolation from neighbors, violence, firearms

Community hazards: Unavailability of grocery stores, laundry facilities, drug store, bus line access

Hazard of maintaining a driver's license: Traffic accidents may occur due to slow reaction time, decreased vision, difficulty turning torso, walking too slowly for traffic signals.

SITUATIONAL VARIATIONS IN THE HEALTH HISTORY

PREGNANT WOMEN

The history of the pregnant client is similar to that of the adult. The general physical and psychologic health of the mother and the management of chronic diseases could affect her health and that of the fetus. Prenatal visits are recommended every 4 weeks up to 28 weeks gestation, every 2 weeks from 28 to 36 weeks gestation, and weekly after 36 weeks gestation.

Biographic Data.

- Age: Note if woman is "elderly primipara" (over 35 years of age).

- Cultural, especially beliefs about child bearing

- Occupation, socioeconomic factors, including health insurance information

- Persons living in home; name of support persons for labor, delivery, child rearing

- Means of transportation, if pertinent

Reason for Seeking Care. Prenatal visits are needed to monitor the health of the mother and growth of the fetus, as well as to educate the mother and family about the care of mother and neonate during the delivery process and neonatal period.

Present Health Status. Data specific to the pregnant woman; include her present nutritional status, motherhood coping abilities, and general physical and psychologic well-being.

Past Health History. A pregnant woman's gravida (number of previous pregnancies), parity (number of children born alive), abortions (both spontaneous "miscarriages" and "therapeutic" pregnancy interruptions), and information about her live and deceased offspring should be noted. Data about previous labor patterns should be explored. History of sexually transmitted diseases, other gynecologic problems, or history of sexual assault are needed.

Family History. A pregnant woman's history should include the childbearing history of her mother and sister(s). Questions should be asked about family history of diabetes mellitus, renal disease, and hereditary diseases.

Review of Systems. An assessment of body systems includes data obtained during an adult examination, plus findings pertinent to pregnancy or after delivery.

Fetal Assessments
Report of fetal movements
Integumentary System
Skin marks, lines, varicosities
Nose and Mouth
Nose bleeding
Nasal stuffiness
Gum bleeding
Ears
Hearing loss
Eyes
Visual changes
Respiratory System
Shortness of breath
Cardiovascular System
Palpitations
Edema of extremities
Orthostatic hypotension
Breasts
Enlargement, engorgement, tenderness
Gastrointestinal System
First trimester: Nausea, vomiting
Heartburn, esophageal reflux
Constipation
Hemorrhoids

Genitourinary System
Urinary frequency and urgency
Vaginal discharge
Musculoskeletal System
Backache
Leg cramps
Ankle edema

Psychosocial History. Adjustment to parenthood should be assessed. Emotional stability data should be collected, which would include the incidence of excessive crying, social withdrawal, or decisions related to infant care.

Environmental Health. Environmental factors are particularly important during childbearing because of risks of teratogens. Exposure to toxins should be assessed and preventive steps taken.

SUMMARY

Collecting a thorough history accomplishes several goals. It establishes a therapeutic relationship with the client. It also provides a picture of the client and identifies problems mentioned by the client that you can confirm or refute during the physical examination.

Once data are collected they must be organized, synthesized, and documented. When you collect health history data in an organized manner, the documentation becomes easier. See the following example of a health history documentation for an adult.

SAMPLE ADULT HEALTH HISTORY DOCUMENTATION

Biographic Data

Name Megan S. Dabney

Address 5410 Cypress Hill, Irving, Texas 75062

Telephone numbers (214) 999-9999-home; (214) 444-4444-work

Birthdate 10-13-54 (40 years old)

Birth place Houston, Texas

Race Caucasian

Culture American female

Religion Methodist

Marital status Married, 15 years

Family Lives with spouse, two sons, and mother in a four bedroom home in a suburban area

Social security number 123-45-6789

Occupation Counselor in a high school

Contact person Kyle Dabney, spouse

Advanced directive Yes, spouse has power of attorney

Source of referral Colleague at work

Type of insurance Network Health

Megan S. Dabney is a 40-year-old, white woman in no acute distress.

Reason for Seeking Care cc: "need Pap smear and something for these allergies"

Present Health Status

Health has been good during last 5 years; during past year has had sneezing, watery eyes, nasal congestion with clear nasal drainage. (Symptom analysis) Symptoms worse in the spring months, slow onset. Nasal congestion interferes with sleep and sometimes eating. Sneezing "fits" interfere with activity at the time; may sneeze 10-15 times in succession. Sneezing "fits" occur every 2-3 days at unpredictable times, at home rather than at work. Tearing of eyes occurs with sneezing. Takes over-the-counter allergy relief medicine, which gives temporary relief. Working in the yard makes symptoms worse.

Current health promotion activities include walking 1.5 miles 2-3 times/week; performs breast self-exam each month.

Diet

Usual breakfast—muffin, 1% milk, fruit juice, coffee
Usual lunch—eats at school; meat, 1 vegetable, salad, tea
Usual dinner—meat (turkey, chicken, pork, rarely beef); fruit or tossed salad; 1 green or yellow vegetable; potato, pasta, or rice; dessert; 1% milk.
Snacks—crackers with salsa or peanut butter

Current medications: Multiple vitamin plus vitamin C 1000 mg; zinc 50 mg; vitamin E 400 units; aspirin 325 mg; over-the-counter allergy medications

SAMPLE ADULT HEALTH HISTORY DOCUMENTATION—*cont'd*

Past Health History

Allergies: Seasonal allergies, does not know what she is allergic to. Denies allergies to drugs or food

Childhood diseases: 1956-1966 measles, mumps, rubella, chicken pox, streptococcal throat, otitis media. Denies complications

Surgeries: 1958 Brachial cleft cyst removed Houston, Texas, Dr. Skylar

1979 appendectomy Irving, Texas Dr. Reed

Hospitalizations: See obstetric below

Accidents/injuries: Denies

Immunizations: Childhood immunizations for school, denies tetanus immunization since high school

Last examinations:

  Physical, pap smear—March, 1993

  Dentist—December, 1994

  Vision—September, 1990

  Hearing—high school

  ECG—denies

  Mantoux test—September, 1994

  Mammogram—denies

Obstetric history: Gravida 2, Para 2, Abortions 0

  1978 vaginal delivery 6 lb 14 oz. healthy boy, no complications

  1982 vaginal delivery, 7 lb healthy boy, no complications

  1985 tubal ligation, no complications

Family History

Review of Systems

General: Client considers herself in "good health" except for allergies. Denies fatigue. Feels rested after sleep periods.

Nutritional: Reported height = 5 ft. 9 in. (27 cm), reported weight = 140 lbs (63 kg). Weight consistent

Integumentary system

  Skin: Denies lesions, masses, discolorations, rashes. Some pruritus during winter months, clears with lotion.

  HP: Uses sun screen when outside >1 hour

  Hair: Denies texture changes or loss, uses hair color monthly to cover gray; no scalp irritation reported from hair coloring

  Nails: Denies changes in texture, color, shape. Manicures nails weekly

Head: Denies scalp itching, headache, trauma, vertigo, syncope

Eyes: Wears glasses/contacts for nearsighted vision. Eyes water during "allergy attacks" Denies discharge, pruritus, pain, visual disturbances

Ears: Has pierced ears—1970. Cleans ears with cotton-tipped applicator after shower. Denies pain, discharge, tinnitus

Nose, nasopharynx, paranasal sinuses: Clear nasal discharge, sneezing, nasal congestion during "allergy attacks", Denies epistaxis, olfactory deficit, snoring

Mouth and oropharynx: Denies sore throat, lesions, gum irritation, chewing or swallowing difficulties, hoarseness, voice changes

  HP: Brushes teeth twice daily followed by flossing

Neck: Denies tenderness or range of motion difficulties

Breasts: Tenderness before menstrual periods, takes vitamin E to prevent fibrocystic breast disease; denies discharge lumps, masses

Cardiovascular system: Denies chest pain, shortness of breath and palpitations; feet frequently feel cold; denies discoloration and peripheral edema

Respiratory system: Denies breathing difficulties, chronic cough and shortness of breath

Gastrointestinal system: Denies eating and digestion problems; denies hematemesis, jaundice, ascites; daily bowel movement is formed, brown; denies hemorrhoids

Urinary system: Describes urine as yellow and clear; voiding frequency 4-5 times daily; denies voiding difficulties, dysuria, urgency and flank pain; infrequent nocturia. Denies polyuria and oliguria.

Genitalia: LMP 4-28-95; menses every 28-30 days, regular intervals, light to medium flow; cramps controlled with ibuprofen; has premenstrual syndrome (PMS) most months; denies genital lesions, discharge, STD history; sexually active, satisfied with sexual activity

Musculoskeletal system: Denies muscular weakness, twitching and pain, gait difficulties and extremity deformities, joint swelling pain, stiffness and crepitus.

Central nervous system: Denies changes in cognitive function, coordination, and sensory deficits

Endocrine system: Denies changes in skin pigment, change in weight, polyuria, polydipsia, polyphagia, anorexia, weakness. Family history of diabetes mellitus.

Continued

SAMPLE ADULT HEALTH HISTORY DOCUMENTATION—*cont'd*

Psychosocial Status

Client states she feels good about herself most of the time. She experiences episodes of frustration integrating her mother into the life of her family. She considers her husband her best friend, but also speaks of two other very close female friends. She counts on her friends to help her "talk through" stress periods. Considers family very close, communication channels are open most of the time. Her oldest teenage son resists sharing what is going on in his life, but has been told that his parents are available if he needs them.

Client's activities include maintaining a home, raising two teenage boys, working full time. Her mother helps to maintain the home and prepare meals. Client is active in a community organization and church activities. A current family demand is disagreements she has with her mother about how to discipline her sons. She would like more time for herself.

She has a Master's degree in counseling. She enjoys her job as a high school counselor which she has held for 12 years. She gets frustrated with the lack of parenting skills of some of her students' parents.

Recent change in her life is a new principal who has just joined the school. She is not sure how well they will interact.

Client denies previous psychiatric counseling or feelings of anxiety or nervousness that she could not cope with. Methods of coping with stress are exercise and talking with her friends. To relax client enjoys drawing, playing piano, and gardening. Client and her spouse have had marriage counseling on two different occasions, which she feels was beneficial.

Drug/Alcohol: Denies drug use; 1-2 glasses wine per week.

Smoking: Denies.

Coffee/tea: 2 cups coffee and 1 glass tea daily.

Financial Status: Feels there is adequate money for their activities and saving for college and retirement.

Environmental Health

Client believes her home and neighborhood environment are safe and without hazards.

Subjective problem list

1. Needs Pap smear
2. Seasonal allergies: Wants more effective medication treatment
3. Needs tetanus immunization
4. Dysmenorrhea monthly controlled with ibuprofen
5. Concerned about fibrocystic disease for which she takes vitamin E
6. Conflict with her mother about discipline of sons
7. Concerned about relation with new principal at work

(Final problem list is developed and priorities are established after physical examination)

??????? STUDY QUESTIONS ???????

1. What is the primary purpose of taking a health history?

2. What general information is obtained when taking a health history.

3. What are the American Nurses Association Standards of Practice and how do they relate to health assessment?

4. List four factors that may affect the outcome of a health assessment interview.

5. What can you do to increase an individual's comfort level during an interview?

6. Distinguish between a focused and a comprehensive assessment. Give an example of a situation where each is appropriate.

7. Identify factors that will enhance communication with the client.

8. List at least five techniques that you may employ to enhance the information you receive when asking questions.

9. Give two examples of an open-ended question that you might use to start a health assessment interview.

10. When are closed-ended questions appropriate? What are directive questions used for?

11. List and give examples of five techniques that can enhance data collection.

12. List six techniques that may interfere with data collection in an interview.

13. Clients are often curious about the health care provider. How should you handle personal questions about yourself?

14. Why do you need to be sensitive to an individual's culture when conducting an assessment?

15. How would you handle a situation in which the individual cries during the interview? What if the person were to suddenly become angry?

16. Define the term *biographic data* and explain why such data would be helpful to you as a health care provider.

17. How would your approach to collecting information about present health status vary based on the reason for seeking care?

18. Describe the components included in a symptom analysis.

19. What is the purpose of collecting data about an individual's past health status?

20. Outline the components of the past health history.

21. Why is a family history important? How many generations should you ask about?

22. What is the purpose of the review of systems?

23. Select four body systems and outline the specific areas that need to be explored in a review of that system.

24. What types of habits need to be assessed? Describe the various aspects of environmental health that need to be reviewed.

25. List at least two areas of health history that are specific to each of the following groups: (a) pregnant women; (b) infants; (c) young children; (d) adolescents; (e) older adults.

26. List the important aspects of the maternal history that are needed in relation to the newborn.

27. How does the health history of a child differ from that of an adult?

28. What are some health promotion areas that need to be explored for the child?

29. How is the health history of an adolescent different from that of an adult?

30. How would you communicate with an adolescent as opposed to an adult?

31. Discuss the information that you might collect from an adolescent during the psychosocial history review.

32. Identify four needs that are unique to the older adult.

33. When should a child receive his or her first rubella vaccine? Polio vaccine? DPT vaccine?

34. Identify health promotion and safety issues specific to the older adult.

35. When should pregnant women schedule prenatal visits? What are the purposes of prenatal visits?

CHAPTER 5

Equipment for Physical Assessment

Many of the techniques of physical assessment require the use of instruments to objectively measure or evaluate clinical signs or health status. This chapter describes the equipment most frequently used for physical assessment, as well as the personal protective clothing that may be required during the examination.

Use of these instruments is found either in Chapter 6, "Techniques of Physical Assessment," or in the clinical chapters where the instruments are most frequently used.

THERMOMETERS (TEMPERATURE MEASUREMENT)

Purpose: *To assess the functional status of the body's tissues and cells.*

Four types of thermometers are commonly in use to evaluate body temperature: mercury-in-glass, electronic, tympanic, and disposable. The most inexpensive, the *mercury thermometer* (Fig. 5-1, *A*), consists of a glass tube sealed at one end with a mercury-filled bulb at the other. Exposure of the bulb to heat causes the mercury to expand and rise in the enclosed tube. These thermometers may be calibrated in either Fahrenheit or Celsius, and may be designed for oral, axillary, or rectal use.

The *electronic thermometer* (Fig. 5-1, *B*) consists of a battery-powered display unit, a thin wire cord, and a temperature-sensitive probe. The probe must be covered with a disposable sheath before use. The probes are color-coded (blue or white for oral and red for rectal) for proper use. The advantage of the electronic thermometer over the mercury thermometer is speed. The electronic thermometer calculates and displays the temperature on a digital screen within 15 to 30 seconds. Many electronic thermometers have a switch on the unit to permit the reporting of temperature in either Fahrenheit or Celsius.

The *tympanic thermometer* (Fig. 5-1, *C*) is becoming very popular in all clinical settings. Taking the client's temperature with this device requires less than 5 seconds and is very easy. The device works when the temperature-sensitive probe, covered with a disposable sheath, is inserted into the client's ear; the probe measures the temperature of the blood flowing near the tympanic membrane. Tympanic thermometers may be programmed to report in either Fahrenheit or Celsius.

Disposable, single-use thermometer strips (Fig. 5-1, *D*) are thin strips of plastic with chemically impregnated paper. They are frequently used for temperature evaluation in children. Chemical dots on the strip change color, representing the highest temperature. The strips are configured so that the examiner can identify the highest colored dot and correlate that with the temperature reading.

STETHOSCOPE

Purpose: *To hear sounds within the body that are not easily heard with the naked ear.*

There are several types of stethoscopes: the acoustic stethoscope, the magnetic stethoscope, the electronic stethoscope, and the stereophonic stethoscope. For routine health assessment, the acoustic stethoscope is most commonly used (Fig. 5-2).

The *acoustic stethoscope* is a closed cylinder that transmits sound waves from the source through the tube to the examiner's ears. It does not magnify sound, but, by blocking out extraneous room noise, it permits difficult-to-hear sounds to be more easily heard. The stethoscope consists of three components: the ear pieces, the tubing, and the end piece. The *ear pieces,* which may be hard or soft, should fit snugly and completely fill the ear canal. When the ear pieces are correctly placed in the ears, they should point toward the nose. This alignment fits the contour of the ear canal. The *tubing* of the stethoscope should be made of thick, firm rubber that is no longer than 12 to 18 inches (30 to 40 cm) in length. If the tubing is longer than 18 inches, the sounds may become distorted. The *head* of the stethoscope consists of two components: the diaphragm and the bell. The head of the stethoscope should be heavy enough to lie firmly on the body surface without being held. This piece is configured by a closure valve so that only the diaphragm or the bell may be activated at any one time. The *diaphragm* consists of a flat surface with a rubber or plastic ring edge. It is used to hear

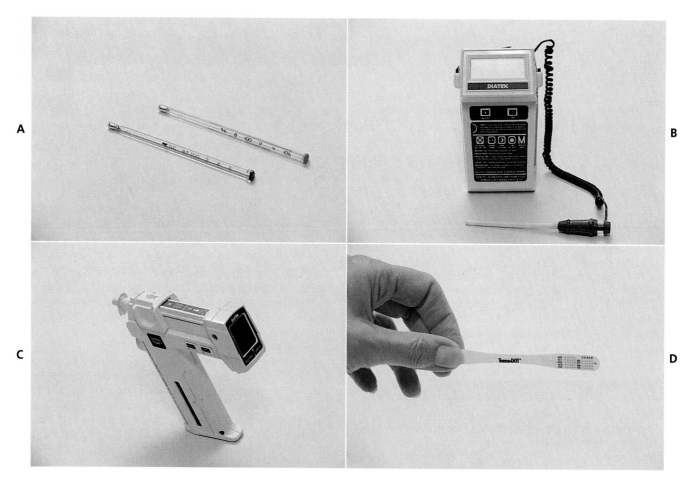

Fig. 5-1   **A,** Mercury thermometer (*rectal*, red tip; *oral*, blue tip). **B,** Electronic thermometer. **C,** Tympanic thermometer. **D,** Disposable, single-use thermometer strips.

high-pitched sounds such as breath sounds, bowel sounds, and normal heart sounds. Its structure screens out low-pitched sounds. The *bell* of the stethoscope is constructed in a concave shape. It should be used to hear soft, low-pitched sounds such as extra heart sounds or vascular sounds (bruits). When using the bell, the examiner should hold it lightly in place to ensure that a complete seal exists around the bell. If the bell is firmly placed on the skin and the concave surface is filled with skin, the bell will convert and function as a diaphragm.

Stethoscopes have varying sizes of end pieces, which are interchangeable. When examining an infant or young child, the diaphragm and bell should be sized accordingly. Ideally, the diaphragm and the bell should span one intercostal space.

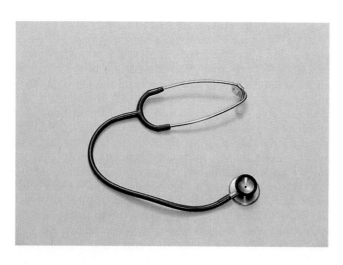

Fig. 5-2   Acoustic stethoscope.

BLOOD PRESSURE MEASUREMENT EQUIPMENT

Purpose: *To assess cardiovascular function by measurement of peripheral blood flow.*

Blood pressure measurement requires three pieces of equipment—the sphygmomanometer, the cuff, and the stethoscope. Together they may be used to measure blood pressure.

There are three types of *sphygmomanometers.* Two types, aneroid and mercury, attach to a blood pressure cuff bladder and require manual cuff inflation. A stethoscope must be used in conjunction with these devices to actually assess the blood pressure. The third type is electronic and assesses the blood pressure without the use of a stethoscope.

1. An *aneroid* sphygmomanometer is a glass-enclosed circular gauge containing a needle that registers in millimeter calibrations. The gauge is attached to the blood pressure cuff bladder (Fig. 5-3, *A*). This gauge needs periodic calibration to ensure accurate measurement.

2. A *mercury* sphygmomanometer is an upright manometer tube containing mercury. The pressure created in the bladder of the cuff moves the column of mercury up against the force of gravity. Millimeter calibrations mark the height of the mercury column (Fig. 5-3, *B*).

3. An *electronic* sphygmomanometer operates by sensing circulating blood flow vibrations and converting these vibrations into electric impulses. These impulses in turn are translated to a digital readout. The readout generally consists of blood pressure, mean arterial pressure, and pulse rate. The device is not capable of determining quality of the pulse, such as rhythm or intensity. The device may be programmed to repeat the measurements on a scheduled periodic basis and to alarm if the measurements are outside of the precalculated limits. No stethoscope is required when the electronic device is used (Fig. 5-3, *C*).

A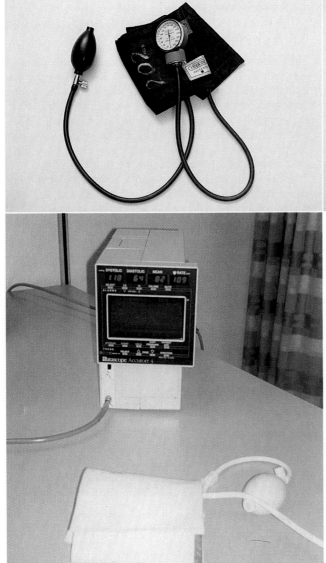

B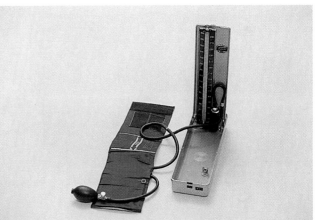

C

Fig. 5-3 A, Aneroid sphygmomanometer. **B,** Mercury manometer tube. **C,** Electronic blood pressure measurement.

Blood pressure cuffs are either disposable and made of a latex substance or reusable and made of a textured fabric (Fig. 5-4). Which type is used depends on the clinical situation. All cuffs have a bladder that inflates during blood pressure measurement and a cuff that secures the bladder on the arm. When selecting a blood pressure cuff it is important to select the correct size for the client. Ideally the bladder of the cuff should be 40%, or ⅓ to ½, of the circumference of the limb. Adult cuffs come in two widths. The standard cuff (4⅔ to 5⅙ inches) is adequate for most adults. If the adult is large or obese, an oversized cuff (6 to 6⅓ inches) may be used. If the adult has an extremely obese arm, a thigh cuff can be used. For children, there are many different sizes or cuffs. The width of the cuff should cover ⅔ of the child's or infant's upper arm. For both children and adults, if the cuff is too wide, it will underestimate the blood pressure; if it is too narrow, it will overestimate the blood pressure.

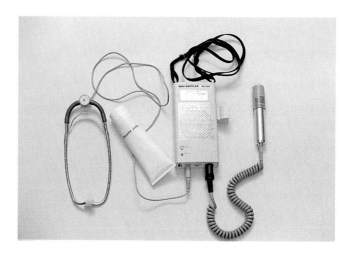

Fig. 5-5   Doppler.

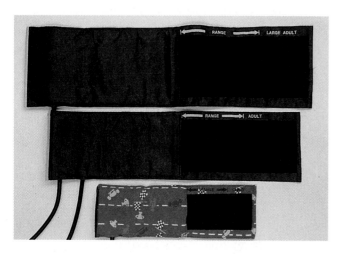

Fig. 5-4   Blood pressure cuffs.

PULSE OXIMETRY

Purpose: *To estimate the arterial oxygen saturation in the blood.*

Pulse oximetry is a noninvasive measurement of arterial oxygen saturation in the blood (Fig. 5-6). This fiber-optic procedure, first developed in Japan, is becoming commonly used as a screening device to determine oxygen saturation. The fiberoptic beam reflects off of the circulating red blood cells. This reflection is used to calculate an estimation of the percentage of oxygen saturation in arterial blood. The oximeter consists of a cutaneous sensor probe that may be taped or clipped to the client's ear, finger, toe, foot, or wrist. The procedure is accurate and precise for saturation in the 50% to 100% range, but may not be reliable for lower saturations (Spyr and Preach, 1990).

DOPPLER

Purpose: *To amplify sounds that are difficult to hear with an acoustic stethoscope.*

The Doppler uses ultrasonic waves to detect difficult-to-hear vascular sounds, such as fetal heart tones or peripheral pulses (Fig. 5-5). To use the device, a gel is applied to the probe; then the probe is slid over the skin surface until the blood flow source is heard in the examiner's earpieces. As blood in the vessels ebbs and flows, the probe on the distal end of the Doppler picks up and amplifies the subtle changes in pitch. The resulting sound that the examiner hears is a swishing, pulsating sound. Most Dopplers have a sound volume control to amplify the sound. In prenatal clinics the Doppler often is attached to speakers so that the expectant parents may also hear the fetal heart sounds.

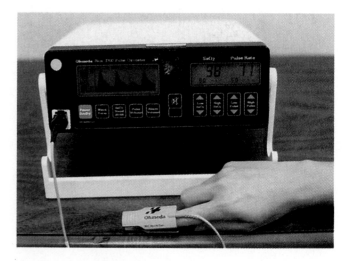

Fig. 5-6   Pulse oximeter.

SNELLEN VISUAL ACUITY CHART

Purpose: *Used as a screening examination for far, or distant, vision.*

The Snellen chart is a large wall chart hung at a distance of 20 feet from the client (Fig. 5-7, *A*). The chart consists of eleven lines of letters of decreasing size. The letter size indicates the degree of visual acuity when read from a distance of 20 feet. The client should be tested one eye at a time. Beside each line of letters is the corresponding acuity rating that should be recorded (e.g., 20/40, 20/100). The top number of the recording indicates the distance between the client and the chart and the bottom number indicates the distance at which a person with normal vision should be able to read that line of the chart.

For young children or non–English-speaking individuals, the "E" chart may be used (Fig. 5-7, *B*). The examiner describes the "E" as a table with legs and asks the client to point in the direction that the legs of the table point. The scoring of the "E" chart is the same as that of the Snellen chart.

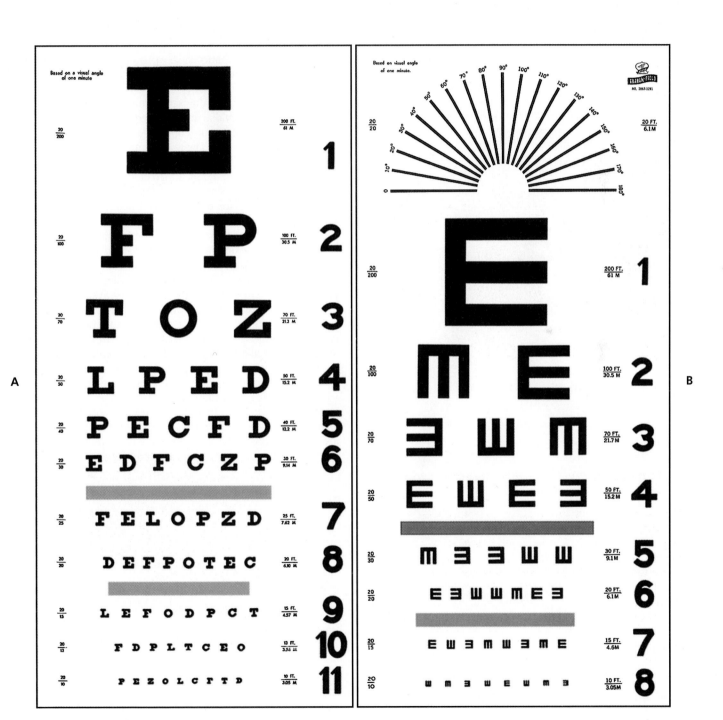

Fig. 5-7   A, Snellen visual acuity chart. **B,** "E" chart.   *(From Seidel et al, 1995.)*

NEAR VISION CHART

Purpose: *To assess the client's near, or close-up, vision.*

Two charts, the Jaeger and Rosenbaum, are commonly used to evaluate near vision. The Rosenbaum chart consists of a series of numbers, Es, Xs, and Os in graduated sizes (Fig. 5-8). The client should hold the chart 14 inches from the face. Each eye should be individually evaluated for visual acuity. Visual acuity is measured in the same distance equivalents as the far vision acuity charts, such as 20/20. The Jaeger equivalent is also shown on the Rosenbaum card. The Jaeger equivalent for 20/20 is Jaeger 2.

Each eye should be evaluated separately. If a Rosenbaum card is not available, near vision may be approximated by holding a newspaper at a distance of 14 inches from the client's face. The client should be able to read the newsprint without difficulty.

OPHTHALMOSCOPE

Purpose: *To examine the internal structures of the eye.*

The ophthalmoscope is a system that consists of a series of lenses, mirrors, and light apertures that, when focused correctly, permits the examiner to inspect the detailed internal structures of the (Fig. 5-9). The instrument itself consists of the ophthalmoscope head and the handle, which either contains batteries or connects to a wall-mounted electrical source. The head and power source fit together by a turn-and-lock system.

The head of the ophthalmoscope consists of two moveable parts, the lens selector dial and the aperture setting. The lenses (diopters) of the ophthalmoscope have varying magnification ranging from −20 to +40. The positive numbers on the lens are shown in black and the negative numbers are shown in red. When the *lens selector dial* is turned clockwise, the positive or black-number-sphere lenses are brought into place. Likewise, when the lens selector disk is turned counterclockwise, the negative or red-number-sphere lenses are brought into place. The plus and minus lenses compensate for myopia or hyperopia in either the examiner's or client's eyes, and also permit focusing at different places within the client's eye. When the nurse begins to examine the client's eye at the cornea, the lens focus setting should be at about a black 20. As the examiner evaluates each area of the internal eye, moving from the anterior surface to the back of the eye, the lens focus must be adjusted downward to maintain clarity. By the time the examiner reaches the macula at the posterior wall of the back of the eye, the focus setting should be approximately at black 0.

The *aperture setting* has several settings that permit light variations during the examination. If the client's pupils have been dilated, the *large light* may be used for the internal eye examination. The *small light* may be used if the client's pupils are very small or if the pupils have not been dilated. The *red-free filter* actually shines a green beam of light. The filter fa-

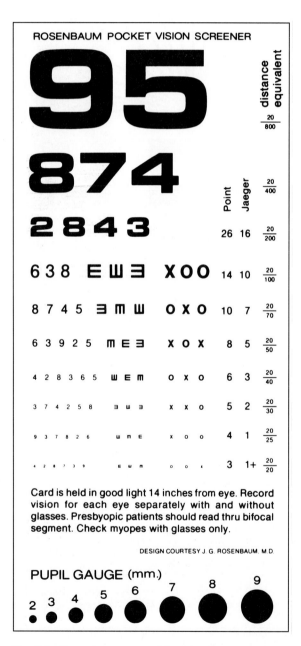

Fig. 5-8 Rosenbaum near vision chart. *(From Seidel et al, 1995.)*

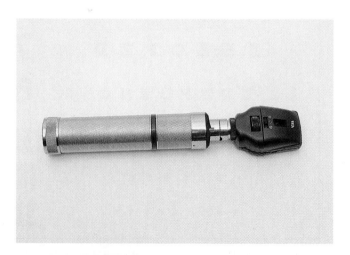

Fig. 5-9 Ophthalmoscope.

cilitates the identification of pallor of the disc and permits the recognition of retinal hemorrhages by making the blood appear black. The *slit light* permits easy examination of the anterior of the eye, as well as determination of elevation or depression of a lesion. The *grid light* permits the examiner to estimate the size, location, or pattern of a fundal lesion.

OTOSCOPE

Purpose: *To provide illumination and magnification for the examination of the external auditory canal and tympanic membrane.*

The otoscope consists of two and sometimes three components: the head, the handle, and sometimes the pneumatic attachment (Fig. 5-10). The *head* of the otoscope consists of a magnification lens, a light source, and a speculum that is inserted into the auditory canal. Specula come in various sizes. Choose the largest size speculum that will fit into the client's ear canal. The *handle* of the otoscope either contains batteries or connects to a wall-mounted electrical source. The *pneumatic attachment* for the otoscope is used to evaluate the fluctuation of the tympanic membrane in children. The attachment consists of a small rubber tube that is attached to the head of the otoscope and a bulb that is attached to the other end of the tubing. When the bulb is squeezed, it produces small puffs of air against the tympanic membrane, causing the membrane to move. No fluctuation of the membrane may indicate pressure behind the membrane.

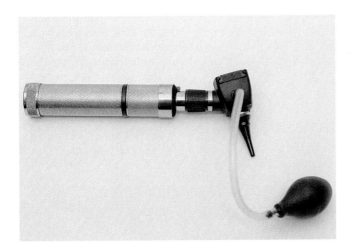

Fig. 5-10　Otoscope with pneumatic bulb.

NASAL SPECULUM

Purpose: *To spread the opening of the nares so the internal surfaces of the nose may be examined.*

Two instruments may be used as a nasal speculum. The *simple nasal speculum* is used in conjunction with a penlight to visualize the lower middle and lower turbinates of the nose (Fig. 5-11). The instrument is used by gently squeezing the handle of the speculum, causing the blades of the speculum to open and spread the nares, which permits internal inspection of the nose. The second type of nasal speculum is a broad-tipped, cone-shaped device that is placed on the end of an otoscope. The nasal cavity may be inspected by using the light source and viewing lens of the otoscope.

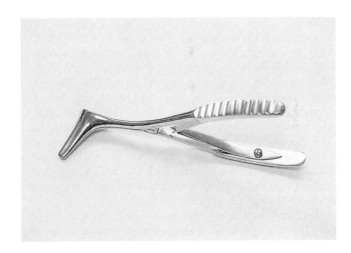

Fig. 5-11　Nasal speculum.

TUNING FORK

Purpose: *The tuning fork has two purposes in physical assessment: (1) auditory screening and (2) assessment of fibratory sensation during the neurologic examination.*

The tuning fork is used during the physical examination for both sound and vibratory sensation evaluation (Fig. 5-12). For *auditory evaluation,* a high-pitched tuning fork with a frequency of 500 to 1000 Hz should be used. This frequency fork can estimate hearing loss in the range of normal speech (300 to 3000 Hz). If a lower-frequency fork were used, overestimation of hearing ability could result. For *neurologic vibratory evaluation* a tuning fork with a pitch between 100 and 400 Hz should be used.

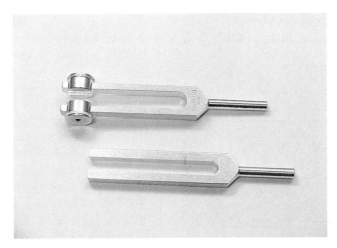

Fig. 5-12　Tuning forks for vibratory sensation *(top)* and auditory screening *(bottom).*

AUDIOMETER

Purpose: *To perform basic screening for hearing acuity.*

The audiometer produces pure tones of simple sound waves. Sound is described by the number of vibrations that occur per second. Cycles per second (cps) or hertz (Hz) represent the vibrations. A young healthy person can hear frequencies from 16 to 20,000 Hz, but hearing is most sensitive from 500 to 4000 Hz; most speech sounds lie between 500 and 3000 Hz. A *decibel* measures the intensity or strength of sound ranging from 0 dB to 140 dB, with 0 being the softest. The intensity of sound required to make any frequency barely audible to the average ear is 0 dB. *Threshold* refers to the signal level at which pure tones are detected. A whisper is 20 dB; normal conversation is 40 to 65 dB. A 40 to 46 dB loss in all frequencies (Hz) causes moderate difficulty in hearing normal speech. A client with a 15 to 20 dB loss in only high frequencies such as 4000 Hz would have difficulty hearing high-pitched consonants (Lewis and Collier, 1992).

The hand-held, battery-operated audiometer (Fig. 5-13) provides a fast, simple test to detect hearing problems. Remove the audiometer from the charging unit. Select the ear speculum that best fits the client's ear canal; a snug fit is desired to screen out surrounding noise. Attach the ear speculum to the audiometer with a clockwise turn. Instruct clients to respond when they hear the tone. Often the client is asked to respond by raising an index finger to indicate hearing a tone. Set the audiometer to 20 dB and push the start button. The audiometer systematically and au-tomatically creates tones at the different frequencies: 1000, 2000, 4000, and 5000. A light appears on the audiometer when the specific tone at a given frequency is sounded. The client's raised index finger, indicating perception of a tone, should correspond to the light seen by the examiner on the audiometer. The client should hear the four tones in each ear. If any of the tones is not heard, increase the dB to 25 and repeat the test procedure at the different frequencies. If any of these tones is not heard, use 40 dB. When these tones are not heard at 40 dB, refer the client for further evaluation.

PERCUSSION OR REFLEX HAMMER

Purpose: *To test deep tendon reflexes.*

The percussion, or reflex, hammer consists of a triangular rubber component on the end of a metal handle (Fig. 5-14). The hammer is configured so that either flat or pointed surfaces may be used to elicit the reflex response. The flat surface is most commonly used when striking the tendon directly. The pointed surface may be used either to strike the tendon directly or to strike the examiner's finger, which is placed on a small tendon such as the client's biceps tendon. A neurologic hammer can also be used to test deep tendon reflexes. It is similar to a percussion hammer, but the rubber striking end is rounded on both sides.

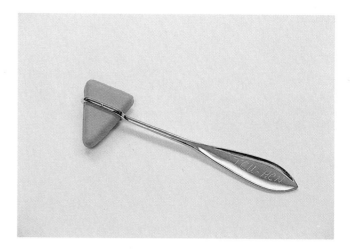

Fig. 5-14   Percussion hammer.

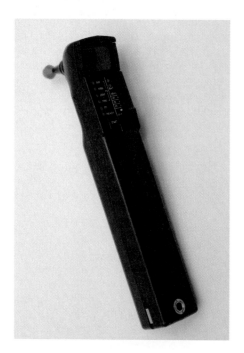

Fig. 5-13   Audiometer.

GONIOMETER

Purpose: *To determine the degree of flexion or extension of a joint.*

The goniometer is a two-piece ruler that is jointed in the middle with a protractor-type measuring device (Fig. 5-15). The goniometer is placed over a joint and, as the individual extends or flexes the joint, the degrees of flexion and extension are measured on the protractor.

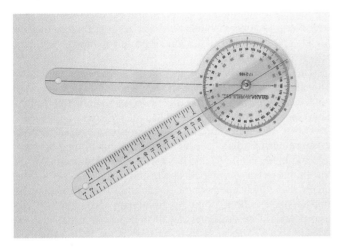

Fig. 5-15   Goniometer.

PENLIGHT

Purpose: *To provide a focused light source during the assessment at any point at which the examiner desires one.*

The penlight has many uses during a physical assessment (Fig. 5-16). It may be used to illuminate the inside of the mouth or nose, highlight a lesion, or evaluate pupillary constriction. It is most important that the penlight have a bright light source. If the examiner does not have a penlight, the light transmitted from the otoscope may be substituted as a focused light source.

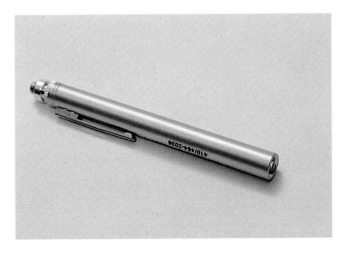

Fig. 5-16   Penlight.

RULER

Purpose: *To measure lesions or other marks on the skin.*

A small metric ruler that has both millimeter and centimeter markings is useful for measuring lesions or other marks on the skin (Fig. 5-17). It is helpful if the ruler is transparent.

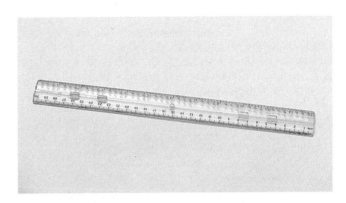

Fig. 5-17   Centimeter ruler.

TAPE MEASURE

Purpose: *To measure circumference and length.*

A tape measure is convenient when measuring the length of an infant, the circumference of a client's head or chest, and in other situations. A tape measure that has inches on one side and centimeters on the reverse side is ideal. To ensure accuracy of measurement, it is imperative that the tape measure be nonstretchable.

CALIPERS FOR SKINFOLD THICKNESS

Purpose: *To measure the thickness of subcutaneous tissue in order to determine an estimate of the amount of body fat.*

Different models of calipers (e.g., Lang or Herpendem) may be used to measure the thickness of subcutaneous tissue at different points on the body (Fig. 5-18). The most frequent location for thickness evaluation is the posterior aspect of the triceps.

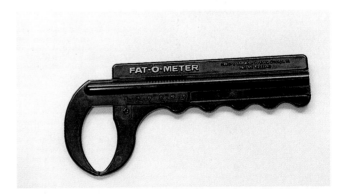

Fig. 5-18   Skinfold thickness calipers.

TRANSILLUMINATOR

Purpose: *To differentiate the characteristics of tissue, fluid, and air within a specific body cavity.*

A transilluminator consists of a strong light source with a narrow beam at the distal section of the light (Fig. 5-19). When the examination room is darkened and the light is placed directly against the skin over a body cavity such as a sinus area or the scrotum, the transilluminator disseminates its light source under the surface of the skin. Depending on whether the area under the skin surface is air, fluid, or tissue, the light is transmitted differentially and provides different glowing red tones of light.

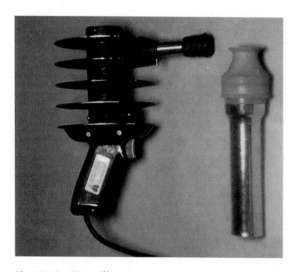

Fig. 5-19 Transilluminator. *(From Seidel et al, 1995.)*

WOOD'S LAMP

Purpose: *To detect fungal infections of the skin or, used with fluorescein dye, to detect corneal abrasions.*

The Wood's lamp produces a black light that, when shined on a fungal infection or corneal abrasion, makes the lesion appear as fluorescent yellow-green (Fig. 5-20). The examination room should be darkened to enhance the clinical interpretation of the lesion color.

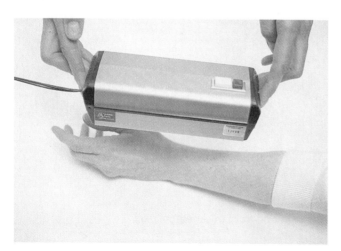

Fig. 5-20 Woods lamp. The purple color on the skin indicates no fungal infection is present.

VAGINAL SPECULUM

Purpose: *To spread the walls of the vaginal canal so the examiner can visualize the vaginal tissue and the cervix.*

There are three types of vaginal specula: the Graves' speculum, the Pederson speculum, and the pediatric or virginal speculum. All of the specula are composed of two blades and a handle, and may be available as either reusable metal or disposable plastic models (Fig. 5-21). The *Graves' speculum* is available in a variety of sizes, with blades ranging from 3.5 to 5.0 inches in length and 0.75 to 1.25 inches in width. The bottom blade is approximately 0.25 inches longer than the top blade. This conforms to the longer posterior vaginal wall and aids with visualization.

The *Pederson speculum* has blades that are as long as the Graves' speculum but are much narrower and flatter.

The *pediatric* or *virginal speculum* is smaller in all dimensions of width and length.

Plastic and metal specula differ slightly in ease of use and positioning. The metal speculum has two positioning devices. The top blade is hinged and has a thumb lever attached. When the thumb lever is pressed down, the distal end of the top blade rises, thus opening the speculum. The blade may be locked open at that point by tightening the screw on the thumb lever. The proximal end of the speculum may also be opened wider if necessary by loosening and then tightening another thumbscrew on the handle.

The disposable plastic speculum differs from the metal type in that the bottom blade is fixed to a posterior handle and the upper blade is fixed to the anterior lever handle. When the lever is pressed, the distal end of the top blade opens and, at the same time, the base of the speculum widens. As the speculum opens it goes through a series of clicking sounds until it actually snaps into the desired position. The client should be forewarned about the clicking and snapping sounds. In addition, some of the plastic models have a port where a light source may be inserted directly into the speculum.

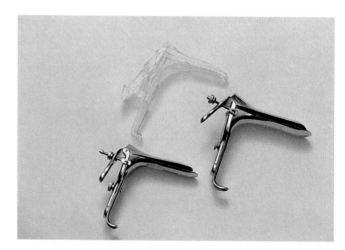

Fig. 5-21 Vaginal specula.

Personal Protective Equipment

It is important that the examiner use appropriate personal protective clothing to protect himself or herself from possible contamination and infection. The Centers for Disease Control and Prevention (1987) have issued Universal Precautions to be taken to protect health care workers from blood and body fluid contamination. The nurse must be informed about sources of infection and methods for personal protection. In addition to using appropriate personal protective equipment, the nurse should always scrupulously wash hands with a germicidal soap both before and after direct contact with the client.

Universal Blood and Body Fluid Precautions

1. *All* health care workers should use appropriate barrier precautions to prevent skin and mucous membrane exposure when contact with blood or body fluids of *any* patient is anticipated. Examples: starting an IV, drawing blood, performing CPR or other emergency procedures, handling soiled linen and waste, performing genital or rectal examination.

2. Gloves should be worn for touching blood and body fluids, mucous membranes, or nonintact skin of all patients, for handling items or surfaces soiled with blood or body fluids, and for performing venipuncture and other vascular access procedures. Gloves should be changed after contact with each patient.

3. Hands and other skin surfaces should be washed immediately and thoroughly if contaminated with blood or other body fluids. Hands should be washed immediately after gloves are removed.

4. Masks and protective eyewear or face shields should be worn during procedures that are likely to generate droplets of blood or other body fluids. Examples: arterial punctures, endoscopies, insertion of arterial lines. Do not rely on eyeglasses; they do not offer complete protection.

5. Gowns or aprons should be worn during procedures that are likely to generate splashes of blood or other body fluids. Example: hemodialysis. Remember, too, that gowns that get wet are not protective when they are saturated.

6. Needles should not be recapped, purposely bent or broken by hand, removed from disposable syringes, or otherwise manipulated by hand. After use, disposable syringes and needles, scalpel blades, and other sharp items should be placed in a puncture-resistant container for transport to the reprocessing area.

7. Although saliva has not been implicated in HIV transmission, pocket masks, resuscitation bags, or other ventilation devices should be available for use in areas in which the need for resuscitation is predicatable.

8. Health care workers who have exudative lesions or weeping dermatitis should refrain from all direct patient care and from handling patient-care equipment until the condition resolves.

9. Pregnant health care workers are not known to be at greater risk of contracting HIV infection than nonpregnant workers; however, if a pregnant worker develops HIV infection, the infant is at risk for perinatal transmission. Pregnant health care workers should strictly adhere to precautions.

10. Invasive procedures (such as surgical entry into tissues, cavities, or organs) or repair of major traumatic injuries carries a risk of splattering of blood and fluids, and requires the use of gloves, masks, protective eyewear or face shield, and gowns or aprons made of materials that provide an effective fluid barrier.

11. During an invasive procedure, if a glove is torn or a needlestick or other injury occurs, the glove should be removed and a new glove used as promptly as patient safety permits; the needle or instrument involved in the incident should be removed from the sterile field.

Modified from Centers for Disease Control and Prevention, 1987.

??????? STUDY QUESTIONS ???????

1. Address the following points about thermometers:
   a. What is the primary purpose of the thermometer?
   b. List and describe four types of thermometers.
   c. List one advantage for use of each thermometer type.
2. Address the following points about stethoscopes:
   a. What is the primary purpose of the stethoscope?
   b. List and describe the three components of the stethoscope most commonly used in health assessment.
   c. How do you know if the stethoscope is the right size for the patient?
3. Address the following points about blood pressure measurement:
   a. What is the primary purpose of measuring blood pressure?
   b. List and describe three types of sphygmomanometers.
   c. List the criteria for selecting the proper size blood pressure cuff.
   d. Why is it important for the cuff to be the right size?
4. When would you use a Doppler instead of an acoustic stethoscope?
5. What is the purpose of pulse oximetry? Under what conditions is it reliable?
6. Which visual acuity chart is appropriate for screening for distant vision? Near vision?
7. If a person has a far vision reading of 20/200 and a near vision reading of 20/15, what does that mean? Does he or she need glasses to read? To drive?
8. Address the following points about the ophthalmoscope:
   a. What function do the diopters serve?
   b. When is it best to use the small aperture setting for the light?
   c. For what is the red-free filter used?
   d. What light is used to examine the anterior eye?
9. Address the following points about the otoscope:
   a. What is the purpose of an otoscope?
   b. List the criteria for selecting the proper size speculum.
   c. When would you use the pneumatic attachment?
10. When is the use of a nasal speculum appropriate? Under what circumstances might you attach a nasal speculum to the end of an otoscope?
11. Address the following points about the tuning fork:
    a. List two purposes for use of the tuning fork.
    b. When is a 750 Hz fork used? A 300 Hz fork?
    c. What can happen if you use the wrong frequency fork?
12. When using an audiometer to screen for hearing acuity, when do you refer the person for further evaluation?
13. Match the equipment to the correct purpose:

Reflex hammer	Measure size of a mole
Goniometer	Measure reflexes in the knee
Caliper	Measure percent of body fat
Ruler	Measure flexion of the knee
Tape measure	Measure size of a waist

14. Match the equipment to the correct purpose:

Penlight	Examine a sore throat
Wood's lamp	Examine a blocked sinus
Grid light	Examine a corneal abrasion
Transilluminator	Examine a fundal lesion

15. What is the purpose of a vaginal speculum? When would you choose a Pederson rather than a Graves' speculum?
16. Which barrier precautions (gloves, masks, gowns, protective eyewear) should be used when performing or assisting with the following procedures:
    a. Surgery
    b. Drawing blood
    c. Cleaning up feces
    d. Arterial punctures
    e. Cleaning bloody equipment
    f. Resuscitation
17. How do you dispose of used needles?
18. What should you do to protect yourself if you have an open skin lesion while at work?
19. What special universal precautions should you take if you are pregnant?

CHAPTER 6

Techniques of Physical Assessment

Data for physical assessment are collected using the techniques of inspection, palpation, percussion, auscultation, and positioning. These techniques are described in this chapter together with assessment of vital signs—pulse, respiration, blood pressure, and temperature—and general assessment techniques of weight and height. Use of selected equipment described in Chapter 5 also is described in this chapter.

TECHNIQUES

INSPECTION

The definition of inspection is "to look at; to examine critically." This includes all data obtained by looking at the client. (Data obtained by smell are included as a part of inspection, even though it falls outside the definition.) Inspection begins the moment the examiner meets the client, and it requires attention to detail. For example, data about the neuromuscular system are obtained by observing the client's gait and ease of movement from standing to sitting. Data about emotional and mental status are collected by noting facial expressions, tone of voice, and affect. Does the client maintain eye contact during the history taking? Are the facial expressions and body language appropriate for the conversation? Is the clothing appropriate for the weather? The skin assessment begins by noticing the color of the client's skin. Are any odors detected? When unpleasant odors are detected, examiners must try to suppress reactions that may be communicated through facial expressions. These preliminary observations can be important clues to data needed during the remainder of the examination.

Inspection is a part of assessment in every body system and is hindered by any preconceived assumptions examiners may have about clients. Observe the client thoroughly with a critical eye, comparing the right and left sides to find and explain variations noted during the examination. By concentrating on the client without being distracted, the examiner will not overlook potentially important data about the client.

During inspection, the client is draped appropriately to maintain modesty but provide sufficient exposure. Adequate lighting is essential and should be direct enough to allow examiners to see color, texture, and mobility without distortions or shadows. Shadows can be useful, however, for observing contour and variations in body surface. Shadows are created with *tangential lighting* by directing the light from a penlight or adjustable lamp at right angles to the area being inspected. At times instruments, such as an otoscope, ophthalmoscope, or vaginal speculum, are used to enhance inspection. Use of these instruments is described in subsequent chapters on assessment of specific body systems. While inspection at first may *seem* like an easy assessment technique to master, examiners must practice to develop this skill, as with any other.

PALPATION

Palpation is the use of sensation of the examiner's hands to feel texture, size, shape, consistency, and location of certain parts of the client's body, and also to identify areas the client reports as being tender or painful. This assessment technique requires the examiner to move into the client's personal space. It is important that the touch is gentle, hands are warm, and nails are short to prevent discomfort or injury to the client. Touch has cultural significance and symbolism. Each culture has its own understanding about the uses and meanings of touch. As a result, it is of utmost importance that examiners tell clients the purpose of their touch (e.g., "I'm feeling for lymph nodes now") and manner and location of touch (e.g., "I'm going to press deeply on your abdomen to feel the organs"). Gloves are worn when palpating mucous membranes or any other area where contact with body fluids is likely.

The palmar surface of fingers and finger pads are more sensitive than fingertips and are used to determine position, texture, size, consistency, masses, fluid, and crepitus. The ulnar surface of hands and fingers is more responsive to vibration. The dorsal surface of hand is best for assessing temperature.

Uses of palpation for specific body systems are discussed in subsequent chapters. Palpation using the palmar surfaces of the fingers may be light or deep and is controlled by the amount of pressure applied with hands or fingers. For example, the following technique is used to assess the abdomen. *Light palpation* is accomplished by pressing to a depth of 1 cm (0.4 inches) and is used to assess skin, pulsations, and tenderness. *Deep palpation* is done by using one or both hands to press in about 4 cm (1.6 inches) and is used to determine organ size and contour. Light palpation should always precede deep palpation because palpation may cause tenderness or disrupt fluid, which would interfere with collecting data by light palpation.

One of the purposes of palpation is to determine the size of tissue such as lymph nodes or nodules. To accomplish this purpose, examiners need to know the width of their fingers to use them as approximate measures as needed.

A bimanual technique of palpation uses both hands, one anterior and one posterior, to entrap an organ or mass between the fingertips to assess size and shape. This technique is used to assess the kidneys and uterus.

PERCUSSION

Percussion is performed to evaluate the size, borders, and consistency of some internal organs, to detect tenderness, and to determine the extent of fluid in a body cavity. There are two percussion techniques, direct and indirect. *Direct percussion* involves directly striking a specific area of the body using a fingertip, lateral aspect of the fist, or reflex hammer. Direct percussion is used to percuss an infant's chest or the adult's sinuses. Fist percussion is used over the costovertebral angle (CVA) to elicit tenderness of the kidney (Fig. 6-1). A reflex hammer used to assess deep tendon reflexes also is a form of percussion and is described in Chapter 22.

Indirect percussion requires both hands, and is done by different methods depending on which body system is being assessed. Indirect fist percussion of the kidney is performed by placing the nondominant hand palm down, fingers together over the CVA and gently striking the fingers with the lateral aspect of the fist of the dominant hand (Fig. 6-2).

Indirect percussion of the thorax or abdomen is performed by placing the distal phalanx of the middle finger of the nondominant hand against the skin over the organ being percussed. This finger is sometimes referred to as the *pleximeter*. The other fingers of that hand are spread apart and slightly elevated off the client's skin so that they do not dampen the vibration. With the *tip* of the middle finger of the dominant hand (plexor), the examiner strikes the distal interphalangeal joint that lies against the client's skin. The tip of the striking finger hits the middle finger, which is against the skin, between the cuticle and first joint. Some examiners use both the index and the middle fingers as plexors. The force of the downward snap

of the striking finger(s) comes from rapid flexion of the wrist. The wrist must be relaxed and loose while the forearm remains stationary (Fig. 6-3). The nail of the plexor must be trimmed to avoid piercing the client with long fingernails. Rebound the plexor finger as soon as it strikes the pleximeter so that the vibration is not muffled. Listen for the vibrations created by one finger striking another. The tapping produces a vibration 1½ to 2 inches (4 to 5 cm) deep in body tissue and subsequent sound waves. Percuss two or three times in one location before moving to another. Stronger percussion will be needed for obese or very muscular clients, since thickness of tissue can impair the vibrations. The denser the tissue, the quieter the percussion tones. The percussion tone over air is loud, over fluid is less loud, and over solid areas is soft. Five percussion tones are described in Table 6-1. *Tympany* is a loud, high-pitched sound heard over the abdomen. *Resonance* is heard over normal lung tissue, while *hyperresonance* is heard in overinflated lungs (as in emphysema). *Dullness* is heard over the liver and *flatness* is heard over muscle. Detecting sound changes is easier when moving from resonance to dullness (e.g., from the lung to the liver). Indirect percussion is an awkward technique at first, but can be mastered with practice.

AUSCULTATION

Auscultation is the act of listening for sounds. The examiner uses auscultation without any assistive devices when evaluating sounds such as coughing, speech, and percussion tones. A stethoscope is an assistive device used in auscultation to block out extraneous sounds when evaluating the condition of the heart, blood vessels, lungs, pleura, and intestines.

Examiners should warm the stethoscope before placing it on clients. If clients become cold and shiver, the involuntary muscle contractions could interfere with normal sounds. The bell or diaphragm of the stethoscope is placed directly against the skin, since clothes obscure or alter sounds. Auscultating a hairy chest can seem to produce an abnormal lung sound (crackles) when actually the sound is the friction of the chest hair against the diaphragm. When this occurs, examiners should moisten the hair before auscultating.

The bell of the stethoscope is used to hear soft, low-pitched (low-frequency) sounds such as vascular sounds,

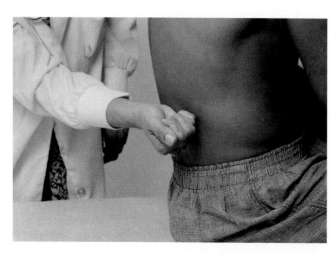

Fig. 6-1 Hand position for direct fist percussion of kidney.

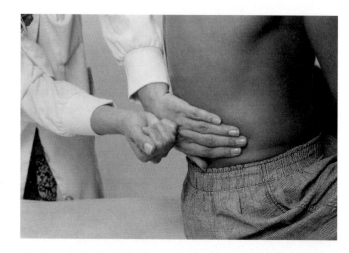

Fig. 6-2 Hand position for indirect fist percussion of kidney.

TABLE 6-1	Percussion Tones				
AREA PERCUSSED	**TONE**	**INTENSITY**	**PITCH**	**DURATION**	**QUALITY**
Lungs	Resonant	Loud	Low	Long	Hollow
Bone and muscle	Flat	Soft	High	Short	Extremely dull
Viscera and liver borders	Dull	Medium	Medium-High	Medium	Thudlike
Stomach and gas bubbles in intestines	Tympanic	Loud	High	Medium	Drumlike
Air trapped in lung (abnormal in adults)	Hyperresonant	Very loud	Very low	Longer	Booming

extra heart sounds, bruits, or murmurs, while the diaphragm is used to hear high-pitched (high-frequency) sounds such as breath, bowel, and normal heart sounds. Avoid pressing the bell too firmly against the skin, because this will stretch the skin so that it acts like the diaphragm of the stethoscope and thus inhibits vibrations. The diaphragm is held firmly against the client's skin, stabilizing it between the index and middle fingers (Fig. 6-4). Listen for sound as well as its characteristics: intensity, pitch, duration, and quality (see box on p. 76). Examiners concentrate as they listen because sounds may be transitory or subtle. Closing the eyes may improve listening because it reduces distracting visual stimuli. Examiners try to isolate the specific sounds, such as sounds of air during inspiration or a single heart sound.

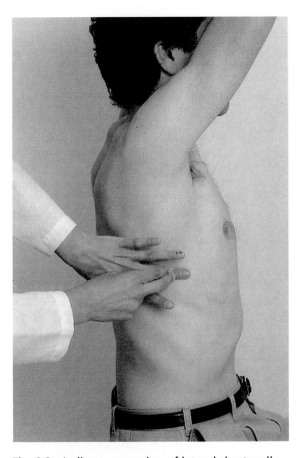

Fig. 6-3 Indirect percussion of lateral chest wall.

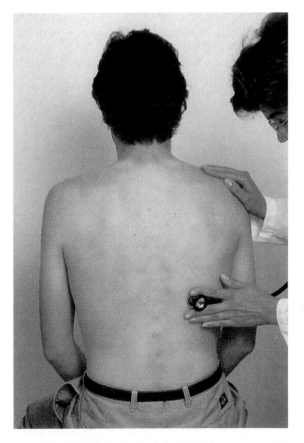

Fig. 6-4 The diaphragm of the stethoscope is stabilized between the index and middle fingers.

Characteristics of Sounds Heard by Auscultation

- *Intensity* is the loudness of the sound, described as *soft, medium,* or *loud.*
- *Pitch* is the frequency or number of sound waves generated per second. High-pitched sounds have high frequencies. Expected high-pitched sounds are breath sounds, while cardiac sounds are low-pitched.
- *Duration* of sound vibrations is short, medium or long. Layers of soft tissue dampen the duration of sound from deep organs.
- *Quality* refers to the description of the sounds (e.g., hollow, dull, crackle).

POSITIONING

The sitting and supine positions are the most common for the client during the physical examination. These plus other positions used in an examination are shown in Table 6-2. The inability of a client to assume a position not only may require use of an alternate examination position, but also may be a significant finding about the client's physical status. For example, a client who is short of breath may not be able to lie supine. To assess the abdomen of this client, the examiner may need to use an examining table that has an elevated headrest or defer the abdominal examination (if it is not an urgent problem) until the respiratory condition is treated. The client is draped appropriately in the various positions to provide for modesty, while allowing exposure needed for the examination.

VITAL SIGNS

The temperature, pulse, respiration, and blood pressure are often referred to as vital signs because they are baseline indicators of a client's health status. They are measured early in the physical examination or integrated into the examination.

TEMPERATURE

Body temperature is maintained by a thermostat located in the hypothalamus. Heat is gained through the processes of metabolism and exercise and lost through radiation, convection, conduction, and evaporation. The expected temperature ranges from 35.8° to 37.3° C (96.4° to 99.1° F) with an average of 37° C (98.6° F). This is the stable core temperature at which cellular metabolism is most efficient.

Temperature changes occur due to normal variations and activities. Diurnal variations of 0.37° to 0.56° C (1° to 1.5° F) occur with the lowest temperature early in the morning and the highest in the late afternoon and early evening. During menstrual cycles a woman's temperature increases 0.5° to 1.0° F at ovulation and remains elevated until menses ceases. This elevation is due to progesterone secretion. Moderate to hard exercise increases temperature.

Temperature can be measured by several routes: oral, tympanic, axillary, and rectal.

Conversion of Fahrenheit to Centigrade

Degrees C = ⅝ (degrees F − 32)
Degrees F = ⅝ (degrees C + 32)

Oral temperature. Oral temperature is the most accurate and convenient to assess. Delay taking the oral temperature 20 to 30 minutes if the client has smoked or ingested hot or cold liquids or food. To take a temperature with a *mercury-in-glass thermometer,* shake the thermometer to move the mercury down to 35.5° C (96° F). Place the thermometer under the client's tongue in the right or left posterior sublingual pocket, which receives its blood supply from the carotid artery that reflects inner core temperature. Ask the client to keep the mouth closed while temperature is being recorded. Leave the thermometer in place for 2 minutes, then remove and read the temperature at the mercury level on the scale.

When using an *electronic thermometer,* cover the blue or white probe with a disposable sheath. Place the probe under the client's tongue as just described. Ask the client to keep the mouth closed while temperature is being recorded. An electronic oral thermometer remains in place for 15 to 30 seconds until the audible signal occurs and the temperature registers on the display screen.

Tympanic membrane temperature. Electronic thermometers that measure temperature from the tympanic surface are convenient. The probe is covered with a protective sheath and placed inside the external ear canal with firm but gentle pressure. The probe must come in contact with all sides of the ear canal. (The probe does not extend all the way to the tympanic membrane.) The thermometer is removed after the audible signal occurs and the temperature reading is displayed, about 2 to 3 seconds.

Axillary temperature. Axillary temperature measurement is safe and accurate for infants and children and for adults who are not candidates for other methods of measurement. Prepare the mercury-in-glass thermometer by shaking down the mercury as described previously. Place the thermometer in the axilla and hold the arm against the body for 5 to 10 minutes. Withdraw the thermometer and read the level of mercury on the scale.

Electronic thermometers also can be used for measuring axillary temperatures. The probe is held in the middle of the axilla until the audible signal occurs and the temperature appears on the screen.

Rectal temperature. Rectal temperatures are taken less frequently with the advent of methods such as the tympanic thermometer. Rectal temperatures may be used when other routes are not possible, such as when the client is unconscious. Appropriate privacy is provided for clients. The Sims' position with upper leg flexed is frequently used. When using a *rectal mercury-in-glass thermometer,* prepare it by shaking down the mercury as described above. A water-soluble lubricant is applied before the thermometer is inserted into the rectum 1 to 1.5 inches (2.5 to 3.5 cm) and held in place 2 minutes. A *rectal electronic thermometer* is used by covering the red probe with a disposable sheath, inserting it into the rectum 1.5 inches (3.5 cm), and holding it in place until the audible signal occurs and the temperature is displayed on the screen.

TABLE 6-2   Positions for Examination

POSITION		AREAS ASSESSED	RATIONALE	LIMITATIONS
Sitting		Head and neck, back, posterior thorax and lungs, anterior thorax and lungs, breasts, axillae, heart, vital signs, and upper extremities	Sitting upright provides full expansion of lungs and provides better visualization of symmetry of upper body parts.	Physically weakened client may be unable to sit. Examiner should use supine position with head of bed elevated instead.
Supine		Head and neck, anterior thorax and lungs, breasts, axillae, heart, abdomen, extremities, pulses	This is the most normally relaxed position. It provides easy access to pulse sites.	If client becomes short of breath easily, examiner may need to raise head of bed.
Dorsal recumbent		Head and neck, anterior thorax and lungs, breasts, axillae, heart, abdomen	This position is used for abdominal assessment because it promotes relaxation of abdominal muscles.	Clients with painful disorders are more comfortable with knees flexed.
Lithotomy*		Female genitalia and genital tract	This position provides maximal exposure of genitalia and facilitates insertion of vaginal speculum.	Lithotomy position is embarrassing and uncomfortable, so examiner minimizes time that client spends in it. Client is kept well draped.
Sims'		Rectum and vagina	Flexion of hip and knee improves exposure of rectal area.	Joint deformities may hinder client's ability to bend hip and knee.
Prone		Musculoskeletal system	This position is used only to assess extension of hip joint.	This position is poorly tolerated in clients with respiratory difficulties.
Lateral recumbent		Heart	This position aids in detecting murmurs.	This position is poorly tolerated in clients with respiratory difficulties.
Knee-chest*		Rectum	This position provides maximal exposure of rectal area.	This position is embarrassing and uncomfortable.

Clients with arthritis or other joint deformities may be unable to assume this position.
From Potter PA, Perry AG: Basic nursing: theory and practice, *ed 3, St. Louis, 1995, Mosby.*

PULSE

Palpation of arterial pulses provides valuable information about the cardiovascular system. Pulses are palpated using the finger pads of the index and middle fingers. Firm pressure is applied over the pulse, but not so hard that the pulsation is occluded. If pulses are difficult to locate, then the amount of pressure is varied and the area around the pulse is palpated.

Each pulse is assessed for rate, rhythm, amplitude, and contour. The *rate* is the number of times in a minute the pulsation is felt. The *rhythm* is the regularity of the pulsations, e.g., the time between each beat. The *amplitude* or strength is rated on a scale from 0 to 4+, with 2+ being normal. A pulse of 1+ is diminished, 3+ is full volume, and 4+ is bounding. (Some authors describe a 0 to 3 scale.) *Contour* is the outline or shape felt during pulsation. Normally it is smooth and rounded, with a sharp upstroke and more gradual downstroke. Large bounding pulses may be felt during exercise, hypertension, or fluid excess, while small, weak pulses may be felt in clients with a fluid deficit or with left ventricular failure. Compare the upper and lower extremity pulses on the same side to detect variations. Likewise, compare pulses on the right and left extremities to detect variations. Expected pulse rates are listed in Table 6-3.

The nine arterial pulses from head to toe are the temporal, carotid, apical, brachial, radial, femoral, popliteal, posterior tibial, and dorsalis pedis. Pulses used in assessing vital signs are the radial, brachial, and perhaps the popliteal arteries (when blood pressure is taken in the leg). Palpation of the other pulses is described in Chapter 15. The *brachial* pulse is located in the groove between the biceps and triceps muscle just medial to the biceps tendon at the antecubital fossa (in the bend of the elbow) (Fig. 6-5). The *radial* pulse is found at the radial or thumb side of the forearm at the wrist (Fig. 6-6). The *popliteal* pulse is located behind the knee in the popliteal fossa (Fig. 6-7).

When pulses cannot be palpated, use alternate techniques such as a Doppler ultrasonic stethoscope to hear the arterial pulsations (see Chapter 5). Ancillary data about the circulation of the extremity can be obtained by inspecting the color of the extremity and palpating for temperature. Fingers and toes should be warm and pink or brown, depending on the client's usual skin tone. Also, capillary circulation can be assessed by timing the capillary refill. Gently squeeze the fingernail, toenail, or pad of the extremity until it turns white (blanches). Release the pressure and note how many seconds it takes for the finger or toe to resume its former color; normally it takes 3 to 5 seconds.

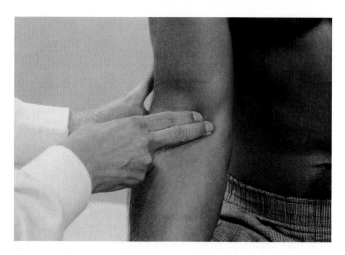

Fig. 6-5   Brachial pulse.

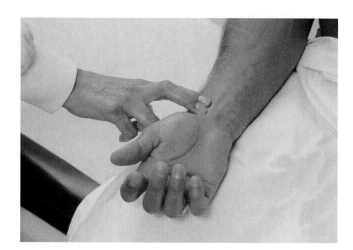

Fig. 6-6   Radial pulse.

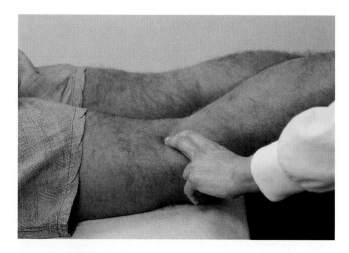

Fig. 6-7   Popliteal pulse.

TABLE 6-3	Normal Heart Rates

AGE	HEART RATE (BEATS/MIN)
Infants	120-160
Toddlers	90-140
Preschoolers	80-110
School agers	75-100
Adolescents	60-90
Adults	60-100

Modified from Potter PA, Perry AG: Basic nursing: theory and practice, ed 3, St. Louis, 1995, Mosby.

RESPIRATION

After assessing pulses, examiners leave their fingers on the pulse (e.g., radial pulse) while they count the client's respirations. Using inspection, they count the number of breaths per minute without the client's knowledge of their assessment. This will prevent the client from becoming self-conscious because of the assessment and perhaps changing the rate or depth of breathing.

This assessment technique is called "assessing respiration." However, it only involves assessing ventilation. *Respiration* is the mechanism used to exchange gases between atmosphere and cells. The total process of respiration involves *ventilation* (movement of gases in and out of the lungs), *diffusion* (movement of gases between the alveoli and pulmonary capillaries), and *perfusion* (the flow of blood to and from the pulmonary capillaries). Assess breathing for rate, rhythm, and depth. *Rate* is the number of times the client completes one ventilatory cycle (inhalation and exhalation) each minute. Respiration rates vary with age (Table 6-4). Other factors that increase respiratory rate are fever, anxiety, exercise, and increased altitude. *Rhythm* is the regularity of breathing; the expected finding when the client is sitting or lying quietly is equal spacing between breaths. Rhythm is described as *regular* or *irregular*. *Depth* is assessed by observing the excursion or movement of the chest wall. Depth is described as *deep* (full lung expansion with full exhalation), *normal,* or *shallow* (small amount of air moves in and out of lungs and may be difficult to observe). Men usually breathe diaphragmatically, which increases the movement of the abdomen, whereas women breathe thoracically with movement of the thoracic cage. Table 6-5 lists alterations in breathing patterns.

BLOOD PRESSURE

Blood pressure is the force of blood against the arterial walls. It reflects the relationship between cardiac output and peripheral resistance. The cardiac output is the volume of blood ejected from the heart each minute. Peripheral resistance is the force that opposes the flow of blood through vessels. For example, when the arteries are narrow, the peripheral resistance to bloodflow is high, which is reflected in an elevated blood pressure. Blood pressure is dependent on the velocity of the blood, intravascular blood volume, and elasticity of the vessel walls.

Blood pressure is measured in millimeters of mercury (mm Hg). The measurement indicates the height to which the blood pressure can raise a column of mercury. *Systolic blood pressure* is the maximum pressure exerted on arteries when the ventricles eject blood from the heart. When the ventricles relax, the blood remaining in arteries exerting a minimum pressure is called the *diastolic blood pressure.* Blood pressure is recorded with the systolic pressure written on top of the diastolic pressure (e.g., 130/76), but it is not a fraction. The difference between the systolic and diastolic pressures is called the *pulse pressure,* which normally ranges from 30 to 40 mm Hg.

The pulmonary blood pressure is the force exerted on the walls of the pulmonary arteries during contraction and relaxation of the *right* ventricle. This blood pressure is measured directly (invasively) by floating a catheter through the heart to measure pressures, and requires continuous monitoring in acute care settings. In contrast, when the *left* ventricle ejects

TABLE 6-4	**Ranges of Expected Respiratory Rates by Age**
AGE	**VENTILATION RATES PER MINUTE**
Newborn	30-50
1 year	20-40
3 years	20-30
6 years	18-26
10 years	16-22
16 years	14-20
18 years and over	12-20

blood into the aorta, the maximum pressure exerted is called the *systemic systolic blood pressure.* Systemic blood pressure can be measured directly or indirectly. Direct measurement is accomplished by inserting a small catheter into an artery that provides continuous blood pressure measurements and arterial waveforms. This direct measurement creates a risk of blood loss from the artery and requires close monitoring available in acute care units.

The most commonly used method of indirect systemic blood pressure measurement is the auscultatory method using a sphygmomanometer and a stethoscope. Two types of sphygmomanometers are used: mercury and aneroid (see Chapter 5). The mercury sphygmomanometer is considered the more accurate and reliable indirect measure of systemic blood pressure.

Procedure for assessing blood pressure. With the client sitting or lying down, position the client's upper arm at heart level with the palm turned up. Palpate either brachial pulse (in the antecubital space) and apply the blood pressure cuff 1 inch (2.5 cm) above the site of brachial pulsation. Center the bladder of the cuff over the artery (Fig. 6-8). Wrap the deflated cuff evenly and snugly around the upper arm. Position the manometer at eye level no more than 1 yard (1 m) away. Close the valve on the pressure bulb clockwise until it is tight but easily releasable with one hand. Palpate the brachial or radial pulse with fingertips of one hand while inflating the cuff rapidly to 30 mm Hg above the point where the pulse disappears. Release the valve slowly to deflate the cuff and note the point when the pulse reappears; this is the palpated systolic pressure. Deflate the cuff and wait 30 seconds. Place the diaphragm over the brachial pulse (Fig. 6-9). Close the valve on the pressure bulb again and inflate the cuff to 30 mm Hg above the palpated systolic pressure. Slowly release the valve and allow the mercury to fall at a rate of 2 to 3 mm Hg per second. Note the manometer pressure reading when the first clear sound (first Korotkoff sound) is heard; this is the systolic pressure. Continue to deflate the cuff, noting the point at which the sound disappears; this is the diastolic pressure. Deflate the cuff and remove from client's arm. If this is the first blood pressure assessment, repeat the procedure on the other arm. Also, the blood pressure often is taken while clients are lying, sitting, and standing so that comparisons can be made. Examiners tell clients the blood pressure measurement, record the data, and compare it with previous readings. Expected blood pressures are found in Table 6-6.

TABLE 6-5   Alterations in Breathing Patterns

PATTERN	DESCRIPTION	ASSOCIATED CONDITIONS
	Normal: smooth and even at a rate of 12-20 per minute	
	Tachypnea: shallow breathing at a rate of >20 per minute	Anxiety, pain, massive liver enlargement, abdominal ascites
	Bradypnea: <12 per minute	Neurogenic disorders, electrolyte imbalance, infection, protective response to pain or pleurisy or other discomfort aggravated by breathing
	Hyperpnea or hyperventilation: deep breathing at a rate of >20 per minute	Exercise, acute anxiety, panic reactions, metabolic disorders
	Kussmaul: fast (>20 per min), deep, sighing breaths without pauses; labored breathing	Renal failure, metabolic acidosis
	Central neurogenic hyperventilation: hyperpnea over a sustained period	Lesions in lower midbrain or upper pons, often secondary to transtentorial herniation
	Cheyne-Stokes: alternating hyperpnea and apnea	In adults, bilateral lesions in cerebral hemisphere, basal ganglia, midbrain, pons, or cerebellum. In infants this pattern is normal
	Biot's or cluster: disorganized sequence of breaths with irregular periods of apnea	Lesions of lower pons or upper medulla
	Ataxic breathing: irregular breathing patterns with both deep and shallow breaths occurring randomly	Lesions of medulla

TABLE 6-6   Normal Blood Pressures

AGE	SYSTOLIC	DIASTOLIC
Infants	60-96 mm Hg	30-62 mm Hg
Age 2	78-112 mm Hg	48-78 mm Hg
Age 8	85-114 mm Hg	52-85 mm Hg
Age 12	95-135 mm Hg	58-88 mm Hg
Adult	100-140 mm Hg	60-90 mm Hg

Systolic pressure in the thigh can be higher by 10 to 40 mm Hg as compared with brachial artery pressure. Diastolic pressure remains the same.
From Canobbio MM: Cardiovascular disorders, *St. Louis, 1990, Mosby.*

Mechanism of blood pressure measurement.

Blood flows freely through the artery until the inflated cuff occludes the artery enough to interrupt bloodflow. As the cuff pressure is slowly released, the examiner listens for the sound of the blood pulsating through the artery again. This sound indicates the return of bloodflow and the systolic blood pressure. This sound is called the first Korotkoff sound, named for the Russian physician who first described it. The first Korotkoff sound is a clear, rhythmic tapping corresponding to the pulse rate that gradually increases in intensity (Fig. 6-10). The pressure reading at which this sound is heard is noted and indicates the systolic pressure. The swishing sound heard as the cuff continues to deflate is the second Korotkoff sound. The third Korotkoff sound is a crisper and more intense tapping. The fourth Korotkoff sound becomes muffled and low-pitched as the cuff is further deflated. The fifth Korotkoff sound occurs at the pressure at which there is no sound, indicating the artery is completely open. In adolescents and adults the manometer pressure noted at the fifth Korotkoff sound is the diastolic pressure.

Systolic blood pressure can be taken in the leg when the arms cannot be used or when assessing adolescents or young adults for a congenital anomaly called *coarctation of the heart.* With the client in the prone position, wrap a large cuff (18 to 20 cm) around the lower third of the thigh, centering the bladder of the cuff over the popliteal artery. Follow the

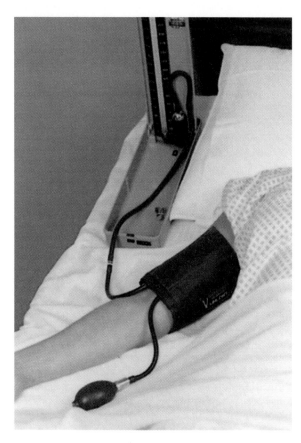

Fig. 6-8 Center the bladder of the blood pressure cuff over artery. *(From Potter and Perry, 1995.)*

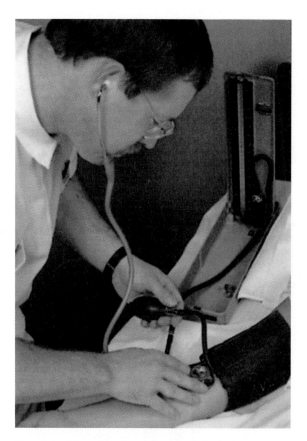

Fig. 6-9 Listening for Korotkoff sounds to assess blood pressure. *(From Potter and Perry, 1995.)*

same procedure for taking a blood pressure in the arm. Normally the systolic blood pressure is 10 to 40 mm Hg higher in the leg than in the arm. The diastolic pressures of arms and legs are similar.

Factors that affect blood pressure measurements.

1. Characteristics of clients that may *alter* blood pressure:
   - *Age.* From childhood to adulthood there is a gradual rise.
   - *Gender.* After puberty, females usually have a lower blood pressure than males; however, after menopause, women's blood pressure is often higher than men's.
   - *Race.* The incidence of hypertension is twice as high in African Americans as in whites.
   - *Diurnal variations.* Blood pressure is lower in the early morning and peaks in later afternoon or early evening.
   - *Emotions.* Feeling anxious, angry, or stressed may stimulate the sympathetic nervous system to increase the blood pressure.
   - *Pain.* Experiencing pain can increase blood pressure.
   - *Personal habits.* Ingesting caffeine or smoking a cigarette within 30 minutes before measurement may increase blood pressure.
   - *Weight:* Obese clients tend to have higher blood pressures than nonobese clients.
2. Examiner error causing falsely high blood pressures:
   - Positioning client's arm above the level of the heart
   - Examiner's eyes not level with the manometer—looking up at the meniscus
   - Using a cuff that is too narrow
   - Wrapping cuff too loosely or unevenly
   - Deflating the cuff too slowly
3. Examiner error causing falsely low blood pressures:
   - Positioning client's arm below the level of the heart
   - Examiner's eyes not level with the manometer—looking down at the meniscus
   - Positioning the manometer higher than the client's heart
   - Using a cuff that is too wide
   - Not inflating the cuff enough
   - Deflating the cuff too rapidly
   - Pressing the diaphragm too firmly on the brachial artery

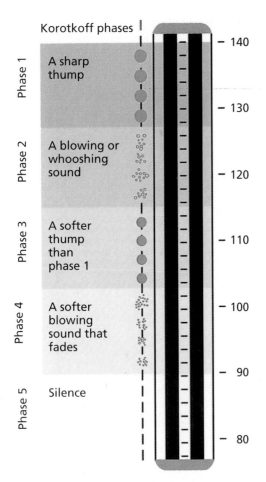

Fig. 6-10   Sounds auscultated during blood pressure measurement can be differentiated into five Korotkoff phases. In this example the blood pressure is 140/90.   *(From Potter and Perry, 1995.)*

GENERAL ASSESSMENT

WEIGHT

The amount of one's body weight or mass is determined by genetics, dietary intake, exercise, and fluid volume. Genetics influence height and body size, including bone structure, muscle mass, and gender. A diet high in fat may increase body weight, particularly when clients do not exercise regularly. Fat distribution varies by gender and age. In men total body fat is evenly distributed, while in women additional fat is distributed over the shoulders, breasts, buttocks, and lateral aspects of thighs and pubic symphysis, which can dramatically alter body shape. Why females deposit fat in specific locations is unknown, but the fat in breasts protects the mammary glands and provides energy for future gestation and lactation needs (Rofles and DeBruyne, 1990).

An unintentional change in weight can be a significant finding. For example, an increase in weight may be the first sign of fluid retention. For every liter of fluid retained (1000 ml or about 1 quart), weight increases 1 kilogram (2.2 lb). Also, unexplained weight loss may be one indication of suspected malignancy or disease process.

Measure weight by asking clients to stand in the middle of the scale platform while the large and small weights are balanced. The scale uses a counterbalance system of adding or subtracting weights in increments as small as 0.25 pound (0.1 kg) to achieve a level horizontal balance beam on the scale. Move the larger weight to the 50-lb (10-kg) increment less than the client's weight. Adjust the smaller weight to balance the scale. Read the weight to the nearest ¼ lb (0.1 kg).

Electronic scales provide a digital reading of the client's weight seconds after the client steps on the scale.

HEIGHT

One's height is determined by genetics and dietary intake. Genetics influence height and body size, including bone structure, muscle mass, and gender. Dietary factors influence bone and muscle growth. Height is measured on a platform scale with a height attachment. The height attachment is pulled up and the horizontal head piece extended before the client steps on the scale to avoid poking the client as the head piece is extended. The attachment then is lowered until the horizontal head piece touches the client's crown. The vertical measuring scale can be in inches or centimeters. Height peaks during the adolescent growth spurt, which is highly variable from adolescent to adolescent. Adult height is attained between ages 18 and 20 (Neinstein, 1991). Height for an adult usually is measured as a baseline only. For adults, a standard source for average weight for height and body frame size is the Metropolitan Life Tables, 1983 (see Table 7-1).

SKINFOLD THICKNESS

Skinfold calipers are used to measure skinfold or fatfold thickness of fat in the subcutaneous tissue to estimate the extent of overnutrition or undernutrition. Measures of body fat are useful in determining nutritional status. About half the body fat is directly beneath the skin and its thickness reflects total body fat.

Three measurements are taken and the two closest measurements are averaged. The most common site for measuring fat folds is the triceps, using a vertical fold on the back of the arm between the shoulder and the elbow. Examiners use their thumb and index finger to grasp and lift a fold of skin and fat about ½ inch (1 cm) on the posterior aspect of the client's arm halfway between the olecranon process (tip of the elbow) and acromial process on the lateral aspect of the scapula. Opened caliper jaws are placed horizontally to the raised skinfold; then the examiner releases the lever of the calipers to make the measurement to the nearest ¼ inch (0.5 cm) (Fig. 6-11).

Another skinfold site is the thigh (a vertical fold on the anterior thigh midway between the iliac crest and patella). Additional sites for men are the chest (diagonal fold midway between the shoulder crease and nipple) and abdomen (vertical fold just to the side of the umbilicus). Another site for women is the supraileum (just above the iliac crest at the midaxillary line). Expected fatfold measurements for men and women are shown in Tables 6-7 and 6-8. Repeated fatfold measurements over time document the increase or decrease in fat stores in the body (Rolfes and DeBruyne, 1990). Body fat percentage can be more precisely determined by water displacement analysis.

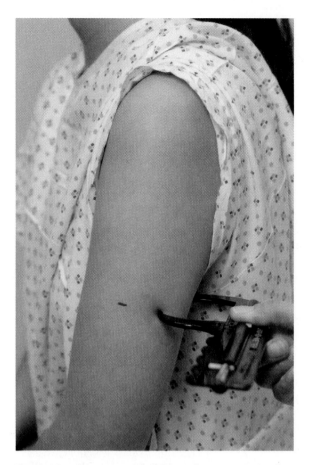

Fig. 6-11 Placement of calipers for triceps skinfold thickness measurement.

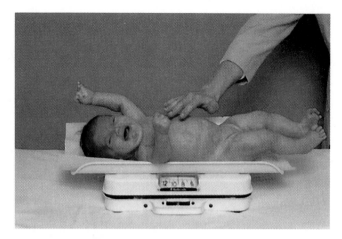

Fig. 6-12 Weighing an infant. *(From Wong, 1995.)*

AGE-RELATED VARIATIONS

NEWBORNS AND INFANTS

In addition to measuring weight and height (length) of an infant, measurements of head circumference and, when necessary, chest circumference are taken to assess growth and development. Monitoring growth of infants is important and can easily be accomplished by plotting the height and weight by age on growth charts at each visit.

Weight. The platform scale is used for weighing newborns, infants, and small children (Fig. 6-12). The scale has curved sides to prevent the infant from rolling. A paper is placed on the scale and the unclothed newborn is laid on the paper. The newborn is weighed by balancing the scale just as for the adult. The weight is recorded to the nearest ½ ounce or 10 grams.

The weight is plotted on the appropriate growth chart for age and gender comparing the newborn's weight to the population standard. The percentile in which the infant's height and weight fall is identified and explained to the caregiver. Healthy newborns weigh between 5 lb 8 oz and 8 lb 13 oz (2500 and 4000 g). Newborns commonly lose 10% of their birth weight in the first week but regain it in 10 to 14 days. In general, they double their birth weight by 4 to 5 months of age and triple their birth weight by 12 months of age.

Height (length). Height of newborns and infants can be measured by using an infant measuring mat, consisting of a soft rubber graduated mat attached to a plastic footboard. The infant lies on the mat with the head against the headboard. The infant's knees are held together and pressed gently against the mat with one hand, while the foot-board is moved against the heels. The height can be recorded in inches or centimeters.

Another device for measuring height of infants has a rigid headboard and movable footboard. The measuring board can be placed horizontally on a table. Barefoot infants lie supine on the measuring board until their head touches the headboard. The footboard is then moved until it touches the bottom of the infant's feet.

When height-measuring devices are not available, the examiner improvises. Using a safety pin at one end of the blanket, the examiner lays the infant's head at the pin, extends the infant's body as just described, and marks the location of the foot on the blanket with another pin. The distance between pins is measured to determine the infant's height. Also, the examiner can place the infant on a piece of paper and mark at the head and feet with a pen.

Head circumference. Head circumference should be measured at every well-child visit up to age 36 months. The measuring tape is wrapped snugly around the infant's head at the largest circumference, usually just above the eyebrows, pinna of the ears, and the occipital prominence at the back of the skull (Fig. 6-13). The tape measure is read to the nearest ⅛ inch (0.5 cm). Head circumference is measured at least twice to check for accuracy.

Expected head circumference for term newborns averages from 13 to 14 inches (33 to 35 cm). The head circumference is plotted on a growth curve appropriate for age and gender and compared with the population standard (Table 6-9). Head circumference should be about 1 inch (2 to 3 cm) larger than chest circumference. Head and chest circumferences are equal at about 1 to 2 years of age. A head circumference that is rapidly increasing suggests increased intracranial pressure. A head circumference below the fifth percentile suggests microcephaly.

Chest circumference. Chest circumference is usually not assessed unless an abnormal head or chest size is suspected.

TABLE 6-7   Selected Percentiles of Weight and Triceps Skinfold Thickness for U.S. Men Ages 25 to 54 Years*

HEIGHT		5TH	15TH	50TH	85TH	95TH	5TH	10TH	15TH	50TH	85TH	90TH	95TH
IN	CM	WEIGHT (KG)†					TRICEPS (MM)‡						
Small Frames, Men													
62	157	46	52	64	71	77				11			
63	160	48	53	61	70	79			6	10	17		
64	163	49	55	66	76	80		5	5	10	16	18	
65	165	52	58	66	77	84	4	5	6	11	17	19	21
66	168	56	59	67	78	84	5	6	6	11	18	18	20
67	170	56	62	71	82	88	5	6	6	11	18	20	22
68	173	56	62	71	79	85	5	6	6	10	15	16	20
69	175	57	65	74	84	88		6	6	11	17	20	
70	178	59	67	75	87	90			7	10	17		
71	180	60	70	76	79	91			7	10	16		
72	183	62	67	74	87	93				10			
73	185	63	69	79	89	94							
74	188	65	71	80	90	96							
Medium Frames, Men													
62	157	51	58	68	81	87				15			
63	160	52	59	71	82	89				11			
64	163	54	61	71	83	90		6	6	12	18	20	
65	165	59	65	74	87	94	5	7	8	12	20	22	25
66	168	58	65	75	85	93	5	6	7	11	16	18	22
67	170	62	68	77	89	100	5	7	7	13	21	23	28
68	173	60	66	78	89	97	4	5	7	11	18	20	24
69	175	63	68	78	90	97	5	6	7	12	18	20	24
70	178	64	70	81	90	97	5	6	7	12	18	20	23
71	180	62	70	81	92	100	4	5	7	12	19	21	25
72	183	68	74	84	97	104	5	7	7	12	20	22	26
73	185	70	75	85	100	104	6	7	8	12	20	24	27
74	188	68	77	88	100	104		6	9	13	21	23	
Large Frames, Men													
62	157	57	66	82	99	108							
63	160	58	67	83	100	109							
64	163	59	68	84	101	110							
65	165	60	69	79	102	111				14			
66	168	60	75	84	103	112			9	14	30		
67	170	62	71	84	102	113		7	10	11	23	27	
68	173	63	76	86	101	114		9	10	14	22	23	
69	175	68	74	89	103	114	6	7	8	15	25	29	31
70	178	68	74	87	106	114	7	7	7	14	23	25	30
71	180	73	82	91	113	123	6	8	10	15	25	27	31
72	183	73	78	91	109	121	5	6	7	12	20	22	25
73	185	72	79	93	106	116	5	6	7	13	19	22	31
74	188	69	82	92	105	120		8		12	19		

*Data from National Center for Health Statistics, 1981.

†1 kg = 2.2 lb.

‡1 mm = 0.0394 inch of ½₅ inch

From Seidel et al: Mosby's guide to physical examination, ed 3, St. Louis, 1995, Mosby.

The chest circumference is measured at the nipples, pulling the tape measure firmly without causing an indentation in the skin. The measurement is noted between inspiration and expiration and recorded to the nearest ⅛ inch (0.5 cm) (Fig. 6-14).

At birth the infant's chest circumference may be equal to or slightly less than the head circumference. Between 1 and 2 years of age, the infant's chest circumference should closely approximate the head circumference (Table 6-9).

Vital signs. **Temperature.** Wide variations are found in temperatures of newborns and infants because they have less effective heat-control mechanisms. Temperature can be measured at several sites in the body. The safest ways to mea-

TABLE 6-8	Selected Percentiles of Weight and Triceps Skinfold Thickness for U.S. Women Ages 25 to 54 Years*

| HEIGHT | | 5TH | 15TH | 50TH | 85TH | 95TH | 5TH | 10TH | 15TH | 50TH | 85TH | 90TH | 95TH |
IN	CM	WEIGHT (KG)†					TRICEPS (MM)‡						
Small Frames, Women													
58	147	37	43	52	58	66		12	13	24	30	33	
59	150	42	44	53	63	72	8	11	14	21	29	36	37
60	152	42	45	53	63	70	8	11	12	21	28	29	33
61	155	44	47	54	64	72	11	12	14	21	28	31	34
62	157	44	48	55	63	70	10	12	14	20	28	31	34
63	160	46	49	55	65	79	10	11	13	20	27	30	36
64	163	49	51	57	67	74	10	13	13	20	28	30	34
65	165	50	53	60	70	80	12	13	14	22	29	31	34
66	168	46	54	58	65	74		12		19	30		
67	170	47	52	59	70	76				18			
68	173	48	53	62	71	77				20			
69	175	49	54	63	72	78							
70	178	50	55	64	73	79							
Medium Frames, Women													
58	147	41	50	63	77	79			20	25	40		
59	150	47	52	66	76	85	15	19	21	30	37	40	40
60	152	47	52	60	77	85	14	15	17	26	35	37	41
61	155	47	51	61	73	86	11	14	15	25	34	36	42
62	157	49	52	61	73	83	12	14	16	24	34	36	40
63	160	49	53	62	77	88	12	13	15	24	33	35	38
64	163	50	54	62	76	87	11	14	15	23	33	36	40
65	165	52	55	63	75	89	12	14	15	22	31	34	38
66	168	52	55	63	75	83	11	13	14	22	31	33	37
67	170	54	57	65	79	88	12	13	15	21	29	30	35
68	173	58	60	67	77	87	10	14	15	22	31	32	36
69	175	49	60	68	79	87		11	12	19	29	31	
70	178	50	57	70	80	87				19			
Large Frames, Women													
58	147	56	67	86	105	117							
59	150	56	67	78	105	116				36			
60	152	55	66	87	104	116				38			
61	155	54	66	81	105	115		25	26	36	48	50	
62	157	59	65	81	103	113	16	19	22	34	48	48	50
63	160	58	67	83	105	119	18	20	22	34	46	48	51
64	163	59	63	79	102	112	16	20	21	32	43	45	49
65	165	59	63	81	103	114	17	20	21	31	43	46	48
66	168	55	62	75	95	107	13	17	18	27	40	43	45
67	170	58	65	80	100	114	13	16	17	30	41	43	49
68	173	51	66	76	104	111		16	20	29	37	40	
69	175	50	68	79	105	111			21	30	42		
70	178	50	61	76	99	110				20			

*Data from National Center for Health Statistics, 1981.

†1 kg = 2.2 lb.

‡1 mm = 0.0394 inch or ¹/₂₅ inch

From Seidel et al: Mosby's guide to physical examination, ed 3, St. Louis, 1995, Mosby.

sure temperature in newborns are at tympanic or axillary sites. Rectal temperatures are contraindicated in newborns because of the risk of rectal perforation.

Pulse and respirations. Pulse and respirations are assessed for the same qualities as in the adult, but at a time when the infant is quiet. If the infant is quiet at the beginning of the assessment, the examiner listens to the apical pulse and counts the respirations before proceeding to other parts of the assessment. Expected heart rates for infants and children are listed in Table 6-3.

Respiratory rates are counted using the same procedure as for adults; however, infants usually breathe diaphragmatically,

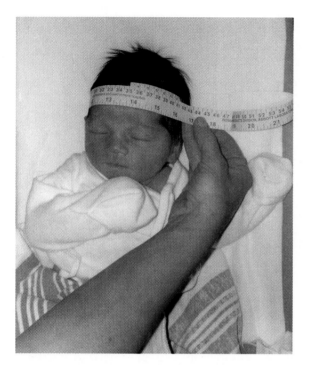

Fig. 6-13   Measuring head circumference of a neonate.

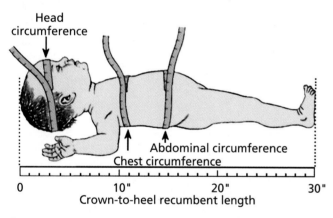

Fig. 6-14   Measurement of head, chest, and abdominal circumference and crown-to-heel (recumbent) length.   *(From Wong, 1995.)*

which requires observation of the abdominal movement. Respirations are counted for a full minute because an infant's respiratory rate may be irregular as a normal variation.

CHILDREN

Height and weight.   To measure height of a child who can stand but is too short for the adult scale, the examiner uses a platform with a moveable headboard. The child stands erect on the platform and the headboard is lowered until it touches the child's head. Height is recorded in inches or centimeters on the growth chart appropriate for the child's age and gender (Fig. 6-15). A tape measure also can be attached to a wall so that the child's height can be measured by having the child stand against the wall.

Monitoring the weight of children is essential. Continuing the graph of height and weight begun in infancy is a

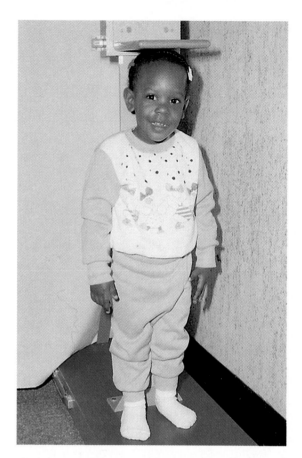

Fig. 6-15   Measuring the height of a child.
(From Seidel et al, 1995.)

valuable screening tool to track the child's growth in comparison with the population standard (Fig. 6-16). The percentile in which the child's height and weight falls is noted and shared with the caregiver. Height and weight measurements continue until the end of the growth spurt between ages 18 to 20.

Head and chest circumference.   Head circumference should be measured at every well-child visit until the age of 2, and then annually until age 6. By 2 years of age the infant's head circumference is ⅔ its adult size. The head circumference is measured as described previously and plotted on the growth chart to compare the growth of the child with a population standard.

Between 5 months and 2 years of age, the infant's chest circumference should closely approximate the head circumference. After 2 years of age the chest circumference should exceed the head circumference.

Vital signs.   Temperature.   Temperatures can be taken safely in children using electronic thermometers or tympanic membrane sensors. Mercury-in-glass thermometers should not be used until the child is at least 5 years old and can be trusted to keep the thermometer under the tongue with the mouth closed without biting the thermometer. Before this age, taking an axillary temperature using mercury-in-glass thermometer is safe and accurate.

Rectal temperatures should be taken as a last resort. A convenient position for taking a rectal temperature is with the

| | | HEAD CIRCUMFERENCE (CM/IN) | |
| | | MALES | FEMALES |
AGE	CHEST CIRCUMFERENCE (CM/IN)		
Birth	35/13.75	35.3/14	34.7/13.63
3 months	40/15.75	40.9/16	40.0/15.75
6 months	44/17.38	43.9/17.25	42.8/16.75
12 months	47/18.5	47.3/18.63	45.8/18
18 months	48/19	48.7/19.25	47.1/18.5
2 years	50/19.5	49.7/19.5	48.1/19
3 years	52/20.5	50.4/19.63	49.3/19.5

TABLE 6-9 Average Chest and Head Circumference for U.S. Children

From Seidel et al: Mosby's guide to physical examination, *ed 3, St. Louis, 1995, Mosby.*

child side-lying with knees flexed toward the abdomen. This position is maintained with one of the examiner's hands while the lubricated thermometer is held in the rectum a maximum of 1 inch (2.5 cm).

Blood pressure. The American Heart Association (AHA) recommends that blood pressure be measured annually in children from age 3 through adolescence. For an accurate reading the appropriate cuff size must be used (see Chapter 5). Show the equipment to be used to the child and explain the procedure before applying the cuff to help enlist the child's cooperation. The AHA recommends using the fourth Korotkoff sound as an indication of the diastolic pressure in children (Report of the Second Task Force, 1987).

ADOLESCENTS

Weight and height. These measurements should be obtained at least annually. Before puberty, the differences in male and female body composition are minimal. Sex differences in the skeletal system, lean body mass, and fat stores become apparent during the adolescent growth spurt. Just before the growth spurt, body fat begins to increase.

OLDER ADULTS

Weight and height. Older adults tend to weigh less and become shorter. For those in their 80s and beyond, body weight may decrease due to muscle wasting or chronic diseases. Also, total body water declines, which contributes to weight loss. Subcutaneous fat distribution shifts from the face and extremities to abdomen and hips. This age group also has decreased bone formation, which may result in reduced height due to shortening of the vertebra and thinning of the vertebral disks. If kyphosis or flexion of knees or hips occurs, arms and legs look longer and out of proportion.

Vital signs. Older adults tend to have lower *normal temperatures,* with an average of 97.2° F (36.2° C). Those who have arteriosclerosis tend to have higher *blood pressures.* As the aorta becomes rigid, the systolic blood pressure increases. Those with diabetes mellitus may have reduced compliance of vessels, resulting in high systolic blood pressures.

SITUATIONAL VARIATIONS

PREGNANT WOMEN

Assessment of pregnant clients is the same as for the adult, with the exception of the variations discussed below.

Weight. Weight gain of between 25 and 35 lbs (11.4-16 kg) is expected during pregnancy as the fetus grows, with 3 lbs expected in the first trimester, 12 lbs in the second, and 12 lbs in the third. The weight gain is attributed to the fetus (7.5 lbs), placenta and membranes (1.5 lbs), amniotic fluid (2 lbs), uterus (2.5 lbs), breast enlargement (3 lbs), increased blood volume (2 to 4 lbs), and extravascular fluid volume and fat reserves (4 to 9 lbs).

Vital signs. Pulse rate increases in the pregnant adult. The heart rate of the fetus is auscultated using a *Doppler ultrasonic stethoscope* from 12 to 20 weeks gestation, then with a *fetoscope* from 20 weeks until delivery. The fetal heart rate is expected to be heard over the lower abdomen for fetuses who are in a head-down position. The expected fetal heart rate ranges from 100 to 160 beats per minute.

Respirations are modified as the breathing pattern changes from abdominal to costal or lateral; likewise, the respiratory rate increases. During the third trimester, the growth of the fetus pushes up against the diaphragm and can cause shortness of breath, especially when the pregnant woman is lying down.

During the first half of the pregnancy, both the systolic and diastolic blood pressure decrease by about 5 to 10 mm Hg. This decrease is probably due to vasodilation from hormonal changes during pregnancy. Maternal position affects blood pressure readings. Brachial blood pressure is highest when the pregnant woman is sitting and lowest when she is lying in the left lateral recumbent position. The blood pressure rises slowly during the third trimester (Bobak and Jensen, 1991). Any marked increase in blood pressure is a cause for concern and should be evaluated.

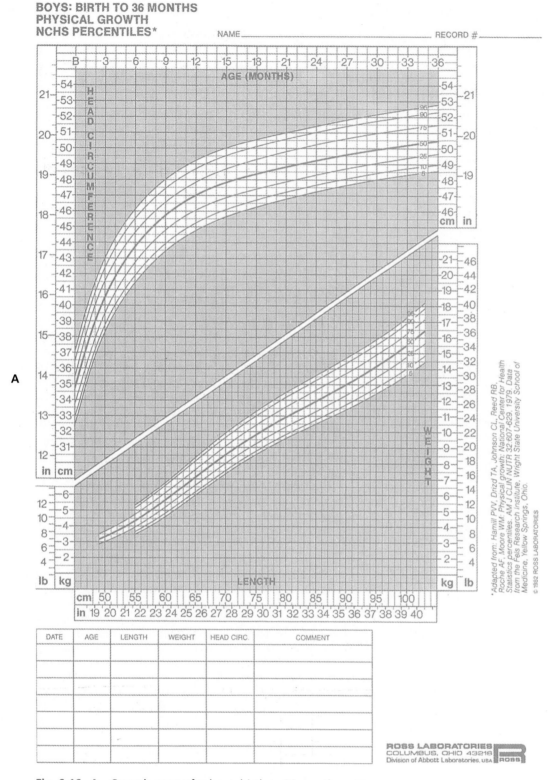

Fig. 6-16, A Growth curves for boys: birth to 36 months.   *(Courtesy Ross Laboratories, Columbus, Ohio.)*

**BOYS: BIRTH TO 36 MONTHS
PHYSICAL GROWTH
NCHS PERCENTILES***

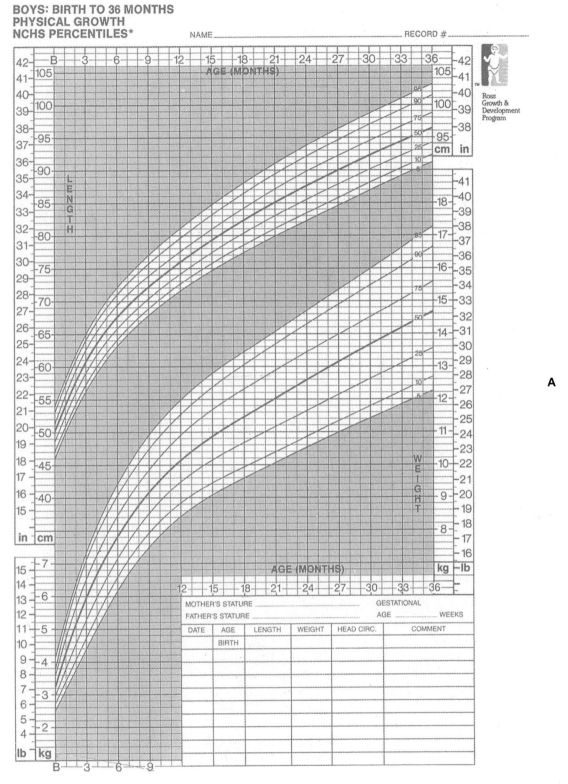

Fig. 6-16, A Growth curves for boys: birth to 36 months. *(Courtesy Ross Laboratories, Columbus, Ohio.)*

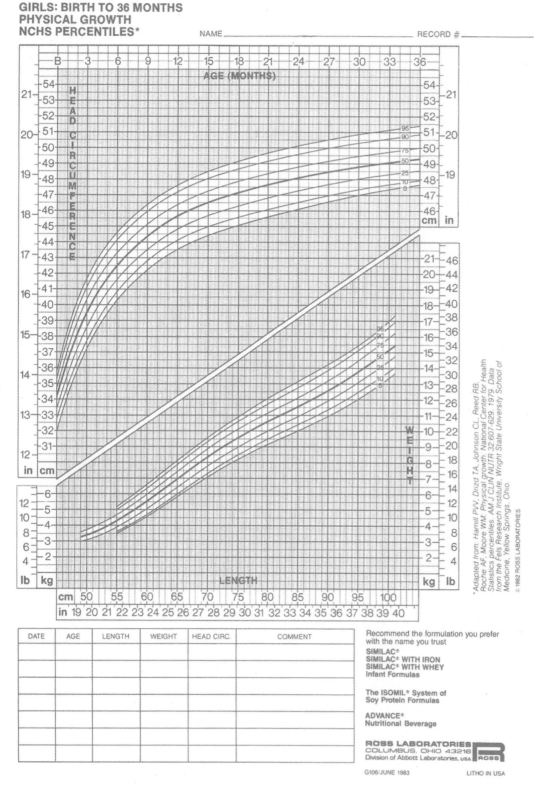

B

DATE	AGE	LENGTH	WEIGHT	HEAD CIRC.	COMMENT

Fig. 6-16, B   Growth curves for girls: birth to 36 months.   *(Courtesy Ross Laboratories, Columbus, Ohio.)*

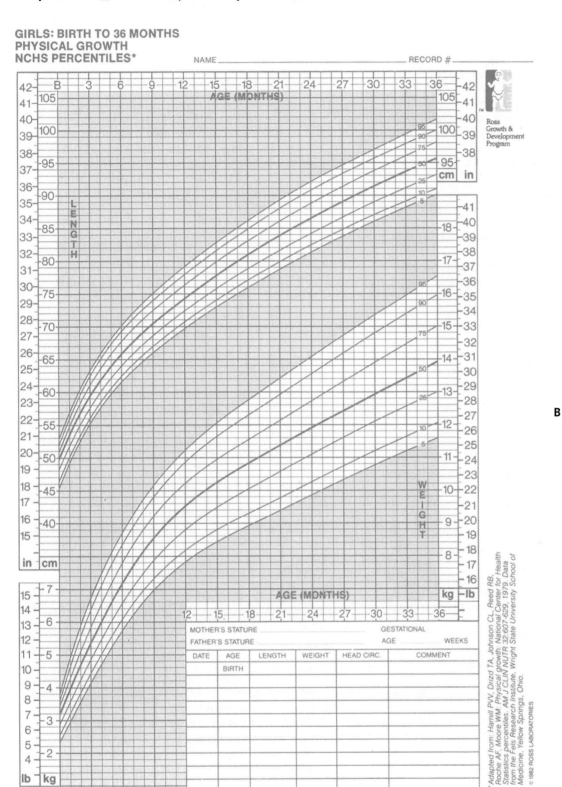

GIRLS: BIRTH TO 36 MONTHS
PHYSICAL GROWTH
NCHS PERCENTILES*

NAME _____ RECORD # _____

*Adapted from: Hamill PVV, Drizd TA, Johnson CL, Reed RB, Roche AF, Moore WM: Physical growth: National Center for Health Statistics percentiles. AM J CLIN NUTR 32:607-629, 1979. Data from the Fels Research Institute, Wright State University School of Medicine, Yellow Springs, Ohio.

© 1982 ROSS LABORATORIES

Fig. 6-16, B Growth curves for girls: birth to 36 months. *(Courtesy Ross Laboratories, Columbus, Ohio.)*

??????? STUDY QUESTIONS ???????

1. List and define the five techniques used for data collection in physical assessment.

2. What role does lighting play in the assessment process? For what technique is adequate lighting essential? What problem is created with tangential lighting? How do you solve that problem?

3. What two characteristics of your hands should you ensure are present before you touch a client when doing an assessment?

4. What should you tell a client as you are palpating a part of his or her body? Why is this important?

5. Match the surface of the hand to the appropriate assessment use.

Palmar finger pads	Crepitus and fluid
Ulnar finger surface	Masses
Dorsal hand surface	Vibration
Palmar finger surface	Temperature

6. Differentiate between light and deep palpation. Which should be done first?

7. Differentiate between direct and indirect percussion. Give an example of each.

8. Match the body system with the most appropriate percussion tones.

Lungs	Tympany
Bone	Resonance
Liver	Flatness
Stomach	Dullness

9. Match the tone with the appropriate sound quality.

Tympany	Hollow
Resonance	Thudlike
Hyperresonance	Drumlike
Dullness	Booming

10. Identify and describe the characteristics of sounds heard by auscultation.

11. What are the uses of the bell and the diaphragm? What should you do to the stethoscope before using it? Why? Can you use a stethoscope over clothing? Why or why not?

12. What are the common positions that the client will assume during a physical assessment? What position is used for a rectal exam? What position allows you to check extension of the hip?

13. Make a chart of the "normal" parameters for temperature, pulse, respiration, and blood pressure in the neonate, child, adult, older adult, and pregnant woman.

14. Identify the four sites for taking a temperature. What type of thermometer can be used for each site? What site might you use for an infant? Someone in a coma?

15. Describe how you would palpate pulses. Define *rate, rhythm, amplitude,* and *contour.*

16. Describe the procedure for assessing ventilation. Define *rate, rhythm,* and *depth of respiration.* How do men and women differ in their breathing patterns?

17. Match the pattern of respiration with the appropriate description.

Tachypnea	< 12 breaths min
Bradypnea	> 20 shallow breaths min
Hyperpnea	
Prolonged hyperpnea	Extended deep breaths > 20 min
	Hyperventilation > 20 min

18. Match the respiratory pattern with the appropriate description.

Kussmaul	Alternating apnea and
Cheyne-Stokes	hyperpnea
	Disorganized breathing/apnea
Ataxic	Continual labored sighing
Cluster	Random shallow and deep breathing

19. Differentiate between systolic and diastolic blood pressure. Describe the physiologic mechanism that creates these readings.

20. List and describe the five Korotkoff sounds.

21. List the factors that influence blood pressure. Give an example of how blood pressure is influenced by each factor.

22. Describe the factors that determine the weight of an individual. What are the difference in body fat distribution in males and females?

23. Describe the process used to weigh an individual using counterbalance scales. How is height measured?

24. For what are skinfold calipers used? Describe the procedure for using skinfold calipers.

25. Describe the procedures used to determine weight and height in infants. What other measures are taken in infants during assessment? Describe the normal variations expected in these measurements.

26. Why are graphs of a child's height and weight important?

27. How do vital signs, height, and weight change over time in the older adult?

28. What is the expected weight gain during pregnancy? Where does the weight gain come from?

29. How is blood pressure expected to change during pregnancy? When is an elevated blood pressure problematic in pregnancy?

CHAPTER 7

Nutritional Assessment

A nutritional assessment of the client is an integral part of the total physical assessment. The most commonly used method for organizing data collection is the acronym *ABCD*, which describes the four types of data collected during nutritional assessment. All types of data collected are equally important; they are anthropometric, biochemical, clinical, and dietary aspects. A brief description of each type of data follows.

Once the client is assessed, data are interpreted, and appropriate interventions are initiated. Although data collection will vary with age group, the general approach is consistent throughout the life cycle.

Anthropometrics: Common assessment tools include evaluation of weight for height and body mass index. Other tools include triceps skinfold measurement and mid-arm circumference. Use of these tools is described later in the chapter.

Biochemical tests: Biochemical data of nutritional significance are most often obtained during routine blood tests. Complete blood counts (CBCs) and routine chemistries (serum glucose, sodium, potassium, chloride, carbon dioxide, phosphorous, magnesium, calcium, albumin, cholesterol, triglycerides, and liver function tests) provide valuable information regarding the client's nutritional status.

Clinical evaluation: A careful physical examination and history may provide the first indication of nutrition-related prob-

lems. Examination of skin, hair, nails, and mouth is an important part of the nutritional assessment.

Dietary assessment: There are multiple methods for assessing dietary intake. Some methods may be more appropriate than others for individual clients. Therefore familiarity with the different approaches is beneficial.

24-hour recall: The examiner asks the client or client's caregiver to describe the foods eaten during the previous 24-hour period or a typical 24-hour day.

Food records: The examiner may ask the client or client's caregiver to record food intake for a specified period (usually 3 to 7 days). Although fairly accurate, this approach is time-consuming and the data are more difficult to analyze.

Food-frequency questionnaire: The examiner asks the client or the client's caregiver how frequently he or she consumes various foods from a number of food groups. Several standardized forms may be helpful with this type of assessment. Food frequency data give the clinician an overview of the client's diet, but the information is difficult to quantify.

ADULTS

ANTHROPOMETRICS

The anthropometric assessment of an adult client should begin with an evaluation of the client's weight. A common method used to assess whether a client's weight is appropriate is to compare his or her body weight and height to published standards (Table 7-1). If the tables are not available, the examiner can calculate desirable body weight using the formulas below:

Female: 100 lbs (45.5 kg) for the first 5 feet + 5 lbs (2.27 kg) for each inch greater than 5 feet ± 10%.

Male: 105 lbs (47.6 kg) for the first 5 feet + 6 lbs (2.73 kg) for each inch greater than 5 feet ± 10%. (Zena, 1991)

To evaluate the client's weight, express the current weight as a percentage of desirable body weight (DBW) (Grant, 1985).

$$\frac{\text{Current weight}}{\text{Desirable weight}} \times 100 = \% \text{ DBW}$$

Variation from desirable body weight may be categorized into the following percentage ranges (Kraus, 1984): greater than 120% DBW, obese; less than 80% DBW, underweight. In general, clients increase their risk of developing nutrition-related problems the further their weight varies from the

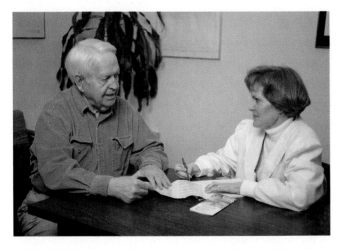

Patient education is vital for improving the nutritional status of a client.

TABLE 7-1   1983 Metropolitan Height and Weight Tables for Adults

| | | | MEN (INDOOR CLOTHING*) | | | | | |
| | | | SMALL FRAME | | MEDIUM FRAME | | LARGE FRAME | |
Feet	Inches	Cm.	Pounds	Kilograms	Pounds	Kilograms	Pounds	Kilograms
5	1	154.9	128-134	58.2-60.9	131-141	59.5-64.1	138-150	62.7-68.2
5	2	157.5	130-136	59.1-61.8	133-143	60.4-65.0	140-153	63.6-69.5
5	3	160.0	132-138	60.0-62.7	135-145	61.4-65.9	142-156	64.5-70.9
5	4	162.6	134-140	60.9-63.6	137-148	62.3-67.2	144-160	65.5-72.7
5	5	165.1	136-142	61.8-64.5	139-151	63.2-68.6	146-164	66.4-74.5
5	6	167.6	138-145	62.7-65.9	142-154	64.5-70.0	149-168	67.7-76.4
5	7	170.2	140-148	63.6-67.2	145-157	65.9-71.4	152-172	69.1-78.2
5	8	172.7	142-151	64.5-68.6	148-160	67.2-72.7	155-176	70.5-80.0
5	9	175.3	144-154	65.5-70.0	151-153	68.6-74.1	158-180	71.8-81.8
5	10	177.8	146-157	66.4-71.4	154-166	70.0-75.5	161-184	73.2-83.6
5	11	180.3	149-160	67.7-72.7	157-170	71.4-77.3	164-188	74.5-85.5
6	0	182.9	152-164	69.1-74.5	160-174	72.7-79.1	168-192	76.4-87.3
6	1	185.4	155-168	70.5-76.4	164-178	74.5-80.9	172-197	78.2-89.5
6	2	188.0	158-172	71.8-78.2	167-182	75.9-82.7	176-202	80.0-91.8
6	3	190.5	162-176	73.6-80.0	171-187	77.7-85.0	181-207	82.3-94.1

Allow 5 pounds.

| | | | WOMEN (INDOOR CLOTHING*) | | | | | |
| | | | SMALL FRAME | | MEDIUM FRAME | | LARGE FRAME | |
Feet	Inches	Cm.	Pounds	Kilograms	Pounds	Kilograms	Pounds	Kilograms
4	9	144.8	102-111	46.4-50.0	109-121	49.5-55.0	118-131	53.6-59.5
4	10	147.3	103-113	46.8-51.4	111-123	50.0-55.9	120-134	54.5-60.9
4	11	149.9	104-115	47.3-52.3	113-126	51.4-57.2	122-137	55.5-62.3
5	0	152.4	106-118	48.2-53.6	115-129	52.3-58.6	125-140	56.8-63.6
5	1	154.9	108-121	49.1-55.0	118-132	53.6-60.0	128-143	58.2-65.0
5	2	157.5	111-124	50.5-56.4	121-135	55.0-61.4	131-147	59.5-66.8
5	3	160.0	114-127	51.8-57.7	124-138	56.4-62.7	134-151	60.9-68.6
5	4	162.6	117-130	53.2-59.0	127-141	57.7-64.1	137-155	62.3-70.5
5	5	165.1	120-133	54.5-60.5	130-144	59.0-65.5	140-159	63.6-72.3
5	6	167.6	123-136	55.9-61.8	133-147	60.5-66.8	143-163	65.0-74.1
5	7	170.2	126-139	57.3-63.2	136-150	61.8-68.2	146-167	66.4-75.9
5	8	172.7	129-142	58.6-64.5	139-153	63.2-69.5	149-170	67.7-77.3
5	9	175.3	132-145	60.0-65.9	142-156	64.6-70.9	152-173	69.1-78.6
5	10	177.8	135-148	61.4-67.3	145-159	65.9-72.3	155-176	70.5-80.0
5	11	180.3	138-151	62.7-73.6	148-162	67.3-73.6	158-179	71.8-81.4

Allow 3 pounds.
The weights presented are those associated with the lowest mortality. They are not necessarily the weights at which people are healthiest,
perform their jobs optimally, or even look their best. Three weight ranges were determined for each sex on each size and attributed to a
small, medium, or large frame.
These tables correct the 1983 Metropolitan tables to height without shoe heels.

norm. Therefore clients who are either underweight or obese are at increased risk.

An alternative method for evaluating the appropriateness of a client's weight-to-height ratio is the Body Mass Index (BMI). Many professionals believe the BMI is a more objective indicator of the presence of obesity than life insurance tables (Fig. 7-1).

$$BMI = \frac{Weight\ (kg)}{Height\ (m^2)}$$

Although assessment of body weight and height are necessary and most commonly used, certain clients require a more accurate measure of their percentage of body fat. Evaluation of a client's triceps skinfold is perhaps the easiest method for measuring body fat. Measurements are made with skinfold calipers at the midpoint between the acromial process and the olecranon of the nondominant arm (see Fig. 6-11). The layer of skin and subcutaneous fat, excluding the underlying muscle, is firmly pinched and measured. Three measurements should be made

Women

Height, m (in.)

Weight kg(lb)	1.47 (58)	1.50 (59)	1.52 (60)	1.55 (61)	1.57 (62)	1.60 (63)	1.63 (64)	1.65 (65)	1.68 (66)	1.70 (67)	1.73 (68)	1.75 (69)	1.78 (70)	1.80 (71)	1.83 (72)	1.85 (73)	1.88 (74)	1.90 (75)	1.93 (76)
39 (85)	17.8	17.2	16.6	16.1	15.5	15.1	14.6	14.1	13.7	13.3	12.9	12.6	12.2	11.9	11.5	11.2	10.9	10.6	10.3
41 (90)	18.8	18.2	17.6	17.0	16.5	15.9	15.4	15.0	14.5	14.1	13.7	13.3	12.9	12.6	12.2	11.9	11.6	11.2	11.0
43 (95)	19.9	19.2	18.6	18.0	17.4	16.8	16.3	15.8	15.3	14.9	14.4	14.0	13.6	13.2	12.9	12.5	12.2	11.9	11.6
45 (100)	20.9	20.2	19.5	18.9	18.3	17.7	17.2	16.6	16.1	15.7	15.2	14.8	14.3	13.9	13.6	13.2	12.8	12.5	12.2
48 (105)	21.9	21.2	20.5	19.8	19.2	18.6	18.0	17.5	16.9	16.4	16.0	15.5	15.1	14.6	14.2	13.9	13.5	13.1	12.8
50 (110)	23.0	22.2	21.5	20.8	20.1	19.5	18.9	18.3	17.8	17.2	16.7	16.2	15.8	15.3	14.9	14.5	14.1	13.7	13.4
52 (115)	24.0	23.2	22.5	21.7	21.0	20.4	19.7	19.1	18.6	18.0	17.5	17.0	16.5	16.0	15.6	15.2	14.8	14.4	14.0
54 (120)	25.1	24.2	23.4	22.7	21.9	21.3	20.6	20.0	19.4	18.8	18.2	17.7	17.2	16.7	16.3	15.8	15.4	15.0	14.6
57 (125)	26.1	25.2	24.4	23.6	22.9	22.1	21.5	20.8	20.2	19.6	19.0	18.5	17.9	17.4	17.0	16.5	16.0	15.6	15.2
59 (130)	27.2	26.3	25.4	24.6	23.8	23.0	22.3	21.6	21.0	20.4	19.8	19.2	18.7	18.1	17.6	17.2	16.7	16.2	15.8
61 (135)	28.2	27.3	26.4	25.5	24.7	23.9	23.2	22.5	21.8	21.1	20.5	19.9	19.4	18.8	18.3	17.8	17.3	16.9	16.4
64 (140)	29.3	28.3	27.3	26.5	25.6	24.8	24.0	23.3	22.6	21.9	21.3	20.7	20.1	19.5	19.0	18.5	18.0	17.5	17.0
66 (145)	30.3	29.3	28.3	27.4	26.5	25.7	24.9	24.1	23.4	22.7	22.0	21.4	20.8	20.2	19.7	19.1	18.6	18.1	17.7
68 (150)	31.4	30.3	29.3	28.3	27.4	26.6	25.7	25.0	24.2	23.5	22.8	22.2	21.5	20.9	20.3	19.8	19.3	18.7	18.3
70 (155)	32.4	31.3	30.3	29.3	28.4	27.5	26.6	25.8	25.0	24.3	23.6	22.9	22.2	21.6	21.0	20.4	19.9	19.4	18.9
73 (160)	33.4	32.3	31.2	30.2	29.3	28.3	27.5	26.6	25.8	25.1	24.3	23.6	23.0	22.3	21.7	21.1	20.5	20.0	19.5
75 (165)	34.5	33.3	32.2	31.2	30.2	29.2	28.3	27.5	26.6	25.8	25.1	24.4	23.7	23.0	22.4	21.8	21.2	20.6	20.1
77 (170)	35.5	34.3	33.2	32.1	31.1	30.1	29.2	28.3	27.4	26.6	25.8	25.1	24.4	23.7	23.1	22.4	21.8	21.2	20.7
79 (175)	36.6	35.3	34.2	33.1	32.0	31.0	30.0	29.1	28.2	27.4	26.6	25.8	25.1	24.4	23.7	23.1	22.5	21.9	21.3
82 (180)	37.6	36.4	35.2	34.0	32.9	31.9	30.9	30.0	29.1	28.2	27.4	26.6	25.8	25.1	24.4	23.7	23.1	22.5	21.9
84 (185)	38.7	37.4	36.1	35.0	33.8	32.8	31.8	30.8	29.9	29.0	28.1	27.3	26.5	25.8	25.1	24.4	23.8	23.1	22.5
86 (190)	39.7	38.4	37.1	35.9	34.8	33.7	32.6	31.6	30.7	29.8	28.9	28.1	27.3	26.5	25.8	25.1	24.4	23.7	23.1
88 (195)	40.8	39.4	38.1	36.8	35.7	34.5	33.5	32.4	31.5	30.5	29.6	28.8	28.0	27.2	26.4	25.7	25.0	24.4	23.7
91 (200)	41.8	40.4	39.1	37.8	36.6	35.4	34.3	33.3	32.3	31.3	30.4	29.5	28.7	27.9	27.1	26.4	25.7	25.0	24.3
93 (205)	42.8	41.4	40.0	38.7	37.5	36.3	35.2	34.1	33.1	32.1	31.2	30.3	29.4	28.6	27.8	27.0	26.3	25.6	25.0
95 (210)	43.9	42.4	41.0	39.7	38.4	37.2	36.0	34.9	33.9	32.9	31.9	31.0	30.1	29.3	28.5	27.7	27.0	26.2	25.6
98 (215)	44.9	43.4	42.0	40.6	39.3	38.1	36.9	35.8	34.7	33.7	32.7	31.8	30.8	30.0	29.2	28.4	27.6	26.9	26.2
100 (220)	46.0	44.4	43.0	41.6	40.2	39.0	37.8	36.6	35.5	34.5	33.5	32.5	31.6	30.7	29.8	29.0	28.2	27.5	26.8
102 (225)	47.0	45.4	43.9	42.5	41.2	39.9	38.6	37.4	36.3	35.2	34.2	33.2	32.3	31.4	30.5	29.7	28.9	28.1	27.4
104 (230)	48.1	46.5	44.9	43.5	42.1	40.7	39.5	38.3	37.1	36.0	35.0	34.0	33.0	32.1	31.2	30.3	29.5	28.7	28.0
107 (235)	49.1	47.5	45.9	44.4	43.0	41.6	40.3	39.1	37.9	36.8	35.7	34.7	33.7	32.8	31.9	31.0	30.2	29.4	28.6
109 (240)	50.2	48.5	46.9	45.3	43.9	42.5	41.2	39.9	38.7	37.6	36.5	35.4	34.4	33.5	32.6	31.7	30.8	30.0	29.2
111 (245)	51.2	49.5	47.8	46.3	44.8	43.4	42.1	40.8	39.5	38.4	37.3	36.2	35.2	34.2	33.2	32.3	31.5	30.6	29.8
113 (250)	52.3	50.5	48.8	47.2	45.7	44.3	42.9	41.6	40.4	39.2	38.0	36.9	35.9	34.9	33.9	33.0	32.1	31.2	30.4
116 (255)	53.3	51.5	49.8	48.2	46.6	45.2	43.8	42.4	41.2	39.9	38.8	37.7	36.6	35.6	34.6	33.6	32.7	31.9	31.0
118 (260)	54.3	52.5	50.8	49.1	47.6	46.1	44.6	43.3	42.0	40.7	39.5	38.4	37.3	36.3	35.3	34.3	33.4	32.5	31.6
120 (265)	55.4	53.5	51.8	50.1	48.5	46.9	45.5	44.1	42.8	41.5	40.3	39.1	38.0	37.0	35.9	35.0	34.0	33.1	32.3
122 (270)	56.4	54.5	52.7	51.0	49.4	47.8	46.3	44.9	43.6	42.3	41.1	39.9	38.7	37.7	36.6	35.6	34.7	33.7	32.9
125 (275)	57.5	55.5	53.7	52.0	50.3	48.7	47.2	45.8	44.4	43.1	41.8	40.6	39.5	38.4	37.3	36.3	35.3	34.4	33.5
136 (300)	62.7	60.6	58.6	56.7	54.9	53.1	51.5	49.9	48.4	47.0	45.6	44.3	43.0	41.8	40.7	39.6	38.5	37.5	36.5
159 (350)	73.2	70.7	68.4	66.1	64.0	62.0	60.1	58.2	56.5	54.8	53.2	51.7	50.2	48.8	47.5	46.2	44.9	43.7	42.6
181 (400)	83.6	80.8	78.1	75.6	73.2	70.9	68.7	66.6	64.6	62.6	60.8	59.1	57.4	55.8	54.3	52.8	51.4	50.0	48.7

A

Fig. 7-1 **A,** Body mass index (weight [kilograms]/height [meters] squared) for women. Weight and heights shown are for adults without shoes and clothing. *(Ross Products Division, Abbott Laboratories, Columbus, Ohio; from Rowland, 1989.)*

☐ Underweight ▨ Overweight
☐ Acceptable weight ▨ Severe overweight
☐ Marginal overweight ▨ Morbid obesity

Body Mass Index Assessment

19-25	Appropriate weight (19-34 years)
21-27	Appropriate weight (>35 years)
27.5-30	Mild obesity
30-40	Moderate obesity
>40	Morbid obesity

(Data from Hopkins, 1993)

and the results averaged. Tables 6-7 and 6-8 contain the normal values for comparison. Values significantly higher than normal indicate increased fat mass. Values significantly lower than normal can indicate decreased fat mass secondary to either an increase in lean mass or depleted fat stores.

BIOCHEMICAL TESTS

Several laboratory values can be helpful with nutritional assessment. As previously stated, serum albumin is a reliable indicator of protein status (Grant, 1985). Albumin measures circulating protein status. Normal values in the adult are 3.5 to 5 g/dl. Interpretation of albumin must be made cautiously because albumin is sensitive to several other factors unrelated to protein status. For instance, albumin is sensitive to fluid status, blood loss, liver function, and trauma. Also, the fluctuation in albumin levels occurs over a 3- to 4-week period (Zeman, 1991). Changes in nutritional status produce slow changes in serum albumin (Grant, 1985). Rapid changes are most likely due to factors other than nutrition.

Several other indicators of protein status are more sensitive to recent protein fluctuations. Serum prealbumin reflects protein and calorie intake for the previous 2 to 3 days (Grant, 1985). A deficiency of either nutrient causes prealbumin to

Men

Weight kg (lb)	1.47 (58)	1.50 (59)	1.52 (60)	1.55 (61)	1.57 (62)	1.60 (63)	1.63 (64)	1.65 (65)	1.68 (66)	1.70 (67)	1.73 (68)	1.75 (69)	1.78 (70)	1.80 (71)	1.83 (72)	1.85 (73)	1.88 (74)	1.90 (75)	1.93 (76)
39 (85)	17.8	17.2	16.6	16.1	15.5	15.1	14.6	14.1	13.7	13.3	12.9	12.6	12.2	11.9	11.5	11.2	10.9	10.6	10.3
41 (90)	18.8	18.2	17.6	17.0	16.5	15.9	15.4	15.0	14.5	14.1	13.7	13.3	12.9	12.6	12.2	11.9	11.6	11.2	11.0
43 (95)	19.9	19.2	18.6	18.0	17.4	16.8	16.3	15.8	15.3	14.9	14.4	14.0	13.6	13.2	12.9	12.5	12.2	11.9	11.6
45 (100)	20.9	20.2	19.5	18.9	18.3	17.7	17.2	16.6	16.1	15.7	15.2	14.8	14.3	13.9	13.6	13.2	12.8	12.5	12.2
48 (105)	21.9	21.2	20.5	19.8	19.2	18.6	18.0	17.5	16.9	16.4	16.0	15.5	15.1	14.6	14.2	13.9	13.5	13.1	12.8
50 (110)	23.0	22.2	21.5	20.8	20.1	19.5	18.9	18.3	17.8	17.2	16.7	16.2	15.8	15.3	14.9	14.5	14.1	13.7	13.4
52 (115)	24.0	23.2	22.5	21.7	21.0	20.4	19.7	19.1	18.6	18.0	17.5	17.0	16.5	16.0	15.6	15.2	14.8	14.4	14.0
54 (120)	25.1	24.2	23.4	22.7	21.9	21.3	20.6	20.0	19.4	18.8	18.2	17.7	17.2	16.7	16.3	15.8	15.4	15.0	14.6
57 (125)	26.1	25.2	24.4	23.6	22.9	22.1	21.5	20.8	20.2	19.6	19.0	18.5	17.9	17.4	17.0	16.5	16.0	15.6	15.2
59 (130)	27.2	26.3	25.4	24.6	23.8	23.0	22.3	21.6	21.0	20.4	19.8	19.2	18.7	18.1	17.6	17.2	16.7	16.2	15.8
61 (135)	28.2	27.3	26.4	25.5	24.7	23.9	23.2	22.5	21.8	21.1	20.5	19.9	19.4	18.8	18.3	17.8	17.3	16.9	16.4
64 (140)	29.3	28.3	27.3	26.5	25.6	24.8	24.0	23.3	22.6	21.9	21.3	20.7	20.1	19.5	19.0	18.5	18.0	17.5	17.0
66 (145)	30.3	29.3	28.3	27.4	26.5	25.7	24.9	24.1	23.4	22.7	22.0	21.4	20.8	20.2	19.7	19.1	18.6	18.1	17.7
68 (150)	31.4	30.3	29.3	28.3	27.4	26.6	25.7	25.0	24.2	23.5	22.8	22.2	21.5	20.9	20.3	19.8	19.3	18.7	18.3
70 (155)	32.4	31.3	30.3	29.3	28.4	27.5	26.6	25.8	25.0	24.3	23.6	22.9	22.2	21.6	21.0	20.4	19.9	19.4	18.9
73 (160)	33.4	32.3	31.2	30.2	29.3	28.3	27.5	26.6	25.8	25.1	24.3	23.6	23.0	22.3	21.7	21.1	20.5	20.0	19.5
75 (165)	34.5	33.3	32.2	31.2	30.2	29.2	28.3	27.5	26.6	25.8	25.1	24.4	23.7	23.0	22.4	21.8	21.2	20.6	20.1
77 (170)	35.5	34.3	33.2	32.1	31.1	30.1	29.2	28.3	27.4	26.6	25.8	25.1	24.4	23.7	23.1	22.4	21.8	21.2	20.7
79 (175)	36.6	35.3	34.2	33.1	32.0	31.0	30.0	29.1	28.2	27.4	26.6	25.8	25.1	24.4	23.7	23.1	22.5	21.9	21.3
82 (180)	37.6	36.4	35.2	34.0	32.9	31.9	30.9	30.0	29.1	28.2	27.4	26.6	25.8	25.1	24.4	23.7	23.1	22.5	21.9
84 (185)	38.7	37.4	36.1	35.0	33.8	32.8	31.8	30.8	29.9	29.0	28.1	27.3	26.5	25.8	25.1	24.4	23.8	23.1	22.5
86 (190)	39.7	38.4	37.1	35.9	34.8	33.7	32.6	31.6	30.7	29.8	28.9	28.1	27.3	26.5	25.8	25.1	24.4	23.7	23.1
88 (195)	40.8	39.4	38.1	36.8	35.7	34.5	33.5	32.4	31.5	30.5	29.6	28.8	28.0	27.2	26.4	25.7	25.0	24.4	23.7
91 (200)	41.8	40.4	39.1	37.8	36.6	35.4	34.3	33.3	32.3	31.3	30.4	29.5	28.7	27.9	27.1	26.4	25.7	25.0	24.3
93 (205)	42.8	41.4	40.0	38.7	37.5	36.3	35.2	34.1	33.1	32.1	31.2	30.3	29.4	28.6	27.8	27.0	26.3	25.6	25.0
95 (210)	43.9	42.4	41.0	39.7	38.4	37.2	36.0	34.9	33.9	32.9	31.9	31.0	30.1	29.3	28.5	27.7	27.0	26.2	25.6
98 (215)	44.9	43.4	42.0	40.6	39.3	38.1	36.9	35.8	34.7	33.7	32.7	31.8	30.8	30.0	29.2	28.4	27.6	26.9	26.2
100 (220)	46.0	44.4	43.0	41.6	40.2	39.0	37.8	36.6	35.5	34.5	33.5	32.5	31.6	30.7	29.8	29.0	28.2	27.5	26.8
102 (225)	47.0	45.4	43.9	42.5	41.2	39.9	38.6	37.4	36.3	35.2	34.2	33.2	32.3	31.4	30.5	29.7	28.9	28.1	27.4
104 (230)	48.1	46.5	44.9	43.5	42.1	40.7	39.5	38.3	37.1	36.0	35.0	34.0	33.0	32.1	31.2	30.3	29.5	28.7	28.0
107 (235)	49.1	47.5	45.9	44.4	43.0	41.6	40.3	39.1	37.9	36.8	35.7	34.7	33.7	32.8	31.9	31.0	30.2	29.4	28.6
109 (240)	50.2	48.5	46.9	45.3	43.9	42.5	41.2	39.9	38.7	37.6	36.5	35.4	34.4	33.5	32.6	31.7	30.8	30.0	29.2
111 (245)	51.2	49.5	47.8	46.3	44.8	43.4	42.1	40.8	39.5	38.4	37.3	36.2	35.2	34.2	33.2	32.3	31.5	30.6	29.8
113 (250)	52.3	50.5	48.8	47.2	45.7	44.3	42.9	41.6	40.4	39.2	38.0	36.9	35.9	34.9	33.9	33.0	32.1	31.2	30.4
116 (255)	53.3	51.5	49.8	48.2	46.6	45.2	43.8	42.4	41.2	39.9	38.8	37.7	36.6	35.6	34.6	33.6	32.7	31.9	31.0
118 (260)	54.3	52.5	50.8	49.1	47.6	46.1	44.6	43.3	42.0	40.7	39.5	38.4	37.3	36.3	35.3	34.3	33.4	32.5	31.6
120 (265)	55.4	53.5	51.8	50.1	48.5	46.9	45.5	44.1	42.8	41.5	40.3	39.1	38.0	37.0	35.9	35.0	34.0	33.1	32.3
122 (270)	56.4	54.5	52.7	51.0	49.4	47.8	46.3	44.9	43.6	42.3	41.1	39.9	38.7	37.7	36.6	35.6	34.7	33.7	32.9
125 (275)	57.5	55.5	53.7	52.0	50.3	48.7	47.2	45.8	44.4	43.1	41.8	40.6	39.5	38.4	37.3	36.3	35.3	34.4	33.5
136 (300)	62.7	60.6	58.6	56.7	54.9	53.1	51.5	49.9	48.4	47.0	45.6	44.3	43.0	41.8	40.7	39.6	38.5	37.5	36.5
159 (350)	73.2	70.7	68.4	66.1	64.0	62.0	60.1	58.2	56.5	54.8	53.2	51.7	50.2	48.8	47.5	46.2	44.9	43.7	42.6
181 (400)	83.6	80.8	78.1	75.6	73.2	70.9	68.7	66.6	64.6	62.6	60.8	59.1	57.4	55.8	54.3	52.8	51.4	50.0	48.7

B

☐ Underweight   ◼ Overweight
☐ Acceptable weight   ◼ Severe overweight
◻ Marginal overweight   ◼ Morbid obesity

Fig. 7-1 B, Body mass index (weight [kilograms]/height [meters] squared) for men. Weight and heights shown are for adults without shoes and clothing. *(Ross Products Division, Abbott Laboratories, Columbus, Ohio; from Rowland, 1989.)*

decline. Refeeding can produce subsequent rises in prealbumin and therefore may be of more benefit in the acute care setting. Normal values for prealbumin in the adult are 15.7 to 29.6 mg/ml.

Blood glucose levels should be a routine laboratory value assessed to screen for diabetes mellitus. It is estimated that the prevalence of diabetes mellitus is 2% to 4% of the U.S. population (Olefsky, 1992). If a fasting blood glucose level is 140 mg/dl or greater, a glucose tolerance test should be done before a diagnosis is made (Olefsky, 1992).

Other routine laboratory tests used for nutrition screening include hemoglobin, hematocrit, total cholesterol, and triglycerides. Hemoglobin and hematocrit values are used to assess the presence of anemia (Zemen and Ney, 1988). Values significantly below normal can indicate anemia. The causes of anemia are numerous, but iron, B_{12}, or folate deficiency are a few possible causes. Further tests should be conducted to determine the cause of the anemia. Total cholesterol and triglyceride lev-

els assess the client's risk for cardiovascular disease. Values equal to or greater than 200 mg/dl for either indicate the client is at increased risk. A complete lipid profile and cardiovascular risk assessment are recommended for clients with total cholesterol or triglycerides above 200 mg/dl (Grundy, 1993).

CLINICAL EVALUATION

A good clinical evaluation of the client is an essential part of nutritional assessment. All of the various indicators can be observed during a routine physical examination. Physical signs of malnutrition include protruding bones and a pale, gaunt appearance. Severe malnutrition is usually apparent due to the client's prominent cheek and clavicle bones or wasted-appearing limbs. When using the process of subjective global assessment, the examiner palpates the back of the upper arm, upper back, and shoulder areas for evidence of fat and muscle wasting. The examiner then subjectively ranks clients as normal, with moderate wasting, or with severe wasting (Detsky, 1987). If muscle wasting is observed, the client should be referred to a dietitian or physician for further evaluation and treatment of malnutrition. Increased adipose tissue indicates overnutrition or obesity. The most objective measure of overnutrition is weight-to-height assessment.

The ability to consume food is directly related to the condition of the client's oral cavity. Poor dentition will negatively impact the client's ability to chew foods and often decreases food intake. Painful oral lesions or sores will also negatively affect food intake. A careful examination of the oral cavity will enable the nurse to identify potential food intake difficulties.

Examining skin quality is another important aspect of the physical nutritional assessment. The presence of edema indicates fluid retention. Skin breakdown increases nutritional needs for calories and protein. Dry skin with decreased elasticity may indicate dehydration.

Table 7-2 lists other clinical signs of nutritional deficiency. Alcoholics are at increased risk for B-vitamin deficiencies, especially thiamin deficiency.

DIETARY ASSESSMENT

A variety of dietary assessment tools may be used to assess the client's eating habits. A combination of a 24-hour recall and food-frequency questionnaire is the most efficient and effective approach. Ask the client to recount the previous 24-hour intake. Then ask how often the client eats each of the food groups listed in the food pyramid. A questionnaire can be given to the client to complete. Alcohol consumption should also be addressed. The examiner should ask the client about type, quantity, and frequency of alcohol consumed. Professionals believe alcohol consumption is underreported by 50% in clients with alcoholic histories (Zemen and Ney, 1988).

Once the client's eating habits have been established, there are two methods to evaluate the adequacy of the diet. The most accurate approach is to compare the client's intake with the recommended dietary allowances (RDAs). A 24-hour recall can be analyzed by hand using a reference book, such as Bowes and Church, or by entering the recall into a diet-analysis computer program (Pennington, 1994). When using a handbook, the nutrient values for each food eaten are written down and added together. Total nutrient intake is compared to the RDA values. If a computer program is available, the 24-hour recall can be entered into the program, and the computer can analyze the nutrient intake. Note that vitamin C needs are increased in smokers (National Research Council, 1989) and should be considered when analyzing the recall (Table 7-3, p. 100). This approach is time-consuming and will not be practical in all situations.

Comparing diet intake against the food pyramid is another approach. The USDA food pyramid (Fig. 7-2) gives recommended servings for each of six food groups. Determine the number of servings per day for each of the six groups and compare food intake with the recommended number of servings. Although less accurate, this method can provide quick feedback to the client and help the nurse identify specific areas of concern.

Healthy eating guidelines. In general, American adults have a high intake of fat, oils, sweets, protein and animal products, and a low intake of bread and cereals, fruit, and vegetables. The daily guidelines for healthy eating are (1) eat 6 to 11 servings of *whole grain* breads and cereals, rice, and pasta; (2) eat 3 to 5 servings of a variety of vegetables (include dark green leafy vegetables several times per week); (3) eat 2 to 4 servings of fruit (include 1 serving of either fruit or vegetable

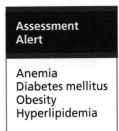

Assessment Alert

Anemia
Diabetes mellitus
Obesity
Hyperlipidemia

high in vitamin C); (4) eat 2 servings of low-fat dairy products such as 1% or skim milk, low-fat yogurt, or cheese; (5) eat 2 to 3 servings of meat, poultry, fish, or a protein alternative such as beans (legumes) or peanut butter; and (6) use fats, oils, and sweets sparingly in the diet.

The National Cholesterol Education Program (NCEP) Guidelines specify that no more than 30% of total calories should be from fat. Ten percent or less of total calories should be saturated fat. Total cholesterol intake should be 300 mg/day or less (Grundy, 1993).

- Many adults eat vegetables only at their evening meal. Adding vegetable servings throughout the day, especially at the noon meal, can help increase the total number of vegetable servings consumed.
- Using the visual image of meat as a "side dish" and grains and vegetables as the "main course" can enhance the client's understanding of portions.
- Meat, poultry, and fish portions can be described as the size of a deck of cards (3 oz). Healthy eating guidelines recommend only 4 to 6 oz of meat, poultry, and fish per day.
- It is important to assess the literacy of the client and tailor recommendations to his or her level. Low-literacy clients would benefit from handouts with pictures or video education tools.
- When discussing various types of fat, remember that saturated fat is solid at room temperature, whereas monounsaturated and polyunsaturated fats are liquid at room temperature. Saturated fats should be minimized. In small quantities, monounsaturated and polyunsaturated fats are preferred.
- Consider the client's cultural food choices when teaching healthy eating.

PREGNANT WOMEN

A woman's preconception nutritional status and diet during pregnancy affect maternal and fetal health. Weight gain during pregnancy is a marker of adequate energy intake. An expected weight gain goal of 25 to 35 pounds is associated with positive pregnancy outcome for normal prepregnancy weight females (a range of 15 to 40 pounds is recommended for obese and underweight women, respectively) (Institute of Medicine, 1990). To achieve weight gain goals, an extra 300 calories per day is recommended for the second and third trimesters of pregnancy. An additional 10 g of protein per day is also recommended. Most other nutrient needs are also increased during pregnancy (Table 7-4, p. 103). All pregnant women should be screened for nutritional risks and counseled on the nutritional needs of pregnancy. Generally, the food guide pyramid is a useful tool for nutritional counseling and is appropriate for many diet variations (see Fig. 7-2).

TABLE 7-2   Clinical Signs and Laboratory Findings in the Malnourished Child and Adult*

CLINICAL SIGN	SUSPECT NUTRIENT	SUPPORTIVE OBJECTIVE FINDINGS
Epithelial		
Skin		
Xerosis, dry scaling	Essential fatty acids	Triene/tetraene ratio >0.4
Hyperkeratosis, plaques around hair follicles	Vitamin A	↓ Plasma retinol
Ecchymoses, petechiae	Vitamin K Vitamin C	Prolonged prothrombin time ↓ Serum ascorbic acid
Hair		
Easily plucked, dyspigmented, lackluster	Protein-calorie	↓ Total protein ↓ Albumin ↓ Transferrin
Nails		
Thin, spoon-shaped	Iron	↓ Serum Fe ↑ TIBC
Mucosal		
Mouth, lips, and tongue	**B vitamins**	
Angular stomatitis (inflammation at corners of mouth)	B_2 (riboflavin)	↓ RBC glutathione reductase
Cheilosis (reddened lips with fissures at angles)	B_2 B_6 (pyridoxine)	See above ↓ Plasma pyridoxal phosphate[†]
Glossitis (inflammation of tongue)	B_6 B_2 B_3 (niacin)	See above See above ↓ Plasma tryptophan ↓ Urinary N-methyl nicotinamide[†]
Magenta tongue	B_2	See above
Edema of tongue, tongue fissures	B_3	See above
Gums		
Spongy, bleeding	Vitamin C	↓ Plasma ascorbic acid
Ocular		
Pale conjunctivae secondary to anemia	Iron Folic acid Vitamin B_{12} Copper	↓ Serum Fe, ↑ TIBC, ↓ serum folic acid, or ↓ RBC folic acid ↓ Serum B_{12} ↓ Serum copper
Bitot's spots (grayish, yellow, or white foamy spots on the whites of the eye)	Vitamin A	↓ Plasma retinol
Conjunctival or corneal xerosis, keratomalacia (softening of part or all of cornea)	Vitamin A	↓ Plasma retinol
Musculoskeletal		
Craniotabes (thinning of the inner table of the skull); palpable enlargement of costochondral junctions ("rachitic rosary"); thickening of wrists and ankles	Vitamin D	↓ 25-OH-vit D ↑ Alkaline phosphatase ±↓ Ca, ↓ PO_4 Long bone films

TABLE 7-2 Clinical Signs and Laboratory Findings in the Malnourished Child and Adult*—cont'd

CLINICAL SIGN	SUSPECT NUTRIENT	SUPPORTIVE OBJECTIVE FINDINGS
Scurvy (tenderness of extremities, hemorrhages under periosteum of long bones; enlargement of costochondral junction; cessation of osteogenesis of long bones)	Vitamin C	↓ Serum ascorbic acid Long bone films
Skeletal lesions	Copper	↓ Serum copper X-ray film changes similar to scurvy since copper is also essential for normal collagen formation
Muscle wasting, prominence of body skeleton, poor muscle tone	Protein-calorie	↓ Serum proteins ↓ Arm muscle circumference
General		
Edema	Protein	↓ Serum proteins
Pallor 2° to anemia	Vitamin E (in premature infants)	↓ Serum vitamin E ↑ Peroxide hemolysis Evidence of hemolysis on blood smear
	Iron	↓ Serum Fe, ↓ TIBC
	Folic acid	↓ Serum folic acid Macrocytosis on RBC smear
	Vitamin B_{12}	↓ Serum B_{12} Macrocytosis on RBC smear
	Copper	↓ Serum copper
Internal systems		
Nervous		
Mental confusion	Protein	↓ Total protein, ↓ albumin, ↓ transferrin
	Vitamin B_1 (thiamine)	↓ RBC transketolase
Cardiovascular		
Beriberi (enlarged heart, congestive heart failure, tachycardia)	Vitamin B_1	Same as above
Tachycardia 2° to anemia	Iron Folic acid B_{12} Copper Vitamin E (in premature infants)	See above
Gastrointestinal		
Hepatomegaly	Protein-calorie	↓ Total protein, ↓ albumin, ↓ transferrin
Glandular		
Thyroid enlargement	Iodine	↓ Total serum iodine: inorganic, PBI[†]

* Fe, iron; PBI, protein-bound iodine; RBC, red blood cells; TIBC, total iron-binding capacity.
† Bio Science Laboratories, 7600 Tyrone Avenue, Van Nuys, CA 91405.
From Kerner A, ed: Manual of Pediatric Parenteral Nutrition, 1983, John Wiley and Sons, pp.22-23.

TABLE 7-3	Food and Nutrition Board, National Academy of Sciences—National Research Council Recommended Dietary Allowances,[a] Revised 1989

Designed for the maintenance of good nutrition of practically all healthy people in the United States.

		WEIGHT[b]		HEIGHT[b]			FAT-SOLUBLE VITAMINS				WATER-SOLUBLE VITAMINS		
CATEGORY	AGE (YEARS) OR CONDITION	(kg)	(lb)	(cm)	(in)	PROTEIN (g)	VITA-MIN A (µg RE)[c]	VITA-MIN D (µg)[d]	VITA-MIN E (µg α-TE)[e]	VITA-MIN K (µg)	VITA-MIN C (mg)	THIA-MIN (mg)	RIBO-FLAVIN (mg)
Infants	0.0-0.5	6	13	60	24	13	375	7.5	3	5	30	0.3	0.4
	0.5-1.0	9	20	71	28	14	375	10	4	10	35	0.4	0.5
Children	1-3	13	29	90	35	16	400	10	6	15	40	0.7	0.8
	4-6	20	44	112	44	24	500	10	7	20	45	0.9	1.1
	7-10	28	62	132	52	28	700	10	7	30	45	1.0	1.2
Males	11-14	45	99	157	62	45	1,000	10	10	45	50	1.3	1.5
	15-18	66	145	176	69	59	1,000	10	10	65	60	1.5	1.8
	19-24	72	160	177	70	58	1,000	10	10	70	60	1.5	1.7
	25-50	79	174	176	70	63	1,000	5	10	80	60	1.5	1.7
	51+	77	170	173	68	63	1,000	5	10	80	60	1.2	1.4
Females	11-14	46	101	157	62	46	800	10	8	45	50	1.1	1.3
	15-18	55	120	163	64	44	800	10	8	55	60	1.1	1.3
	19-24	58	128	164	65	46	800	10	8	60	60	1.1	1.3
	25-50	63	138	163	64	50	800	5	8	65	60	1.1	1.3
	51+	65	143	160	63	50	800	5	8	65	60	1.0	1.2
Pregnant						60	800	10	10	65	70	1.5	1.6
Lactating	1st 6 months					65	1,300	10	12	65	95	1.6	1.8
	2nd 6 months					62	1,200	10	11	65	90	1.6	1.7

From National Research Council: Recommended dietary allowances, *ed 10, Washington, DC, 1989, National Academy Press.*

[a] *The allowances, expressed as average daily intakes over time, are intended to provide for individual variations among most normal persons as they live in the United States under usual environmental stresses. Diets should be based on a variety of common foods in order to provide other nutrients for which human requirements have been less well defined.*

[b] *Weights and heights of Reference Adults are actual medians for the U.S. population of the designated age, as reported by NHANES II. The median weights and heights of those under 19 years of age were taken from Hamill et al. (1979). The use of these figures does not imply that the height-to-weight ratios are ideal.*

ANTHROPOMETRICS

Prenatal weight may give the clinician insight into the client's prenatal nutritional status. A weight-for-height assessment will help determine if the client's prenatal weight was within normal limits or outside of the normal weight range. Using prenatal weight and height values, a body mass index value can be calculated (see Fig. 7-1). Based on the client's body mass index, an appropriate weight gain goal for the pregnancy can be determined.

A weight history should be obtained and assessed. It is important to compare actual weight change to the correct body mass index graph throughout the pregnancy. Although weight gain is not linear, a constant weight increase throughout the pregnancy is optimal. Rate of weight change should be evaluated by the examiner at each prenatal visit in addition to assessment of overall weight change. A rapid weight increase or significant weight decrease indicates the need for additional evaluation by the examiner. A rapid weight increase could indicate a multiple gestation, preeclampsia, or gestational diabetes with a large infant. Poor weight gain or weight loss may indicate placental dysfunction, fetal death in utero, or poor caloric intake. Ultrasound, biophysical profile test, nonstress test, oxytocin challenge test, or amniocentesis may further as-

sist the examiner in assessing maternal and fetal health. An assessment of social resources also may be beneficial, as the client's access to food directly impacts weight changes. The presence of an erratic weight change pattern may be an indication for more in-depth evaluation of the client's clinical status.

Weight changes that are less than expected for the weeks of gestation may reflect intrauterine growth retardation of the fetus. Weight changes that are greater than expected may indicate that the fetus is large for gestational age. Aggressive nutritional intervention can positively affect both of these diagnoses if the mother is compliant with the prescribed medical nutritional therapy.

BIOCHEMICAL TESTS

The client's hematocrit and hemoglobin should be assessed to screen for iron deficiency anemia. A client is considered anemic if the hemoglobin is less than 11.0 g/dl and hematocrit is less than 33 g/dl in the first and third trimesters. Cutoff values for anemia in the second trimester are less than 10.5 g/dl hemoglobin and less than 32 g/dl hematocrit. Normal values vary slightly for smokers and people living at high altitudes.

A normal value for serum albumin is greater than or equal to 3.0 g/dl in pregnancy. Lab values below normal may reflect

WATER-SOLUBLE VITAMINS				MINERALS						
Niacin (mg NE)f	Vitamin B6 (mg)	Folate (µg)	Vitamin B12 (µg)	Calcium (mg)	Phosphorus (mg)	Magnesium (mg)	Iron (mg)	Zinc (mg)	Iodine (µg)	Selenium (µg)
5	0.3	25	0.3	400	300	40	6	5	40	10
6	0.6	35	0.5	600	500	60	10	5	50	15
9	1.0	50	0.7	800	800	80	10	10	70	20
12	1.1	75	1.0	800	800	120	10	10	90	20
13	1.4	100	1.4	800	800	170	10	10	120	30
17	1.7	150	2.0	1,200	1,200	270	12	15	150	40
20	2.0	200	2.0	1,200	1,200	400	12	15	150	50
19	2.0	200	2.0	1,200	1,200	350	10	15	150	70
19	2.0	200	2.0	800	800	350	10	15	150	70
15	2.0	200	2.0	800	800	350	10	15	150	70
15	1.4	150	2.0	1,200	1,200	280	15	12	150	45
15	1.5	180	2.0	1,200	1,200	300	15	12	150	50
15	1.6	180	2.0	1,200	1,200	280	15	12	150	55
15	1.6	180	2.0	800	800	280	15	12	150	55
13	1.6	180	2.0	800	800	280	10	12	150	55
17	2.2	400	2.2	1,200	1,200	320	30	15	175	65
20	2.1	280	2.6	1,200	1,200	355	15	19	200	75
20	2.1	260	2.6	1,200	1,200	340	15	16	200	75

c Retinol equivalents. 1 retinol equivalent = 1 µg retinol or 6 µg β-carotene.

d As cholecalciferol. 10 µg cholecalciferol = 400 IU if vitamin D.

e α-Tocopherol equivalents. 1 mg d-α tocopherol = 1 α-TE.

f 1 NE (niacin equivalent) is equal to 1 mg of niacin or 60 mg of dietary tryptophan.

protein calorie malnutrition. Causes of decreased albumin are multifactorial. Low albumin should be interpreted cautiously as a reflection of malnutrition. Fluid status may affect the accuracy of the lab value because excess fluid causes hemodilution, which lowers the albumin.

Between 24 and 28 weeks gestation, a fasting 50-g glucose tolerance test is recommended to screen for gestational diabetes. If this value is abnormal, a 3-hour glucose tolerance test may be done. Two abnormal values on this test definitively diagnose gestational diabetes.

Ketones in urinalysis testing may reflect inadequate caloric intake or diabetes. Protein in urine reflects kidney function, but may also help the examiner determine the need for protein replacement in the diet if excessive protein is lost.

Alterations in lipoprotein metabolism occur normally with pregnancy. Elevated cholesterol and triglyceride values do not require dietary intervention during pregnancy.

CLINICAL EVALUATION

The physical and clinical evaluation is an important part of the nutrition assessment. Skin tone and appearance should be noted for anything outside the normal changes associated with pregnancy. Women with edema, not associated with preeclampsia or normal lower extremity swelling, should be evaluated for adequate protein intake. Women with petechia, bruising, and scaly dry skin should be evaluated for possible vitamin deficiencies (see Table 7-2). Dental erosion and/or callused knuckles should be noted as possible signs of bulimia. Low subcutaneous fat, a cachexic appearance, excessive exercise, and amenorrhea may indicate anorexia nervosa. (See Table 7-5 for additional information.)

The physical examination should also include a complete breast assessment. Breast tenderness, enlargement, darkening of the areolas, prominent Montgomery glands, and some breast secretions are normal changes in pregnancy (Lawrence, 1994). In preparation for breast-feeding, assessment of the nipples should be done in the third trimester (preferably between 6 and 7 months of pregnancy). Prenatal breast-feeding education is essential for all pregnant women who want to breast-feed, and is especially important for women with non-protrusive nipples.

Gastrointestinal (GI) complaints of morning sickness, food aversions, heartburn, and constipation are common in pregnancy. In the first trimester, morning sickness is the most frequently reported GI-related complaint due to elevated levels of human chorionic gonadotropin hormone. The morning

Fig. 7-2 Food guide pyramid. *(Table from* Oklahoma Diet Manual, *ed 9, 1993.)*

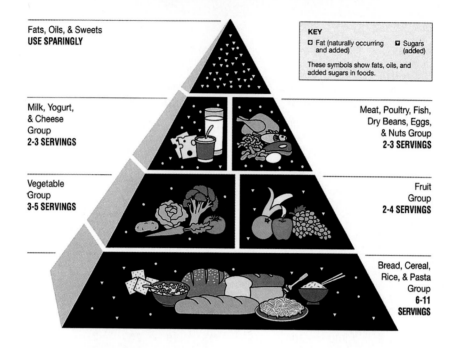

Food Group	Suggested Daily Servings	What Counts as a Serving?
Breads, cereals, and other grain products Whole-grain Enriched	**6–11** servings from entire group *(Include several servings of whole-grain products daily.)*	▪ 1 slice of bread ▪ ½ hamburger bun or english muffin ▪ a small roll, biscuit, or muffin ▪ 3 to 4 small or 2 large crackers ▪ ½ cup cooked cereal, rice, or pasta ▪ 1 ounce of ready-to-eat breakfast cereal
Fruits Citrus, melon, berries Other fruits	**2–4** servings from entire group	▪ a whole fruit such as a medium apple, banana, or orange ▪ a grapefruit half ▪ a melon wedge ▪ ¾ cup of juice ▪ ½ cup of berries ▪ ½ cup cooked or canned fruit ▪ ½ cup dried fruit
Vegetables Dark-green leafy Deep-yellow Dry beans/peas (legumes) Starchy Other vegetables	**3–5** servings from entire group *(Include all types regularly: use dark-green leafy vegetables and dry beans and peas several times a week.)*	▪ ½ cup of cooked vegetables ▪ ½ cup of chopped raw vegetables ▪ 1 cup of leafy raw vegetables, such as lettuce or spinach
Meat, poultry, fish and alternates (eggs, dry beans and peas, nuts and seeds)	**2–3** servings from entire group	Amounts should total 5 to 7 ounces of cooked lean meat, poultry, or fish a day. Count 1 egg, ½ cup cooked beans, or 2 tablespoons peanut butter as 1 ounce of meat.
Milk, cheese, and yogurt	**2** servings from entire group *(3 servings for women who are pregnant or breast-feeding and for teens; 4 servings for teens who are pregnant or breast-feeding)*	▪ 1 cup of milk ▪ 8 ounces of yogurt ▪ 1½ ounces of natural cheese ▪ 2 ounces of process cheese
Fats, sweets, and alcoholic beverages	Avoid too many fats and sweets. If you drink alcoholic beverages, do so in moderation	

TABLE 7-4   Indications for Nutrient Supplementation

REPRODUCTIVE PERIOD AND CONDITION	LOW-DOSE (30 MG) IRON*,†	60-120 MG OF IRON†,‡	LOW-DOSE MULTIVITAMIN/ MINERAL PREPARATION	600 MG OF CALCIUM
Preconception, interconception				
Iron deficiency anemia		✓	✓	
Pregnancy				
Normal	✓			
Complete vegetarian			✓	
Multiple gestation			✓	
Poor-quality diet and resistant to change			✓	
Heavy cigarette smoking			✓	
Alcohol abuse			✓	
Under age 25, consuming no calcium-rich milk products, and resistant to change			✓§	✓
Iron deficiency anemia		✓	✓	
Lactation				
Low energy intake			✓	
Low intake of milk products			✓§	✓
Iron deficiency anemia		✓	✓	

From Institutes of Medicine: Nutrition during prenancy and lactation: an implementation guide, *Washington, DC, 1993, National Academy Press.*

* Begin routine iron supplementation for all pregnant women by the 12th week of gestation.

† Iron should be taken with juice or water, apart from meals.

‡ Therapeutic doses of iron should be taken apart from other supplements.

§ The vitamin supplement is indicated to supply vitamin D. Regular exposure to sunshine reduces the need for this supplement.

sickness usually resolves by the end of the first trimester or early in the second trimester. Generally, the client's nutritional status does not suffer significantly with morning sickness. Nausea and vomiting leading to weight loss require nutritional intervention. Extreme nausea and vomiting may indicate hyperemesis gravidarum (see Table 7-5).

Food aversions often are reported throughout pregnancy. Usually, avoiding a particular food or several foods is not a problem nutritionally. If the client is avoiding an entire food group, she may be at risk for nutrient deficits. Extensive nutritional counseling may be necessary to ensure that nutritional needs are met.

Problems with constipation and heartburn generally occur in the second and third trimesters. It is important to determine how the woman is coping with these GI problems. Constipation may be secondary to a general slowing of the GI tract associated with increased progesterone with pregnancy. Additionally, the enlarging fetus may cause physical difficulties with bowel movements. Prescribed iron supplements also can be constipating. Heartburn may cause mild to severe discomfort with meals or between meals. In some cases, the pain may be so intense that the patient avoids eating in an effort to avoid heartburn. An assessment of over-the-counter antacid use is necessary. Aluminum-containing antacids should be avoided, because aluminum is contraindicated due to concerns with fetal development.

The clinical evaluation should include a discussion of possible street-drug usage. Many drugs are known teratogens.

Stimulants may affect the client's appetite and, therefore, lead to decreased nutrient intake. Barbiturates and opiates may impair the client's desire and ability to obtain food. In some cases the client's resources for food may be used to obtain drugs. Clients should be counseled and referred to a drug treatment program.

It is advisable to assess caffeinated beverage and alcohol intake as part of the diet history. Clients should be counseled to take caffeinated beverages in moderation, defined as 2 to 3 servings or fewer daily (IOM, 1993). No safe level of alcohol ingestion has been identified for pregnant women (Cerrato, 1992). It is therefore best to avoid drinking alcoholic beverages entirely while pregnant. Women with heavy drinking habits should be referred for professional intervention.

Tobacco use should be assessed. Tobacco increases the need for vitamin C, which is already increased in pregnancy. Smokers have babies with low birthweight more often than nonsmokers.

The clinical assessment should include a discussion of the client's current use of nutritional supplements and recommendations on appropriate use of supplements with pregnancy. The Committee on Nutritional Status during Pregnancy and Lactation (CNSPL), published recommendations on nutrient supplementation in *Nutrition During Pregnancy: Part II, Nutrient Supplements.* The committee consensus is that supplements should not be used to replace a well-balanced diet and nutritional counseling. Prescription of nutrient supplements should be based on evidence of benefit as well as lack of harm.

TABLE 7-5	High-Risk Nutritional Conditions

HIGH-RISK NUTRITIONAL CONDITIONS	CLINICAL AND PHYSICAL INDICATIONS
Hyperemesis gravidarum	Persistent nausea and vomiting Significant weight loss Acidosis—urine ketones, decreased serum pH Dehydration—concentrated urine, increased serum sodium
Preeclampsia	Hypertension Albuminuria Edema/Rapid weight increase Headache
Eating Disorders:	

Anorexia nervosa	Self-inflicted weight loss
	Disturbance in body image perception
	Cachectic appearance
	Cardiovascular symptoms
	  Bradycardia
	  Arrhythmias
	Fluid and electrolyte imbalances
	  Overhydration—diluted serum and urine electrolytes
	  Dehydration—concentrated serum and urine electrolytes
	Hypothermia
	Hypoglycemia
	Lanugo
	Amenorrhea

Bulimia	2 binge eating episodes per week for a 3-month period (American Psychiatric Association, 1987) Self-inflicted vomiting Laxative abuse Dehydration—concentrated serum and urine electrolytes Fluid retention/edema Dental caries/enamel erosion Hypokalemia/hypomagnesesmia
Mixed eating disorder	Combination of anorexia nervosa and bulimia
Multiple gestation	Confirmed by ultrasound Number of fetuses
Vegans (complete vegetarian)	By diet history—avoids meats, fish, dairy products, and eggs Supplement use
Pregnancy with lactation	Number of children nursing Frequency of nursing
Pregnant adolescent	Maternal age Age of menarche

The National Academy of Sciences (NAS) does not advocate routine prenatal vitamin administration (IOM, 1990).

Currently the Centers for Disease Control and Prevention (CDC) recommends that all women of childbearing age consume 400 mcg of folic acid per day to decrease the chance of neural tube defects (NTD) (Centers for Disease Control and Prevention, 1992). The CDC recommends that women should keep their total daily folate consumption under 1 mg to avoid potential risks associated with oversupplementation. Increased folate intake in pregnant women may cause problems ranging from nausea to serious neurologic damage secondary to the masking of B_{12} deficiency (Giotta, 1993). The CDC further advises that women who have had a previous NTD-related pregnancy consult a physician on folate supplementation when planning to become pregnant again (Rush, 1994). If these women are seen in the first trimester, 4 mg of folic acid per day through the first 3 months of pregnancy may be prescribed under physician supervision. After the third month, folate supplementation does not protect against NTD (IOM, 1992).

The RDA for iron during pregnancy is 30 mg/day, twice the RDA for nonpregnant women. Adequate iron intake is difficult to achieve by diet alone. To prevent iron deficiency anemia, the NAS recommends a 30-mg ferrous iron supplement daily for all pregnant women in the second and third trimester in addition to a well-balanced diet (IOM, 1990).

Women should be cautioned on the use of vitamin A supplements during pregnancy. Hypervitaminosis A can result in spontaneous abortion, fetal heart defects, abnormalities of the central nervous system, and malformation of craniofacial features (IOM, 1990).

DIETARY ASSESSMENT

The *Nutrition During Pregnancy and Lactation: an Implementation Guide* advocates the use of a nutrition questionnaire as a screening tool for dietary assessment (Fig. 7-3). Food recall for 24 hours, food frequency, food checklists, and diet records are all useful tools for obtaining nutrient intake information.

Clients should be interviewed regarding food allergies or intolerance. Development of an individualized meal pattern may be necessary to ensure nutrient needs are met if the client must avoid particular foods or food groups. Lactose intolerance is a commonly reported problem.

Cultural diversity should be taken into account with dietary assessment. An understanding of how different foods are viewed is important. Specific foods may be considered healthful or harmful during pregnancy and lactation by some cultures. The state health department or state Women, Infant and Children (WIC) office may provide useful information on local ethnic dietary practices.

Dietary assessment should also include questions regarding ingestion of nonnutritive substances or pica. Clay, starch, baking soda, and dirt are some of the items women "crave" during pregnancy. An assessment of what, how much, and how often these items are ingested is important to determine potential harmful effects.

Nondietary factors may affect a woman's ability to obtain adequate nutrition. A complete dietary assessment includes review of the client's socioeconomic status and access to re-

NUTRITION QUESTIONNAIRE

What you eat and some of the lifestyle choices you make can affect your nutrition and health now and in the future. Your nutrition can also have an important effect on your baby's health. Please answer these questions by circling the answers that apply to you.

Eating Behavior

1. Are you frequently bothered by any of the following? (Circle all that apply):

   Nausea   Vomiting   Heartburn   Constipation

2. Do you skip meals at least 3 times a week?   No   Yes

3. Do you try to limit the amount or kind of food you eat to control your weight?   No   Yes

4. Are you on a special diet now?   No   Yes

5. Do you avoid any foods for health or religious reasons?   No   Yes

Food Resources

6. Do you have a working stove?   No   Yes
   Do you have a working refrigerator?   No   Yes

7. Do you sometimes run out of food before you are able to buy more?   No   Yes

8. Can you afford to eat the way you should?   No   Yes

9. Are you receiving any food assistance now? (Circle all that apply):   No   Yes

   Food stamps   School breakfast   School lunch
   WIC   Donated food/commodities   CSFP
   Food from a food pantry, soup kitchen, or food bank

10. Do you feel you need help in obtaining food?   No   Yes

Food and Drink

11. Which of these did you drink yesterday? (Circle all that apply):

    Soft drinks   Coffee   Tea
    Fruit drink   Orange juice   Grapefruit juice
    Other juices   Milk   Kool-Aid
    Beer   Wine   Alcoholic drinks
    Water   Other beverages (list)_____

12. Which of these foods did you eat yesterday? (Circle all that apply):

    Cheese   Pizza   Macaroni and cheese
    Yogurt   Cereal with milk
    Other foods made with cheese (such as tacos, enchiladas, lasagna, cheeseburgers)

    Corn   Potatoes   Sweet potatoes
    Green salad   Carrots   Collard greens
    Spinach   Turnip greens   Broccoli
    Green beans   Green peas   Other vegetables
    Apples   Bananas   Berries
    Grapefruit   Melon   Oranges
    Peaches   Other fruit

    Meat   Fish   Chicken
    Eggs   Peanut butter   Nuts
    Seeds   Dried beans

    Cold cuts   Hot dog   Bacon
    Sausage   Cake   Cookies
    Doughnut   Pastry   Chips
    French fries
    Other deep-fried foods, such as fried chicken or egg rolls

    Bread   Rolls   Rice
    Cereal   Noodles   Spaghetti
    Tortillas
    Were any of these whole grain?   No   Yes

13. Is the way you ate yesterday the way you usually eat?   No   Yes

Lifestyle

14. Do you exercise for at least 30 minutes on a regular basis (3 times a week or more)?   No   Yes

15. Do you ever smoke cigarettes or use smokeless tobacco?   No   Yes

16. Do you ever drink beer, wine, liquor, or any other alcoholic beverages?   No   Yes

17. Which of these do you take? (Circle all that apply):

    Prescribed drugs or medications

    Any over-the-counter products (such as aspirin, Tylenol, antacids, or vitamins)

    Street drugs (such as marijuana, speed, downers, crack, or heroin)

---

sources. The nutrition questionnaire may include questions to help determine need for intervention and referral to food assistance programs, income support programs, or both.

POSTPARTUM AND LACTATING WOMEN

Women who choose to formula-feed their infants should continue to maintain healthy eating habits in the postpartum period. The mother's diet is important for her health maintenance and provision of the infant's nutrient needs. For nursing mothers, nutrient needs are actually greater with lactation than with pregnancy (see Table 7-4 and dietary section on p. 106).

ANTHROPOMETRICS

Assessment of weight change in the lactating woman is important. An expected weight loss of 0.6 to 0.8 kg/month may occur in the first 4 to 6 months of lactation. Weight loss may occur at a slower rate for the following 6 to 12 months (IOM, 1991; Dewey, 1993). Some women do not lose weight with lactation. Rapid weight loss is not advisable.

BIOCHEMICAL TESTS

Nutritional screening by normal biochemical standards is inaccurate because of a lack of reference standards for lactation.

CLINICAL EVALUATION

Screening criteria for nutrient deficiency in the lactating population are not available. See adult section for general assessment information. Care should be taken to document over-the-counter drug use, street-drug use, and caffeine and tobacco use since many substances are transmitted to the infant via the breast milk.

DIETARY ASSESSMENT

Collection of nutrient intake information should be done and analyzed for adequacy. The RDAs for lactating women are 2700 kcal/day or an additional 500 kcal/day (see Table 7-4). An additional 15 g of protein per day is recommended for the first 6 months of lactation, then 12 g/day after 6 months (see Table 7-4). Nutrients likely to be suboptimal in women consuming less than 2700 kcal/day are calcium, zinc, magnesium, B$_6$, folate, E, and thiamin (IOM 1991). Fluid intake should be assessed. Women are encouraged to drink to satisfy thirst. Generally 2 quarts/day is adequate.

Many mothers verbalize food myths and taboos regarding proper diet while breast-feeding. No foods should be routinely eliminated from the diet while lactating. If the mother suspects a certain food bothers her infant, she may consider eliminating it from her diet and trying it again later.

Socioeconomic resources should be evaluated to determine if the woman has adequate access to food. Referral to assistance programs may be necessary.

Assessment Alert

Age <17 years
Economic deprivation
Eating disorders/unsound dietary practices/vegetarians
On special diet for systemic disease
Heavy smoker
Multiple gestation
Weight <85% suggested for height
Rapid weight loss
Poor weight gain with pregnancy resulting in LBW infant
Pregnant while lactating (IOM, 1991)

LBW, low birthweight.

NEONATES AND INFANTS (UP TO 12 MONTHS)

The nutritional status of the neonate, whether preterm or full term, is determined by multiple, cumulative health, hereditary, and dietary factors. Consistent clinical examinations throughout infancy and childhood will promote optimal growth and development of the individual. Whether the clinical setting is the hospital, home, or outpatient facility, the basic "ABCD" methodology of nutritional assessment easily can be adapted and utilized (Barkauskas et al, 1994).

ANTHROPOMETRICS

Weight, length, and circumference.   Within moments after birth, the most common initial anthropometric measurements include body weight, height (length), and circumference of head (frontal occipital circumference, or FOC) and chest. The measurements obtained not only provide baseline parameters of the newborn's nutritional status at birth, but also reflect overall intrauterine growth and development. The importance of accurate metric measuring tools, such as scales, right-angle length boards (Nichols, 1992), and nonstretchable cloth or fiberglass tapes, as well as competent clinical assessment of gestational age, cannot be overemphasized (see Chapter 6).

AGA/LGA/SGA: definition of terms.   Infants having birth measurements that fall between the 5th and 95th percentile of the intrauterine growth chart may be considered as having appropriate growth for gestational age (AGA).

Large-for-gestational-age (LGA) infants will exhibit macrosomia with growth parameters greater than the 95th percentile, and these infants should be closely monitored during the first 24 hours for hypoglycemia. (Carlson, 1993; Wong, 1993). Hypoglycemia is a plasma glucose level of less than 90 mg/dl in all newborns less than 24 hours of age (Cornblath and Schwartz, 1993). Further discussion of clinical manifestations of hypoglycemia will follow in the clinical assessment.

Small for gestational age (SGA) refers to those infants born weighing less than the 5th percentile on the intrauterine growth charts (Carlson, 1993; Metcoff, 1994). If length and FOC are appropriate, the infant has asymmetric growth, and the weight deficit may be attributed to a short-term deficiency of nutrients in utero secondary to maternal preeclampsia, hypertension, or other disease states (see the discussion of maternal assessment). When all growth parameters are less than the 5th percentile, the infant manifests symmetric growth retardation and reflects a long-term lack of adequate intrauterine nutrition as seen with maternal substance abuse or congenital infections or abnormalities.

Frequency of measurements.   The "well baby" may be nutritionally assessed at 2 to 4 weeks, bimonthly until 6 months, at 9 months, and 1 year postnatally according to American Academy of Pediatrics (AAP) recommendations (Unti, 1994). After the initial expected weight loss (5% to 10%) in the first week of life because of shifts in body water, growth parameters over time are important to monitor. Incremental growth of preterm infants should approximate 15 to 20 g/day (intrauterine rate), and should be plotted against corrected gestational postnatal age.

Skinfold determinations.   Although skinfold measurements are not currently recommended for routine nutritional assessment, they may clarify the status of infants and children above or below the 90th and 10th percentiles of weight for stature, respectively.

Circumferences/lengths.   In the first year of life, monthly measurements of head circumference (FOC), mid-arm circumference (MAC), and length can provide pertinent information about the infant's nutritional status (Georgieff and Sasanow, 1986). An increased FOC-to-MAC ratio may be indicative of head sparing in nutritional deprivation. Because of the direct correlation between brain growth and FOC, it is important to measure the head circumference of infants and young children routinely until the age of 36 months (Barkauskas, 1994).

If developmental delay or neurologic problems such as microcephaly or hydrocephalus are suspected, an FOC measurement may provide important information at any age (Barkauskas, 1994).

BIOCHEMICAL TESTS

Although serum and urine indices for nutritional status are not routinely evaluated in the well newborn, or during the first year of life, the examiner should make use of the most common biochemical tests if an abnormality is suspected. The following laboratory measurements summarize the most common nutrient levels to evaluate and the rationale for their evaluation (Barkauskas, 1994).

CLINICAL EVALUATION

After the neonates have adjusted to extrauterine existence, their initial physical examination reflects prenatal as well as immediate postnatal nutritional status. As anthropometric measurements are being evaluated, skin color; turgor; texture; and presence of bruising, edema, or rashes should be noted. Maternal history of disease states such as poor or excessive weight gain, diabetes, preeclampsia, or hypertension may substantiate clinical findings of poor growth, presence of neonatal disease, or abnormal serum glucose or other electrolytes. Physical activity may be indicative of a transient imbalance of serum glucose, calcium, or magnesium, causing symptoms of lethargy or jitteriness, depending on the electrolyte abnormality.

The infant's neurologic integrity may be ascertained by suck, swallow, and rooting behaviors and may determine the infant's ability to successfully nurse, whether by breast or bottle. Other important physical assessments that may influence immediate nutritional status include the presence of active bowel sounds in all quadrants with a soft, nondistended abdomen. Passage of meconium and time of first voiding should be documented. Frequency, amount, color, and consistency of subsequent stools should be evaluated, especially in the first 24 to 48 hours of life. Urine output during the first 24 to 48 hours should be measured for low birthweight infants (less than 2000 g) and estimated per diaper change in the

TABLE 7-6	Common Biochemical Measurements to Assess Nutritional Status	
AGE OF INFANT	**BIOCHEMICAL MEASUREMENT**	**RATIONALE**
All neonates before hospital discharge	PKU, Galactose, T4, TSH	Law requires identification of inborn errors of metabolism
Preterm, septic, asphyxiated, or total parenteral nutrition (TPN)–dependent neonates	Serum chemistries*	Immature renal function with labile sodium/fluid balance At risk for electrolyte imbalances
Newborn birthweight ≤2000 g; SGA, LGA, or IODM	Serum glucose	At risk for hypoglycemia or hyperglycemia
Newborn to 12 months, especially after age 3 months	Hemoglobin and hematocrit	At risk for anemia, especially if twin gestation, preterm or low birthweight, maternal blood loss, poor iron intake, use of sulfa antibiotics (Roberts, 1984)
Infants and toddler	Albumin Prealbumin Retinol binding protein Serum transferrin	Labs may be indicative of visceral protein stores combined with physical assessment for malnutrition
All ages	Urinalysis	Initial screen for suspected protein or sugar spilling into urine
	24-hour urea nitrogen[†]	Evaluate degree of nitrogen balance (Barkauskas, 1994)

* Initial electrolyte screens include serum glucose, sodium, chloride, potassium, carbon dioxide, and blood urea nitrogen.

[†] Nitrogen balance = dietary protein/6.25 − (urinary urea nitrogen + 4)

larger newborn with at least 6 to 8 wet diapers per 24 hours (Breastfeeding Task Force, St. Louis Model, 1991).

DIETARY ASSESSMENT

During the first year of life, a comprehensive diet history of the infant's feeding habits, types of and tolerance to foods and formula, and an estimate of amounts consumed will give valuable information to the examiner in addition to the anthropometric examination. Assessment of adequate health and growth will be made, as previously described, by a complete physical examination and growth measurements. A common feeding problem observed is formula intolerance with symptoms of constipation, diarrhea, emesis, dermatitis, and even respiratory distress. Suck/swallow coordination and bottle or breast-feeding technique and frequency are especially critical during the first 24 to 72 hours of life. With current trends of early hospital discharge, the home health care nurse may be responsible for giving the initial support and feeding instructions to the new mother. Unsuccessful breast-feeding or incorrectly mixed infant formulas are examples of feeding problems that may be avoided with knowledgeable and timely follow-up of mothers in the initial postpartum period. The support, encouragement, and nutritional information a new mother receives may positively affect the success or failure of her ability to nurture and nourish her baby for months and even years. Early identification and interventions of all feeding problems will prevent weight loss and assume optimal growth and development during the first year.

TODDLER TO PRESCHOOL (12 TO 36 MONTHS)

ANTHROPOMETRICS

The rapid growth that has been monitored monthly during the first year typically slows down during the toddler years. Weight-for-age still remains the most reliable indicator of growth, but weight-for-height indices such as body mass index (BMI) may be important indicators of body fat after the first year (Barkauskas et al, 1994).

$$BMI = \frac{Wt\ (kg)}{Ht\ (m)^2}$$

In malnourished edematous children, however, the triceps skinfold (described in section on Infants) and mid-arm circumference (MAC) provide a more reliable indicator of nutritional status than height for weight (Peterson, 1993).

The identification and management of the malnourished or failure-to-thrive (FTT) child is a high priority in this age group, as children are being weaned from the breast or bottle. During this transition from infancy to childhood, the potential for FTT or undernutrition is defined as less than the 5th percentile of the NCHS growth in age and weight for height (Peterson, 1993). Inadequate intake of nutrients such as calcium, iron, and vitamins A and C is common and physical assessment for acute weight loss is especially important.

BIOCHEMICAL TESTS

During the life cycle of toddlerhood (12 to 36 months), iron deficiency is the most common cause of anemia as determined most typically by serum hemoglobin and hematocrit. Reference ranges for this age for hemoglobin and hematocrit are 11 g/100 ml and 33%, respectively (Pipes and Trahms, 1993).

Development of Iron Deficiency Anemia

Decreased iron intake

↓

Plasma ferritin

↓

Iron deficient normocytic red blood cells (RBCs) with decreased transferrin saturation (<15%)

↓

Iron deficiency anemia
(Microcytic and hypochromic RBCs with hemoglobin <11 g/dl and hematocrit <33%)

Modified from Pipes and Trahms.

If FTT is suspected, a comprehensive laboratory screen may include hemoglobin and hematocrit, total protein, albumin, and a liver enzyme profile, in addition to a complete health and social history and clinical examination (Peterson, 1993).

CLINICAL EVALUATION

Evaluation of the toddler's physical health status includes assessment of skin for color, rashes, turgor, muscle tone, and presence of subcutaneous fat, in addition to examination of mouth, gums, and teeth for bleeding and dental caries. "Baby-bottle tooth decay" or dental caries of primary teeth can result from intake of carbohydrate-containing beverages such as juice or milk before nap or bedtime. During sleep, the sweet liquid ferments, providing energy for plaque-forming bacteria.

Neuromuscular coordination and developmentally appropriate behaviors should be assessed. Any delays or abnormal oral or neuromotor patterns should be referred to a pediatrician.

Overall activity level and appetite should be evaluated, with food likes and dislikes noted. During the physical examination, a thorough history of illness (frequency and duration), especially nausea and vomiting or elimination problems such as diarrhea or constipation, should be made as well as any history of acute or recurring infections. Signs of abuse and neglect should be documented, especially if associated with FTT as defined earlier.

Evidence of parental ability to care and nourish the toddler child is essential, and the examiner should observe evidence of eye and physical contact between parent and child with mutual exchange and understanding of nonverbal communication. Family and social history may be significant if abnormal growth of a toddler is observed, especially if seen with poor or excessive weight gain for length or age.

DIETARY ASSESSMENT

As infants grow into upright toddlers, not only do they discover the limitless boundaries of the physical world about them, but they also experience the new tastes, textures, and smells of solid foods. Although many new foods such as pureed cereals, teething cookies, fruits, and vegetables may have been introduced in the latter half of the first year, the main source of food should still be the milk component to ensure adequate calcium and protein intakes.

Although a 3- to 7-day diet history provides the most reliable method of ensuring nutrient intake, a 24-hour diet recall will provide the examiner with sufficient information to approximate adequacy of nutrient intake. Assessment of the information may be completed by hand or by computer calculations, then compared to the Recommended Dietary Allowances for the specific age as seen on Table 7-3 (Pipes and Trahms, 1993).

PRESCHOOL AND SCHOOL-AGE CHILDREN (36 MONTHS TO 12 YEARS)

The preschool and school-age period is typically characterized by a slowing in the child's growth rate. The child should, however, continue to grow approximately 4½ to 8½ lbs (2 to 4 kg)/year until adolescence. Anticipated height change is 2⅜ to 3 inches (6 to 8 cm)/year at age 4 and decreases to 2 to 2⅜ inches (5 to 6 cm)/year around age 6 years (Chumlea, 1993).

ANTHROPOMETRICS

An evaluation of body growth is determined by height (stature) and weight measurements. Stature is a reflection of linear growth of the bone or skeleton. Weight is a measurement of muscle, adipose tissue, and bone. The measured values are plotted in National Center for Health Statistics (NCHS) growth grids (see Fig. 6-15). These values are compared to those of other American children at the same age. Plotted values should be used cautiously when determining nutrition risk. Children who fall at less than the 5th percentile or greater than the 95th percentile of weight for age should be further evaluated. (Ethnic group differences are not accounted for on current NCHS growth grids.) Weight for stature may be a useful indicator of nutritional status for a particular child.

A weight-for-stature index can be calculated to further evaluate nutritional status. It is calculated by dividing the 50th percentile weight-for-length value (from the NCHS growth grids in Chapter 6) by the child's actual weight. An index value of 1.1, or 110%, reflects an overweight or obese individual. An evaluation for protein energy malnutrition (PEM) is recommended for children with an index below 0.9, or 90% (Krug-Wispe, 1993).

Other anthropometric measurement tools include skinfold thickness measurements and upper arm measurements. Skinfold measurements are not usually included in a nutrition screening. The measurement indicates percent body fat and is most useful in long-term assessment. The mid-arm anthropometric data are used to assess lean mass and body fat stores.

BIOCHEMICAL TESTS

Routine biochemical evaluation is usually not necessary for nutritional assessment of healthy children. Hemoglobin and hematocrit may be used as a screening tool to assess iron status. Serum proteins, such as albumin and prealbumin, are helpful in diagnosing nutritional depletion.

Children who are considered at risk for developing premature cardiovascular disease should have their blood cholesterol measured as part of their nutritional assessment. If values are elevated, the child and family should be referred for diet counseling according to National Cholesterol Education Program (NCEP) guidelines (U.S. Department of Health and Human Services, 1991).

CLINICAL EVALUATION

Nutritional assessment of the preschool or school-age child should include a complete clinical and physical assessment. Skin should be examined for signs of appropriate hydration. Note dry, scaling skin and pigmentation for possible indications of nutrient deficiencies (see Table 7-2).

A clinical review of the child's hair is important. Easily plucked, lackluster hair may indicate protein calorie deficit. Fingernails should be examined. Thin, spoon-shaped nails may indicate iron deficiency. Additional hematologic tests are necessary to confirm the iron-deficient state.

The child's oral cavity should be reviewed for dentition. If the child has a history of baby-bottle tooth decay, dental caries, missing teeth, or evidence of gum inflammation, the effect on oral intake should be noted with the diet history and assessment. Abnormal oral cavity findings may indicate vitamin deficiencies (see Table 7-2).

DIETARY ASSESSMENT

Several methods exist for determining nutritional needs in a child of this age. The RDAs provide a guideline for estimating nutrient needs in healthy children (see Table 7-3). Energy estimation is based on a reference weight for each age group in the RDA. Calories per centimeter of height can also be used to assess and estimate energy needs (Table 7-7). A rule of thumb for estimating kcal needs is 1000 kcal for the first year and 100 kcal/year up to age 12. Physical activity level should be assessed. Adjustments in energy and nutrient needs may be necessary for varying activity levels in individual children.

The child's diet should also be compared to NCEP recommendations. The NCEP guidelines for children over 2 years of age are the same as for the general population, a low–saturated fat, low-cholesterol diet (U.S. Department of Health and Human Services, 1991).

Cultural influence on food selection and intake should be reviewed for the effect it may have on adequate nutritional intake. If counseling is necessary, care should be taken to respect cultural beliefs whenever possible while still promoting optimal nutrition.

TABLE 7-7	Energy Intake per Centimeter of Height*				
	MALES (PERCENTILES)			**FEMALES (PERCENTILES)**		
AGE	**10TH**	**50TH**	**90TH**	**10TH**	**50TH**	**90TH**
1	10.3	14.1	18.8	10.6	13.6	17.6
2-3	11.6	15.0	20.2	10.5	13.5	17.9
4-6	12.3	15.2	20.4	10.7	13.8	18.6
7-10	12.8	16.7	22.3	10.4	14.1	18.4
11-14	12.4	16.8	22.2	9.0	13.0	18.2
15-16	11.4	15.9	21.1	7.4	11.8	17.3

From Lucas B: Normal nutrition from infancy through adolescence. In Queen PM, Lang CE, editors: Handbook of pediatric nutrition, Gaithersburg, Maryland, 1993, Aspen Publishers, Inc.

* These energy intakes are means of the age groups listed. The data were collected on normal, healthy children involved in a prospective study.

An assessment of eating behavior and patterns should be done. Parents of preschool age children often report finicky eating behavior or "food jags." Reduced intake may be related to a decline in growth rate. Satter states, "Appropriate eating behavior for a preschooler is sitting at the table with the rest of the family, being pleasant, and being able to handle utensils reasonably well" (Satter, 1987).

School-age children may tend to eat less frequently. The habit of skipping breakfast may begin in this age group (Lucas, 1993). Children in this age group are developing a sense of autonomy, but Satter emphasizes the importance of maintaining division of responsibility at mealtime between parent and child: the parent decides what food is served, the child decides how much to eat (Satter, 1987).

Assessment Alert

Obesity
Failure to thrive
Vegetarian children
Multiple food allergies
Parent with eating disorder

While assessing eating behaviors, be mindful of the influences of family, media, and peers on food intake. It is not too early to explore body-image issues and food behaviors in the school-age child if restrictive or eating disorder–type behavior is suspected.

Finally, a socioeconomic assessment should be done if concerns about family resources are suspected to affect nutritional adequacy.

ADOLESCENTS

Adolescence is defined as starting before puberty and ending with growth and sexual maturation. Generally, girls are thought to have completed growth by age 16 and boys by age 18 (Chumlea, 1993).

ANTHROPOMETRICS

Anthropometric assessment of the adolescent is similar to that for the preschool and school-age child (see previous section for details). Adolescence is a time of rapid growth. If the adolescent's growth is outside the expected growth channel, closer follow-up may be warranted to track growth pattern and provide nutrition intervention to maintain optimal growth.

The Expert Committee on Clinical Guidelines for Overweight in Adolescent Preventive Services recommends that individuals with a BMI (kg/m^2 greater than 30, or 95% for age and sex), be referred for medical treatment (Himes, 1994). Youths with BMIs of 30 or greater than 85% but less than 95% for age should be considered at risk for obesity and should be screened.

BIOCHEMICAL TESTS

As with preschool and school-age children, routine biochemical evaluations are not necessary in healthy adolescents. (See previous section for information on common biochemical tests for nutritional screening.)

The menstruating female is at increased risk for iron-deficiency anemia. If signs and symptoms of anemia are present, a hemoglobin and hematocrit should be drawn. Since adolescence is a time of rapid growth, increased risk of nutrient deficiencies occurs. If the clinical assessment indicates the need for more in-depth assessment, more biochemical tests may be necessary (see Table 7-6).

CLINICAL EVALUATION

A complete clinical and physical assessment of skin, hair, nails, and oral cavity should be done as part of the nutrition assessment of the adolescent (see previous section for details.)

Girls generally reach puberty 2 years before boys. (See Tanner Stages in Tables 18-2 and 19-1.) During maximum height velocity, girls may grow 3 to 3½ inches (8.4 to 9.0 cm)/yr, whereas boys grow 3.7 to 4 inches (9.5 to 10.3 cm)/yr (Chumlea, 1993). Changes in body composition are also seen in adolescence.

Questions relating to menstrual history are important for assessing the female adolescent. If the adolescent is pregnant, referral for intensive nutritional counseling is necessary. Tanner stage at time of pregnancy influences nutritional needs and should be part of the assessment.

Obesity can be diagnosed by anthropometrics and confirmed by physical examination. Obese adolescents or those at risk for obesity should be referred for medical intervention (Himes, 1994). Additionally, further biochemical assessment may be indicated for cholesterol screening.

Some high school students are on a restrictive diet, suffer from bulimia, or both. Physical appearance; decreased weight/height; reported excessive exercise; food rituals and patterns; amenorrhea; and reported dread of being fat, help the examiner identify anorexia nervosa. Episodes of binging and purging large amounts of food, use of laxatives and diuretics, dieting and exercise patterns, and erratic weight change assist in diagnosing bulimia. Dental caries and tooth enamel decay may be caused by prolonged vomiting (Barkauskas, 1994). The consequences of continued eating disorder behavior can be severe, and these patients should be referred to a specialized multidisciplinary team for treatment. (See Assessment Alert box, p. 106, for assessment information.)

Assessment of alcohol and substance use should be made. Use of tobacco products should be noted.

DIETARY ASSESSMENT

Collection of diet intake information should be accomplished by previously mentioned methods. Methods of determining nutritional needs in adolescents are similar to methods of determining childhood needs. RDAs are separated by sex at age 11 years (see Table 7-3). Adolescents are at greatest risk for inadequate intake of calcium, iron, zinc, and vitamin D during growth spurts. Comparison to recommendations for NCEP guidelines should also be done. Refer to p. 99 for guidelines.

In assessing dietary behavior, it is important to be aware that adolescents are striving to attain autonomy and identity (Satter, 1987). Eating patterns often reflect these themes. Meal skipping is seen more frequently in this age group than any other (Lucas, 1993). Snacking and eating at fast-food restaurants are common dietary behaviors. Cultural food choices and socioeconomic resources should also be assessed, as mentioned in the previous section.

Assessment Alert

Eating disorders (see Table 7-5)
Obesity
Vegetarian
Pregnant adolescent

OLDER ADULTS

Older adults are frequently defined as those adults over 60 years of age. The elderly are at increased risk for developing malnutrition due to a combination of physical and social factors. Physically, older adults require fewer calories, have decreased taste sensation, and decreased absorption from the GI tract. Socially, many older adults live alone and have limited access to foods (Valassi, 1992).

Early identification of possible nutrition problems can help prevent malnutrition in this group. Two important factors to monitor are changes in serum albumin and activities of daily living (Baden, 1993).

ANTHROPOMETRICS

Evaluation of the geriatric client's weight is similar to that of the adult, but desirable body weight is slightly increased in the geriatric population. The geriatric tables for approximate weight and height are presented in Table 7-8. Calculating the client's percentage of desirable body weight and comparing the result to the ranges on p. 93 is useful in this population as well. As previously mentioned, clients who vary the greatest from the norm are at the greatest risk for nutrition-related problems.

Recent weight history is helpful in many age groups, but can be especially indicative of nutritional status in the elderly. Reports of a slow, gradual weight loss may indicate chronic undernutrition. The client's social situation may have changed, limiting his or her access to or desire for food. A rapid decrease of body weight can indicate either a change in the client's social situation or the presence of illness. To evaluate the significance of recent weight changes, calculate the client's percent of usual body weight using the formula below:

$$\frac{\text{Current body weight}}{\text{Usual body weight}} \times 100 = \% \text{ UBW}$$

TABLE 7-8 Average Height/Weight Table for Persons Aged 65 Years and Older

MEN

HEIGHT (IN)	AGES 65-69	AGES 70-74	AGES 75-79	AGES 80-84	AGES 85-89	AGES 90-94
61	128-156	125-153	123-151			
62	130-158	127-155	125-153	122-148		
63	131-161	129-157	127-155	122-150	120-146	
64	134-164	131-161	129-157	124-152	122-148	
65	136-166	134-164	130-160	127-155	125-153	117-143
66	139-169	137-167	133-163	130-158	128-156	120-146
67	140-172	140-170	136-166	132-162	130-160	122-150
68	143-175	142-174	139-169	135-165	133-163	126-154
69	147-179	146-178	142-174	139-169	137-167	130-158
70	150-184	148-182	146-178	143-175	140-172	134-164
71	155-189	152-186	149-183	148-180	144-176	139-169
72	159-195	156-190	154-188	153-187	148-182	
73	164-200	160-196	158-192			

WOMEN

HEIGHT (IN)	AGES 65-69	AGES 70-74	AGES 75-79	AGES 80-84	AGES 85-89	AGES 90-94
58	120-146	112-138	111-135			
59	121-147	114-140	112-136	100-122	99-121	
60	122-148	116-142	113-139	106-130	102-124	
61	123-151	118-144	115-144	109-133	104-128	
62	125-153	121-147	118-144	112-136	108-132	107-131
63	127-155	123-151	121-147	115-141	112-136	107-131
64	130-158	126-154	123-151	119-145	115-141	108-132
65	132-162	130-158	126-154	122-150	120-146	112-136
66	136-166	132-162	128-157	126-154	124-152	116-142
67	140-170	136-166	131-161	130-158	128-156	
68	143-175	140-170				
69	148-180	144-176				

From Journal of the American Medical Association *172:658, 1960.*

% UBW values can be interpreted using the following % change ranges:

TIME	SIGNIFICANT WEIGHT LOSS %	SEVERE WEIGHT LOSS %
1 week	1-2	>2
1 month	5	>5
3 months	7.5	>7.5
6 months	10	>10

(Blackburn, 1977)

Clients with significant or severe weight loss should be referred to the appropriate dietitian or physician for evaluation and treatment of malnutrition.

BIOCHEMICAL TESTS

As in adults, serum albumin is an important indicator of protein status in the elderly. In fact, the ASPEN guidelines suggest that serum albumin and activities of daily living are the most important indicators for nutrition status of the geriatric client (Baden, 1993). One study demonstrated that low serum albumin levels predicted increased risk for medical complications in a rehabilitation program (Glenn, 1985).

The degree of depletion with low serum albumin is often categorized as follows:

Mild	2.8-3.5 g/dl
Moderate	2.1-2.7 g/dl
Severe	<2.1 g/dl

(Grant, 1985)

Routine screening of serum glucose, hemoglobin, and hematocrit, as discussed on pp. 95-96, is also recommended in the elderly. One laboratory value of possible decreased significance in older adults is total cholesterol. A recent study found that elevated serum cholesterol in clients over 70 years of age, with no other risk factors for cardiovascular disease (CVD), does not increase risk for cardiovascular events (Krumholz, 1994). It is important to note that the presence of other risk factors, such as a previous myocardial infarction (MI) or stroke or a positive family history of CVD or diabetes, in conjunction with an elevated cholesterol level does increase the client's risk, and the client should therefore be referred to the appropriate health professional for treatment.

CLINICAL EVALUATION

The clinical assessment of the elderly client should include all the evaluations of the adult client with some additional considerations. All geriatric patients should be evaluated for obvious signs of muscle wasting and malnutrition (see section on clinical evaluation of the adult, pp. 96-97). Special attention should be given to the examination of the oral cavity and skin quality. The elderly often have a decreased sense of taste and smell, accompanied by a loss of teeth (Burke, 1992). The result is decreased food and fluid intake, which can lead to malnutrition and dehydration.

Dehydration is the most common fluid and electrolyte disorder among the elderly and is responsible for a large number of hospitalizations in this population (Weinberg, 1994; Burke, 1992). Warm, dry skin and dry oral mucosa are indications of dehydration. Other indications include decreased urinary output, confusion, and elevations in serum, sodium, hematocrit, and blood urea nitrogen (BUN) (Valassi, 1992).

Older adults frequently have difficulties chewing or swallowing. Many elderly clients have dentures, missing teeth, or periodontal disease. During a clinical evaluation, the nurse should examine the oral cavity and ask the client about chewing problems. Ill-fitting dentures and missing teeth will decrease the client's ability to chew meats and fresh fruits and vegetables. Observing the client while he or she eats can aid in determining swallowing ability. The examiner should notice any choking or coughing with eating. Clients with swallowing difficulties frequently have more problems swallowing thin liquids such as water than thicker liquids such as pudding or milkshakes.

Potential food and drug interactions should be evaluated during a nutritional clinical assessment of the elderly patient. Older adults take more prescription medications than any other age group (Valassi, 1992). Assessment of common over-the-counter medications is also important. Older adults frequently take vitamin or mineral supplements or protein/amino acid supplements. Some foods decrease the absorption of various medications, as dairy products do with tetracycline. Some medications have negative effects on nutritional status by decreasing appetite or increasing excretion of nutrients. Table 7-9 lists common drugs taken by the elderly and possible nutritional deficiencies that may develop.

Past medical history may also affect the elderly client's nutrition status today. History of a cerebral vascular accident (CVA) with hemiparesis or dysphagia may decrease the client's ability to take in food. Decreased ability to ambulate may limit the client's ability to obtain and prepare food. A history of diabetes, renal insufficiency, or cardiovascular disease may require special diet modifications. All of these factors should be considered when evaluating the client's needs.

DIETARY ASSESSMENT

A dietary assessment should begin with an evaluation of the client's food habits. Again, a combination of a 24-hour recall and food frequency questionnaire is an effective approach. The client's food habits can then be compared to the RDAs by analyzing the 24-hour recall (see p. 93). The RDAs for the elderly are similar to those for the adult. The largest difference is a decreased energy requirement as age increases (Valassi, 1992). As total calorie needs decrease but other nutrient needs plateau, elderly clients need to make wise, nutrient-dense food choices.

When analyzing an elderly client's diet, several nutrients are of particular concern. Diets of older adults are frequently inadequate in calcium and iron (Valassi, 1992). Vitamins that tend to be underconsumed include thiamin, riboflavin, and pyridoxine (Valassi, 1992). If the client is lactose-intolerant, as many older adults are, a calcium supplement may be necessary. Several recent studies indicate that older adults consume adequate amounts of zinc and vitamin A, two nutrients previously thought to be deficient in the elderly diet (Swanson, 1988; Garry, 1987).

TABLE 7-9	Nutritional Deficiences Caused by Common Drugs Taken by the Elderly

DRUG AND DRUG GROUP	DEFICIENCY
Cardiac glycosides Digitalis	Anorexia→ protein energy malnutrition Zinc and magnesium deficiency

Diuretics
  Thiazides→
  Furosemide
  Ethacrynic acid
  Triamterene→
	Potassium, zinc, and magnesium depletion
	
	Folacin deficiency

Antiinflammatory drugs
  Aspirin
  Indomethacin→
 	
  Colchicine→
	GI blood loss→ iron deficiency
	Malabsorption of fat-soluble and water-soluble vitamins

Antacids (antacid abuse)	Phosphate depletion; osteomalacia
Laxatives (laxative abuse) Mineral oil→	Deficiency of vitamins A, D, and K Phenollphthalein (potassium deficiency) Multiple nutrient deficiencies due to malabsorption Folacin and vitamin D deficiency

Modified from Roe D: Geriatric nutrition, *ed 2, Englewood Cliffs, NJ, 1987, Prentice-Hall.*

Many social and economic factors affect the dietary habits of older adults. Several studies indicate social isolation, loneliness, and living alone are significant factors that decrease the quality of the elderly person's food intake. For instance, elderly persons who had reported loneliness previously and then experienced increased social interactions had increased nutrient intakes (Walker, 1991). Likewise, elderly participants in congregate meal programs were less likely to skip meals than elderly clients with meals delivered to their homes (Frongillo, 1992). Apparently, elderly men 75 years of age or older are at the greatest risk of consuming poor quality diets. Conversely, elderly women living alone did not have decreased dietary adequacy (Davis, 1990). The most important variable associated with decreased dietary adequacy and living alone was energy intake. Elderly persons living alone consumed less food rather than foods of poorer quality (Davis, 1990). Low income increases the risk of poor dietary intake. The examiner should assess the client's living situation and refer the client to the appropriate assistance program if necessary.

??????? STUDY QUESTIONS ???????

1. What does the acronym *ABCD* stand for in the context of a nutrition assessment? Define each term.
2. Describe three methods that may be used for dietary recall. List an advantage and disadvantage of each.
3. A woman is 19 years old, weighs 102 pounds, and is 5'2" tall. Evaluate and interpret this individual's weight using (a) current weight as a percentage of desirable body weight and (b) BMI. Which is more objective?
4. Make a table of laboratory values that are useful in nutrition assessment. Include the test, the normal findings, and what the test indicates.
5. Describe what you would expect to find on clinical examination if an individual were malnourished. List supportive objective findings that would be expected in malnourishment.
6. What is the most accurate method to evaluate the adequacy of the client's dietary intake?
7. Describe the recommended dietary intake in each food group for healthy eating. How does the typical American diet tend to deviate from these guidelines?
8. What is the recommended weight gain during pregnancy? What does a rapid increase or decrease in weight indicate?
9. What biochemical analysis should be completed during pregnancy? What biochemical alterations are expected in pregnancy?
10. What are common nutritional changes that occur during pregnancy?
11. Explain the nutritional adjustments that need to be made for a nursing mother.
12. Define AGA, LGA, and SGA. What problems might LGA or SGA be indicative of in neonates?
13. What is the recommended frequency of well-baby nutrition and growth assessments for the first year of life?
14. List and give the rationale for the recommended biochemical measurements used to assess the nutrition status of the newborn, infant, and toddler.
15. List the common feeding problems that occur during infancy.
16. How do you identify a failure-to-thrive child?
17. Outline the steps of development in iron deficiency anemia in toddlers. What laboratory values assist in diagnosis of iron deficiency anemia?
18. What nutrition assessment areas are specific to the toddler during clinical assessment?
19. Describe common changes that occur in the dietary intake of toddlers, preschoolers, and school-age children.
20. Describe the indicators that may signal nutritional problems in children.
21. Identify behaviors and nutrition patterns that are commonly seen with adolescents. What indicators signal potential nutritional problems?

22. Identify factors that place the older adult at risk for developing malnutrition.

23. What is the importance of a weight history in older adults? What does a serum albumin level indicate?

24. What is a common result of decreased fluid intake in the elderly? What are indicators of this condition?

25. What nutrients are frequently lacking in the diets of the elderly?

CHAPTER 8

Skin, Hair, and Nails

ANATOMY AND PHYSIOLOGY

The skin is an elastic, self-regenerating, protective cover for the entire body, protecting against microbial and foreign substance invasion and minor physical trauma while keeping vital body fluids and components safely contained. Protection is its most important function, but it is not the only one. The skin and its appendages provide the body with its primary contact with the outside world, providing sensory input about the environment; its sensitive surface detects and reports—via nerve endings and specialized receptors—comfort factors such as temperature and surface textures, enabling the body to adapt through either temperature regulation or position changes. This regulation of body temperature is accomplished continuously through radiation, conduction, convection, and evaporation. Other functions of the skin include production of vitamin D; excretion of sweat, urea, and lactic acid; expression of emotion (e.g., blushing); and even repair of its own surface wounds by exaggerating the normal process of cell replacement.

The skin is composed of three layers that are functionally related: the epidermis, the dermis, and the hypodermis. The main components of each of these layers and their functional and spatial relationships are shown in Fig. 8-1.

EPIDERMIS

The outermost layer, the epidermis, has an exposed, cornified layer that serves as a protective barrier and regulates water loss. The underlying epidermal layers fold into the dermis and contain hair roots, apocrine sweat glands, eccrine sweat glands, and sebaceous glands. Hair and nails arise from these underlying layers and are composed primarily of keratin (produced by keratin cells, which are generated in the epidermis). Melanocytes, located in the base epidermal layer, secrete melanin, which provides pigment for the skin and hair and serves as a shield against ultraviolet radiation. The epidermis is avascular and is shed and replaced with new cells about every 30 days.

DERMIS

The dermis is made up of highly vascular connective tissue. The blood vessels dilate and constrict in response to external heat and cold and to internal stimuli such as anxiety or hemorrhage, resulting in the regulation of body temperature and blood pressure. The dermal blood nourishes the epidermis, and the dermal connective tissue provides support for the outer layer. The dermis also contains sensory fibers that react to touch, pain, and temperature. The arrangement of connective tissue enables

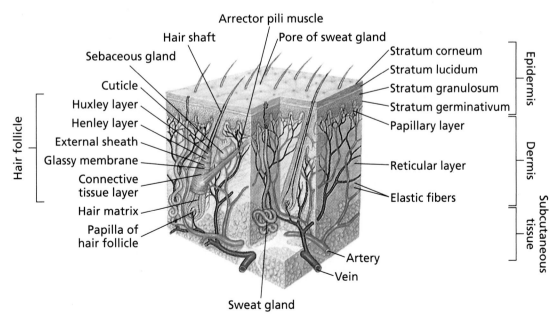

Fig. 8-1 Anatomic structures of the skin. *(From Seidel et al, 1995.)*

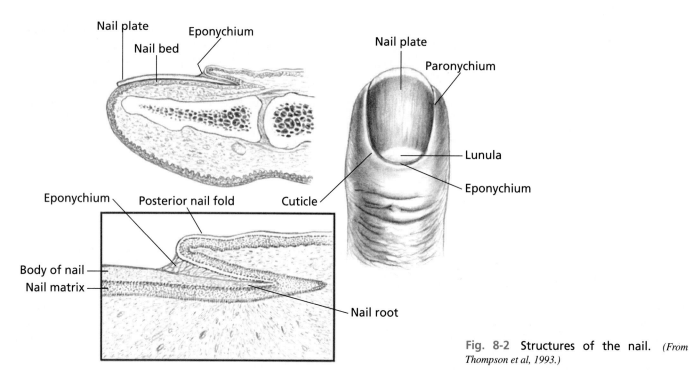

Fig. 8-2 Structures of the nail. *(From Thompson et al, 1993.)*

the dermis to stretch and contract with body movement. Dermal thickness varies from 1 to 4 mm in different parts of the body.

HYPODERMIS

The hypodermis is composed primarily of loose connective tissue interspersed with subcutaneous fat. These fatty cells help to retain heat and to provide a protective cushion and a storage for calories.

APPENDAGES

At junctions between the epidermis and the dermis, the hair, nails, and several glands are formed; the skin glands include the eccrine sweat glands, the apocrine sweat glands, and the sebaceous glands.

Hair.   Hair is formed by epidermal cells in the dermis. Each hair consists of a root, a shaft, and a follicle (the root and its covering). At the base of the follicle, the papilla—a loop of capillaries—supplies nourishment for growth. Melanocytes in the shaft provide color.

Nails.   Nails are really epidermal cells converted to hard plates of keratin. Their pink color comes from the vascular nail bed beneath the plate, but the true site of nail growth occurs at the white crescent-shaped area extending beyond the proximal end of the nail (Fig. 8-2).

 Racial Variation

Normal nail color can range from pink in those with white skin to yellow or brown as skin hue darkens.

Eccrine sweat glands.   These glands regulate body temperature by water secretion through the skin's surface. They are distributed almost everywhere throughout the skin's surface.

 Racial Variation

American Indians, Alaskan Natives, Pacific Islanders, and Asian Americans have fewer apocrine glands than whites. They sweat less and produce a milder body odor. In Alaskan Natives, most eccrine glands are located in the face. Chloride concentrations in sweat decrease as skin color darkens.

Apocrine sweat glands.   These structures are much larger, deeper, and not nearly as widely spread as the eccrine glands; they are found only in the axillae, nipples, areolae, anogenital area, eyelids, and external ears. In response to emotional stimuli, the glands secrete an odorless fluid containing protein, carbohydrates, and other substances. Decomposition of apocrine sweat produces what we associate with body odor.

Sebaceous glands.   These glands secrete a lipid-rich substance, sebum, that keeps the skin and hair from drying out. The secretion, which is stimulated by sex hormone activity, varies throughout the life span, according to hormone levels at different stages of the life span.

DEVELOPMENTAL CONSIDERATIONS

INFANTS AND CHILDREN

The smoother texture of a child's skin is due in part to its lack of exposure to the elements and in part to its lack of the coarser adult hairs, called terminal hairs. A newborn may have some desquamation, varying from flakiness to shedding of large strips of cornified epidermis. A white, waxy coating called vernix caseosa, a mixture of sebum and cornified epidermis, covers the newborn's body, and the shoulders and back may be covered

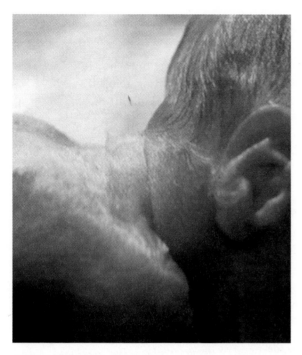

Fig. 8-3 Newborn with vernix caseosa and fine, silky body hair (lanugo). *(From Zitelli and Davis, 1992.)*

with fine silky hair called lanugo, which is shed within 10 to 14 days after birth. (Fig. 8-3). The infant may be bald or have unusually thick scalp hair. In either case, the hair is usually shed within 2 to 3 months and is replaced by more permanent hair, which may or may not have the same color.

Temperature regulation is not well developed in the newborn. For one thing, the subcutaneous fat layer is poorly developed in newborns, so they are subject to hypothermia. The eccrine sweat glands begin functioning after the first month of life, but apocrine glands will not be active until adolescence. Until then, the skin will have a less oily texture and a milder, inoffensive perspiration odor.

ADOLESCENTS

The apocrine glands enlarge and become active during adolescence, and increased sebaceous gland activity, in response to increased hormone levels, heightens sebum production. As a result, the teen will have oilier skin and possibly some acne.

In response to increased androgen levels, the axillae and pubic areas of both males and females will develop coarse terminal hair; males will develop coarser facial hair as well.

PREGNANT WOMEN

During pregnancy, a woman experiences increased blood flow to the skin, especially in her hands and feet, increasing vasodilation and number of capillaries. Sweat and sebaceous gland activities also increase to help relieve the extra heat caused by increased metabolic activity. All this activity may increase the size of vascular spiders and angiomas.

During pregnancy, the skin thickens and the subdermal layers receive more fat. As the skin stretches, connective tissues may separate, causing characteristic "stretch marks" (striae). Finally, hormonal changes may cause increased pigmentation of the face (melasma, or the "mask of pregnancy"), nipples, areolae, axillae, and vulva.

OLDER ADULTS

Older adults may notice that their skin is drier or that they seem to produce less perspiration. Both changes are due to decreased sebaceous and sweat gland activity. The thin, parchment-like appearance of the skin is caused by decreased dermal vascularity. Increased permeability of the epidermis results in a less efficient barrier of the stratum corneum.

Several factors contribute to the characteristic folding and wrinkled appearance of the skin in later life: the dermis loses elasticity, collagen, and mass. Joints and bony prominences take on a sharp, angular appearance, and there is a deepening in the hollows of the thoracic, axillary, and supraclavicular regions. These changes are due to a decrease in cutaneous tissue.

A number of hormonal changes affect hair in various parts of the body. For instance, a decrease in melanin production tends to produce gray hair. Scalp, axillary, and pubic hair thin because of reduced hormonal functioning. Because the size of hair follicles also changes, there is a progressive transition of the coarse, terminal scalp hair into the finer, vellus hair. This causes the characteristic age-associated baldness in both men and women. The opposite change, from vellus to terminal, occurs in the hair of the nares and on the tragus of men's ears. Higher androgen-to-estrogen ratios cause women to produce increased coarse facial hair. Both genders experience a loss of hair from the trunk and extremities, axillary, and pubic areas. Decreased peripheral circulation slows nail growth. The nails also become thicker, brittle, hard, and yellowish; they also develop ridges and are prone to splitting into layers.

HEALTH HISTORY | Skin, Hair, and Nails

The history related to the assessment of the skin, hair, and nails involves not only investigation of a potential underlying disease state or condition, but also exploration related to prior skin, hair, and nail problems and care patterns, as well as exposure to environmental irritants and communicable diseases. The question areas include disease, care, and risk.

QUESTIONS

RATIONALE

SKIN

RASH

- How long have you had the rash? When did it start? What makes it better? Worse? What have you done to treat it? (Describe medications, oils, lotions, creams, etc.)
- Do you have any known allergies to pets, foods, drugs, plants, soaps, deodorants, etc? Are you currently taking any medications, either prescription or over the counter? If so, what?
- Have you been exposed to anyone else who has a similar rash?
- Did the rash start when you were in the sun? Does the sunshine make it worse?
- Describe what the rash looked like initially: Flat? Raised? Does the rash itch or burn?
- Do you have any joint pains? Fatigue? Fever?
- Does anyone else in your family or other people you are around have a similar rash?
- If so, have they been seen or treated for their problem? Is it a communicable disease?
- Do you have or have you recently had any flea bites or been exposed to any environmental irritants?

◄ *Rashes are not generally a disease in themselves, but rather a symptom of an allergic response, skin disorder, or systemic illness. The questions asked should try to differentiate between these three entities.*

- *Systemic illnesses: Examples are Rocky Mountain spotted fever, rheumatic fever, and meningococcemia.*
- *Allergic responses: hives, eczema, and psoriasis.*
- *Communicable diseases: measles, rubella, and chicken pox.*

◄ *If the client has flea bites, he or she should be evaluated for plague. A confirmation of diagnosis is determined by elevated serum plague antibodies. Prevalence of the disease is highest in the western states of Arizona, New Mexico, Colorado, and California.*

ITCHING (PRURITUS) AND HIVES

- Do you have any known allergies to pets, foods, drugs, plants, etc?
- What were the circumstances when you first noticed the itching? Taking medications? Contact with possible allergens?
- Is the itching associated with any body rash or lesions? Does perspiration make the itching worse?
- Do you have dry or sensitive skin?
- Do you have any chronic or systemic diseases?

◄ *Pruritus is also a symptom of an allergic response or an illness process. Systemic diseases such as biliary cirrhosis and some types of cancer such as lymphoma may cause pruritus.*

◄ *Itching may occur secondary to an infestation of scabies, lice, or insect bites.*

DRY SKIN/OILY SKIN

- Do you have excessive dry (xerosis) or oily (seborrhea) skin? If so, is it seasonal, intermittent, or continuous? What do you do to treat it?

◄ *A history of dry skin may provide information about an existing systemic disease (e.g., thyroid disease) or it may be related to an environmental condition such as low humidity or hard water. Dry skin may also occur secondary to poor skin lubrication.*

TECHNIQUES and NORMAL FINDINGS

ABNORMAL FINDINGS

■ *Moles* (pigmented nevi): May be tan to dark brown in color and may be raised or flat (Fig. 8-6). See the box below for warning signs related to changes in moles.

A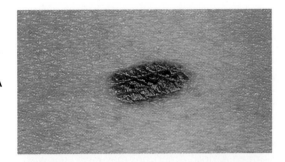

B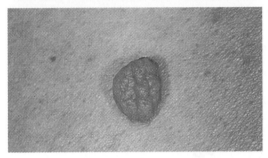

Fig. 8-6 Moles (nevi). **A,** Flat. **B,** Raised. *(From Habif, 1990.)*

■ Pallor: In *light skin* it will appear as a loss of "rosy glow" in skin, appearing pale instead; in *dark skin* pallor will appear as an ashen or gray appearance of black skin, more yellowish-brown in brown skin, with loss of the underlying red tones. Pallor is easiest to see in the mucous membranes, lips, nail beds, and the palpebral conjunctiva.

Warning Signs for Changes in Moles and Other Pigmented Lesions

The following changes in skin moles or lesions are considered to be risk factors for carcinoma and require further medical investigation:

■ A sudden enlargment or change in shape.

■ Irregular borders of a mole that previously had a regular border.

■ A change in color or variegated coloring.

■ A mole or lesion that has maldistribution of color.

■ Itching, tenderness, pain, or bleeding

■ A change in surface characteristics, such as flaking, scaling, or oozing.

■ A change in the surrounding skin, such as redness or swelling.

■ *Freckles:* Small, flat macules that may appear anywhere on the body. The most common locations are on the face, arms, and back.

■ *Birthmarks:* May be tan, reddish, or brown in color and are generally flat. Types of birthmarks include port-wine stains (nevus flammeus), strawberry mark (immature hemangioma), cavernous hemangioma, and Mongolian spots (see section on infant/newborn age-related variations).

■ Jaundice: In *light skin* the skin will have a yellowish color, seen most clearly in the sclera of the eyes, oral mucosa, palms of hands, and soles of feet; *dark-skinned clients* will also have a yellowing of the sclera of the eyes, oral mucosa, palms of hands, and soles of feet.

TABLE 8-1   Special Considerations for Examining Dark-Skinned Clients

CLINICAL SIGN	LIGHT SKIN	DARK SKIN
Cyanosis	Grayish blue tone especially in nail beds, ear-lobes, lips, mucous membranes, and palms and soles of feet.	Ashen-gray color most easily seen in the conjunctiva of the eye, oral mucous membranes, and nail beds.
Ecchymosis (bruise)	Dark red, purple, yellow, or green color, depending on age of bruise.	Deeper bluish or black tone, difficult to see unless it occurs in an area of light pigmentation.
Erythema	Reddish tone with evidence of increased skin temperature secondary to inflammation.	Deeper brown or purple skin tone with evidence of increased skin temperature secondary to inflammation.
Jaundice	Yellowish color of skin, sclera of eyes, fingernails, palms of hands, and oral mucosa.	Yellowish-green color most obviously seen in sclera of eye (don't confuse with yellow eye pigmentation, which may be evident in dark-skinned clients), palms of hands, and soles of feet.
Pallor	Pale skin color that may appear white.	Skin tone will appear lighter than normal. Light-skinned African Americans may have yellowish brown skin; dark-skinned African Americans may appear ashen. Specifically evident is a loss of the underlying healthy red tones of the skin.
Petechiae	Lesions appear as small, reddish-purple pinpoints.	Difficult to see; may be evident in the buccal mucosa of the mouth or sclera of the eye.
Rash	May be visualized as well as felt with light palpation.	Not easily visualized but may be felt with light palpation.
Scar	Generally heals, showing narrow scar line.	Frequently has keloid development, resulting in a thickened, raised scar.

 Racial Variation

Those with darker skin may have lighter areas of pigmentation on palms, soles, nail beds, and lips, and darker areas of pigmentation on knuckles and around elbows and knees. Lips and gums in darker-skinned individuals may have a bluish hue.

TECHNIQUES and NORMAL FINDINGS

ABNORMAL FINDINGS

The skin should also be observed for evidence of tattoos and needle-track marks. If a tattoo is present, its location and the characteristics of the surrounding areas should be examined and noted on the chart.

INSPECT the skin for Vascularity or Bruising. Bruising on the extremities is generally considered to be a normal finding secondary to the activities of daily living. However, if bruising is noted on areas of the body where no history of bumping or injury has occurred, it may be considered abnormal and warrants further investigation including blood studies. Normal vascularity variations may include:

- *Cherry/strawberry angioma:* As adults get older, small, slightly raised red areas may appear on the trunk (Fig. 8-7). These normal variations may increase in appearance and number as the individual ages.
- *Spider nevus or spider angioma:* A small, red, branching arteriole. With direct pressure, it will blanch. The most common locations are the face, neck, arms, and upper trunk.
- *Telangiectasia:* Permanent dilation of a group of superficial capillaries and venules. Blanches with direct pressure. The most common locations are on the lips, tongue, nose, palms, and fingers.

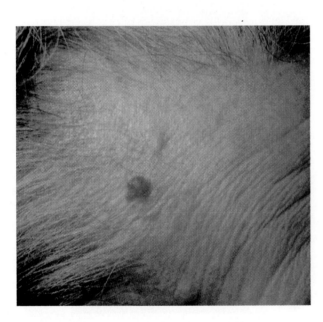

Fig. 8-7 Cherry angioma. *(From Baran et al, 1991.)*

INSPECT and PALPATE the skin for Texture and Lesions. The skin should be smooth, soft, and intact. There should be no rough spots or callouses. Note bruises, scars, or lesions. Carefully examine the skin texture in body creases such as under breasts, under skin folds on the obese abdomen, and in the inguinal area looking for rashes, discoloration, or areas of maceration. If a lesion is found, it is important to note its distribution and characteristics. Use a small ruler to measure the size of lesions. A flashlight may be helpful to determine the exact color, elevation, and borders. Transillumination may be used to determine the presence of fluid in cysts and masses.

Text continued on p. 131

- Needle-track marks are generally indicative of intravenous drug use.

- Vascular abnormalities include such findings as:
  - Petechiae: In *light skin* these appear as purple pinpoints that are most easily seen on buttocks, abdomen, and inner surface of arms and legs; in *dark skin* they are difficult to see except in the oral mucosa and conjunctiva. Petechiae will not disappear (blanch) with direct palpation (Fig. 8-8).

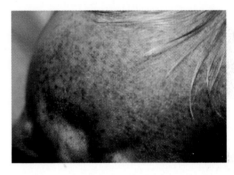

Fig. 8-8 Petechiae. *(From Weston and Lane, 1991.)*

  - Ecchymoses: In *light skin* these appear as purple to yellowish-green areas; in *dark skin* they are very difficult to see except in the mouth or conjunctiva.
  - Purpura: Brownish-red or purple discolorations on the skin as a result of hemorrhage into the tissue or a disorder such as idiopathic thrombocytopenic purpura (ITP).

- The common characteristics of primary and secondary lesions are described in Table 8-2.
- Reddened areas or open lesions may be monilia. Clients with diabetes are at increased risk for epidermal monilia.

TABLE 8-2   Primary and Secondary Skin Lesions

PRIMARY SKIN LESIONS	EXAMPLES		
Macule A flat, circumscribed area that is a change in the color of the skin; less than 1 cm in diameter	Freckles, flat moles (nevi), petechiae, measles, scarlet fever	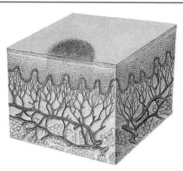	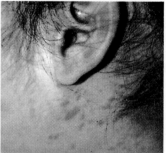 Macules. *(From Farrar et al, 1992.)*
Papule An elevated, firm, circumscribed area less than 1 cm in diameter	Wart (verruca), elevated moles, lichen planus	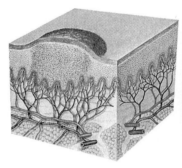	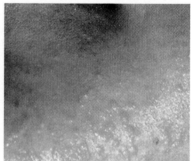 Flat warts. *(From Farrar et al,, 1992; courtesy Dr. E. Sahn.)*
Patch A flat, nonpalpable, irregular-shaped macule more than 1 cm in diameter	Vitiligo, port-wine stains, mongolian spots, café au lait spot	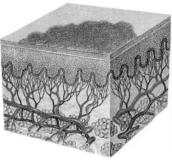	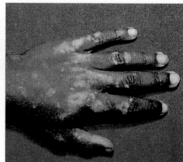 Vitiligo. *(From Weston and Lane, 1991.)*
Plaque Elevated, firm, and rough lesion with flat top surface greater than 1 cm in diameter	Psoriasis, sebor-rheic and actinic keratoses	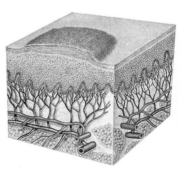	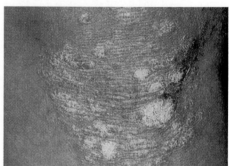 Plaque. *(From Habif, 1990.)*

TABLE 8-2 Primary and Secondary Skin Lesions—*cont'd*

PRIMARY SKIN LESIONS	EXAMPLES		
Wheal Elevated irregular-shaped area of cutaneous edema; solid, transient; variable diameter	Insect bites, urticaria, allergic reaction	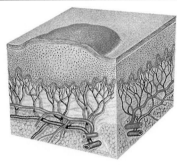	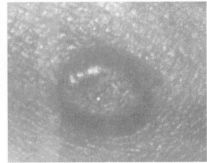
Nodule Elevated, firm, circumscribed lesion; deeper in dermis than a papule; 1 to 2 cm in diameter	Erythema nodosum, lipomas	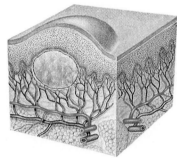	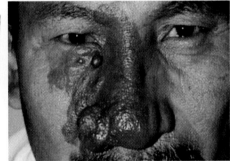
Tumor Elevated and solid lesion; may or may not be clearly demarcated; deeper in dermis; greater than 2 cm in diameter	Neoplasms, benign tumor, lipoma, hemangioma	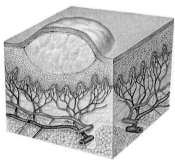	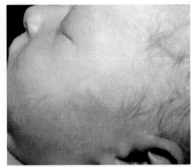
Vesicle Elevated, circumscribed, superficial, not into dermis; filled with serous fluid; less than 1 cm in diameter	Varicella (chicken pox), herpes zoster (shingles)	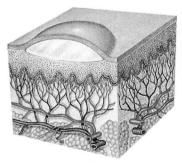	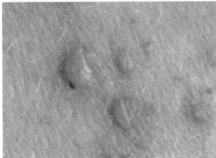

Wheal. *(From Farrar et al, 1992.)*

Hypertrophic nodule. *(From Goldman and Fitzpatrick, 1994.)*

Hemangioma. *(From Weston and Lane, 1991.)*

Vesicles. *(From Farrar et al, 1992.)*

Continued

TABLE 8-2   Primary and Secondary Skin Lesions—*cont'd*

PRIMARY SKIN LESIONS	EXAMPLES

Bulla
Vesicle greater than 1 cm in diameter

Blister, pemphigus vulgaris

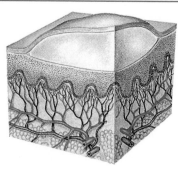 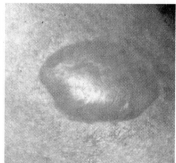

Bulla. *(From Farrar et al, 1992; courtesy Dr. K.A. Riley.)*

Pustule
Elevated, superficial lesion; similar to a vesicle but filled with purulent fluid

Impetigo, acne

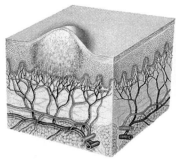 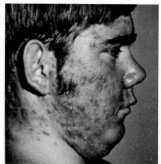

Acne. *(From Weston and Lane, 1991.)*

Cyst
Elevated, circumscribed, encapsulated lesion; in dermis or subcutaneous layer; filled with liquid or semi-solid material

Sebaceous cyst, cystic acne

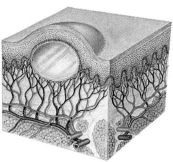 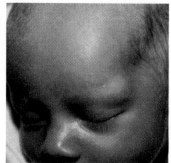

Sebaceous cyst. *(From Weston and Lane, 1991.)*

Telangiectasia
Fine, irregular red lines produced by capillary dilation

Telangiectasia in rosacea

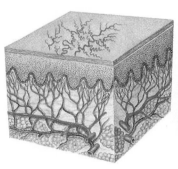 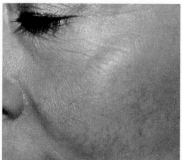

Telangiectasia. *(From Goldman and Fitzpatrick, 1994.)*

TABLE 8-2   Primary and Secondary Skin Lesions—*cont'd*

SECONDARY SKIN LESIONS	**EXAMPLES**		

Scale
Heaped-up keratinized cells; flaky skin; irregular; thick or thin; dry or oily; variation in size

Flaking of skin with seborrheic dermatitis following scarlet fever, or flaking of skin following a drug reaction; dry skin

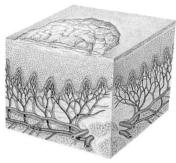 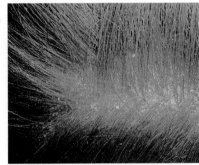

Fine scaling.   *(From Baran et al, 1991.)*

Lichenification
Rough, thickened epidermis secondary to persistent rubbing, itching, or skin irritation; often involves flexor surface of extremity

Chronic dermatitis

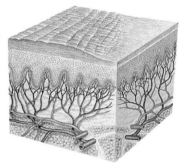 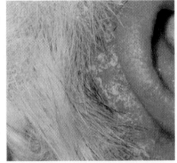

Stasis dermatitis in an early stage.
(From Marks and DeLeo, 1992.)

Keloid
Irregular-shaped, elevated, progressively enlarging scar; grows beyond the boundaries of the wound; caused by excessive collagen formation during healing

Keloid formation following surgery

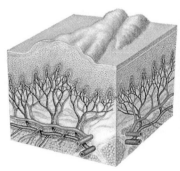 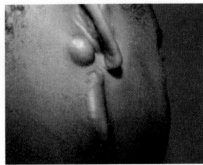

Keloid.   *(From Weston and Lane, 1991.)*

Scar
Thin to thick fibrous tissue that replaces normal skin following injury or laceration to the dermis

Healed wound or surgical incision

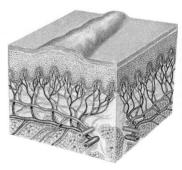 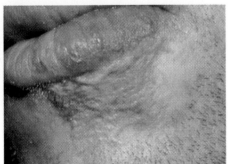

Hypertrophic scar.   *(From Goldman and Fitzpatrick, 1994.)*

Continued

TABLE 8-2   Primary and Secondary Skin Lesions—*cont'd*

SECONDARY SKIN LESIONS	EXAMPLES		
Excoriation Loss of the epidermis; linear hollowed-out crusted area	Abrasion or scratch, scabies	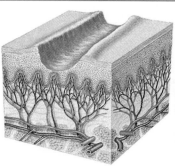	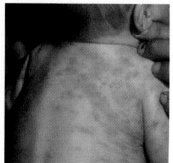 Scabies. *(From Weston and Lane, 1991.)*
Fissure Linear crack or break from the epidermis to the dermis; may be moist or dry	Athlete's foot, cracks at the corner of the mouth	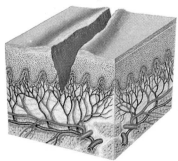	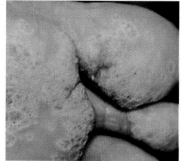 Fissures. *(From Goldman and Fitzpatrick, 1994.)*
Erosion Loss of part of the epidermis; depressed, moist, glistening; follows rupture of a vesicle or bulla	Varicella, variola after rupture	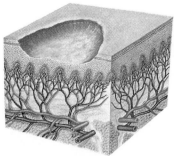	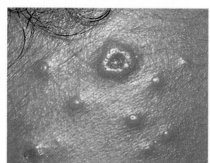 Erosion. *(From Cohen, 1993.)*
Ulcer Loss of epidermis and dermis; concave; varies in size	Decubiti, stasis ulcers	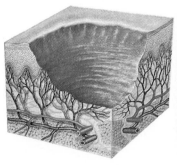	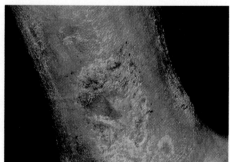 Stasis ulcer. *(From Habif, 1990.)*

TECHNIQUES and NORMAL FINDINGS   ## ABNORMAL FINDINGS

| TABLE 8-2 | Primary and Secondary Skin Lesions—*cont'd* |

SECONDARY SKIN LESIONS	EXAMPLES	
Atrophy Thinning of the skin surface and loss of skin markings; skin appears translucent and paper-like	Aged skin, striae	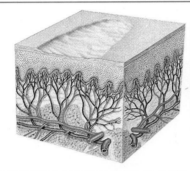 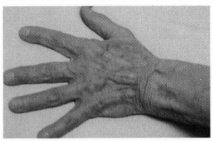

Aged skin. *(From Seidel et al, 1995.)*

The box below summarizes the characteristics of a lesion that should be described.

Lesion Characteristics to Be Noted during Examination

- Note the **location and distribution** of the lesion. Is the lesion generalized over the entire body or section of the body, or is it localized to a specific area such as around the waist, under a piece of jewelry, or just in the hair?
- Describe the **color** of the lesion and describe how this lesion may be different in color from other lesions noted on the body (e.g., a mole or freckle). Has the patient noticed a change in the color of the lesion?
- What is the **pattern** of the lesion? Are the lesions clustered? Are they in a line? How does the patient describe the development of the pattern of the lesion?
- What are the **edges** of the lesion like? Is the edge of the lesion regular or irregular? Has the patient noticed a change in the shape of the lesion?
- Is the lesion **flat, raised, or sunken**?
- What is the current **size** of the lesion? Measure using a centimeter ruler. Has the patient noticed a change in the size of the lesion?
- What are the **characteristics** of the lesion? Is it hard, soft, or fluid-filled? If there is an exudate, what is the color of the drainage fluid? Does the exudate have an odor? Note both the color and odor if present. Has the patient noticed a change in either the characteristics or drainage of the lesion? If so, how and when?

A Wood's lamp can be used to distinguish fluorescing lesions. Darken the room and shine the light on the area to be examined. Look for the characteristic blue-green fluorescence that indicates the presence of fungal infection. If there is no fungal infection, the light tone on the skin will appear soft violet.

PALPATE the skin for Temperature, Moisture, Mobility, and Turgor.
Temperature and Moisture: The skin should be warm and dry without being hot. There should be minimal perspiration or oiliness. Increased perspiration may be associated with anxiety, environmental temperatures, body weight or activity. The skin should be intact without cracking, flaking, or scaling.

■ Dryness, flaking, or cracking of the skin may occur secondary to environmental conditions, or they may be signs of systemic disease.

TECHNIQUES and NORMAL FINDINGS

ABNORMAL FINDINGS

Mobility and turgor: The skin should be assessed by picking up and slightly pinching the skin under the clavicle. The skin should move easily when lifted and should return to place immediately when released. Fig. 8-9 shows the technique and normal skin turgor.

■ Fig. 8-10 shows *poor skin turgor.* This may be associated with dehydration or aging.

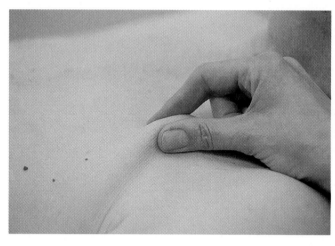

A

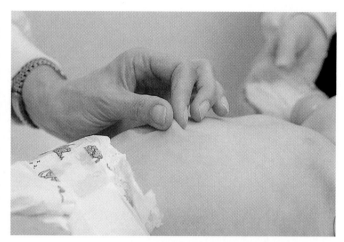

B

Fig. 8-9   Normal skin turgor in **A,** an adult and **B,** an infant.

Fig. 8-10   Poor skin turgor.   *(From Kamal, 1991.)*

HAIR

While some characteristics of the hair may have been noted during the examination of the skin, take time to specifically examine the characteristics of all body hair. The areas of hair to be examined include not only the hair on the head, but also axillary, pubic, and facial hair, as well as body hair.

INSPECT and PALPATE the scalp and hair for Surface Characteristics, Hair Distribution, Texture, Quantity, and Color. The scalp should be smooth to palpation and should show no evidence of flaking, scaling, redness, or open lesions. The hair should be shiny and soft. The texture of the hair may be fine or coarse. Note the quantity and distribution of the hair for balding patterns and isolated areas of hair loss. If there are areas of isolated hair loss, note whether the hair shaft is broken off or whether it is absent completely. Men may show a gradual, symmetric hair loss on the scalp due to genetic disposition and elevated androgen levels.

■ Hair bleaching or coloring may cause the hair to become abnormally coarse and brittle.
■ Lice or nits (eggs) may be found on the scalp at the base of the hair shaft.
■ *Alopecia* (hair loss) may be due to a variety of causes, such as chemicals, secondary to hair products and bleaching; cicatrical, or hair loss secondary to scarring; radiation, or secondary hair loss to antineoplastic agents; and syphilitic, a generalized thinning of the hair or mucous patches without hair.
■ Asymmetric hair loss may indicate underlying pathology.

TECHNIQUES and NORMAL FINDINGS

ABNORMAL FINDINGS

INSPECT facial and body hair for Hair Distribution, Quantity, and Texture. Examine the quantity and distribution of facial and body hair. *Men* most generally have noticeable hair present on the lower face, neck, nares, ears, chest, axilla, back, shoulders, arms, legs, and pubic region. The noticeable hair distribution in *women* is most commonly limited to the arms, legs, axillae, pubic region, and around the nipples. Women may also have fine or light-colored hair on the back, face, and shoulders. The women in some cultural groups may also have facial or chin hair. Note hair distribution patterns and areas of hair loss. Fine vellus hair covers the body, whereas coarser hair is found on the eyebrows and lashes, pubic region, axillary area, male beards, and to some extent on the arms and legs. The male pubic hair configuration is an upright triangle, with the hair commonly extending midline to the umbilicus (Fig. 8-11). The female pubic hair configuration forms an inverse triangle; the hair may also extend midline to the umbilicus (Fig. 8-12).

■ *Hirsutism* (in women) is hair growth in a male distribution pattern with an increase of hair on the face, body, and pubic area. Hirsutism may be a sign of an underlying endocrine disorder.
■ Pubic hair distribution in either the male or the female that does not follow the designated patterns may indicate a hormonal imbalance.

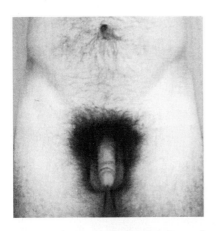

Fig. 8-11 Normal distribution of male pubic hair. *(From Bowers and Thompson, 1992.)*

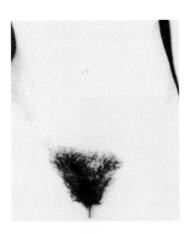

Fig. 8-12 Normal triangular distribution of female pubic hair. *(From Bowers and Thompson, 1992.)*

🌐 Racial Variation

Hair texture varies widely across races. African Americans may have fine, thick, and very curly or kinky hair. Asian Americans, Pacific Islanders, American Indians, and Alaskan Natives often have coarse, straight hair. African American men often have curly facial hair that tends to ingrow, producing a condition known as "razor bumps." Body and facial hair is sparse or absent in many American Indians and Alaskan Natives. Female balding patterns are frequently seen in American Indian women. Baldness is rare in American Indian men.

TECHNIQUES and NORMAL FINDINGS

ABNORMAL FINDINGS

NAILS

INSPECT and PALPATE the nails for Shape, Contour, Consistency, Color, Thickness, and Cleanliness. Inspect the edges of the nails to determine if they are smooth and rounded. Examine the curvature of the nail surface. It should be flat and slightly curved. The normal angle of the nail base is 160°. Inspect the nail surface itself to determine its smoothness. Note grooves, depressions, pitting, and ridges. Transverse grooves may be secondary to repeated injury to the nail. Examine the thickness of the nail itself. The nail should be smooth and have a uniform thickness. Finally, palpate the nail to ensure that the nail base feels firms and adheres to the nail bed.

🌐 Racial Variation

Pigment bands in the nails beds of individuals with dark skin may be present as a normal finding (Fig. 8-14). Pigment bands that suddenly appear in light-skinned individuals should be considered an abnormal finding and may be an indicator of melanoma.

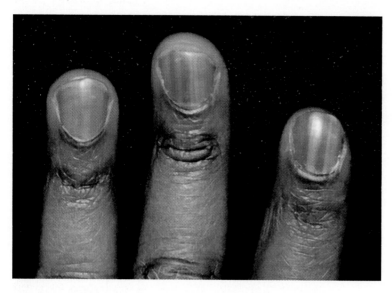

Fig. 8-14 Nail bed color of a dark-skinned person (pigmented bands occur as a normal finding in over 90% of African Americans). *(From Habif, 1990.)*

■ *Clubbing* is present when the angle of the nail base exceeds 180°. Clubbing may be associated with respiratory or cardiovascular problems, cirrhosis, colitis, and thyroid disease (Fig. 8-13).

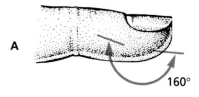

A   160°

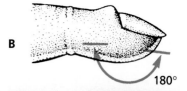

B   180°

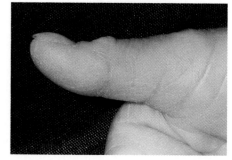

C

Fig. 8-13 Finger clubbing. **A,** Normal angle of the nail. **B,** Abnormal angle of the nail seen in late clubbing. **C,** Distal phalange is enlarged to a rounded bulbous shape. *(A and B from Barkauskus, 1994; C from Beaven, Brooks, 1994.)*

TECHNIQUES and NORMAL FINDINGS

ABNORMAL FINDINGS

- A thickening or hypertrophy of the nail is usually secondary to repeated trauma, fungal infection, or decreased vascular circulation. Thinning or brittleness of the nail may be secondary to poor peripheral circulation or inadequate nutrition.
- *Koilonychia (spoon nails)* is present when the nail is thin and depressed and the lateral edges of the nail turn upward (Fig. 8-15). This finding may be congenital or may be associated with anemia.
- *Paronychia* is an inflammation, swelling, and induration of the folds of the finger tissue near the base of the nail (Fig. 8-16). There is usually pain and tenderness associated with paronychia.
- *Lichen planus* is an inflammation of the matrix of the nail resulting in adherence of the proximal nail fold to the scarred matrix (Fig. 8-17).
- *Pitting of the nail* is commonly associated with psoriasis. Minor degrees of pitting may also be seen in individuals with no other health care problems.

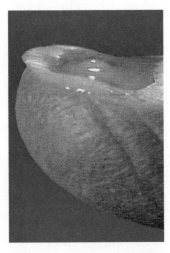

Fig. 8-15　Severe spooning with some thinning of the nail. *(From Beaven and Brooks, 1994.)*

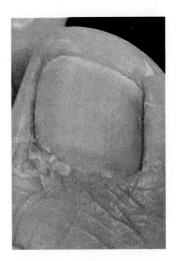

Fig. 8-16　Acute lateral paronychia. *(From Beaven and Brooks, 1994.)*

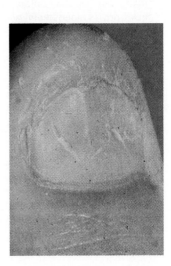

Fig. 8-17　Lichen planus. *(From Beaven and Brooks, 1994.)*

INFANTS

■ APPROACH

The techniques of the examination for the infant are the same as for the adult. To adequately examine the skin, the infant should be completely undressed. The examiner may want to keep the diaper in place until ready to examine the buttocks and genitalia area. Because many birthmarks and skin lesions may be in the diaper area, it is imperative that the diaper be removed at some point to conduct the comprehensive skin examination.

Care must also be taken to ensure that the infant remains warm during the examination period. If the infant becomes chilled, the skin, hands, and feet may take on transient mottling.

■ FINDINGS

Skin

Appearance, Color, and Pigmentation. The skin color in the newborn is partially dependent on the amount of fat present. Preterm infants generally appear to be redder because they have less subcutaneous fat than do full term infants. In addition, the infant may appear to have a red skin tone for a short period because of vasomotor instability. This color tends to fade within the first few days. Also, immediately following birth the neonate's lips, nail beds, and feet may be dusky or appear cyanotic. Once the newborn is adequately warmed, the dusky color should fade and a well-oxygenated pink tone should reappear. Even dark-skinned newborns should have a dark pink tone, which is most evident on the palms of the hands and the soles of the feet.

🌐 Racial Variation

Dark-skinned newborns generally have a lighter skin pigmentation than their parents. The child's actual skin color will take several months to develop. The scrotum in dark-skinned male infants, and the nail beds in all dark-skinned infants, most closely show their full melanotic color.

Physiologic jaundice may be present in the newborn following the third or fourth day of life. The skin, mucous membranes, and sclera will appear to have a yellow tone. This generally normal phenomenon occurs in almost half of all newborns and is secondary to the increased number of red blood cells that hemolyze following birth.

Birthmarks in newborns may be a pigmentation variation (Figs. 8-18 and 8-19) or may be associated with a vascular variation (Figs. 8-20 to 8-23).

- *Mongolian spot:* Is an irregularly shaped darkened flat area over the sacral area and buttock (Fig. 8-18). They are most prevalent in African-American, Hispanic, American Indian, and Asian children and generally disappear by the time the child is 1 or 2 years of age.
- *Café au lait spot:* Is a large round or oval patch of light brown pigmentation that is generally present at birth (Fig. 8-19). Occasionally these spots may be associated with neurofibromatosis.

Vascularity and Bruising. The skin of the neonate should be carefully examined for evidence of vascular-related birthmarks. These birthmarks may be either benign and within normal limits or considered to be deviations from normal. The most common normal vascular birthmark is a "stork bite."

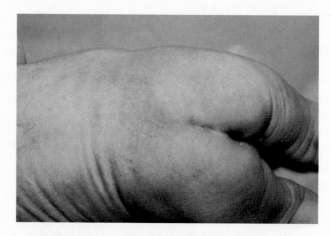

Fig. 8-18 Mongolian spot. *(From Weston and Lane, 1991.)*

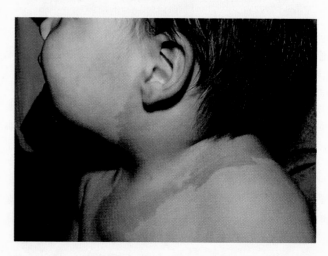

Fig. 8-19 Café-au-lait spot. *(From Weston and Lane, 1991.)*

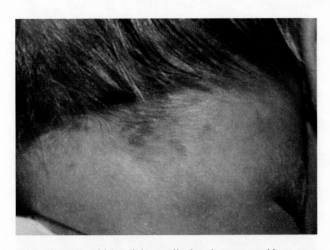

Fig. 8-20 Storkbite (also called *salmon patch*). *(From Weston and Lane, 1991.)*

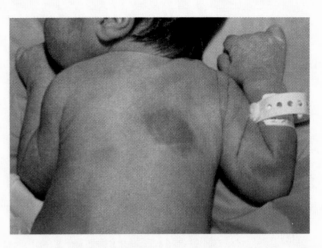

Fig. 8-21 Port-wine stain. *(From Weston and Lane, 1991.)*

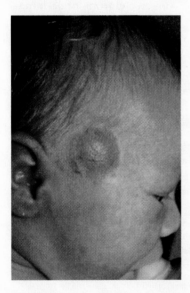

Fig. 8-22 Strawberry mark (hemangioma). *(From Weston and Lane, 1991.)*

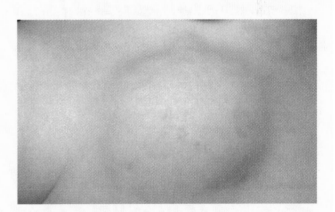

Fig. 8-23 Cavernous hemangioma. *(From Cohen, 1993.)*

- *Storkbite (telangiectases or flat capillary hemangioma):* Small red or pink spots that are often seen on the back of the neck (Fig. 8-20). Storkbites will usually disappear by 5 years of age.

Vascular findings that should be considered deviations from normal include the following:

- *Port-wine stains (nevus flammeus):* Large, flat, bluish-purple capillary areas (Fig. 8-21). They are most frequently found on the face along distribution of the fifth cranial nerve. Port-wine stains do not disappear spontaneously.
- *Strawberry mark (immature hemangioma).* Slightly raised, reddened areas with a sharp demarcation line

(Fig. 8-22). They may be 2 to 3 cm in diameter and will usually disappear by 5 years of age.

- *Cavernous hemangioma:* A reddish-blue round mass of blood vessels (Fig. 8-23). They may continue to grow until the child reaches 10 to 15 months of age. Frequent reassessment should be conducted.

Texture and Lesions. The skin of the infant should be smooth, soft and without lesions. Possible findings include the following:

- *Milia:* Small, whitish papules that may be found on the cheeks, nose, chin, and forehead of newborns (Fig. 8-24). These are benign and generally disappear by the third week of life.

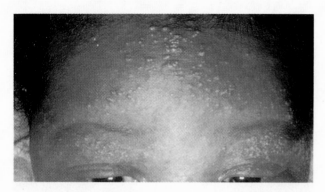

Fig. 8-24 Milia on the forehead of a newborn. *(From Cohen, 1993.)*

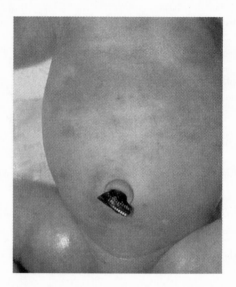

Fig. 8-25 Erythema toxicum on the trunk of an infant. *(From Cohen, 1993.)*

■ *Erythema toxicum:* A very common rash among newborns (Fig. 8-25). It is a self-limited and benign rash of unknown etiology consisting of erythematous macules, papules, and pustules. The rash may appear anywhere on the body except the palms of the hands and the soles of the feet. While it may be present at birth, it most commonly appears by the third or fourth day of life.

The buttocks of the infant should be carefully examined for rashes or lesions. Diaper rashes may be a benign reaction to damp skin or a contact reaction to the diaper, or they may be bacterial or fungal. If a rash is present, a careful history and possible cultures should be obtained.

Temperature, Moisture, Mobility, Thickness, and Turgor. Turgor in the newborn is best evaluated on the abdomen. The examination findings are the same as for the adult.

Hair

Scalp Hair Characteristics, Hair Distribution, Texture, Quality and Color. Scalp hair on the newborn may be present or absent. If present, it is generally fine and soft.

Seborrheic dermatitis (cradle cap) is a scaly crust that commonly appears on the scalp.

Facial and Body Hair Distribution, Quality, and Texture. The newborn's skin may be covered with fine, soft, immature hair called *lanugo hair.* This fine, soft hair may be found anywhere on the body but is most common on the scalp, ears, shoulders, and back. The lumbosacral area of the newborn should be carefully examined for evidence of tufts of hair. Hair in this area is suggestive of spina bifida or a sinus tract.

Nails

Shape, Contour, Consistency, Color, Cleanliness, and Thickness. The nails of the newborn should be examined for presence and texture. Postterm infants may have long fingernails at birth.

YOUNG CHILDREN

■ **APPROACH**

To examine the skin of young children, they should be completely undressed. The examiner may want to have the child leave his or her underpants on during the skin examination. If the child is shy or modest, the examination of the skin in the genital area may be deferred until the actual examination of the buttocks and genitalia.

Any child, regardless of age, who presents with itching of the scalp or pulling of the hair should have the hair and scalp carefully evaluated for the possibility of nits, lice, or scabies. These are common infestations in children and easily spread among peers and siblings.

■ **FINDINGS**

Skin

Vascularity and Bruising. It is important to assess a young child for evidence of bruising that may be inconsistent with the child's developmental level or bruising that may be in an unusual area. As the child becomes mobile, bruising is common on the lower legs and perhaps even the face. Bruising on other areas of the body (e.g., upper arms, back, buttocks, and abdomen) are abnormal and should warrant further investigation. The examiner should have an index of suspicion for possible abuse. In addition to the location of bruising, it is equally important to note bruises that may be at different stages of healing. Bruising on the body in unusual areas or multiple bruises found at different stages of healing should be further investigated to rule out abuse.

Texture and Lesions. The most common lesions found in the young child are associated with communicable diseases and bacterial infections. The common problems and conditions seen in children are presented starting on p. 146. These include:

- Herpes varicella (chicken pox)
- Rubella, rubeola, roseola
- Tinea corporis (ringworm)
- Impetigo
- Pediculosis corporis (body lice)
- Scabies

Temperature, Moisture, Mobility, Thickness, and Turgor. *Dehydration* must be evaluated in the ill young child. In addition to other clinical signs such as sunken eyes, dry mucous membranes, and decreased urinary output, it is important to evaluate the turgor of the skin. A child who is seriously dehydrated (more than 3% to 5% of body weight) will have skin that appears "tented" after the abdominal skin is pinched.

Hair

Scalp Characteristics, Hair Distribution, Texture, Quality and Color. The scalp and hair of the young child should be carefully evaluated for common problems. Common problems associated with the scalp and hair of the young child include such things as *alopecia,* which may be secondary to hair pulling, twisting, or head rubbing, and *lice, nits,* and *scabies,* which are common problems for the young and school-age child.

Facial and Body Hair Distribution, Quality, and Texture. The young child should have little body or facial hair. Indication of such warrants further evaluation.

Nails

Shape, Contour, Consistency, Color, Cleanliness, and Thickness. Nail biting needs careful evaluation. Evidence of cyanosis of the nail bed or nail clubbing require careful evaluation. These may indicate a cardiac problem or systemic disease such as cystic fibrosis.

OLDER CHILDREN AND ADOLESCENTS

■ APPROACH

Although the examination of the skin, hair, and nails is thought to be a benign and straightforward examination, special care must be taken when examining the older child and adolescent. Because of maturational changes and body hair development, the client may be very shy and want privacy. The examiner should provide adequate privacy and draping and should be sensitive to the client's concerns during the examination.

Developmental changes for the older child and adolescent are difficult. It is important for the nurse to take time to listen to the adolescent's concerns regarding acne and body odor and to provide appropriate hygiene and prevention education.

■ FINDINGS

Skin

Appearance. The general examination techniques and findings are the same as for the adult. There should also be a continued evaluation of unusual bruising patterns (see discussion under the young children section). As the child becomes an adolescent, the skin undergoes significant maturational development. The skin texture takes on more adult characteristics. In addition, the skin has increased perspiration, oiliness, and acne secondary to an increase in sebaceous gland activity. The two most common findings and concerns for the adolescent are acne and acne vulgaris.

- *Acne* may appear in children as young as 7 to 8 years of age, but peaks in adolescence at approximately 16 years of age. Although most acne appears on the face (Fig. 8-26), it may also be prevalent on the chest, back, and shoulders. Acne may appear as blackheads (open comedones) or whiteheads (closed comedones) and is generally a benign developmental body change unless it becomes infected or indurated with body hair.

- *Acne vulgaris* is a more serious condition that includes inflamed lesions of acne involving the stagnation of sebum and bacterial invasion (Fig. 8-27).

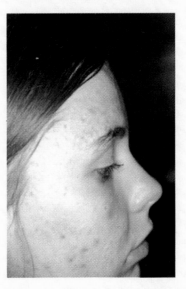

Fig. 8-26 Adolescent acne. Comedones (blackheads) are occasionally inflamed. *(From Weston and Lane, 1991.)*

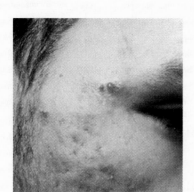

Fig. 8-27   Acne vulgaris with confluent pustules.   *(From Weston and Lane, 1991.)*

Temperature, Moisture, Mobility, Thickness, and Turgor. The most significant maturational change in this area is the development of body odor and axillary perspiration.
Hair
Facial and Body Hair Distribution, Quality, and Texture. The older child and adolescent should be given a

gown, and care should be taken to avoid embarrassment either in front of the parent or during the examination of body hair. The findings are maturationally determined. As the child reaches adolescence, the presence and characteristics of facial hair in boys, and body hair in both boys and girls, changes significantly, and by the end of adolescence has an adult hair distribution pattern. According to Tanner (1962):

- *Boys:* Pubic hair development in boys starts at about age 12 and continues to develop until age 15.
- *Girls:* Pubic hair development in girls begins at about age 8 and continues to develop until about age 13.

A full discussion of secondary sex characteristics development is presented in Chapters 18 and 19.
Nails
Shape, Contour, Consistency, Color, Thickness, and Cleanliness. The examination and findings are the same as for the adult. Although persistent nail biting may be a habit, it may also be an abnormal or coping mechanism for dealing with stress. The nurse should take the time to evaluate why nail biting persists.

OLDER ADULTS

■ APPROACH

Because there are many physiologic skin changes with aging, the examiner must take special care when examining the skin, hair, and nails of the older adult and carefully correlate the client's history of the problem with the physical characteristics of the condition or lesion. Some changes are simply a normal aging process, whereas others may be indicative of a cancerous lesion or systemic disease.

 Racial Variation

Light-skinned individuals wrinkle earlier than darker-skinned individuals. Brown or black hair grays much earlier in light-skinned individuals than in dark-skinned individuals. Graying hair is often not seen in American Indians and Alaskan Natives until they reach their seventies.

■ FINDINGS
Skin
Appearance, Color, and Pigmentation. The examination techniques are the same as for the younger adult. Finding differences may include an increased amount of pigmentation, especially in sun-exposed areas. Likewise, there may be isolated areas of hypopigmentation. Pro-

longed exposure to the sun may cause the skin to take on a thickened, ruddy appearance.
Texture and Lesions. Normal variations in the skin of the older adult include findings such as the following:

- *Senile lentigines (age or liver spots)* are irregularly shaped, flat, deeply pigmented macules that may appear on body surface areas having repeated exposure to the sun. (Fig. 8-28).
- *Seborrheic keratoses* are pigmented, raised, warty-appearing lesions that may appear on the face or trunk (Fig. 8-29). Care must be taken to differentiate these benign lesions from similarly appearing actinic keratoses, which are premalignant lesions.
- *Acrochordons (skin tags)* are small, soft tags of skin that generally appear on the neck and upper chest (Fig. 8-30). These tags may or may not be pigmented.
- *Sebaceous hyperplasia* are yellowish, flattened papules that have a central depression (Fig. 8-31).

Temperature, Moisture, Mobility, Thickness, and Turgor. As the individual ages, the texture and characteristics of the skin change. Changes include (1) an increase in dryness and flaking of the skin, especially over the extremities; (2) thinning of the skin, which may take on a parchment-like appearance, especially over bony prominences, the dorsal surfaces of the hands and feet, the forearms, and lower legs; and (3) appearance of the skin hanging loosely on the frame, secondary to a loss of adipose

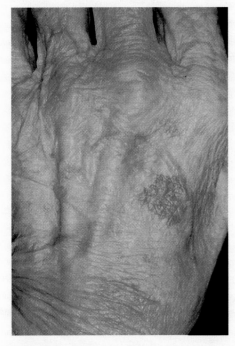

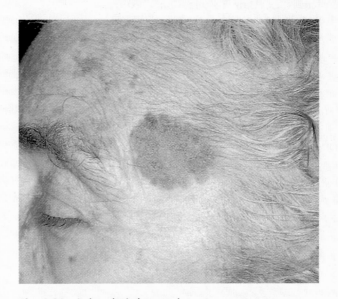

Fig. 8-29 **Seborrheic keratosis.** *(From Habif, 1990.)*

Fig. 8-28 **Senile lentigines (liver spots). Brown macules that appear in chronically sun-exposed areas.** *(From Habif, 1990.)*

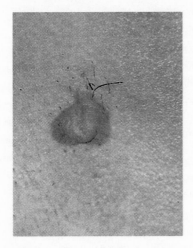

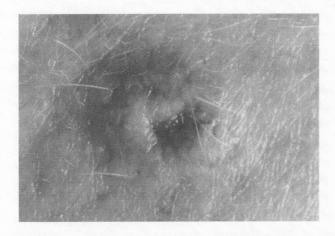

Fig. 8-31 **Sebaceous hyperplasia.** *(From Habif, 1990.)*

Fig. 8-30 **Cutaneous tag in older adult.** *(From Habif, 1990.)*

tissue and loss of elasticity. When evaluating skin turgor, there may be significant tenting of the skin (Fig. 8-32).

Hair

Scalp Characteristics, Hair Distribution, Texture, Quality, and Color. In the older adult, the hair of the head turns gray or white as the melanocytes cease to function. The hair may also become thin and change in texture. Symmetric balding may occur in men.

Facial and Body Hair Distribution, Quality, and Texture. Changes with aging include a decrease in the amount of body, pubic, and axillary hair. Men may have an increase in the amount and coarseness of nasal and eyebrow hair. Women may develop coarse facial hair.

Nails

Shape, Contour, Consistency, Color, Thickness, and Cleanliness. Changes that occur with aging include thickening and increased brittleness of the nails. The nails, especially the toenails, may become slightly deformed, lose their transparency, and may turn a yellowish color.

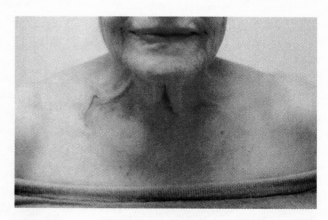

Fig. 8-32   Poor skin turgor in older adult.   *(From Seidel et al, 1995.)*

CLIENTS WITH SITUATIONAL VARIATIONS

PREGNANT WOMEN

■ APPROACH

The variations that occur during pregnancy are transitional and will generally disappear or fade following the child's birth.

■ FINDINGS

Skin

The skin in the pregnant woman undergoes several changes:

- As the abdomen grows with the fetus, *striae gravidarum,* or pinkish to silvery-white stretch lines, appear on the abdomen and occasionally on the buttocks. Following delivery, the striae remain but fade to a light silver color.
- *Linea nigra,* a pigmented dark line from the umbilicus to the mons pubis, may appear. Following delivery, the line fades but a light line may remain.
- *Chloasma, melasma,* or hyperpigmentation mask-type spots, may appear on the face. Following delivery, the hyperpigmentation often disappears.
- *Vascular spiders or varicosities* may appear on the lower legs and thighs. Following delivery, the spiders and varicosities will remain but generally fade.

Hair

Normal hair changes of the pregnant woman include:

- An increase in hair growth about the third month of pregnancy. The change may include an increase in fine, lanugo-type hair on the face and chest.
- The woman's general hair texture may become coarser during pregnancy.
- Following delivery, there may be a transient hair loss for 2 to 4 months secondary to a decrease in thyroid function.

Nails

During pregnancy, the client's nails may become thin and brittle.

■ Women who take prenatal vitamins usually report fast-growing, strong nails.

CLIENTS WITH LIMITED MOBILITY (Hemiplegia, Paraplegia, Quadriplegia)

■ APPROACH

Clients with limited mobility are at special risk for skin breakdown secondary to pressure and body fluid pooling. The nurse should carefully examine the client's skin, especially the areas of the body where there are bony prominences. The nurse may need assistance to move and turn the client so that a complete skin assessment may be performed.

In addition, clients who operate their own wheelchairs are at high risk for developing hand calluses. Therefore special care should be taken to examine the client's hands.

■ FINDINGS

Skin

Carefully assess all contact and skin pressure points for clients who have limited mobility (Fig. 8-33). The examiner should expect areas to have initial pallor when pressure is applied, but when the pressure is removed, the skin tone should quickly become red and then return to its normal color. An abnormal response is prolonged blanching, indicating ischemia, or prolonged redness, indicating that the area is engorged with blood. The stages of actual tissue damage are (1) prolonged redness with unbroken skin; (2) prolonged redness that does not blanch with excoriation; (3) full thickness skin loss with serosanguineous drainage; and (4) invasion of deeper tissue (subcutaneous or muscle), open ulceration, and purulent drainage with peripheral crusting.

 Racial Variation

Pressure areas in darker-skinned individuals are often harder to see in the early stages. Thus extra care should be taken when inspecting common pressure sites. Initially those with dark skin are likely to have a grayish or yellow-brown pallor at the pressure site that becomes purple, then returns to normal color when pressure is removed. A prolonged purple area may be seen as a beginning indication of actual tissue damage.

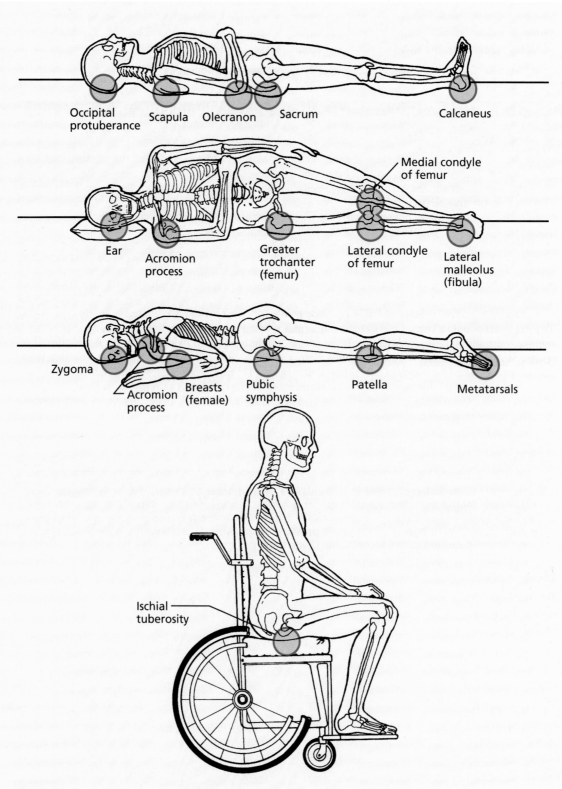

Fig. 8-33   Bony prominences vulnerable to pressure.

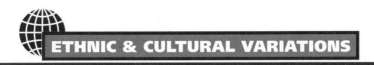

ETHNIC & CULTURAL VARIATIONS

■ FINDINGS

A range of normal differences exists in the physical appearance of skin, hair, and nails. Skin color can range from white to deep brown with yellow, olive, copper, and red overtones. This color is often absent or diminished at birth, developing over months during infancy. Skin often retains its elasticity and tone longer and wrinkles later in the aging process in darker-skinned individuals. Hair texture may range from fine to coarse, thin to thick, straight to kinky. Hair on the face and body may be absent, or range from sparse to abundant. Brown and black hair gray earlier in light-skinned individuals. Sweat glands have different distributions and produce various levels of salt concentrations on the skin. Nail color ranges from pink to dark brown, and pigment bands may be naturally present in darker-skinned individuals.

Certain physical findings also vary by skin color. Cyanosis and pallor are easily observed on the skin of light-skinned individuals, whereas these conditions are often seen only on the lips, tongue, or mucous membranes in dark-skinned individuals. Jaundice and petechiae, while visible on light skin, are best seen in the oral mucosa and sclera/conjunctiva of those with darker skin. Bruising is often purple to yellowish-green in light-skinned individuals and purple to brownish black in dark-skinned individuals. Inspection for pressure areas, which lead to decubitus, may require more careful scrutiny in those with darker skin.

Cultural practices may also affect findings when inspecting the skin. Practices such as coining or cupping may leave skin markings that are common in certain ethnic groups. Various cultural groups are also at higher risk for certain disease processes, such as diabetes mellitus and peripheral vascular disease, that predispose them to skin complications. All of these factors should be considered when examining the skin, hair, and nails.

EXAMINATION SUMMARY
Skin, Hair, and Nails

Skin *(pp. 122-132)*
- Inspect the skin for:
  Appearance
  Color
  Pigmentation
  Vascularity
  Bruising
- Inspect and Palpate the skin for:
  Texture
  Lesions
- Palpate the skin for:
  Temperature
  Moisture
  Mobility
  Turgor

Hair *(pp. 132-133)*
- Inspect and Palpate the scalp and hair for:
  Surface characteristics
  Hair distribution
  Texture
  Quantity
  Color
- Inspect the facial and body hair for:
  Distribution
  Quantity
  Texture

Nails *(pp. 134-135)*
- Inspect and Palpate the nails for:
  Shape
  Contour
  Consistency
  Color
  Thickness
  Cleanliness

COMMON PROBLEMS/CONDITIONS
associated with the Skin, Hair, and Nails

SKIN

DERMATOLOGIC

■ *Eczema:* Erythematous papules and vesicles that may weep, ooze, and become crusted (Fig. 8-34). There is significant pruritus. The lesions are most prevalent on the scalp, forehead, cheeks, back of the knee, at the popliteal flexure, and on the arms, especially the antecubital flexure. Generally there is a family history of allergies. A chronic form of this disease is called *atopic dermatitis.*

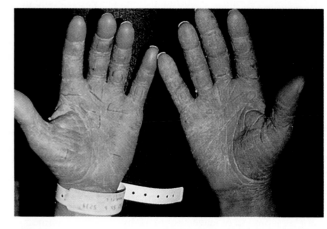

Fig. 8-34   Severe eczema of the hand.   *(From Hill, 1994.)*

■ *Seborrheic dermatitis (cradle cap):* A thick, scaly condition of the scalp and forehead most commonly seen in infants and young children (Fig. 8-35). It resembles eczema, but there is usually no pruritus or family history of allergy.

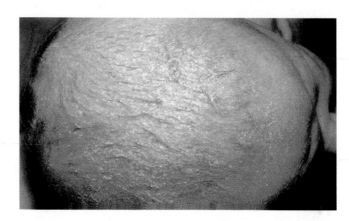

Fig. 8-35   Seborrheic dermatitis (cradle cap).   *(From Cohen, 1993.)*

■ *Contact dermatitis:* A local rash that may have secondary characteristics of swelling, wheals, urticaria, and sometimes papular vesicles or scales (Fig. 8-36). The dermatitis appears secondary to a contact or environmental irritant or allergy.

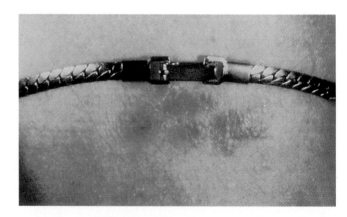

Fig. 8-36   Contact dermatitis. In this case, allergic reaction to nickel.   *(From Cohen, 1993.)*

■ **Stasis dermatitis:** Usually appears in the older adult and consists of areas of erythematous, scaling, and weeping patches (Fig. 8-37). The lesions most commonly appear on the dependent lower legs and are secondary to chronic edema and poor peripheral circulation.

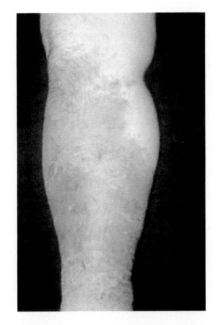

Fig. 8-37 **Stasis dermatitis.** *(From Marks and DeLeo, 1992.)*

■ **Psoriasis:** Appears as a scaly erythematous patch that may be a silver color on the surface (Fig. 8-38). Psoriasis appears most frequently on the scalp, the elbows and knees, and occasionally on the lower back.

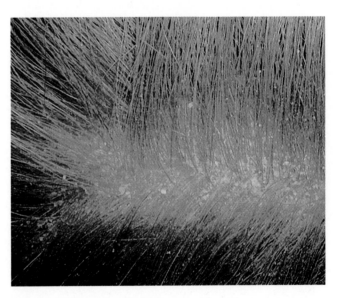

Fig. 8-38 **Psoriasis in the temporal region.** *(From Baden, 1987.)*

■ *Pityriasis rosea:* A common, acute, self-limiting inflammatory disease of unknown origin (Fig. 8-39). It appears as papulosquamous plaques over the trunk. The generalized eruption is preceded by the "herald patch," which is a single lesion resembling tinea corporis. The client generally feels well but may complain of mild itching. Because secondary syphilis may manifest with a similar-appearing rash, it is important to conduct serologic testing for individuals with pityriasis rosea.

A

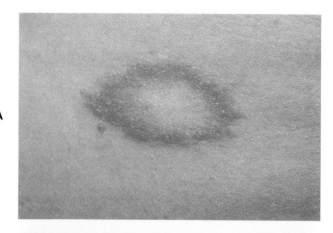

B

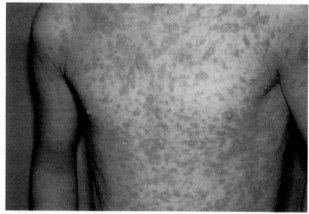

Fig. 8-39   Pityriasis rosea. **A,** Large herald patch shown on chest of a 10-year-old girl. **B,** Many oval lesions seen on the chest of a white teenager.   *(From Cohen, 1993.)*

VIRAL

■ *Herpes simplex (cold sores):* Appear most frequently on the upper lip and occasionally on the genitalia (Fig. 8-40). They start with a feeling of slight stinging and increased sensitivity. As the lesions erupt they move through maturational stages of vesicles, pustule, and finally crusting.

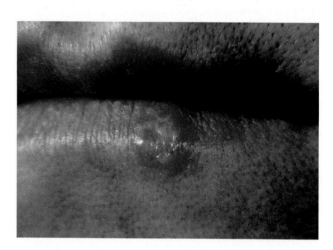

Fig. 8-40   Herpes simplex (cold sore).   *(From Grimes, 1991.)*

■ *Herpes zoster (shingles):* Actually the dormant virus of chicken pox that erupts (Fig. 8-41). It appears as linearly grouped vesicles along a cutaneous sensory nerve line. As the disease progresses, the vesicles turn into pustules, then crusts. This painful condition is generally unilateral and commonly appears on the trunk and face. Pain may preceed lesion eruption by several days.

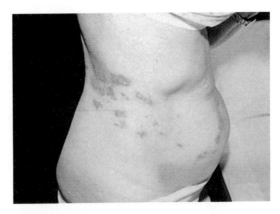

Fig. 8-41 Herpes zoster (shingles). *(From Raj, 1992.)*

■ *Herpes varicella (chicken pox):* Starts as small, isolated vesicles, generally appearing first on the trunk and then spreading to the face, arms, and legs (Fig. 8-42). As the course of the disease progresses, new vesicles erupt and the older vesicles become pustules, then finally become crusts.

A

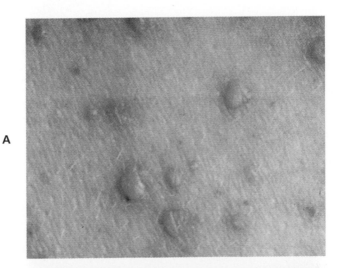

B

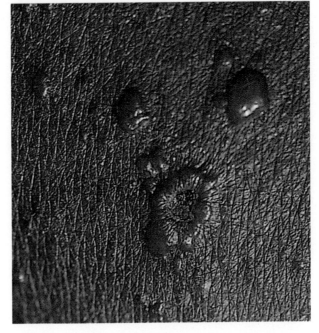

Fig. 8-42 Herpes varicella (chicken pox). Lesions in various stages of development including red papules, vesicles, umbilicated vesicles, and crusts. **A,** Light-skinned person. **B,** Dark-skinned person. *(From Farrar et al, 1992).*

■ *Rubella (German measles):* A pink papular rash that generally starts on the face and then spreads to the trunk, arms, and legs (Fig. 8-43). Concurrent with the rash is the presence of lymphadenopathy.

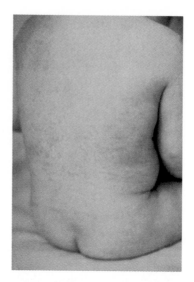

Fig. 8-43   Rubella (German measles).   *(From Grimes, 1991.)*

■ *Rubeola (measles):* Appears as a red-purple, maculopapular, blotchy, nonblanching, slightly raised rash (Fig. 8-44). The rash appears 3 to 4 days after the actual onset of the disease. It generally starts behind the ears and spreads over the face, neck, trunk, arms, and legs. Concurrent with the rash, Koplik's spots are found in the mouth.

A

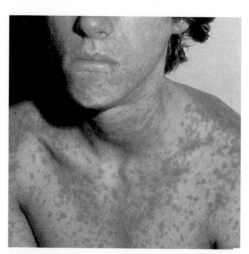

B

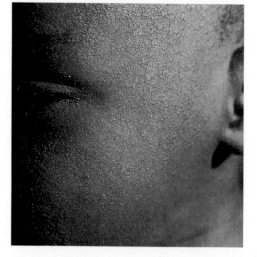

Fig. 8-44   Rubeola (measles). **A,** Blotchy, erythematous, blanching maculopapular eruption on a light-skinned woman. **B,** Slight follicular swelling on a dark-skinned child.   *(A From Cohen, 1993; B from Farrar et al, 1992.)*

FUNGAL

■ *Tinea corporis (ringworm):* Appears as circular, well-demarcated scaly lesions that may have a clear center (Fig. 8-45). They appear to be hyperpigmented in light-colored skin and hypopigmented in dark-skinned individuals.

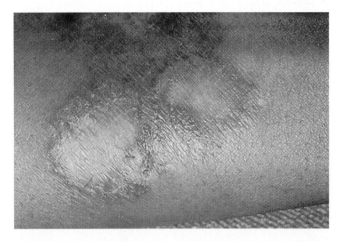

Fig. 8-45   Tinea corporis (ringworm). Classical presentation with central clearing.   *(From Hill, 1994.)*

■ *Tinea pedis (athlete's foot):* Generally appears as small weeping vesicles between the toes and sometimes on the sole of the foot (Fig. 8-46). As the lesions develop, they may become scaly and hard.

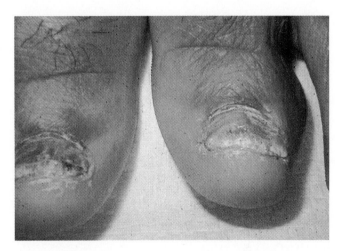

Fig. 8-46   Tinea pedis (athlete's foot).   *(From Beaven and Brooks, 1994.)*

BACTERIAL

■ *Cellulitis:* An acute streptococcal or staphylococcal infection of the skin and subcutaneous tissue (Fig. 8-47). The skin is red, warm to the touch, tender, and appears to be indurated. There may be regional lymphangitic streaks and lymphadenopathy.

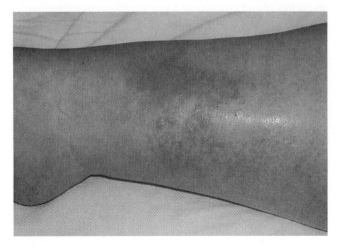

Fig. 8-47   Cellulitis (lower leg).

■ *Impetigo:* Appears as areas of moist vesicles with a thin erythematous base (Fig. 8-48). This is a contagious bacterial infection that is most prevalent in infants and children.

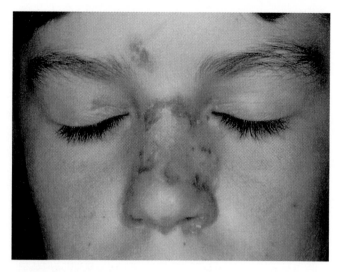

Fig. 8-48   Impetigo.   *(From Habif, 1990.)*

■ *Candidiasis:* Appears as a scalding red rash with sharply demarcated borders (Fig. 8-49). The area is generally a large patch but may have some loose scales. Common locations for the rash are the genitalia and inguinal area and along the gluteal folds. Urine, feces, heat, and moisture aggravate the problem.

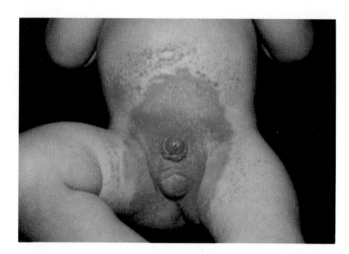

Fig. 8-49   Candidiasis.   *(From Weston and Lane, 1991.)*

■ *Scarlet fever:* Appears as a fine, punctate, erythematous rash that blanches with pressure (Fig. 8-50). It appears most commonly on the face, along skin folds, and on the trunk.

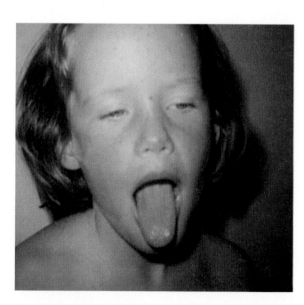

Fig. 8-50   Scarlet fever.   *(From Weston and Lane, 1991.)*

■ *Furuncle or abscess:* A localized bacterial (usually staphylo-coccal) lesion that appears to be red, swollen, tender, and hard (Fig. 8-51). As the lesion develops, the center becomes filled with pus. Common locations for the lesions include the back of the neck and buttocks. The *furuncle* appears secondary to an infected hair follicle. The *abscess,* which is usually larger and deeper, has a variety of precipitating causes.

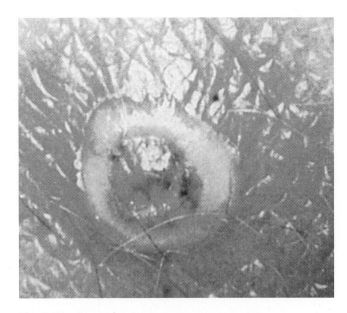

Fig. 8-51   Furuncle.   *(From Zitelli and Davis, 1992.)*

NEOPLASIA

■ *Kaposi's sarcoma:* A neoplasm characterized by dark blue-purple macules, papules, nodules, and plaques (Fig. 8-52). It is most commonly seen on the legs, trunk, arms, neck, and head. The disease is most commonly seen in patients with AIDS.

A

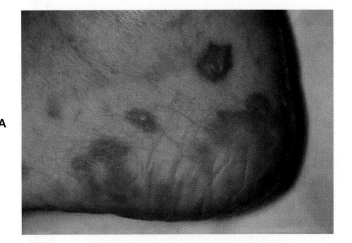

B

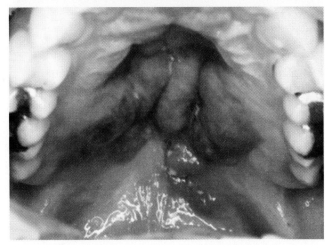

Fig. 8-52   **A,** Kaposi's sarcoma of the heel and lateral foot. **B,** Oral Kaposi's sarcoma.   *(From Grimes et al, 1991; **B** courtesy Sol Silverman, Jr., DDS, University of California, San Francisco.)*

■ *Basal cell carcinoma:* The most common form of skin cancer, commonly found on the face (Fig. 8-53). The lesion has different forms but usually appears as a nodular pigmented lesion. It is most commonly found in areas that have had repeated exposure to the sun or ultraviolet light.

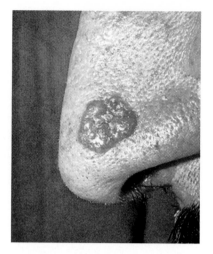

Fig. 8-53 Basal cell carcinoma. *(From Thompson et al 1986; courtesy Gary Monheit, MD, University of Alabama at Birmingham School of Medicine.)*

■ *Squamous cell carcinoma:* Appears as a red, scaly patch that has a sharply demarcated border (Fig. 8-54). The lesion is soft, mobile, and slightly elevated. As the tumor matures, a central ulcer may form with surrounding redness. The most common areas for the lesion to appear include those areas exposed to excessive sun or ultraviolet light.

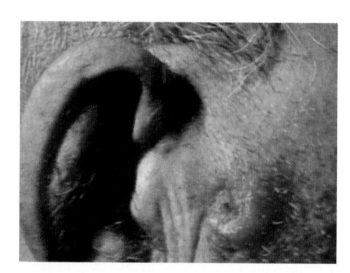

Fig. 8-54 Squamous cell carcinoma. *(From Thompson et al; courtesy Gary Monheit, MD, University of Alabama at Birmingham School of Medicine.)*

■ *Malignant melanoma:* Lesions frequently grow from already present nevi (Fig. 8-55). The border of the melanoma is irregular and the lesion may have a flaking or scaly texture. Its color may vary from brown to pink to purple, or it may have mixed pigmentation.

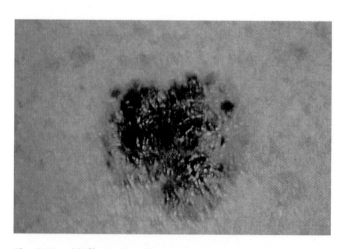

Fig. 8-55 Malignant melanoma. *(From Hill, 1994.)*

HYPERKERATOSIS

■ *Clavus (corn):* A flat or slightly raised, painful lesion that generally has a smooth, hard surface (Fig. 8-56). A "soft" corn is a whitish thickening commonly found between the fourth and fifth toes and is secondary to chronic pressure of a bony prominence against softer tissue. A "hard" corn is clearly demarcated and has a conical appearance. These occur most commonly secondary to chronic pressure from a shoe over a bony prominence.

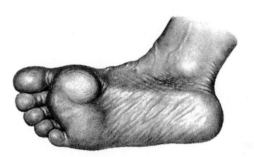

Fig. 8-56   Clavus (corn on foot).   *(From Seidel et al, 1995.)*

■ *Callus:* A superficial "tough skin" nontender area on the hand or foot (Fig. 8-57). The area is well demarcated and develops secondary to repeated pressure or use.

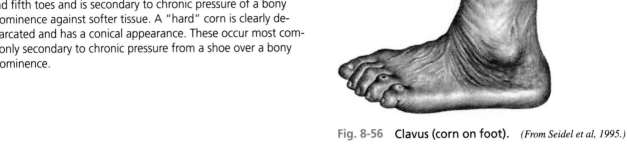

Fig. 8-57   Callus.   *(From Seidel et al, 1995.)*

INFESTATION

■ *Scabies:* A parasitic infection caused by *Sarcoptes scabiei,* which generally affects the hands, wrists, axillae, genitalia, and inner aspects of the thigh (Fig. 8-58). The lesions are small papules, vesicles, and burrows that result from the mite entering the skin to lay eggs. The burrows appear as short irregular marks that look as if they were made by the end of a pencil.

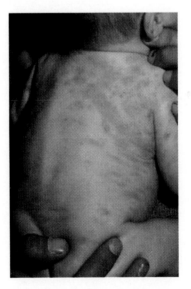

Fig. 8-58   Scabies in infant. Hundreds of lesions present. *(From Weston and Lane, 1991.)*

HAIR

■ *Pediculosis (lice):* Parasites that may invade the scalp, body, or pubic hair regions (Fig. 8-59). The eggs (nits) are visible as small, white particles. The skin underlying the infested area may appear excoriated. Lice on the body are called *pediculosis corporis* and pubic lice are called *pediculosis pubis.*

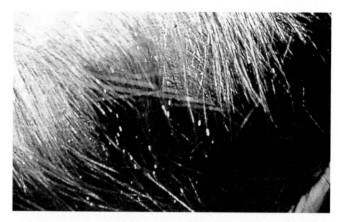

Fig. 8-59   Pediculosis (lice). The eggs, or nits, are visible attached to hair shafts.   *(From Farrar et al, 1992; courtesy Dr. E. Sahn.)*

■ *Alopecia areata:* A sudden patchy loss of scalp or face hair (Fig. 8-60). It is usually due to poorly developed and fragile hair shafts and will generally grow back within 3 to 4 months.

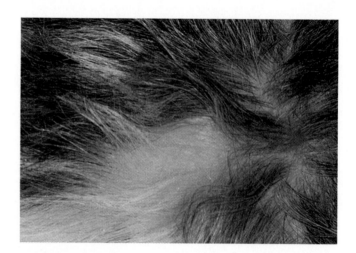

Fig. 8-60   Alopecia.

■ *Folliculitis:* A superficial staphylococcal infection of the hair follicle (Fig. 8-61). Multiple "whitehead" pustules with an erythematous base form around the hair follicles.

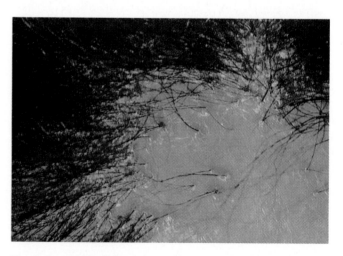

Fig. 8-61   Folliculitis.   *(From Baran et al, 1991.)*

■ **Hirsutism:** An increase in the growth of facial, body, or pubic hair in women (Fig. 8-62). The hair may take on a male distribution pattern and may or may not be associated with other signs of virilization.

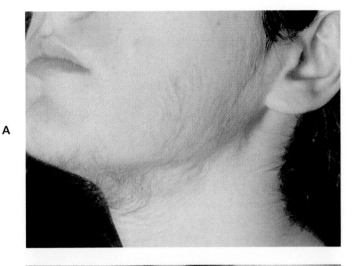

A

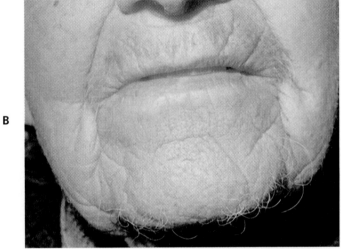

B

Fig. 8-62 Hirsutism. **A,** Hair growth on the jaw line and neck of a young woman. **B,** Hair growth on the chin of a postmenopausal woman. *(From Baran et al, 1991.)*

NAILS

■ **Leukonychia punctata:** White spots that may be seen in the nail plate (Fig. 8-63). The benign and transient lesions are generally secondary to minor trauma or manipulation of the cuticle.

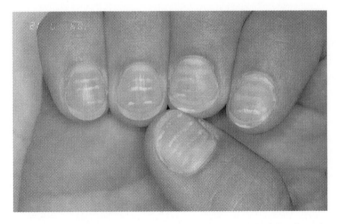

Fig. 8-63 Leukonychia punctata. Transverse white bands resulting from repeated minor trauma to the nail matrix. *(From Baran et al, 1991.)*

■ *Tinea unguium :* A fungal infection of the fingernail (Fig. 8-64). The nail plate most commonly turns yellow or white as hyperkeratotic debris accumulates. As the problem progresses, the nail tends to separate from the nail bed, and the nail plate crumbles.

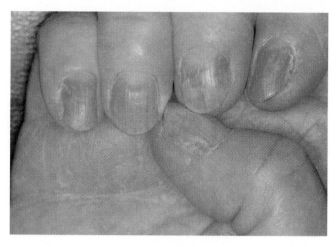

Fig. 8-64   Tinea unguium (fungal infection of the fingernail).   *(From Baran et al, 1991.)*

■ *Ingrown toenail:* Most commonly involves the great toe (Fig. 8-65). As the nail grows, it cuts into the lateral nail fold and actually grows into the dermis, causing pain, redness, and swelling.

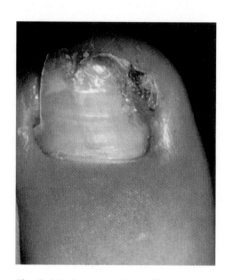

Fig. 8-65   Ingrown toenail.   *(From Baden, 1987.)*

Sample Documentation & Nursing Diagnosis

CASE 1 Healthy 15-year-old male

Subjective

Healthy male with complaints of acne on upper chest, face, and shoulders. Client states acne is becoming worse despite daily face scrubbing with Dial soap. Also applies benzoyl peroxide to face and chest at bedtime.

Objective

Temperature 98.8° F (37° C).

Skin Warm, dry, pink skin tone; elastic skin turgor, without evidence of rash except for mixture of papules and pustule lesions on face, upper chest, and shoulders. Several areas appear inflamed, suggesting possible infection.

Hair Normal scalp and body hair distribution, texture, and quality. Scalp without skin lesions.

Nails Fingernails and toenails intact, without lesions or deformity.

• •

Nursing Diagnosis #1

Risk for impaired skin integrity related to presence of secretions, presence of infective organisms.

Defining Characteristics Papules, pustules on the face, upper chest, and shoulders.

Nursing Diagnosis #2

Body image disturbance related to perceptions of facial lesions.

Defining Characteristics Age of the client, presence of acne, and verbalization of concern about acne.

Nursing Diagnosis

CASE 2   62-year-old woman with change in mole

Subjective

A very worried and anxious 62-year-old woman presents, stating that there has been a "change" in the mole on her forearm. The mole, which has been present for the past 20+ years, has changed in color from light brown to a purple and had grown from a "small dot" to an area that is now "as big as my thumb." Client states that she noticed the changes in the mole approximately 2 months ago.

There is no previous history of skin problems, changes in moles, or history of cancer. She states that she is healthy and currently takes no medications. She provides a history of "spending lots of time in the sun," keeps a good tan year-round, and uses no sunblock or sunscreen lotion. There is no family history of cancer.

Objective

Skin   Warm, dry, dark tan skin tone of leathery appearance with evidence of tanning. No evidence of rash. Multiple light brown nevi noted on shoulders, back, and forearms. The nevus in question appears to be a 2-cm, bluish-purple lesion with an irregular border. The lesion is slightly raised and has a rough, scaling texture. There is no evidence of flaking or oozing. No other nevi on the body has a similar appearance.

Hair   Gray, thinning scalp hair with normal distribution. Thinning pubic and axillary hair with normal female distribution.

Nails   Fingernails and toenails intact and without lesions or deformity.

• •

Nursing Diagnosis #1

Impaired skin integrity related to presence of the lesion secondary to sun exposure.

Defining Characteristics   Change in the mole created a disruption of the skin surface.

Nursing Diagnosis #2

Anxiety related to potential diagnosis of cancer.

Defining Characteristics   Frightened, with reassurance-seeking behavior.

Nursing Diagnosis #3

Altered health maintenance for skin protection related to inadequate knowledge or failure to assume responsibility for primary prevention.

Defining Characteristics   Lack of knowledge regarding basic health practices, lack of health-seeking behavior, or verbalization of inaccurate information.

HEALTH PROMOTION

■ **Immunizations** Clients of all ages should be taught about the benefits of immunizations and the life-time schedules for immunizations. Adults as well as children should maintain current immunizations. Parents of young children should especially be encouraged to immunize their children against communicable diseases, as well as taught to identify common skin lesions related to those diseases. See Table 8-3 for the age-specific immunization schedule.

■ **Sun exposure and protection** Clients of all ages should be taught about the need for careful protection of the skin with the use of sunscreens, avoidance of excessive exposure to the sun, and limited exposure to ionizing radiation. Sun exposure is intensified for clients living in sunny climates and those living near water or at high altitudes (e.g., mountains). Exposure to natural radiation from sunlight is linked directly to skin cancer, and approximately 400,000 cases of this type of cancer each year *(Healthy People 2000).* Teach the client about the various strengths of available sunscreens and sunblocking creams and lotions. The use of sunblocking agents such as paraaminobenzoic acid (PABA) is recommended, since these agents can be chosen on the basis of skin type and sensitivity to burning. Instruct the client to use a sunscreen with a sun protection factor (SPF) of at least 15 (the SPF is shown on the bottle). Children and infants should have an even higher SPF level. All clients should be encouraged to wear hats.

■ **Skin cancer** Young and older adults alike should be taught to perform skin self-assessment and to recognize the cardinal signs of skin changes that may be indicative of a malignancy.

■ **Signs of Basal Cell Carcinoma** Basal cell carcinoma is the most common type of cancer. One out of every four new cancers discovered is basal cell carcinoma, and one in eight Americans develops this type of skin cancer. The cause of 95% of all basal cell carcinomas is chronic overexposure to sunlight. That is why these lesions occur most frequently on exposed parts of the body—the face, ears, neck, scalp, shoulders, and back.

The most common signs of basal cell carcinoma are:

■ A persistent, nonhealing, open sore that bleeds, oozes, or crusts and remains open for 3 or more weeks.

■ A reddish patch or irritated area, usually on the chest, shoulders, or limbs that may or may not itch or hurt.

■ A smooth growth with an elevated, rolled border and indented center.

■ A shiny bump or nodule that is pearly or translucent and that can be pink, red, white, tan, black, or brown.

■ A scarlike area, white, yellow, or waxy, which often has poorly defined borders and loss of normal skin markings.

■ **Early Signs of Melanoma** In the United States, the incidence of malignant melanoma is increasing at an alarming rate. The following signs may indicate the presence of a malignant melanoma. Any one or more of the following changes occurring in a new or existing pigmented (tan or brown) area of the skin or in a mole may indicate the presence of a malignant melanoma:

■ *Change in size:* especially sudden or continuous enlargement.

■ *Change in color:* especially multiple shades of tan, brown, dark brown, black; the mixing of red, white, and blue; or the spreading of color from the edge into the surrounding skin.

■ *Change in shape:* especially development of an irregular, notched border, which used to be regular.

■ *Change in elevation:* especially the raising of a part of a pigmented area that used to be flat or only slightly elevated.

■ *Change in surface:* especially scaliness, erosion, oozing, crusting, ulceration, or bleeding.

■ *Changes in surrounding skin:* especially redness, swelling, or development of colored blemishes next to, but not part of the pigmented area.

■ *Change in sensation:* especially itchiness, tenderness, or pain.

■ *Change in consistency:* especially softening or hardening.

The A, B, C, D Early Signs of Melanoma

A = Asymmetry
B = Border (notched, scalloped, or indistinct)
C = Color (uneven, variegated)
D = Diameter (usually larger than 6 mm)

■ **Ingrown toenails** may, in most cases, be prevented if the nails are trimmed properly. The nail should be trimmed straight across, not curved around the toe.

TABLE 8-3	Recommended Immunization Schedule[a]

Infants and Children Born in the United States

RECOMMENDED AGE[b]	IMMUNIZATION(S)[c]	COMMENTS
Birth	HBV[d]	
1-2 months	HBV[d]	
2 months	DTP, Hib, OPV	DTP and OPV can be initiated as early as 4 weeks after birth in areas of high endemicity or during outbreaks
4 months	DTP, Hib, OPV	2-month interval (minimum of 6 weeks) recommended for OPV
6 months	DTP, (Hib[e])	
6-18 months	HBV,[d] OPV	
12-15 months	Hib, MMR	MMR should be given at 12 months of age in high-risk areas; if indicated, tuberculin testing may be done at the same visit
15-18 months	DTaP or DTP	The fourth dose of diphtheria-tetanus-pertussis vaccine should be given 6 to 12 months after the third dose of DTP and may be given as early as 12 months of age, provided that the interval between doses 3 and 4 is at least 6 months and DTP is given; DTaP is not currently licensed for use in children younger than 15 months
4-6 years	DTaP or DTP, OPV	DTaP or DTP and OPV should be given at or before school entry; DTP or DTaP should not be given at or after the seventh birthday
11-12 years	MMR	MMR should be given at entry to middle school or junior high school unless 2 doses were given after the first birthday
14-16 years	Td	Repeat every 10 years throughout life

Modified from American Academy of Pediatrics, Committee on Infectious Diseases: 1994 Red Book: Report of the Committee on Infectious Diseases, *ed 23, Elk Grove Village, IL, 1994, The Academy.*

[a]*Table is not completely consistent with all package inserts. For products used, also consult manufacturer's package insert for instructions on storage, handling, dosage, and administration. Biologics prepared by different manufacturers may vary, and package inserts of the same manufacturer may change from time to time. Therefore the practitioner should be aware of the contents of the current package insert.*

[b]*These recommended ages should not be construed as absolute. For example, 2 months can be 6 to 10 weeks. However, MMR usually should not be given to children younger than 12 months. If measles vaccination is indicated, monovalent measles vaccine is recommended, and MMR should be given subsequently at 12 to 15 months.*

[c]*Vaccine abbreviations: HBV, hepatitis B virus vaccine; DTP, diphtheria and tetanus toxoids and pertussis vaccine; DTaP, diphtheria and tetanus toxoids and acellular pertussis vaccine; Hib, Haemophilus influenzae type b conjugate vaccine; OPV, oral poliovirus vaccine (containing attenuated poliovirus types 1, 2, and 3); MMR, live measles, mumps, and rubella viruses vaccine; Td, adult tetanus toxoid (full dose) and diphtheria toxoid (reduced dose), for children ≥7 years and adults.*

[d]*An acceptable alternative to minimize the number of visits for immunizing infants of HBsAg-negative mothers is to administer dose 1 at 0 to 2 months, dose 2 at 4 months, and dose 3 at 6 to 18 months.*

[e]*Hib; dose 3 of Hib is not indicated if the product for doses 1 and 2 was PedvaxHIB (PRP-OMP).*

TABLE 8-3	Recommended Immunization Schedule—*cont'd*

Children Not Immunized in the First Year of Life in the United States

RECOMMENDED TIME/AGE	IMMUNIZATION(S)[f,g]	COMMENTS
Younger Than 7 Years		
First visit	DTP, Hib, HBV, MMR, OPV	If indicated, tuberculin testing may be done at same visit If child is 5 years of age or older, Hib is not indicated
Interval after first visit: 1 month	DTP, HBV	OPV may be given if accelerated poliomyelitis vaccination is necessary, such as for travelers to areas where polio is endemic
2 months	DTP, Hib, OPV	Second dose of Hib is indicated only in children whose first dose was received when younger than 15 months
≥8 months	DTP or DTaP[h], HBV, OPV	OPV is not given if the third dose was given earlier
4-6 years (at or before school entry)	DTP or DTaP,[h] OPV	DTP or DTaP is not necessary if the fourth dose was given after the fourth birthday; OPV is not necessary if the third dose was given after the fourth birthday
11-12 Years	MMR	At entry to middle school or junior high school
10 years later	Td	Repeat every 10 years throughout life
7 Years and Older[i,j]		
First visit	HBV,[k] OPV, MMR, Td	
Interval after first visit: 2 months	HBV,[k] OPV, Td	OPV may also be given 1 month after the first visit if accelerated poliomyelitis vaccination is necessary
8-14 months	HBV,[k] OPV, Td	OPV is not given if the third dose was given earlier
11-12 years	MMR	At entry to middle school or junior high
10 years later	Td	Repeat every 10 years throughout life

Modified from Wong DL: Nursing care of infants and children, ed. 5, St. Louis, 1995, Mosby.

[f]*If all needed vaccines cannot be administered simultaneously, priority should be given to protecting the child against those diseases that pose the greatest immediate risk. In the United States these diseases for children younger than 2 years usually are measles and Haemophilus influenzae type b infection; for children older than 7 years, they are measles, mumps, and rubella (MMR).*

[g]*DTP or DTaP, HBV, Hib, MMR, and OPV can be given simultaneously at separate sites if failure of the patient to return for future immunizations is a concern.*

[h]*DTaP is not currently licensed for use in children younger than 15 months of age and is not recommended for primary immunization (i.e., first 3 doses) at any age.*

[i]*If person is 18 years or older, routine poliovirus vaccination is not indicated in the United States.*

[j]*Minimal interval between doses of MMR is 1 month.*

[k]*Priority should be given to hepatitis B immunization of adolescents.*

???????STUDY QUESTIONS???????

1. List five functions of the skin and underline the most important functions.

2. Identify and describe the function of the three skin layers.

3. List at least one difference in the skin of: infants, adolescents, pregnant women, and older adults.

4. List the questions you might pose to gain information about the history of a rash on the forehead.

5. List questions that would be necessary to help you assess someone's risk of skin cancer.

6. Describe how you would distinguish between jaundice, pallor, and cyanosis.

7. Identify the early signs of melanoma.

8. Are pigment bands a normal finding in the nail bed?

9. Describe what you are looking for when you palpate the skin for temperature, moisture, mobility, and turgor.

10. Identify the normal range of characteristics that are possible in hair color, quality, texture, and distribution. Be sure to include how these are affected by race, gender, and age.

11. Identify the normal range of characteristics that are possible in skin color, quality, texture, and vascularity. Be sure to include how these are affected by race, gender, and age.

12. Identify the normal range of characteristics that are possible in nail shape, consistency, thickness, and color. Be sure to include how these are affected by race, gender, and age.

13. Describe the characteristics of the following: eczema, cradle cap, psoriasis, contact dermatitis, pityriasis rosea.

14. Tell how you would distinguish the following viral skin lesions: Herpes simplex, Herpes zoster, and Herpes varicella.

15. Distinguish the appearance of tinea corporis from tinea pedis.

16. Describe the appearance of the following: cellulitis, impetigo, furuncles, abscesses.

17. How would you tell the difference between a basal cell carcinoma and a squamous cell carcinoma?

18. How would you distinguish leukonychia punctata from tinea unguium?

19. At what age should children first be immunized for mumps? Hepatitis B? Typhoid? Polio?

20. What immunizations should be repeated throughout the life span?

21. List seven changes that may occur in moles and pigmented skin lesions that serve as warning signs of cancer.

22. Describe the difference between a macule, papule, plaque, and wheal and give a specific example of each.

23. Describe the differences between a vesicle, bulla, pustule, and cyst and give a specific example of each.

24. Describe the differences between a keloid and a scar.

25. Describe the difference between an excoriation and an ulcer.

CHAPTER 9

Lymphatic System

ANATOMY AND PHYSIOLOGY

Every tissue supplied by blood vessels has lymphatic vessels except for the central nervous system, cornea, and placenta. The lymphatic system is a special vascular system that provides immunity, phagocytizes foreign and abnormal cells, and collects interstitial fluid and returns it to the blood stream. This system is made up of lymph fluid, the collecting ducts, and lymph tissue that includes lymph nodes, spleen, thymus, tonsils, adenoids, and Peyer's patches (Fig. 9-1). Lymph tissue is found within other parts of the body, such as mucosa of the stomach and appendix, bone marrow, and lungs.

LYMPHATIC FLUID CIRCULATION

Lymphatic fluid is clear, composed mainly of water and small amounts of proteins, mostly albumin, that are absorbed from the interstitial spaces. As blood flows from arterioles into venules, fluid is forced out at the arterial capillary bed into the interstitial spaces and then into cells. However, not all of this fluid is reabsorbed by the venous capillaries (Fig. 9-2). The fluid left in the interstitial spaces is reabsorbed by the lymph system and carried on to lymph nodes throughout the body. Flow through lymph nodes is slow to allow the lymphocytes in the node to ingest and destroy foreign substances, thus preventing them from reentering the blood stream. Finally, ducts from the lymph nodes empty into the subclavian veins. The right lymphatic duct drains fluid from the right side of the head and neck, right arm, and right chest into the right subclavian vein. The larger thoracic duct drains the rest of the body into the left subclavian vein (Fig. 9-3). The lymphatic system has no means of pumping this fluid; instead, it depends entirely on arterial pulsation, lymphatic vessel compression by the skeletal muscles, and smooth muscle contraction in the lymphatic vessels, lymph nodes, and collecting ducts. The larger lymphatic vessels have valves similar to the circulatory veins.

LYMPHOCYTES

The most important component of the lymphatic fluid is its lymphocytes, since they are central to the body's immunity. There are two types of lymphocytes. The *B lymphocytes* produce specific antibodies to provide humoral immunity. These antibodies (immunoglobulins A, D, E, G, and M) act by neutralizing bacterial toxins, neutralizing viruses, phagocytizing bacteria, and activating the inflammatory response. The *T lymphocytes* produce several types of lymphocytes to provide cellular immunity, including cytotoxic, helper, and suppressor T cells, as well as cytokines. The functions of T lymphocytes are to kill cells infected by viruses, including tumors and transplanted tissue; activate the inflammatory response; and stimulate production of more B and T lymphocytes.

LYMPH NODES

Lymph nodes are tiny oval clumps of lymphatic tissue, usually occurring in groups along the blood vessels at numerous sites. Those located in subcutaneous connective tissue are called superficial nodes; those beneath the fascia of muscles or within various body cavities are called deeper nodes. Deeper nodes are not accessible to inspection or palpation. However, superficial nodes are accessible and become

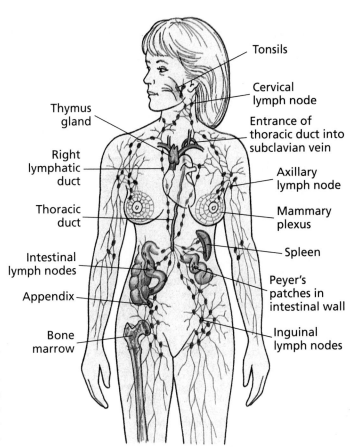

Fig. 9-1 The major organs and vessels of the lymphatic system. *(From Seeley, Stephens, and Tate, 1995.)*

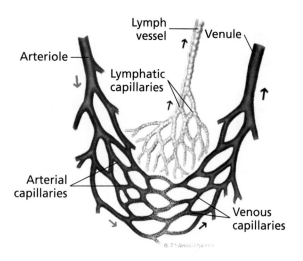

Fig. 9-2 Microcirculation involving blood, interstitial fluid, oxygen, and nutrients. *(From Canobbio, 1990.)*

enlarged and tender, providing early signs of infection or inflammation.

Regional Nodes.   Lymph nodes are widely distributed throughout the body. These locations include the following regions.

Head.   In the head, the lymph nodes are categorized as follows: preauricular, postauricular, occipital, parotid, retropharyngeal, submandibular, and submental (Fig. 9-4). See Table 9-1 for lymphatic drainage pattern for lymph nodes.

Neck.   The cervical nodes are named according to their relation to the sternocleidomastoid muscle and the neck's anterior and posterior triangles: anterior cervical chain; posterior cervical chain; deep cervical chain; and supraclavicular (Fig. 9-5). The internal jugular chain of nodes is located beneath the sternocleidomastoid muscle.

Axilla.   There are five groups of lymph nodes in the axilla, draining upward and medially toward the main lymph-collecting channels. These nodes drain the upper arm and radial surface of the forearm. These are the lateral axillary nodes; the posterior axillary nodes; the central axillary nodes; the anterior axillary nodes; and the apical axillary nodes (Fig. 9-6).

Breast.   Breast lymph drains primarily to the axillary nodes. Lymph nodes receiving drainage from the breast

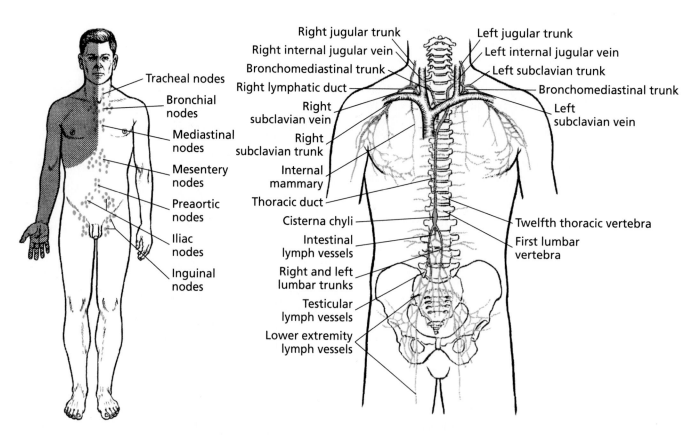

Fig. 9-3 Lymphatic drainage pathways. Shaded area of the body is drained via the right lymphatic duct, which is formed by the union of three vessels: right jugular trunk, right subclavian trunk, and right bronchomediastinal trunk. Lymph from the remainder of the body enters the venous system by way of the thoracic duct. *(From Seidel et al, 1995.)*

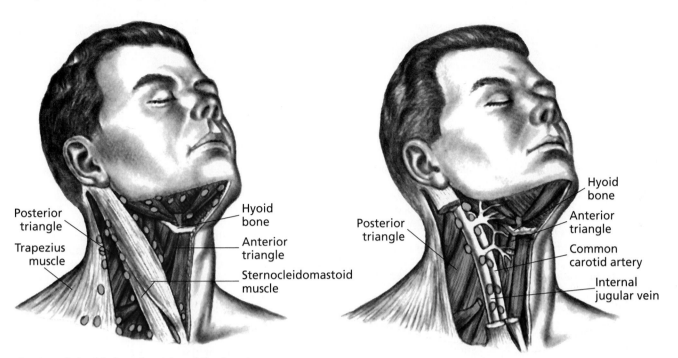

Posterior triangle

Trapezius muscle

Hyoid bone

Anterior triangle

Sternocleidomastoid muscle

Posterior triangle

Hyoid bone

Anterior triangle

Common carotid artery

Internal jugular vein

Fig. 9-4 Palpable lymph nodes of the head. *(From Seidel et al, 1995.)*

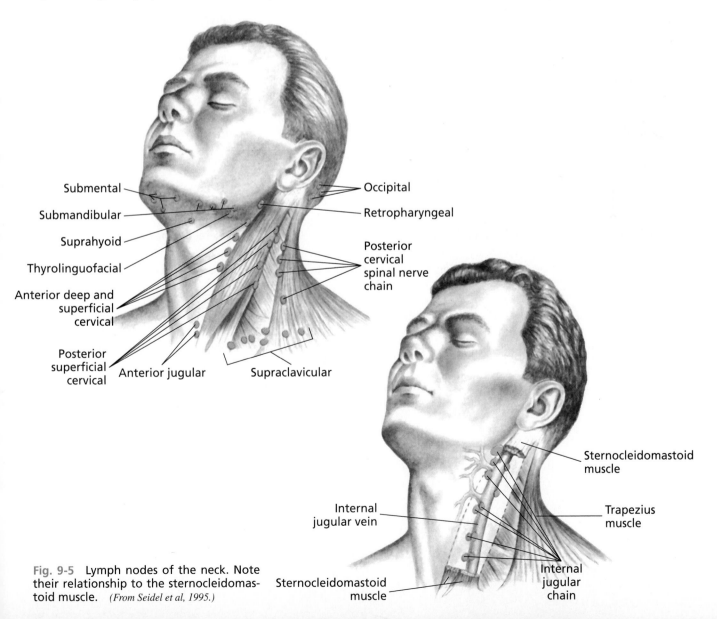

Submental

Submandibular

Suprahyoid

Thyrolinguofacial

Anterior deep and superficial cervical

Posterior superficial cervical

Anterior jugular

Occipital

Retropharyngeal

Posterior cervical spinal nerve chain

Supraclavicular

Internal jugular vein

Sternocleidomastoid muscle

Sternocleidomastoid muscle

Trapezius muscle

Internal jugular chain

Fig. 9-5 Lymph nodes of the neck. Note their relationship to the sternocleidomastoid muscle. *(From Seidel et al, 1995.)*

TABLE 9-1　Lymphatic Drainage Pattern

NODE	LOCATION	RECEIVES DRAINAGE FROM
Head		
Preauricular	In front of tragus of external ear	Scalp, external auditory canal, forehead or upper facial structures, lateral portion of eyelids
Postauricular (mastoid)	Behind ear on mastoid process	Parietal region of scalp, external auditory canal
Occipital	Midway between external occipital protuberance and mastoid process	Parietal region of scalp
Parotid	Near the jaw angle	Eyelids, frontotemporal skin, external auditory meatus, tympanic cavity
Retropharyngeal (tonsillar)	At angle of mandible	Tonsils, posterior palate, thyroid, floor of mouth
Submandibular (submaxillary)	Halfway between angle and tip of mandible	Tongue, submaxillary glands, mucosa of lips and mouth
Submental	In midline behind tip of mandible	Tongue, mucosa of lips and mouth, floor of mouth
Neck		
Anterior cervical chain	Superficial to sternocleidomastoid muscle	Skin of neck, ear
Posterior cervical chain	Along anterior edge to trapezius muscle in the posterior triangle	Posterior scalp, thyroid, posterior skin of neck
Deep cervical chain	Under sternocleidomastoid muscle; includes four separate chains extending over larynx, thyroid gland, and trachea	Larynx, thyroid, trachea, ear, and upper part of esophagus
Supraclavicular	Deep in angle formed by sternocleidomastoid muscle and clavicle	Upper abdomen, lungs, breast, arm
Axilla		
Lateral axillary (brachial)	Axilla	Breast
Posterior axillary (subscapular)	Axilla	Breast
Central axillary (intermediate)	Axilla	Breast
Anterior axillary (pectoral)	Axilla	Breast
Apical axillary (infraclavicular or subclavian)	Inferior to midclavicle	Breast
Breast		
Mammary (Rotter nodes)	Superior central breast	Superior breast
Internal mammary	Medial breast adjacent to sternal border	Medial breast
External mammary	Lateral breast	Lateral and posterior breast
Arm		
Epitrochlear	Depression above and posterior to medial condyle of humerus	Ulnar surface of forearm, fourth and fifth finger
Groin		
Superior and inferior superficial inguinal	Over inguinal canal deep in groin	Upper and lower leg; vulva and lower third of vagina drain into inguinal nodes; penis and scrotal surface; nodes of the testes drain into the abdomen

Modified from Bowers AC and Thompson JM: Clinical manual of health assessment, *ed 4, St. Louis, 1992, Mosby.*

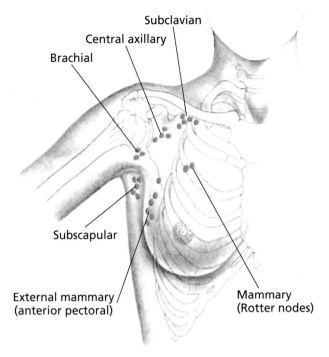

Fig. 9-6 Six groups of lymph nodes may be distinguished in the axillary fossa. *(From Seidel et al, 1995.)*

include mammary (Rotter's nodes), internal mammary, and external mammary (see Fig. 9-6).

Arm. Only the epitrochlear nodes on the medial surface of the arm above the elbow are palpable (Fig. 9-7).

Inguinal area. The superficial nodes in this area are divided into superior and inferior nodes; they receive most of the lymph drainage from the legs. In men, lymph from the penile and scrotal surfaces drains to the inguinal nodes, but nodes of the testes drain into the abdomen (Fig. 9-8).

Leg. The posterior surface of the leg, behind the knee, houses the popliteal nodes, which receive lymph from the medial portion of the lower leg (see Fig. 9-8).

THYMUS

The thymus is located behind the sternum in the superior mediastinum. This gland has its greatest importance in early life, when it produces T lymphocytes, the effector cells for cell-mediated immune reactions. With maturity into adulthood, the thymus atrophies with a loss of function.

SPLEEN

The spleen is a highly vascular organ about the size of a fist, situated in the upper left quadrant of the abdomen between the stomach and diaphragm. It is composed of two systems: the white pulp (consisting of lymphatic nodules and diffuse lymphatic tissue) and the red pulp (consisting of venous sinusoids). As a blood-forming organ early in life, the spleen stores red blood cells and destroys old ones, and filters the

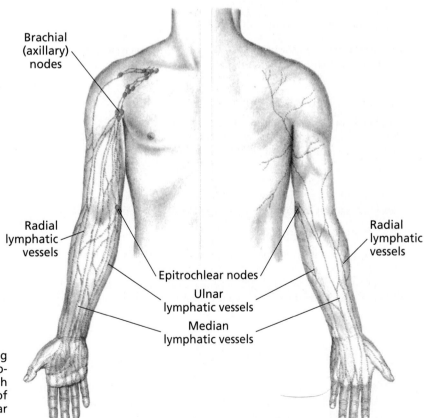

Fig. 9-7 System of deep and superficial collecting ducts, carrying lymph from upper extremity to subclavian lymphatic trunk. The only peripheral lymph center is the epitrochlear, which receives some of the collecting ducts from the pathway of the ulnar and radial nerves. *(From Seidel et al, 1995.)*

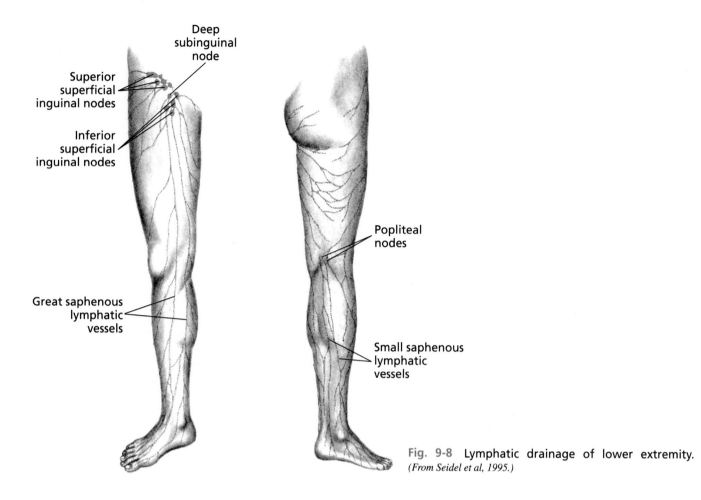

Fig. 9-8 Lymphatic drainage of lower extremity. *(From Seidel et al, 1995.)*

blood through its network of lymphocytes and macrophages to provide immunity against microorganisms and abnormal and foreign cells.

TONSILS AND ADENOIDS

The oropharyngeal tonsils, more prominent in childhood than adulthood, are largely composed of lymphoid tissue with a mucous membrane. They are located between the palatine arches on either side of the larynx, below the base of the tongue. The nasopharyngeal tonsils, also called the adenoids, are located at the nasopharyngeal border. They can obstruct the nasopharyngeal passageway if they become enlarged as a result of infection.

PEYER'S PATCHES

Peyer's patches, groups of clustered lymphoid tissue, are referred to as gut-associated lymphoid tissue (GALT). They are present in the mucosa and submucosa of the small intestine, primarily the ileum.

DEVELOPMENTAL CONSIDERATIONS

INFANTS

At 20 weeks gestation, the lymphoid system usually begins to develop, but the ability to produce antibodies is not present for the first few months of life, making infants particularly susceptible to infection, especially bacterial infection.

CHILDREN

Lymphoid tissue, plentiful in infancy, increases during childhood, especially between 6 and 9 years. The palatine tonsils also reflect this same pattern. Like all lymphoid tissue, they are much larger in early childhood than after puberty.

ADOLESCENTS

In puberty, lymph tissue regresses to adult levels.

OLDER ADULTS

Lymph nodes may decrease in both size and number with advanced age and are more likely to be fibrotic and fatty. This results in an impaired ability to resist infection. The number of lymphocytes is not reduced; however, their function declines with age. The most significant change is the decline of T lymphocyte function due to thymus gland atrophy.

PREGNANT WOMEN

During the second and third trimesters, immunoglobulin G (IgG) concentrations decrease slightly, and maternal defenses are at an increased risk for certain types of infections. IgG crosses the placenta to provide initial immunity to the neonate.

HEALTH HISTORY Lymphatic System

The focus of the history questions includes presence of infections and past history of risk factors.

● ●

QUESTIONS

RATIONALE

INFECTION

■ Do you have any lumps or swelling under the chin, along the lower jaw, in the neck, under the arm, in your arm or leg, or in the groin area? How long did the swelling last? Have you recently had an infection? Do you have difficulty swallowing? Have you noticed any "swollen glands"? How long have you had them? Have there been any recent changes in these lumps? Do they feel hard? Soft? Tender? Painful? Warm? Are they red? Have you felt fatigued or weak? Have you had a weight change? Have you had a fever? What did you do as treatment? Elevation, elastic bandage, or support stockings? Do you have recurrent infections?

◀ *Temporary lumps or swelling and tenderness indicate an acute infection. Persistent lumps indicating chronic infection may be round, rubbery, and mobile. In contrast, persistent lumps indicating a malignancy may be hard and fixed (nonmobile)*

◀ *Recurrent infections may indicate an ineffective immune system and/or increased risk of infectious disease.*

PAST HISTORY

■ Have you had any surgeries that involved removing lymph nodes (e.g., mastectomy)? What was the purpose of the surgery?
■ Have you been diagnosed with a lymphoma (e.g., Hodgkin's disease)?
■ Do you use intravenous (IV) drugs?
■ How many sexual partners do you have?
■ Have you had any blood transfusions?
■ Are you exposed to environmental radiation? Toxic chemicals? Infections?

◀ *Surgery may result in lymphedema.*

◀ *A positive response to these questions may indicate risk factors for AIDS.*

◀ *A positive response to these questions may indicate risk factors for cancer.*

FAMILY HISTORY

■ Is there a history in your family of malignancy? Anemia? Recent infectious disease?

INFANTS

The history questions are the same as for adults.

CHILDREN

The history questions are the same as for adults.

ADOLESCENTS

The history questions are the same as for adults. Be sure to inquire about exposure to infectious disease (including HIV), use of IV drugs, and sexual practices.

OLDER ADULTS

The history questions are the same as for adults, with the addition of the following.
■ Have you recently had an immunization against influenza and pneumonia?

◀ *Older adults are at greater risk for influenza and pneumonia.*

EXAMINATION Procedure and Findings

Guidelines Palpate the lymph nodes with the finger pads, using a gentle circular motion. Move the skin lightly over tissue rather than moving the fingers over the skin. Applying too much pressure may compress the node. Usually, only superficial nodes can be evaluated during the physical examination. Collections of nodes are found in the head and neck, under the arm and surrounding the breast, at the elbow, and alongside the genitalia.

EQUIPMENT   Centimeter ruler (to measure enlarged nodes or alternatively estimate the size by comparing the node to the width of your finger)
Tape measure (to document extent of edema of extremities)

TECHNIQUES and NORMAL FINDINGS

ABNORMAL FINDINGS

HEAD AND NECK

INSPECT superficial lymph nodes for Edema, Erythema, and Red Streaks. Superficial nodes should not be visible.

PALPATE nodes for Size, Consistency, Mobility, Borders, Tenderness, and Warmth. Location of nodes is shown in Fig. 9-4. Lymph nodes usually are not palpable.

Preauricular Nodes. Begin with the preauricular nodes and palpate all nodes in a specific sequence so none are missed (Fig. 9-9). You may want to use both hands, one on each side of the neck, to compare the findings. However, the submental node is easier to palpate with one hand.

■ Infection of the head and throat may be indicated when nodes are palpable bilaterally and feel large, warm, tender, firm, but freely movable.

■ Malignancy may be indicated when nodes are unilateral, hard, discrete, asymmetric, fixed, and nontender. These nodes may be attached to underlying tissue.

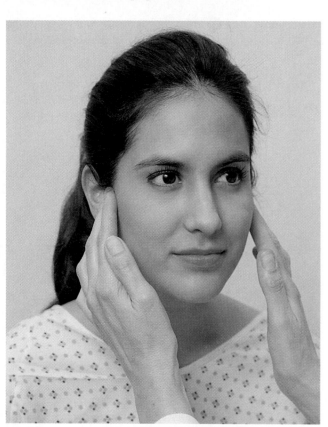

Fig. 9-9 Palpation of the preauricular nodes.

TECHNIQUES and NORMAL FINDINGS

ABNORMAL FINDINGS

Anterior and Posterior Cervical Chain. Examine the anterior and posterior cervical chain by tipping the client's head toward the side being examined, which relaxes these tissues. Palpate these nodes superficially first, then more deeply into soft tissues on either side of the sternocleidomastoid muscle (Fig. 9-10). The deep posterior cervical nodes are palpated at the anterior border of the trapezius muscle.

Supraclavicular nodes. Palpate the supraclavicular nodes by having the client hunch the shoulders forward and flex the chin toward the side being examined, which makes the node more accessible (Fig. 9-11). An alternate approach is to palpate the supraclavicular nodes by standing behind the client. The examiner places fingers into the medial supraclavicular fossa, deep into the clavicle and adjacent to the sternocleidomastoid muscle. Instruct the client to take a deep breath while you press deeply behind the clavicles. As the client inspires, enlarged supraclavicular nodes will be felt.

■ If nodes are enlarged and tender, check the structures they drain for the source of the problem. For example, an enlarged submental node may be caused by facial acne; an enlarged supraclavicular node may indicate thoracic or abdominal pathology such as carcinoma, lymphoma, sarcoidosis, AIDS, syphilis, or tuberculosis.

■ Detection of supraclavicular nodes should always be considered cause for concern.

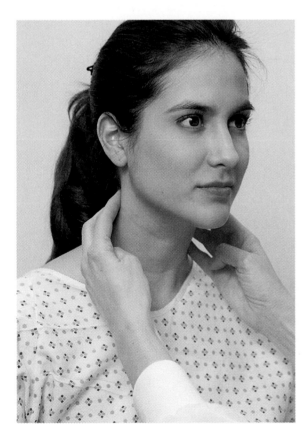

Fig. 9-10 Palpation of the posterior superficial cervical chain nodes.

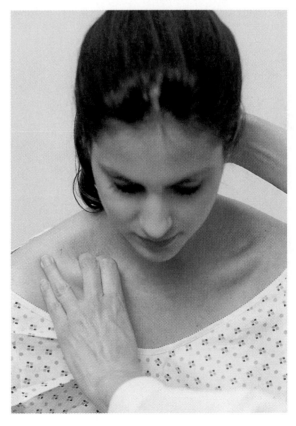

Fig. 9-11 Palpation of the supraclavicular nodes.

TECHNIQUES and NORMAL FINDINGS   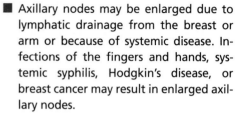 **ABNORMAL FINDINGS**

AXILLARY AND BREAST AREAS

PALPATE axillary nodes.

PALPATE nodes for Size, Consistency, Mobility, Borders, Tenderness, and Warmth. *Palpable* nodes are shown in Fig. 9-6. Support the client's arm on your contralateral arm or, alternatively, flex the client's elbow and lay the forearm across your arm (Fig. 9-12). Then place the palm of your examining hand flat into the axilla. Slightly cup the fingers of the examining hand and insert them high into the axilla. Let the soft tissues roll between your fingers, the chest wall, and muscles as you palpate. Rotate your fingers and palm, feeling the nodes. Also palpate the anterior, posterior, and lateral areas of the axillae. For the ticklish client, use a firm, deliberate, yet gentle touch. Lymph nodes of the breast are normally not palpable.

- Axillary nodes may be enlarged due to lymphatic drainage from the breast or arm or because of systemic disease. Infections of the fingers and hands, systemic syphilis, Hodgkin's disease, or breast cancer may result in enlarged axillary nodes.
- Enlarged nodes can be felt "popping" out from under the fingers.

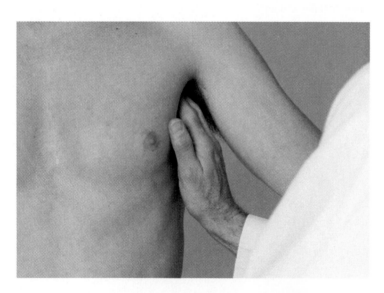

Fig. 9-12   Soft tissues of the axilla are gently rolled against the chest wall and the muscles surrounding the axilla. *(From Seidel et al, 1995.)*

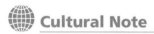 **Cultural Note**

Women of Asian, Hispanic, and American Indian or Alaskan Native origin are frequently quite modest and may be uncomfortable with examination of the breast and groin areas.

TECHNIQUES and NORMAL FINDINGS

ABNORMAL FINDINGS

ARM

PALPATE nodes for Size, Consistency, Mobility, Borders, Tenderness, and Warmth. Flex the client's arm to a 90° angle and palpate below the elbow posterior to the medial condyle of the humerus (Fig. 9-13).

■ Enlargement and tenderness may be associated with infection of the ulnar aspect of the forearm and the fourth and fifth fingers.

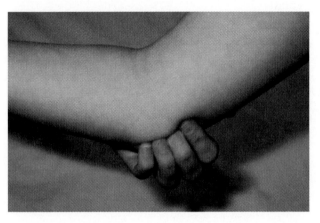

Fig. 9-13 Palpation for epitrochlear lymph nodes is performed in the depression above and posterior to the medial condyle of the humerus. *(From Seidel et al, 1995.)*

GROIN

Inguinal nodes.

PALPATE nodes for Size, Consistency, Mobility, Borders, Tenderness, and Warmth. With client in supine position, lightly palpate with finger pads in the area just below the inguinal ligament and on the inner aspect of the thigh at the groin (Fig. 9-14). The inguinal nodes are small, mobile nodes, some of which may be nontender. It may not be possible to palpate them at all, but they should be smooth and soft if they can be felt. Moving inward toward the genitalia, you can locate the anatomy using the mnemonic NAVEL: *N*, nerve; *A*, artery; *V*, vein; *E*, empty space; *L*, lymph nodes.

■ Enlarged, tender, firm, warm, and freely movable nodes indicate an inflammatory process.

A
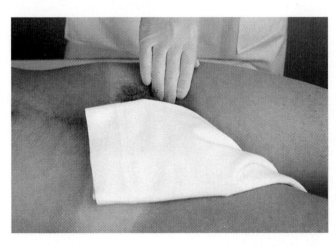

B
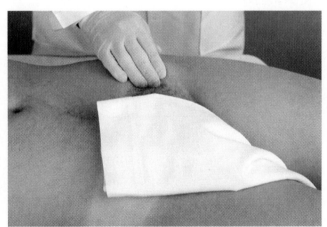

Fig. 9-14 **A,** Palpation of inferior superficial inguinal (femoral) lymph nodes. **B,** Palpation of superior superficial inguinal lymph nodes. *(From Seidel et al, 1995.)*

AGE-RELATED VARIATIONS

NEWBORNS

■ FINDINGS

Normally the newborn's cervical and inguinal lymph nodes are not palpable. The breast tissue itself may be enlarged and secrete a milky substance in response to maternal estrogen, but this resolves over the first few days or weeks after birth. Inguinal nodes may be enlarged due to diaper rash.

CHILDREN

■ APPROACH

Often children are ticklish during assessment of lymph nodes, particularly in the neck and axilla. A firm palpation and assurance that you are not trying to tickle them is needed.

■ FINDINGS

Lymph nodes up to 3 mm may be palpable normally in children and may reach 1 cm in the cervical and inguinal areas, but are discrete, mobile, and nontender. The term "shotty" may be used to describe small, firm, and mobile nodes occurring as a normal variation in children. It is not unusual to find enlarged postauricular and occipital nodes in children under 2 years of age. Likewise, cervical and submandibular nodal enlargements are more frequent in older children. Thus age of the client should be considered in your decision to evaluate further lymph node enlargement. When tender, fixed nodes greater than 1 cm are found, their presence should be correlated with the overall health history of the child. Enlarged, tender nodes may occur after immunizations or upper respiratory infection.

ADOLESCENTS

■ FINDINGS

At puberty lymph tissue begins to atrophy so that nodes are no longer palpable. Multiple discrete or matted nodes should be investigated further, as should nodes that are warm to the touch or in areas where the skin is erythematous (red).

OLDER ADULTS

■ FINDINGS

As with younger adults, the lymph nodes are generally not palpable. The size of lymph nodes decreases with advancing age because of loss of lymphocyte function.

CLIENTS WITH SITUATIONAL VARIATIONS

CLIENTS WHO HAVE HAD A RADICAL MASTECTOMY

■ FINDINGS

Surgical excision of malignant tissue requires the removal of surrounding lymph nodes to prevent metastasis of the cancer to other sites. As a result, edema develops, called *lymphedema,* because lymph nodes are no longer present to drain fluid from the interstitial spaces. After a radical mastectomy, lymphedema may develop in the upper arm on the operative side. Clients with lymphedema should be carefully assessed for adequate peripheral circulation and range of motion. Lymphedema is further discussed in the Common Problems/Conditions section later in this chapter.

IMMUNOSUPPRESSED CLIENTS

■ APPROACH

Immunosuppressed clients are at great risk for developing infections and should be separated from other clients who might be infectious. These clients might include those who are taking large doses of corticosteroids to treat an autoimmune disease or inflammatory condition. Also in this category are clients who have had an organ transplant and are receiving immunosuppressive therapy.

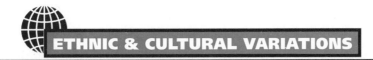

ETHNIC & CULTURAL VARIATIONS

■ APPROACH

Modesty may be an issue for the client undergoing examination of the nodes in the breast or groin areas. This may be a particularly sensitive issue for women in Asian, Hispanic, and American Indian or Alaskan Native cultures and may be ameliorated by use of a female examiner and careful use of draping and privacy.

■ FINDINGS

There is no evidence in the literature to date to indicate that lymph nodes vary in normal character or location among various racial or ethnic groups.

E X A M I N A T I O N S U M M A R Y
Lymphatic System

The lymphatic system is examined region by region during the examination of related body parts (head and neck, breast and axilla, arm, and groin).

Head and Neck *(pp. 172-173)*
- Inspect the visible nodes for:
  Edema
  Erythema
  Red streaks
- Palpate nodes for:
  Size
  Consistency
  Mobility
  Borders
  Tenderness
  Warmth

Axillary and Breast Areas *(p. 174)*
- Palpate nodes for:
  Size
  Consistency
  Mobility
  Borders
  Tenderness
  Warmth

Arm *(p. 175)*
- Palpate nodes for:
  Size
  Consistency
  Mobility
  Borders
  Tenderness
  Warmth

Groin *(p. 175)*
- Palpate nodes for:
  Size
  Consistency
  Mobility
  Borders
  Tenderness
  Warmth

COMMON PROBLEMS/CONDITIONS
associated with the Lymphatic System

IMMUNE DEFICIENCY

■ ***Acquired Immunodeficiency Syndrome (AIDS):*** Caused by human immunodeficiency virus (HIV), resulting in a defect in cell-mediated immunity. Loss of helper T lymphocytes leads to progressive loss of immune competence with development of opportunistic infections, impairment of central nervous system, chronic wasting, and often malignancy. The Centers for Disease Control and Prevention have classified the disease into four groups based on the pathophysiology as immune function declines. The virus can be transmitted to others at all stages of the disease. Group I is the acute infection when the client's body develops antibodies against the HIV. When these antibodies are detected, the client is HIV-positive. This acute infection can occur within 1 to 8 weeks after infection with HIV, and produces flu-like symptoms that resolve completely. Group II is an asymptomatic period when the client is HIV-positive without laboratory indicators of immune deficiency. This stage in the disease has been called the "clinical latency" period due to its lack of symptoms. Group III develops when symptoms of persistent generalized lymphadenopathy (longer than 3 months), fever or diarrhea, and weight loss occur. Group IV includes symptoms such as diarrhea or fever for more than one month as well as dementia, neuropathy, malignancies, and opportunistic infections (Centers for Disease Control and Prevention, 1993). Common opportunistic infections associated with AIDS are pneumocystis carinii pneumonia, cytomegalovirus (CMV), herpes simples, herpes zoster, *Candida albicans, Cryptococcus* organisms, *Toxoplasma gondii, Cryptosporidium* organisms, and *Mycobacterium* tuberculosis. Malignancies often occur, especially Kaposi's sarcoma (Fig. 9-15) and non-Hodgkin's lymphoma. In children, although there is a prolonged clinical latency period, initial signs of AIDS may be indicated by parotid enlargement resembling mumps, anemia, thrombocytopenia, chronic diarrhea, and recurrent infections.

■ ***Lymphedema:*** The excessive collection of fluid in the interstitial spaces due to inadequate drainage from blocked or infected lymphatic channels. Congenital lymphedema (Milroy disease) is the hypoplasia and maldevelopment of the lymph system. Acquired lymphedema results from trauma to the ducts of regional lymph nodes (particularly axillary and inguinal) after surgery or metastasis. Lymphedema is nonpitting, and the overlying skin will eventually thicken and feel tougher than usual.

■ ***Malignant neoplasms:*** Can be spread by lymph that drains from the primary site of malignant neoplastic growth. The lymph node may be hard, fixed to surrounding tissue, and nontender. Malignant lymphomas, including Hodgkin's disease, cause lymph nodes to be large, discrete, nontender, and firm to rubbery. Enlarged nodes usually are unilateral and localized; however, chronic lymphocytic leukemia causes generalized lymphadenopathy. Hodgkin's disease is a malignant lymphoma characterized by a painless, progressive enlargement of lymphoid tissue, usually first evident by the cervical lymph nodes, splenomegaly, and atypical macrophages. It occurs in adolescents and young adults as well as persons over 50 years of age.

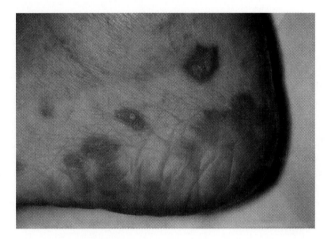

Fig. 9-15 Kaposi's sarcoma of the heel and lateral foot. *(From Grimes, 1991.)*

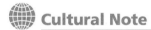 **Cultural Note**

AIDS is the leading cause of death for Hispanic and African-American men age 25 to 44 years and the second leading cause of death for African-American women.

ACUTE INFLAMMATION

■ *Epstein-Barr virus mononucleosis* (infectious mononucle-osis): Occurs at any age but is most common in adolescents and young adults. Mononucleosis is spread person to person by the oropharyngeal route (by saliva). The incubation period is 4 to 6 weeks, and the period of communicability is prolonged; pharyn-geal secretions may persist for a year after the illness. Initial signs and symptoms include pharyngitis with fever, malaise, and fatigue. Splenomegaly, hepatomegaly, and/or maculopapular rash may be noted. The affected nodes may be generalized, but are more commonly palpated in the anterior and posterior cervi-cal chains. The nodes vary in firmness and are generally discrete and occasionally tender.

■ *Acute lymphangitis:* An inflammation of one or more lym-phatic vessels, usually resulting from an acute streptococcal in-fection of one of the extremities. It is characterized by fine red streaks extending from the infected area to the axilla or groin and by fever, chills, headache, and myalgia. Inspect and palpate distal to the inflammation for sites of infection, particularly in-terdigitally.

■ *Acute lymphadenitis:* An inflammatory condition of lymph nodes usually resulting from systemic neoplastic disease, bacter-ial infection, or other inflammatory condition. The involved nodes are enlarged, firm, and tender (Fig. 9-16). The surround-ing tissue becomes edematous and skin appears erythematous, usually within 72 hours. The location of the affected node is in-dicative of the site or origin of disease. Other forms include actinomycotic adenitis resulting from dental disease and cat scratch disease or *Pasteurella multocida* infection at the site of a scratch or bite from a dog or cat. Mycobacterial lymphadenitis in the presence of tuberculosis is characterized by enlarged nodes without warmth that may or may not be slightly tender.

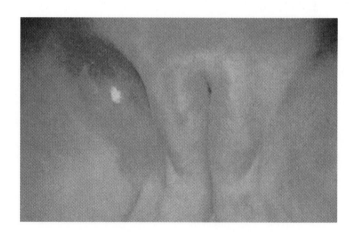

Fig. 9-16   Acute lymphadenitis.   *(From Zitelli, 1992.)*

■ *Streptococcal pharyngitis:* An inflammation of the phar-ynx and surrounding lymph tissue (tonsils). It is commonly seen in school-age children. Anterior cervical nodes are commonly palpated and tend to be firm, discrete, mobile and tender. Ac-companying signs and symptoms include fever greater than 101° F (38.3° C), sore throat with dysphagia, and erythematous tonsils and pharynx with white or yellow exudate.

Sample Documentation & Nursing Diagnosis

CASE 1   16-year-old male with sore throat and fever.

Subjective

States, "I just feel tired all the time." Reports several days of headache and malaise. Unable to attend school or practice sports; sore throat with dysphagia and fever 38.2° to 38.6° C (100.8° to 101.6° F), treated with acetaminophen with temporary relief. Reports no malignancy, chronic illness, recent surgery, or exposure to infectious disease. Does not use street drugs, not sexually active. No family history of malignancy, blood disease, or other chronic diseases.

Objective

Temperature   38.2° C (100.8° F).

Pulse   96.

Respiratory rate   20.

Blood pressure   110/70.

16-year-old male appears tired, but cooperative and reliable.

ENT   Tympanic membranes clear bilaterally, observable landmarks without redness or bulging; turbinates pink, moist without exudate; oropharynx is erythematous, with tonsillar hyperplasia without exudate. Anterior and posterior cervical nodes are enlarged bilaterally, several palpable, 2 × 1.5 cm, discrete, tender, and mobile.

Chest   Lungs clear to auscultation bilaterally.

Skin   Maculopapular confluent rash noted on chest and back. Skin warm and dry with elastic turgor.

Abdomen   Flat, bowel sounds × 4, nontender to palpation. No organomegaly.

• •

Nursing Diagnosis #1

Pain related to infectious process in oropharynx.

Defining Characteristics   Fatigue, verbalized pain in throat.

Nursing Diagnosis #2

Risk for fluid volume deficit related to pain and inability to drink fluids normally.

Defining Characteristics   Factors influencing fluid needs (fever) or pain on swallowing.

Sample Documentation & Nursing Diagnosis

CASE 2   5-year-old Hispanic female who needs a physical examination.

Subjective

Child needs a physical examination before starting kindergarten. Five-year-old Hispanic girl accompanied by mother. Present health status: no allergies, takes no medications on a regular basis; has had diphtheria-tetanus-pertussis (DPT), hepatitis B, and oral poliovirus vaccine; last physical examination was 1 year ago. Passed Denver Developmental Screening Test appropriate for her age.

Past medical history   Child was full-term vaginal delivery without complications. Has had no hospitalizations since birth; had chicken pox at age 3, has annual upper respiratory infection treated with over-the-counter drugs.

Family history   No history of cancer, hypertension, tuberculosis, or diabetes mellitus.

Social history   Only child, attends day care while parents work.

Review of systems   Noncontributory.

Objective

Temperature   36.8° C (98.4° F).

Pulse   86.

Respiratory rate   22.

Blood pressure   94/56

Weight   17 kg (38 lb).

Height   110 cm (44 in).

Lymph system only is documented: Small (about 5 mm), firm, discrete, movable, nontender nodes palpated postauricular and occipital bilaterally; nontender, shotty nodes found along left superficial cervical chain; otherwise no other nodes felt at supraclavicular, axillary, epitrochlear, or inguinal sites.

• •

Nursing Diagnosis

Health-seeking behaviors related to maintaining daughter's health behaviors.

Defining Characteristics   Stated or observed unfamiliarity with wellness community resources, verbalized lack of knowledge in health promotion.

HEALTH PROMOTION

■ **Infection** Risk factors that alter the host response to infectious agents include smoking, alcohol intake, dehydration, and inadequate dietary intake (Grimes, 1991). You can reduce infections by maintaining a healthy immune system. This is accomplished by eliminating modifiable risk factors, eating a balanced diet, getting adequate sleep, and managing your stress.

Selecting your diet from the food pyramid provides all of the essential nutrients. Malnutrition alters the immune system. For example, deficits in vitamin A reduce the number of T lymphocytes, while deficits in vitamins B_6 and E reduce the antibody response to vaccines. Inadequate iron creates ineffective white blood cells. Insufficient zinc causes abnormalities in cellular and humoral immunity (Rolfes and DeBruyne, 1990).

During periods of sleep, rest, relaxation, meditation, or visualization, potent immune-enhancing compounds are released and many immune functions are increased (Murray, 1994). They are also useful in reducing stress. The adrenal gland secretes more glucocorticoid (cortisol) than usual in response to stress as a protective mechanism. One action of prolonged stress, however, is extended release of cortisol, which interferes with immune and allergic responses. For example, cortisol decreases the number of lymphocytes, decreases the rate of antibody formation, and masks the signs of infection. Thus use of stress reduction techniques can help to lower cortisol levels, which improves immune system function.

??????? STUDY QUESTIONS ???????

1. What is the main function of the lymphatic system? Explain the role of the lymphocytes in carrying out this function.

2. Describe the formation and circulation of lymphatic fluid.

3. List and describe the position of the lymph nodes in the head, neck, axilla, breast, arm, leg, and inguinal area.

4. What two age groups are more susceptible to infection? Explain why.

5. What questions would you ask of the client who has enlarged lymph nodes?

6. What past history information should you collect when assessing the lymph system?

7. Describe how to palpate lymph nodes.

8. Describe the sequence used for examination of the nodes.

9. Describe in detail how to examine the lymph nodes in the axillary and breast area.

10. Identify the location of the inguinal lymph nodes. How are they distinguished from other anatomic structures such as arteries or nerves?

11. What does it indicate if head and neck nodes are large, warm, tender, and moveable? What if they are hard, fixed, and nontender?

12. List three conditions that may cause enlarged axillary lymph nodes.

13. What techniques are used for the ticklish child during a lymph node examination?

14. What are the six characteristics that lymph nodes are examined for?

15. Review the effects that HIV and AIDS have on the lymph system.

16. List the characteristics of the following acute inflammatory diseases of the lymph system: Epstein-Barr mononucleosis, acute lymphangitis, acute lymphadenitis, and streptococcal pharyngitis.

17. List and discuss four strategies to assist in maintaining a healthy immune system.

CHAPTER 10

Head and Neck

ANATOMY AND PHYSIOLOGY

The bones of the head and neck house and protect not only the brain but also the components of the special senses of vision, hearing, smell, and taste.

The seven bones of the head are fused together and covered by the scalp. These seven bones include two frontal, two temporal, and one occipital bone (Fig. 10-1). The face consists of eight bones—the nasal, frontal, lacrimal, sphenoid, zygomatic, ethmoid, and maxillary bones and the movable mandible (Fig. 10-2).

The eyes, ears, nose, and mouth are basically symmetric; the facial muscles are innervated by cranial nerves V and VII. The ophthalmic, maxillary, and mandibular sensory branches are innervated by cranial nerve V. Facial expression is controlled through cranial nerve VII.

The neck is formed by the cervical vertebrae, which are supported by ligaments and by the sternocleidomastoid and trapezius muscles; these also give the neck its movement. This mobility is greatest at the level of C4-5 or C5-6.

Major structures of the neck include the sternocleidomastoid muscle, the hyoid bone, the thyroid cartilage, the cricoid cartilage, the thyroid gland, and the trachea. The thyroid gland lies across the trachea and tucks back behind the sternocleidomastoid muscle. The middle section of the thyroid is called the *isthmus* of the thyroid (Fig. 10-3).

The relationships of the neck muscles to each other and to adjacent bones create anatomic landmarks called *triangles.* The anterior triangle is formed by the medial borders of the sternocleidomastoid muscles and the mandible. Inside this triangle lies the hyoid bone, cricoid cartilage, trachea, thyroid, and anterior cervical lymph nodes. The posterior triangle is formed by the trapezius and sternocleidomastoid muscles and clavicle; it contains the posterior cervical lymph nodes (Fig. 10-4, *A*).

Lymph nodes of the head and neck occur in chains and clusters. Superficial nodes are located in subcutaneous connective tissue, and deeper nodes lie beneath the muscles (Fig. 10-4, *B*). The deep cervical chain lies beneath the sternocleidomastoid muscle. Other cervical chains can be palpated. Lymph nodes are round and smooth and normally not palpable.

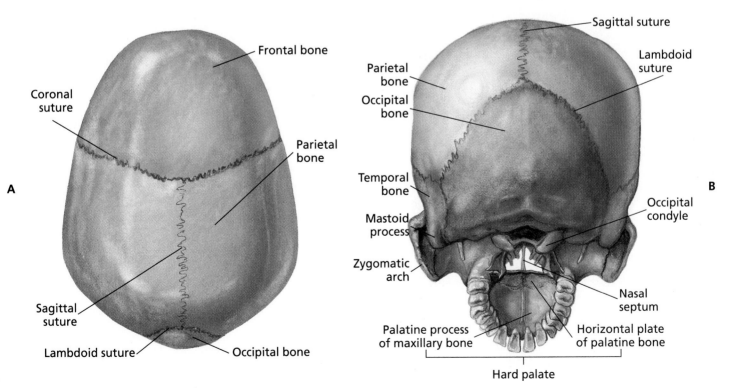

Fig. 10-1   **A,** Bones of the head as seen from the superior view. **B,** Bones of the head as seen from the posterior view.   *(From Seeley, Stephens and Tate, 1995.)*

185

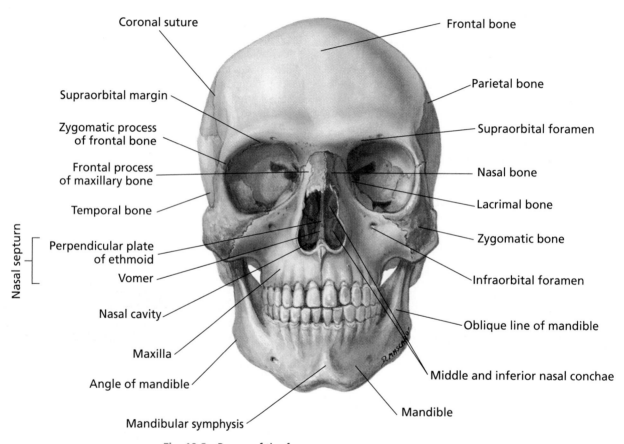

Coronal suture

Frontal bone

Supraorbital margin

Parietal bone

Zygomatic process
of frontal bone

Supraorbital foramen

Frontal process
of maxillary bone

Nasal bone

Temporal bone

Lacrimal bone

Nasal septum

Perpendicular plate
of ethmoid

Zygomatic bone

Vomer

Infraorbital foramen

Nasal cavity

Oblique line of mandible

Maxilla

Middle and inferior nasal conchae

Angle of mandible

Mandible

Mandibular symphysis

Fig. 10-2 Bones of the face. *(From Seeley, Stephens and Tate, 1995.)*

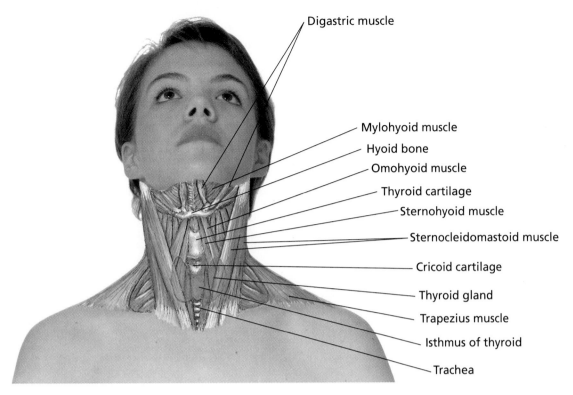

Fig. 10-3   Major structures of the neck.

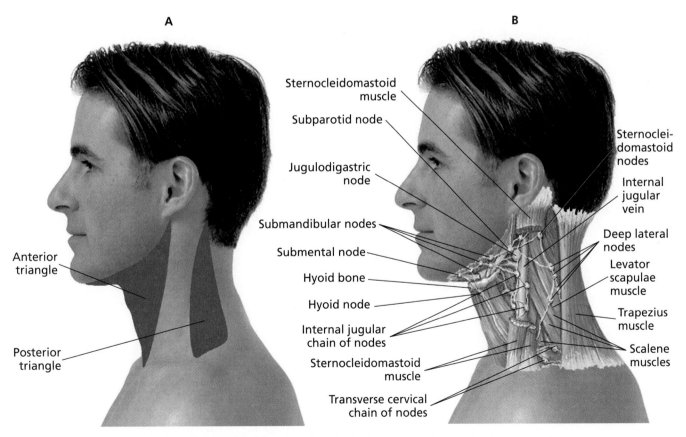

Fig. 10-4   Anatomic landmarks of the lateral head and neck. **A,** Anterior and posterior triangles of the neck. **B,** Major muscles and lymph nodes of the neck.

DEVELOPMENTAL CONSIDERATIONS

INFANTS

The seven cranial bones are soft and separated by the sagittal, coronal, and lambdoid sutures at birth; these intersect at membranous spaces called anterior and posterior fontanels, which permit expansion of the skull to accommodate brain growth (Fig. 10-5). Ossification of the sutures begins at about 6 years of age when brain growth is completed; it is not finished until adulthood. However, the fontanels ossify earlier, the posterior fontanel closing by 2 months, and the anterior fontanel closing by 24 months. Passage through the vaginal canal at birth may temporarily alter the shape of the newborn skull as cranial bones overlap or move to new positions. Within days the skull resumes its appropriate shape and size.

ADOLESCENTS

Subtle changes in facial appearance occur throughout childhood. In the male adolescent the nose and thyroid cartilage enlarge and facial hair develops, emerging first on the upper lip, then the cheeks, lower lip, and chin. Female adolescents may also have increased facial hair. This is most prevalent in women of Eastern European descent.

PREGNANT WOMEN

Glandular tissue hyperplasia and increased vascularity cause a slight enlargement of the thyroid gland. Although thyroid function tests are altered, thyroid function remains unchanged.

OLDER ADULTS

The rate of T_4 production and degradation gradually decreases, and the thyroid gland becomes more fibrotic.

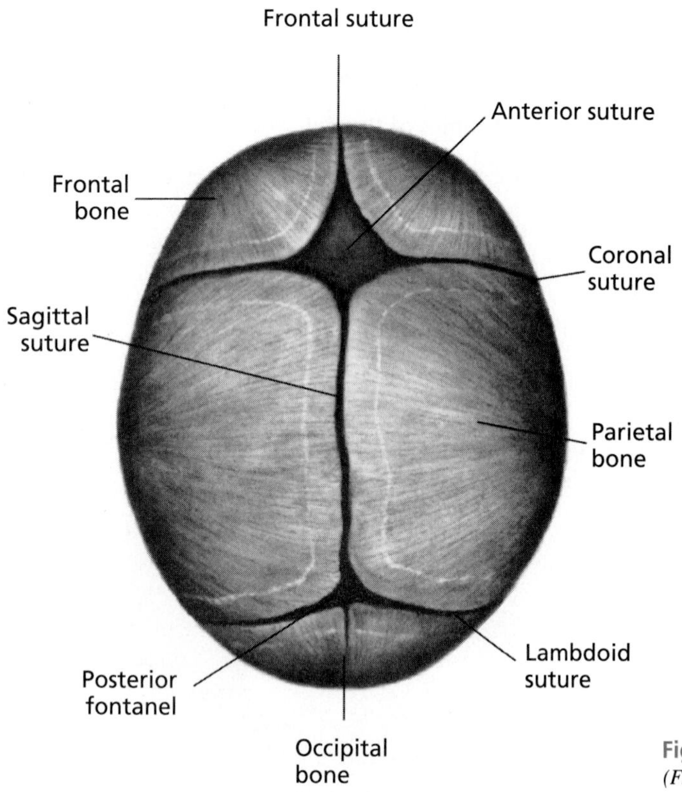

Fig. 10-5   Sutures and fontanels on the infant skull. *(From Wong, 1995.)*

HEALTH HISTORY Head and Neck

The history related to the head and neck should focus primarily on common problems in the area of the head such as headache, dizziness, and head injury. Next, questioning should focus on the neck, including neck pain, stiff neck, or decreased range of motion. Finally, questioning should focus on thyroid function. History questions related to the neck's lymphatic functioning and scalp, hair, and facial characteristics are discussed in Chapters 8 and 11.

● ●

QUESTIONS

RATIONALE

HEAD

HEADACHE

Everyone seems to have an occasional headache, so your questions should focus on headaches that are not usual or headaches that are debilitating to the client.

Pattern

■ Do you have frequent or severe headaches? How often? Do they start gradually or suddenly?

Many times a headache may be a sign of stress. At other times, headaches may be a sign of chemical imbalance in the body or even a sign of a more serious pathologic condition.

■ Where do they generally start? Forehead? Temples? Eye area? Over the sinus? In the back of the neck at the base of the skull?

■ When do you usually get the headache? When does it start? Early morning? During the day? During the night? At work?

Tension headaches *tend to be located in the front or back of the head,* migraines a*re usually in the eye area, and* cluster headaches *produce pain over the eye, temple, forehead, and cheek areas. Some types of headaches occur on only one side of the head and others involve both sides.*

Characteristics

■ What is the pain like? Constant? Throbbing or pounding? Shooting? Dull or nagging ache? Sharp? Is there pressure over a single area or in general? Does it feel like a band around your head? Is it on one side or both? Is the headache aggravated with movement? Does it follow a pattern?

Tension headaches *are described as viselike, whereas migraines and temporal arteritis produce throbbing pain.*

Cluster headaches *may occur with alcohol ingestion or daytime naps. They may occur more than once a day and last for less than an hour to about 2 hours. They may follow this pattern for a couple of months and then disappear for months or years.*

Migraine headaches *may occur at periodic intervals and may last from a few hours to 1 to 3 days. They may be triggered by various factors, including alcohol, stress or relief of stress, menstruation, and eating foods high in tyramine such as chocolate or cheese or drinking red wine.*

QUESTIONS

RATIONALE

 Cultural Note

> African Americans have a high incidence of hypertension, and headaches may be one of the few associated symptoms.

Associated symptoms
- What other associated symptoms do you have? Nausea? Vomiting? Diarrhea?
- Do you have blurred vision? Double vision (diplopia)? Sensitivity to light (photophobia)? Increased lacrimation? Nasal discharge?
- Do you have ringing in the ears (tinnitus)? Feelings of numbness (paresthesia)? *If yes:* Is it always present or just sometimes?
- Do you have high blood pressure? *If yes:* How is it being managed? What kind of medication are you taking? How much? How often?

Migraines may be accompanied by visual disturbances, nausea, and vomiting. Cluster headaches may occur with nasal stuffiness or discharge, red teary eyes, or drooping eyelids. Tension headaches occur with stress and anxiety.

Precipitating factors
- What factors do you feel may bring the headache on? Stress? Fatigue? Food additives? Sudden movement or exercise? Alcohol or medications? Weather? Allergies? Long periods without eating? Menstrual cycle? Do you have other health problems, such as a history of head injury or seizures?

Illnesses that may be associated with headaches include hypertension, hypothyroidism, and vasculitis. Medications that may actually cause headaches include oral contraceptives, estrogen preparations, and bronchodilators.

Movement or rest may increase the headache, with migraines requiring rest for relief and cluster headaches requiring movement. Migraines are frequently associated with menstrual periods.

Efforts to treat
- What do you usually do to treat the headache? Sleep? Take pain medication? *If medication:* What kind? Is the medication effective in relieving the pain? How often do you take the medication?

Knowing what brings relief may help in determining the cause of the headache.

DIZZINESS
- Do you ever feel dizzy or lightheaded, as though you cannot keep your balance and may fall? *If so:* When and how often does this occur?
- What do you do when the dizziness occurs? Does it interfere with your activities of daily living?

First, it is very important to define what the client means when he or she reports a history of dizziness. It may mean different things to different people. Dizziness may be a result of imbalance, loss of balance, medication, an inner ear infection, or a more serious problem such as Meniere's disease.

- Does the dizziness ever occur when you are driving the car or operating machinery? Have you ever fallen as a result of the dizziness?

It is important to ensure client safety and to inquire whether the client is at risk during periods of dizziness.

HEAD INJURY
- What happened? What caused the injury? Did you fall or get hit by something? Did you have a seizure? Feel lightheaded? Black out?

Note any predisposing factors, such as epilepsy or a seizure disorder, a blackout, poor vision, dizziness, cardiac irregularity, or light-headedness. Note also dangerous environmental conditions that may have led to the injury, such as wet floors, an unsecured throw rug, or getting up too fast.

QUESTIONS

RATIONALE

 Cultural Note

> Motor vehicle crashes remain the leading cause of morbidity and mortality among American Indians and Alaskan Natives, with age-adjusted mortality rates three times the U.S. average. Head injuries figure prominently in these statistics.

■ What was your level of consciousness following the injury? (It may be best if someone other than the client answers this question.) Do you remember what happened? Do you have difficulty with thinking or your memory?

■ What were your symptoms following the injury? Did you have head or neck pain? Cuts (lacerations)? A loss of consciousness? Blurred or double vision? Drainage from your nose or ears? Nausea or vomiting? Incontinence?

◄ *If the head injury has just occurred and the client reports a loss of consciousness, he or she should be referred to a physician or hospital for full evaluation of a possible significant head injury such as a skull fracture or subdural or epidural hematoma. If, however, the head injury occurred in the past and the client is now relaying ongoing symptoms to the nurse, a clustering or pattern of the symptoms may be used to determine an ongoing potential problem that the client is having.*

■ Are you currently taking any medications because of your head injury? *If so:* What and how often?

◄ *It is important to assess the client's compliance with medications such as anticonvulsants. If the client is noncompliant, there is an increased risk for seizures.*

NECK

NECK PAIN, STIFF NECK, OR LIMITED MOTION

Symptom onset
■ Do you have any neck pain? Did it occur suddenly or as the result of an injury or fall or from lifting something or twisting? Did the pain start gradually over time?
■ *If there has been no injury, ask:* Have you been ill? Do you have a fever? A rash? A headache?

Characteristics
■ Does the pain radiate to the arm, shoulders, hands? Down the back?
■ Is there a limitation of movement or pain with movement? Is the pain relieved by movement?
■ Do you have any tingling or numbness of the neck, shoulders, arms, or hands?
■ Does the pain or stiffness keep you from sleeping or working?
■ Overall, is the problem getting better? Getting worse? Staying about the same?

Treatment methods
■ What makes the pain better or worse? What have you done to alleviate the pain or stiffness? Medications? Applying heat or cold? Physical therapy?

◄ *It is important to differentiate between neck pain and stiffness caused by sudden injury or the slow onset of pain resulting from stress and strain and neck pain and stiffness secondary to systemic illness. Stiffness that begins suddenly and is accompanied by fever and headache may indicate meningeal inflammation. Likewise, a myocardial infarction may cause radiating pain up into the neck and even the jaw.*

◄ *Pain and tension may create a cycle of further pain and tension, thereby increasing anxiety and causing related problems.*

QUESTIONS

RATIONALE

NECK MASS

- When did you first notice a lump (mass) in your neck? Is this the first time that you have had it examined? *If not:* When and where was it evaluated before? What were you told during that examination?
- Does the lump or mass hurt?
- Has it changed in size? *If so:* How? Does it get large and then small? Does it stay about the same? Or is it getting larger?
- Have you had recent ear infection? An infection of a tooth or in your mouth? A sore throat? Fever?

◀ *A lump or mass in the neck may be a swollen lymph node secondary to an infection or it may be an enlargement of the thyroid or goiter. A careful history may help to isolate the problem.*

◀ *If the mass has had a sudden onset and the client reports a history of infection or fever, the mass is most likely enlarged lymph nodes. If, on the other hand, the mass is midline in position and has been slowly growing or present for months, it is more likely to be a neoplasm, cyst, or goiter.*

- Have you had any hoarseness of your voice since you first noticed the mass?

◀ *Hoarseness in association with an enlarged thyroid may indicate a tumor involving the laryngeal nerve.*

THYROID

There are many questions that the examiner may ask to assess thyroid functioning. The number of questions actually asked should depend on the client's individual situation. *Hyperthyroidism* is hyperactivity of the thyroid gland. The gland is usually enlarged and is secreting greater than normal amounts of thyroid hormones. *Hypothyroidism* is characterized by decreased activity of the thyroid gland. The gland may be normal size or enlarged. *Graves' disease* is pronounced hyperthyroidism associated with an enlarged thyroid gland and exophthalmos. A detailed discussion of all three conditions is presented in the Common Problems section later in this chapter.

- Have you ever been told that you have a thyroid problem? *If so:* Is it overactive or underactive? How has it been treated—surgery, medication, or irradiation?

If the client has not been previously diagnosed with a thyroid problem, ask questions to determine whether there have been changes that indicate possible thyroid problems now.

- Has your sleep pattern or energy level changed? Do you have feelings of fatigue or drowsiness during the day? Inability to sleep well at night? Has there been a change in your weight?
- Have you been feeling moody, maybe irritable or nervous? Have you had increased energy, decreased energy, or lethargy?
- Are you more sensitive to hot and cold? Are you wearing more or less clothing than the rest of your family?
- Have you recently lost more hair than usual? Have your nails become brittle or has your skin texture changed?
- Have you experienced changes in appetite, weight loss, or bowel habits?
- Has your menstrual cycle changed?
- Have you had hoarseness, difficulty swallowing, or pain or tenderness in your neck?
- Have you had difficulty buttoning the collar of your shirt? Does your neck seem to be larger or swollen?

- Do you feel that your pulse is racing (tachycardia) or that your heart pounds (palpitations)?

◀ *Such changes may indicate dysfunction of the thyroid gland. A definitive determination must be confirmed by TSH, T_3, and T_4 laboratory studies.*

◀ *An enlarged thyroid may cause subtle neck swelling that may be noticed as a tight collar.*

◀ *Increased thyroid function causes an increase in metabolism and tachycardia.*

QUESTIONS

RATIONALE

INFANTS

The infant's history should focus on the mother's prenatal history, the infant's birth history, and the current situation. Ask the parent or caregiver the following questions. Reword as appropriate based on whether you are addressing the mother, father, or another caregiver.

- Did the mother use alcohol or recreational drugs while she was pregnant? How much, how often?
- Was the infant's mother treated for either hypothyroidism or hyperthyroidism during the pregnancy?
- Was the delivery vaginal or by cesarean section? Were forceps used? Were there any problems?

- Have you noticed any depression or bulging over the infant's "soft spots" (fontanels)?

- *If the infant is irritable or appears ill:* Does the infant have a fever? Diarrhea? Stiff neck? Vomiting?

◀ *These substances increase the risk for developmental, emotional, and neurologic impairment, including fetal alcohol syndrome.*

◀ *The use of forceps can increase the risk of caput succedaneum, cephalhematoma, and Bell's palsy.*

◀ *A sunken fontanel may be a sign of dehydration. A swollen or bulging fontanel may be a sign of increased cerebral swelling consistent with infection. If the infant is crying, the fontanel may also appear full or bulging.*

◀ *These signs may be consistent with meningitis.*

CHILDREN

History questions for the child focus on developmental issues, infection, and headaches. Ask the parent or caregiver the following questions:

DEVELOPMENT

- Has the child reached growth and development milestones on schedule? Has the child's head grown and the fontanels closed on schedule? Is the child's neck growing along with the body?

◀ *Delay in achieving developmental milestones may indicate some type of developmental or congenital problem. Many times problems will not be identified in young children until they show indications of developmental delay.*

INFECTION

- Have you noticed any swelling of the child's neck or has the child complained of any neck stiffness? *If so:* Does the child have any other signs of infection or illness? Fever? Sore throat? Crying with neck movement? Swollen glands?
- Does the child have headaches? *If so:* How often and how severe? Does the child ever have to stay home from school because of the headache? Has the child ever had a medical evaluation for the headaches?
- Do the headaches seem to be associated with chocolate, cheese, stress, or exercise?

HEAD INJURY RISK

Ask the child:

- Do you have a bicycle helmet? *If so:* Do you wear it when you ride your bicycle? *If so:* How often—always or occasionally?
- Do you wear a helmet or head protection when you rollerblade or play other high-risk sports?

◀ *The most common reasons for a stiff neck or swollen glands in the child is either a localized or systemic infection.*

◀ *Approximately 40% of children have headaches by age 7, 66% by age 12, and 75% by age 15. Most of these headaches are infrequent and nonrecurrent. Any variation from the usual occurrence should be noted.*

◀ *Head injury in children is a leading cause of death and disability. Determine whether the child owns a helmet. If not, provide resource material. If the child does own a helmet but does not wear it, determine the causative factors.*

QUESTIONS

RATIONALE

ADOLESCENTS

The adolescent is more likely to have problems similar to the adult than to the younger child. History questions should therefore focus on the same areas as for the adult. This may be the time of the appearance of headaches, thyroid problems, and risk of head injury.

In addition to the questions in the adult section, ask the following:

HEADACHES

- Do you think that there is a relationship between your headaches and what is going on at either home or school? If so, how do you believe that they are related?
- *For girls:* Are the headaches related to your period?

◀ *Headaches occur with about equal prevalence among males and females until around age 12. At that time headaches become more common in females because of the increasing prevalence of migraine headaches.*

HEAD INJURY RISK

- Do you routinely wear a helmet when you ride your bicycle or engage in sports where a head injury may occur? *If so:* Always or just occasionally?

◀ *Head injury among adolescents is a major cause of morbidity and mortality.*

OLDER ADULTS

The older adult may have many aches and pains and may consider them as part of the aging process. Indeed, some problems are secondary to growing older, but others are indicative of a treatable problem.

In addition to the questions in the adult section, ask the following:

HEADACHE

- Do you have high blood pressure? *If yes:* How is it being managed? What kind of medication do you take? How much? How often?

◀ *High blood pressure may cause headaches and may put the client at risk for an impending stroke.*

DIZZINESS

- Do you have episodes of dizziness? How long has it been going on? When does it most generally occur? Is it related to head or neck movements?
- Does your dizziness interfere with your daily activities? Have you fallen because you lost your balance?

◀ *Self-care and potential for injury must be assessed.*

NECK PAIN OR STIFFNESS

- How long have you had the neck pain? Did you fall or suffer some trauma or injury? Do you have pain radiating to the shoulder, arms, or chest? Have you noticed any numbness or tingling?
- What changes have you made in your daily activities because of the pain? Are you able to drive safely, work, do housework, sleep, look down when you are on the stairs?

◀ *Assess the client's ability to care for himself or herself, as well as the potential for injury.*

EXAMINATION Procedures and Findings

Guidelines The examination of the head and neck may be organized in numerous ways. For clarity, the presentation in this chapter focuses only on the characteristics of the skull and face, the symmetry and motion of the neck, and the thyroid. The presentation of the skin, hair, eyes, ears, nose, mouth, lymphatics, and pulses of the head and neck are presented elsewhere in the text. It is assumed that during the actual complete physical examination, the examiner will integrate the assessment of all sections of the head and neck into a logical sequence of examination. Refer to the following chapters:

Skin and hair: Chapter 8	*Ears:* Chapter 12
Lymphatics: Chapter 9	*Eyes:* Chapter 13
Nose and mouth: Chapter 11	*Vascular:* Chapter 15

The client should be in a gown and seated comfortably. The examination table should be situated so that the examiner can move both in front of and behind the client during the examination. (Ask the client to remove any wig or hairpiece.)

EQUIPMENT   A glass of water (for the thyroid examination)
Gloves (optional for scalp assessment)

TECHNIQUES and NORMAL FINDINGS

ABNORMAL FINDINGS

HEAD

The examination of the head includes the inspection and palpation of the skull, including inspection of the features of the face.

INSPECT the client's head for Characteristics of Facial Features and Appropriateness of Facial Expression. The client should be alert, relaxed, and engaged with the examiner.

- Note evidence of worry, pain, or abnormality in the client's expression.

 Cultural Note

> Many Asian cultures believe that the soul resides in the individual's head. The examiner should therefore ask permission before examining the head. *(Kneisl and Hutchinson, 1988.)*

INSPECT and PALPATE the skull to assess Contour and Intactness. Palpate the skull from front to back using a gentle rotary motion. Note areas of tenderness, marked protrusions, or lumps. The skull should be symmetric and should feel firm and nontender. The frontal, parietal, and bilateral occipital prominences may be felt. *Examination gloves should be worn if the client has scalp lesions, injury, or poor hygiene.*

Normocephalic is the term designating that the skull is symmetric and is appropriately proportioned for the size of the body.

- Lumps, marked protrusions, or tenderness should be differentiated to determine if they are on the scalp or actually part of the skull. Depressions or unevenness of the skull may occur secondary to skull injury.
  - *Microcephaly* is an abnormally small head.
  - *Macrocephaly* is an abnormally large head.

TECHNIQUES and NORMAL FINDINGS	ABNORMAL FINDINGS

INSPECT and PALPATE the bony structures of the face and jaw, noting Size, Symmetry, Intactness, and Tenderness. The eyebrows, palpebral fissures, nasolabial folds, and sides of the mouth should be symmetric (Fig. 10-6). (Sinus assessment is discussed in Chapter 11.) The facial bones should be symmetric and appear proportionate to the size of the head.

■ Abnormal facial structures include coarse facial hair (in women), prominent eyes (exophthalmos), pallor, uneven skin pigmentation, swelling, and abnormal facial movements (tics).
  ■ *Acromegaly* is a chronic metabolic condition that is characterized by a gradual enlargement and elongation of the bones of the face and jaw.

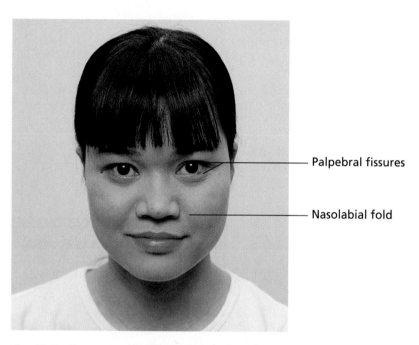

Palpebral fissures

Nasolabial fold

Fig. 10-6   Symmetry of eyebrows, palpebral fissures, nasolabial folds, and the corners of the mouth are normal findings.

 Racial Variation

There is a wide variation in the normal size and shape of the skull, bony structures of the face, and facial features within and across racial and ethnic groups. Jaws and foreheads, for example, may range from receding to prominent. Noses may be flattened or elongated, broad or narrow, large or small, straight or curved, or tilted up or down. Lips may range from full to thin, heart to oval in shape.

NECK

The examination of the neck, as presented in this chapter, includes evaluation of the range of motion of the neck and examination of the thyroid.

INSPECT the neck for Positioning in relation to the head. It should be centered, and the trapezius and sternocleidomastoid muscles should be bilaterally symmetric (Fig. 10-7). Inspect the midline position of the trachea.

■ Observe for jumpy, ratchety movement of the neck and head. Note rhythmic movements or tremor. Observe also for tics or spasms.

TECHNIQUES and NORMAL FINDINGS	ABNORMAL FINDINGS

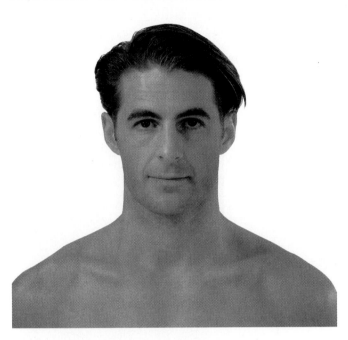

Fig. 10-7 Bilateral symmetry of the neck muscles.

INSPECT the neck for Range of Motion (ROM). Ask the client to:

- Move the chin to the chest. Movement should be 45 degrees.
- Move the head back so that the chin points toward the ceiling. Movement should be 55 degrees.
- Move the head side-to-side so the ear moves close to the shoulder. Movement should be 40 degrees.
- Rotate the head laterally to the right and then to the left. Rotation should be 70 degrees in both directions.

All movements should be controlled and smooth. *Note:* Remind the client to hold the shoulders stationary during the performance of ROM of the head and neck. "Bend your head to your shoulder; do not raise the shoulder to meet the head. Do not force range of motion beyond the range of comfort."

Instruct the client to shrug his or her shoulders. Then instruct the client to turn the head side to side against the resistance of your hands. *(This is a partial evaluation of cranial nerve XI, the spinal accessory nerve.)*

PALPATE the neck for Positioning of the anatomic structures. Palpate the neck and trachea just above the suprasternal notch (see Fig. 10-3). Palpate for the tracheal rings, cricoid cartilage, and thyroid cartilage. All structures should be midline and nontender.

■ Limited ROM or pain during movement may indicate either a systemic infection with meningeal irritation or a musculoskeletal problem.

■ Note pain or weakness of muscles or tremors. Note if the client complains of pain throughout the movement or at particular points.

■ Abnormalities include tenderness upon palpation or location of the structures in a nonmidline position.

| TECHNIQUES and NORMAL FINDINGS | ABNORMAL FINDINGS |

THYROID

INSPECT the anterior neck to Visualize the Thyroid. Instruct the client to raise the chin up as if drinking from a glass and then swallow. The thyroid gland may not be clearly visualized. The lobes of the gland may be seen as a slight thickening as the client swallows (Fig. 10-8).

■ A goiter may be seen as a fullness in the neck (Fig. 10-9).

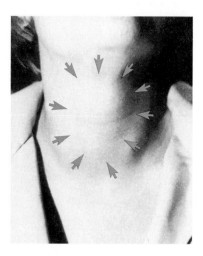

Fig. 10-8 Minimum thyroid enlargement encroaching on the sternocleidomastoid muscle. Note full appearance of the neck.

PALPATE the thyroid gland for Size, Shape, Consistency, Tenderness, and Presence of Nodules. *Caution:* The examiner's fingernails should be well trimmed. The palpation of the thyroid may be done by either an anterior or posterior approach. Although the technique used is the choice of the examiner, the anterior approach is more awkward and generally more difficult for the beginner. The examiner should choose one of the following techniques.

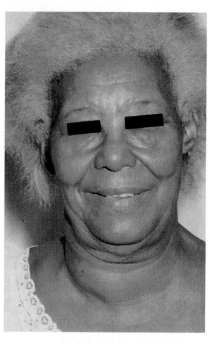

Fig. 10-9 A goiter is a palpable or visible enlargement of the thyroid gland. *(From Bingham, Hawke, and Kwok, 1992.)*

Characteristics of Thyroid Nodules	
Benign Thyroid Nodules	**Malignant Thyroid Nodules**
■ Adult onset	■ Adult onset
■ Prevalent in females	■ Prevalent in males
■ Family history of benign thyroid disease	■ History of multiple x-rays
■ Slow growth of nodule	■ No family history of thyroid problems
■ No change in voice	■ Rapid growth of nodule
■ More than one nodule	■ Voice change (hoarseness)
■ No lymphatic involvement	■ Generally only one nodule
	■ May have lymph node involvement

TECHNIQUES and NORMAL FINDINGS

ABNORMAL FINDINGS

PALPATE the thyroid using the *Posterior Approach* (Fig. 10-10). Stand behind the client. Instruct the client to take a sip of water from the glass and hold the water in the mouth until instructed to swallow. Have the client sit straight with the head slightly extended. Using both hands, reach from behind around the client's neck. Locate the cricoid process with your right hand. The thyroid gland is located directly beneath the cricoid process. Carefully slip the right hand downward and slightly to the right. Use two fingers of the left hand to push the trachea to the right. Instruct the client to swallow while using the finger pads of your right hand to feel for the right lobe of the thyroid gland against the right sternocleidomastoid muscle. Then have the client take and hold another sip of water. Repeat the technique using the right hand to push the trachea to the left. Instruct the client to swallow while your left hand feels for the left lobe of the thyroid.

PALPATE the thyroid using the *Anterior Approach* (Fig. 10-11). Have the client sit facing you. You should be standing in front of the client. Ask the client to take a sip of water from the glass and hold the water in the mouth until instructed to swallow. Ask the client to sit up straight, then bend the head slightly forward and to the right. Place your fingers on the client's neck. Locate the thyroid gland beneath the cricoid process. Your right hand should be used to displace the larynx to the right. Instruct the client to swallow the sip of water. As the sip of water is swallowed, the client's displaced right thyroid lobe should be palpated by the finger pads of your left thumb and index finger. After the right lobe is evaluated, instruct the client to take another sip of water and hold it. Use the same examination techniques with reversed hand position to examine the left thyroid lobe.

The thyroid tissue should feel smooth and soft and the gland should move freely during swallowing. The right side is frequently slightly larger than the left.

The normal thyroid gland is approximately the size of your thumb pad. If the thyroid gland is enlarged, use the bell of the stethoscope to auscultate the thyroid for vascular sounds (see Chapter 15).

■ A tender thyroid may be an indication of acute infection.

■ The presence of nodules or swelling may indicate a thyroid tumor or goiter.

■ A vascular bruit, indicating a hypermetabolic state, sounds like a soft rushing sound.

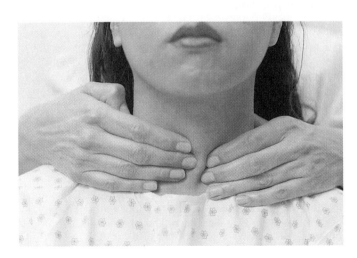

Fig. 10-10 Posterior approach for palpating the thyroid.

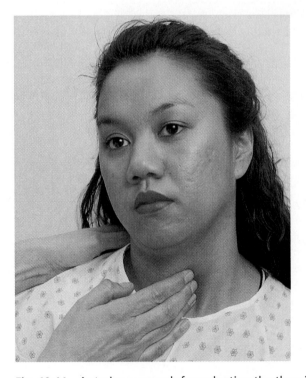

Fig. 10-11 Anterior approach for palpating the thyroid.

AGE-RELATED VARIATIONS

INFANTS

■ APPROACH

As the infant grows, the assessment of the head continues to be an important measure of normal growth and development. Likewise, assessment of the infant's ability to gain head and neck control are continuing measures of developmental progress.

The actual examination of the infant's head and neck is straightforward and direct. Place the infant first in a supine position to examine the head and neck, then have the infant held in a sitting position to examine the fontanels. The thyroid of the infant is not routinely examined.

■ FINDINGS

Head

It is important to carefully assess the infant's head until the child reaches age 2. The circumference of the skull should be measured using a tape measure and placing it around the area just above the ears and the eyes. The normal head circumference of the infant should measure between 27 and 32 cm (Fig. 10-12). The skull diameter usually measures approximately 2 cm greater than the infant's chest diameter. The infant's head circumference (see box below for growth rates) should be remeasured at each visit and plotted on a growth chart.

Head Circumference Growth Rates	
Full-term newborn to 3 months	2.0 cm/month
3 to 6 months	1.0 cm/month
6 months to 1 year	0.5 cm/month

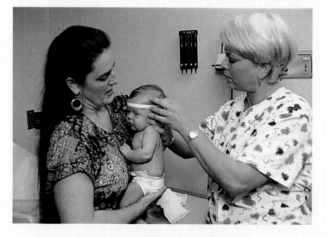

Fig. 10-12   Measuring skull circumference in an infant.

The newborn's head should be inspected for shape and contour. A common finding in newborns is a *cephalhematoma*. This is a subperiosteal hematoma under the scalp that occurs secondary to birth trauma. The area, which appears as a soft, well-defined swelling over the cranial bone, generally is reabsorbed within the first month of life. The hematoma does not cross suture lines.

The newborn's head should also be palpated to evaluate the suture lines and fontanels. *Molding* is a common finding; it is when the cranial bones actually override each other. The molding is secondary to the head passing through the birth canal and generally lasts less than a week. If the infant's suture lines are still palpable when the infant reaches 6 months of age, it may be indicative of hydrocephalus. The newborn's and infant's fontanels should be evaluated when the infant is calm and not crying. The two fontanels to be assessed are the anterior and posterior.

 Cultural Note

American Indian and Alaskan Native infants are often secured to traditional cradle boards from birth, which may cause a cosmetic flattening of the posterior skull.

Both the anterior and posterior fontanels of the infant should also be assessed for fullness and measured for size. To do this, the infant should be held in a sitting position and not be crying. If the infant is lying down or is crying, a false fullness may be felt. The fontanels should be palpated for either depression or bulging. The fontanels should have a slight depression, feel soft, and may have a slight pulsation. A deeply depressed fontanel may be an indication of dehydration. A bulging fontanel may indicate an increase in intracranial pressure. The anterior fontanel in infants less than 6 months of age should not exceed 4 to 5 cm. It should get progressively smaller as the child gets older and should be completely closed by the time the infant reaches 18 to 24 months of age. The infant's posterior fontanel may or may not be palpable at birth. If it is palpable, it should measure no more than 1 cm and it should close by 2 months of age.

If the infant's fontanels are full or the infant has a rapidly increasing head circumference, *transillumination* of the skull may be performed. To do this, darken the room and wait for at least one minute to allow your eyes to adjust to the dark. Place a transluminator or penlight firmly

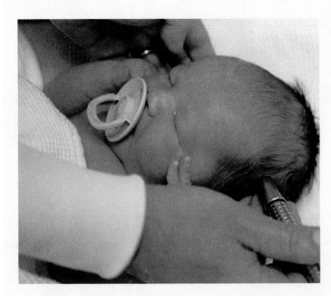

Fig. 10-13 **Transillumination of the infant's scalp.** *(From Seidel et al, 1995.)*

against the infant's skull so that no light escapes (Fig. 10-13). Start the assessment at the midline position of the infant's frontal region and repeat the procedure at one-inch increments over the entire head. The examiner should expect to see a ring of light around the light extending out 1 to 2 cm. The ring of light should be symmetric and even around the transilluminator. If the ring of light is asymmetric or extends beyond 2 cm, excess fluid or decreased brain tissue in the skull should be suspected.

Neck

The infant should be able to turn his or her head from side to side by 2 weeks of age. Head control should be gained by 3 to 4 months of age. A full discussion of the infant's muscular development is presented in Chapter 21.

Begin the infant's neck examination by lifting the infant's shoulders off of the examining table by lifting the infant by the arms. Permit the infant's head to lag back and inspect the infant's neck for a midline trachea, abnormal skin folds, and generalized neck enlargement. If the infant's neck is proportionately short or has webbing (loose, fanlike skin folds), the infant should be evaluated for congenital abnormalities such as Down or Turner syndromes. The neck of the newborn should be palpated for tone, presence of masses, and enlarged lymph nodes (discussed in Chapter 9). Because the infant's neck is short and thick, the examination of the thyroid is extremely difficult. If however, the nurse palpates an enlargement of the infant's anterior neck, the infant should be referred to a physician for further evaluation.

CHILDREN

■ APPROACH

The examination of the head and neck of the child should focus on normal developmental growth and assessment of signs of infection or injury. The most common problems are either infestations of the scalp, as discussed in Chapter 8, or lymphatic enlargements that may result from a head, mouth, ear, or neck infection, as presented in Chapter 9.

■ FINDINGS

Head

The child's fontanels should continue to be evaluated at each assessment visit until they are closed, by at least age 2.

Neck

The thyroid of the child may be assessed using the same techniques as for the adult. The challenge for the nurse is to encourage the child to sit still and swallow the water as described so that an adequate evaluation may be done. If the child is not able to cooperate, the thyroid exam may be deferred.

ADOLESCENTS

■ APPROACH AND FINDINGS

The techniques for examining the head and neck of the adolescent and the clinical findings are the same as for the adult. The most common abnormalities noted by the client's health care provider are those related to simple thyroid abnormalities such as goiter and hypothyroidism or hyperthyroidism.

OLDER ADULTS

■ APPROACH

The examination of the client's head and neck should be conducted the same as for the adult.

■ FINDINGS

A rhythmic movement or slight tremor of the neck may occur with aging. A history should be obtained to determine if the movement has had a new and sudden onset or has developed slowly over time. The client also may have increased concave cervical curvature, causing the positioning of the head and jaw to be in a forward and downward position. The technique of examining the thyroid is the same as for the younger adult. Because the thyroid becomes more fibrotic with aging, the client's thyroid may feel more nodular or irregular.

CLIENTS WITH SITUATIONAL VARIATIONS

PREGNANT WOMEN

■ APPROACH

It is important to gather baseline data from the woman about thyroid functioning before the pregnancy. Women with preexisting hypothyroidism or hyperthyroidism require special monitoring.

■ FINDINGS

The examiner may notice that the woman has blotchy, brownish pigmentation of the face. This is actually chloasma, which is commonly called "the mask of pregnancy." There may also be transient thyroid enlargement that would make the thyroid more predominately palpable. Both of these signs disappear following delivery.

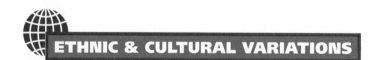

ETHNIC & CULTURAL VARIATIONS

■ APPROACH

Certain cultural belief systems hold that the head serves as a receptacle for the soul. This belief may lead individuals from these cultures to interpret an examination of the head in light of this belief. The examiner needs to seek permission before the examination from these individuals. Various cultural groups are also at higher risk for certain diseases such as hypertension, which may be displayed through headache symptomatology. These factors are essential to consider in history taking.

■ FINDINGS

A wide range of normal differences exists in the physical size and appearance of the skull and facial features within and across racial and ethnic groups. The cosmetic shape of an infant's head may be affected by traditional child-care practices such as the use of a cradle board. It is important to consider this range of normal variation when inspecting for symmetry and size. The varying rate of fetal alcohol syndrome (FAS) among cultural groups is an important factor to consider when examining infant facial features for evidence of FAS.

E X A M I N A T I O N S U M M A R Y
Head and Neck

Head (pp. 195-196)
- Inspect the head for
  Facial features
  Appropriateness of facial expression
  Head size
- Palpate the scalp and skull for
  Contour and intactness
  Tenderness
- Inspect and palpate the face and jaw for
  Size
  Symmetry
  Intactness
  Tenderness

Neck (pp. 196-197)
- Inspect the neck for
  Positioning in relation to the head
  Symmetry of muscles
  Range of motion
  Pain with movement
  Evidence of edema or enlargement of the
    thyroid area
  Deviation of the trachea
- Palpate the neck for
  Positioning of the anatomic structures of the
    neck

Thyroid (pp. 198-199)
- Palpate the thyroid for
  Size
  Shape
  Tenderness
  Presence of nodules or enlargement

C O M M O N P R O B L E M S / C O N D I T I O N S
associated with the Head and Neck

HEAD

■ *Vascular headache*

Migraine headache: A vascular headache that generally begins in childhood, adolescence, or early adult life. It is frequently familial and occurs in approximately 5% of the general population. Women are twice as likely as men to have migraines. Young women are most susceptible. The frequency of the headaches generally decreases with advancing age. The headache most generally starts with an aura caused by a vasospasm of intracranial arteries. Accompanying signs may include feelings of depression, restlessness or irritability, photophobia, and nausea or vomiting. The headache typically lasts 4 to 6 hours.

Cluster headache: Intense episodes of excruciating unilateral pain that last from 1/2 to 1 hour but may repeat over a period of days or weeks. They may be accompanied by ipsilateral lacrimation, nasal stuffiness, and drainage. The only prodromal sign may be slight nausea. Cluster headaches are four times more common in men and generally occur in the third or fourth decade of life.

■ *Tension headache*

Muscle contraction headache: The most common type of headache for persons 20 to 40 years of age. The headache is usually bilateral and may be diffuse or confined to the frontal, temporal, parietal, or occipital area. The onset may be very gradual and may last for several days. The headache may be accompanied by contraction of the skeletal muscles of the face, jaw, and neck.

Traumatic headache: Occurs secondary to a head injury or concussion. It is characterized by a dull, generalized head pain. Accompanying symptoms may be a lack of ability to concentrate, giddiness, or dizziness.

■ *Traction-inflammatory headache*

Traction headache: May result from increased intracranial pressure, cerebral hemorrhage, decreased intracranial pressure (e.g., lumbar pressure), or an infection (e.g., encephalitis).

Temporal headache: A focused headache over the temporal region of the skull that may be caused by temporal arteries. This generally occurs in individuals over 60 years of age and may be accompanied by a decrease in vision.

■ *Acromegaly:* A chronic metabolic condition that is characterized by a gradual enlargement and elongation of the bones of the face and jaw (Fig. 10-14). This condition, which afflicts middle-aged persons, is caused by the overproduction of growth hormone.

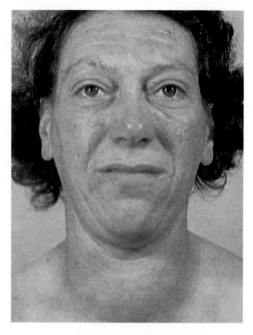

Fig. 10-14 Acromegaly. Note large head, forward projection of jaw, and protrusion of frontal bone. *(From 400 More Self Assessment Picture Tests in Clinical Medicine, 1988.)*

■ *Hydrocephalus:* A condition in which there is an obstruction of the drainage of the cerebrospinal fluid in the head (Fig. 10-15). Because of this drainage problem, fluid accumulates, causing an increase in intracranial pressure and actual enlargement of the head. As the head enlarges, the facial features appear small in proportion to the cranium, the fontanels may bulge, and scalp veins dilate.

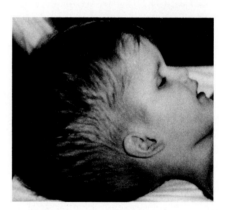

Fig. 10-15 Hydrocephalus. Note characteristic enlarged head, bulging fontanel, dilated scalp veins, and bossing of the skull. *(From Seidel et al, 1995.)*

■ **Microcephaly:** A congenital anomaly characterized by an abnormally small head in relation to the rest of the body and by the underdevelopment of the brain, resulting in some degree of mental retardation (Fig. 10-16).

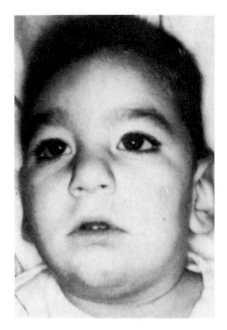

Fig. 10-16 Primary familial microcephaly. *(From Seidel et al, 1995.)*

■ **Macrocephaly:** A congenital anomaly characterized by an abnormally large head and brain in relation to the rest of the body, resulting in some degree of mental and growth retardation.

■ **Down syndrome:** A chromosome abnormality (trisomy-21) characterized by slanted eyes with inner epicanthal folds, a small flat nose with a flat nasal bridge, a protruding thick tongue, ear dysplasia, and a short broad neck with webbing (Fig. 10-17). There are also varying degrees of mental retardation.

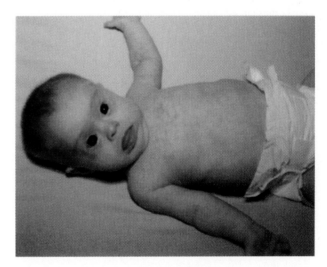

Fig. 10-17 Down syndrom in infant. Note small, square head with upward slant to eyes, flat nasal bridge, protruding tongue, mottled skin, and hypotonia. *(From Wong, 1995.)*

FACE

■ *Parkinson's syndrome:* Caused by a deficiency of the neurotransmitter dopamine and a degeneration of the basal ganglion in the brain, characterized by a "masklike" appearance of the face showing elevated eyebrows, a staring gaze, and sometimes drooling. The neck flexes forward and the eyes gaze upward.

■ *Cushing syndrome:* A metabolic disorder resulting from the chronic and excessive production of cortisol by the adrenal cortex (Fig. 10-18). Clinical signs include such signs as a decreased glucose tolerance, central obesity, a round "moon" face, supraclavicular fat pads, edema, hypokalemia, and some degree of emotional change. There may be excessive facial hair growth.

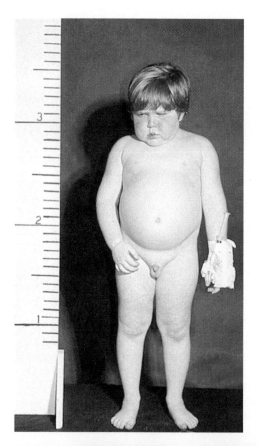

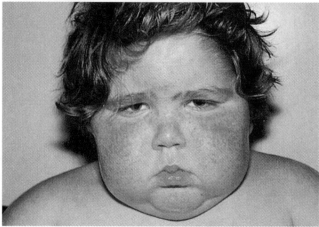

Fig. 10-18   Cushing syndrome.   *(From Zitelli and Davis, 1992.)*

■ **Fetal alcohol syndrome:** Characterized by narrow palpebral fissures, epicanthal folds, and midfacial hypoplasia such as a deformed upper lip (Fig. 10-19). There is also some degree of mental retardation. The mother reports alcohol consumption during pregnancy.

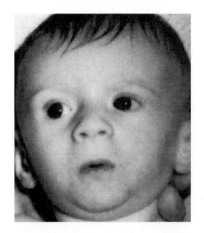

Fig. 10-19 Fetal alcohol syndrome. Note small palpebral fissures, epicanthal folds, hypoplastic philtrum, thinned upper lip, and retrognathia. *(From Goodman and Gorlin, 1977; courtesy Dr. Charles Linder.)*

🌐 **Cultural Note**

The rate of fetal alcohol syndrome is estimated to be six times higher among American Indians and Alaskan Natives than among the general U.S. population.

NECK

■ **Torticollis (wry neck):** Often the result of injury during the birth process. The client's head is tilted and twisted toward the sternocleidomastoid muscle due to the constriction of the muscle on this side of the neck (Fig. 10-20). Torticollis may also occur in older children and adults secondary to neck injury, muscle spasms, infections, or drug ingestion.

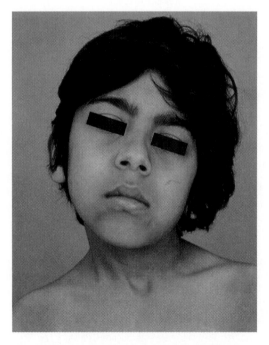

Fig. 10-20 Torticollis (wry neck). Child has tilt of the head to the left. Underlying problem was an inflammatory mass in the left parapharyngeal space. *(From Bingham, Hawke, and Kwok, 1992.)*

■ **Graves' disease:** A disorder characterized by pronounced hyperthyroidism, usually associated with an enlarged thyroid gland and exophthalmos (Fig. 10-21). The disease is five times more common in women than men, occurs most frequently between 20 and 40 years of age, and often arises after an infection or physical or emotional stress. Typical signs are nervousness, a fine tremor of the hands, weight loss, fatigue, shortness of breath, palpitations, heat intolerance, increased metabolic rate, and gastrointestinal motility.

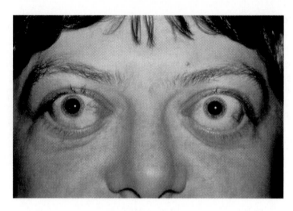

Fig. 10-21 Graves' disease. Client shows characteristic features of endocrine orbitopathy, with peculiar stare produced by retraction of the upper eyelid and the unnatural degree of separation between the margins of the two eyelids. *(From Bingham, Hawke, and Kwok, 1992.)*

■ **Hyperthyroidism:** A condition characterized by increased activity of the thyroid gland.

Signs and Symptoms of Hyperthyroidism	
SYSTEM	**SIGNS AND SYMPTOMS**
General	Preference for the cold Weight loss
Eyes	Prominence of the eyeballs Puffiness of the eyelids Double vision Decreased motility
Neck	Goiter
Cardiovascular	Palpitations Peripheral edema
Gastrointestinal	Increased bowel movements
Genitourinary	Polyuria
Reproductive	Decreased fertility
Neuromuscular	Fatigue Weakness Tremors
Emotional	Nervousness Irritability
Dermatologic	Hair thinning Increased perspiration Change in skin texture Change in pigmentation

Modified from Swartz MH: Textbook of physical diagnosis, *Philadelphia, 1994, Saunders.*

■ **Myxedema:** The most severe form of hypothyroidism. It is characterized by swelling of the hands, face, feet, and puffiness of the eyes. There may also be coarse facial features, dry skin, and dry, coarse head and facial hair. If not treated, death may occur.

■ **Hypothyroidism:** A condition characterized by decreased activity of the thyroid gland (see box below).

SYSTEM	SIGNS AND SYMPTOMS
Signs and Symptoms of Hypothyroidism	
General	Weight gain
	Chilly
	Obesity
Gastrointestinal	Constipation
	Enlarged tongue
Cardiovascular	Fatigue
	Hypotension
	Bradycardia
Neurologic	Speech disorders
	Hyporeflexia
	Short attention span
	Defective abstract reasoning
	Spasticity
	Tremor
	Depressed affect
Musculoskeletal	Lethargy
	Thickened, dry skin
	Hair loss
	Brittle nails
	Legs cramps
	Puffy eyelids
	Puffy cheeks
	Hypotonia
	Puffy face
Reproductive	Heavier menses
	Decreased fertility

Modified from Swartz MH: Textbook of physical diagnosis, *Philadelphia, 1994, Saunders.*

&Nursing Diagnosis

CASE 1   4-month-old male infant for well-baby checkup.

Subjective

Mother reports bringing infant to clinic today for well-baby checkup and immunizations; reports infant healthy at birth, weighing 6 lb 8 oz.; reports child holds head up from prone position and seems to have good head control; mother concerned that it now seems very difficult to pull infant's shirts on over his head.

Objective

Alert, active, healthy-appearing male infant.

Length   24" (61 cm).

Weight   13.1 lb (5.9 kg).

Head   Lifts head from prone position with ease and turns side to side; skull contour smooth, without depressions or bulging; sagittal and coronal suture lines palpable; anterior fontanel 5 cm; posterior fontanel not palpable; head circumference 39 cm (chest circumference 30 cm). (Past visit note: at 3 month visit, head circumference 38 cm.)

Neck   No bulging or deformities; thyroid not palpated.

Denver II appropriate for age.

• •

Nursing Diagnosis #1

Health-seeking behaviors related to expressed desire to ensure health of child.

Defining Characteristics   Mother brings baby for check-up.

Nursing Diagnosis #2

Anxiety and *knowledge deficit* related to normal head size and growth of children.

Defining Characteristics   Mother expresses concern about difficulty of putting on infant's shirt over head.

Nursing Diagnosis

CASE 2 38-year-old woman with complaints of fatigue and weight gain.

Subjective

Complains of 2-month gradual onset of fatigue, inability to stay warm, constipation, and feeling of facial puffiness; denies similar feeling in past; reports dry skin despite daily application of lotion; concerned about areas of scalp hair thinning and menses "heavier than normal"; reports gaining 18 pounds (8.18 kg) over past 4 months; reports no other illnesses or problems; states never had thyroid tested.

Objective

Head Normocephalic with no evidence of lesions or injury; scalp hair thin and fine.

Neck Supple with full range of motion; soft painless thyroid nodule (2 cm) palpated 2 cm from midline in upper portion of right lobe; nodule not fixed to overlying skin or muscles.

• •

Nursing Diagnosis #1

Fatigue related to reduced metabolic rate and blood loss.

Defining Characteristics Expressed fatigue and weight gain; thyroid nodule palpated.

Nursing Diagnosis #2

Hypothermia related to reduced metabolic rate.

Defining Characteristics Complaints of inability to stay warm; thyroid nodule palpated.

Nursing Diagnosis #3

Constipation related to reduced metabolic rate.

Defining Characteristics Complaints of constipation; thyroid nodule palpated.

Nursing Diagnosis #4

Body image disturbance related to changes in physical appearance.

Defining Characteristics Facial puffiness, weight gain, dry skin, thinning hair.

HEALTH PROMOTION

- **Iodine in the Diet** To prevent goiter, the diet should contain iodine in some manner. Many areas of the United States have iodine in the ground. Subsequently, the individual has an adequate iodine intake secondary to the foods grown locally and eaten. Other areas of the country have little iodine in the earth. Individuals living in these areas should supplement their diet with iodine. This may be done easily and inexpensively by using iodized salt.

- **Congenital Hypothyroidism** The American Academy of Pediatrics and the American Thyroid Association (1987) recommend that all neonates be screened for congenital hypothyroidism during the first week of life. Congenital hypothyroidism occurs each year in about one of every 3500 to 4000 newborns. Because many cases go undiagnosed and do not receive prompt treatment they develop irreversible mental retardation and a variety of neuropsychologic deficits comprising the syndrome of cretinism (Postellon et al, 1986).

- **Thyroid Cancer** It is estimated that in the United States, each year 11,300 individuals are diagnosed with thyroid cancer and an additional 1000 people die from thyroid cancer. Individuals who require careful screening include people with a neck mass, hoarseness, a history of multiple endocrine neoplasia syndrome, and multiple exposure to upper body radiation since childhood. Palpation of the thyroid remains the routine screening examination for adults. More invasive screening procedures such as ultrasonography or needle aspiration are reserved for individuals with nodular disease or goiter.

??????? STUDY QUESTIONS ???????

1. List the major structures of (a) skull; (b) face; (c) neck.

2. Describe what a triangle is (in reference to the human body) and identify the structures in the anterior and posterior triangles.

3. What common problems of the head form the primary focus in history taking?

4. List the questions you might pose to gain information about the pattern, characteristics, and associated symptoms of a headache.

5. List questions that would be important in assessment of an individual who came to the clinic and stated that he was lightheaded.

6. What questions would you ask in doing a head and neck assessment of someone who bumped his head after falling off of his bicycle?

7. Why are questions about sleep patterns, energy level, mood, and heat sensitivity relevant in assessment of the thyroid?

8. List the factors that must be considered when inspecting and palpating the head, scalp, skull, face, neck, and thyroid gland.

9. What characteristics distinguish benign and malignant nodules of the thyroid?

10. List three physical findings of the head that could indicate an abnormality in an infant.

11. Define and list the categories and distinguishing characteristics among vascular, tension, and traction-inflammatory headaches.

12. What distinguishes hydrocephalus from macrocephaly?

13. What are the distinguishing facial characteristics of Parkinson's syndrome, Cushing disease, and fetal alcohol syndrome?

14. List the features of the head and neck that distinguish hypothyroidism from hyperthyroidism.

15. What substance prevents goiter formation? What dietary supplement provides easy and inexpensive access to this substance?

16. What are the consequences when infants with congenital hypothyroidism go undiagnosed and untreated?

CHAPTER 11

Nose, Paranasal Sinuses, Mouth, and Oropharynx

ANATOMY AND PHYSIOLOGY

Besides serving as a passageway for inspired and expired air, the nose also serves as a humidifier and filter for the inspired air, warming and cleaning the air before it enters the lungs. Other functions of the nose include identifying odors and giving resonance to laryngeal sounds. The paranasal sinuses are air-filled cavities that make the skull lighter and perform all of the same functions as the nose.

NOSE AND PARANASAL SINUSES

The upper third of the nose is encased in bone, which attaches to the frontal bone (Fig. 11-1). The bone extends to the lower two thirds of the nose, which is composed of cartilage. The septal cartilage maintains the shape of the nose and sepa-

rates the nares (nostrils), which maintain an open passage for air. The interior of the nose—the nasal cavity—is lined with a highly vascular mucous membrane containing cilia (nasal hairs) that trap airborne particles and prevent them from reaching the lungs. The lateral walls of the nasal cavity are lined with the inferior, middle, and superior turbinates, which contain openings, or meatuses. The inferior meatus drains tears from the nasolacrimal duct, and the middle meatus serves as an outlet for paranasal sinus drainage (Fig. 11-2).

The paranasal sinuses extend out of the nasal cavities through narrow openings into the skull bones to form bilateral (paired), air-filled pockets. They are lined with mucous membranes and cilia that move secretions along excretory pathways. (Fig. 11-3). The sphenoid, frontal, ethmoid, and maxillary sinuses constitute the paranasal sinuses. The frontal

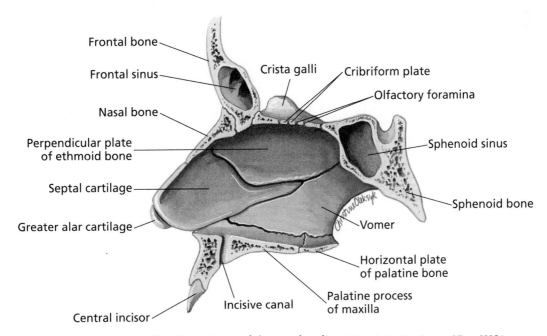

Fig. 11-1 Bones of the nasal cavity. *(From Seeley, Stephens and Tate, 1995.)*

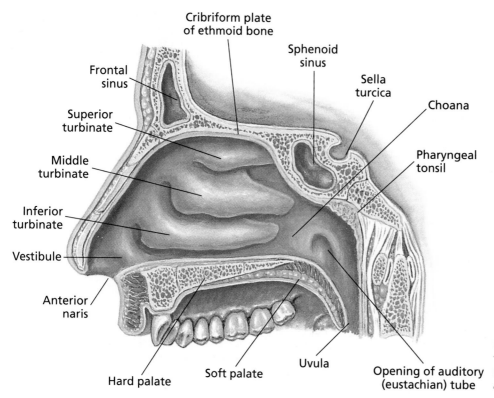

Fig. 11-2 Cross-sectional view of the anatomic structures of the nose and nasopharynx. *(From Seidel et al, 1995.)*

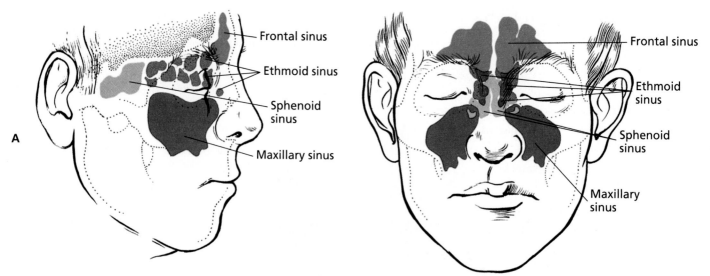

Fig. 11-3 Paranasal sinuses. **A,** Side view. **B,** Front view. *(From Seeley, Stephens and Tate, 1995.)*

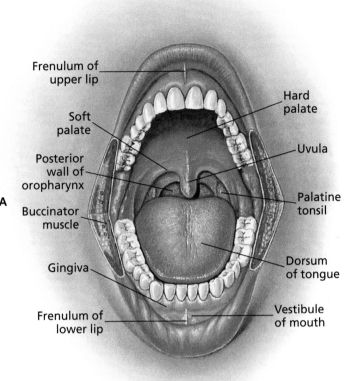

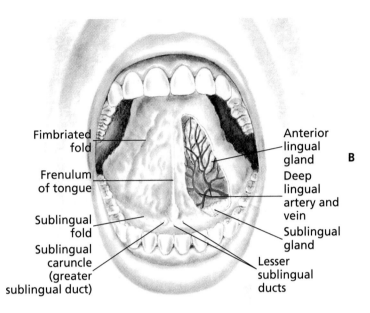

Fig. 11-4 **A,** Dorsal and **B,** ventral surfaces of the tongue. *(From Seidel et al, 1995.)*

sinuses are in the frontal bone superior to the nasal cavities. The ethmoid sinuses lie behind the frontal sinuses and near the superior portion of the nasal cavity. The sphenoid sinuses are deep in the skull behind the ethmoid sinuses.

MOUTH

The mouth contains the tongue, which has hundreds of taste buds (papillae) on its dorsal surface. The taste buds distinguish sweet, sour, bitter, and salty tastes. The ventral surface is smooth and very vascular (Fig. 11-4). Three pairs of salivary glands—the submandibular, the sublingual, and the parotid—release saliva through small openings (ducts) in response to the presence of food particles, to begin the process of digestion (Fig. 11-5). The submandibular glands are tucked under the mandible and lie approximately midway between the chin and the posterior mandibular angle. They are soft, symmetric, and palpable, and are sometimes mistaken for lymph nodes by the beginning examiner. The parotid glands are anterior to the ears, immediately above the mandibular angle. They are not palpable unless they are enlarged. The sublingual glands lie on the floor of the mouth and are not palpable or visible. Wharton's ducts, the openings for the submandibular glands, are visible on both sides of the floor of the mouth under the tongue. Stensen's ducts (parotid gland openings) are visible on both sides of the cheek adjacent to the second molars.

The normal adult has 32 teeth, which are tightly encased in mucous membrane–covered, fibrous gum tissue and rooted in the alveolar ridges of the maxilla and mandible. The third molars are congenitally absent in some adults (Fig. 11-6).

🌐 Racial Variation

About 30% of Asian Americans, 15% of American Indians/Alaskan Natives, and 10% of whites have agenesis of the third molar, displaying a pattern of 28 teeth as adults. This pattern is rare in African Americans.

OROPHARYNX

The oropharynx includes the structures at the back of the mouth that are visible on examination: the uvula, the anterior and posterior pillars, the tonsils, and the posterior pharyngeal wall (Fig. 11-7). The uvula is suspended, midline, from the soft palate, which extends out to either side to form the anterior pillar. The tonsils are tucked between the anterior and posterior pillars and normally may be atrophied in adults to the point of being barely visible. The posterior pharyngeal wall is visible when the tongue is extended and depressed. This wall is highly vascular and may show color variations of red and pink because of the presence of small vessels and lymphoid tissue. The epiglottis, a cartilaginous structure that protects the laryngeal opening, sometimes projects into the pharyngeal area and is visible as the tongue is depressed.

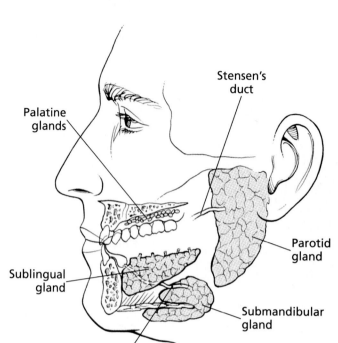

Fig. 11-5 Position of the major salivary glands. *(From Finkbeiner and Johnson, 1995.)*

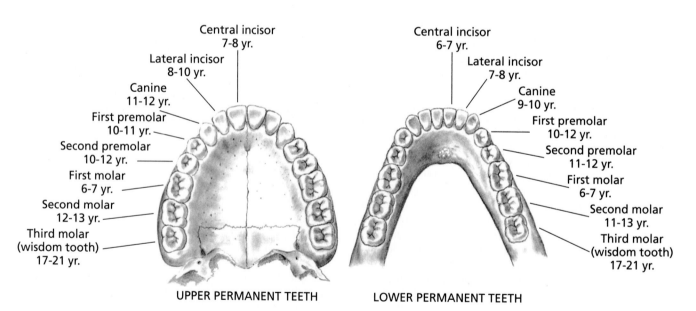

UPPER PERMANENT TEETH   LOWER PERMANENT TEETH

Fig. 11-6 Dentition of permanent teeth and their sequence of eruption. *(From Seidel et al, 1995.)*

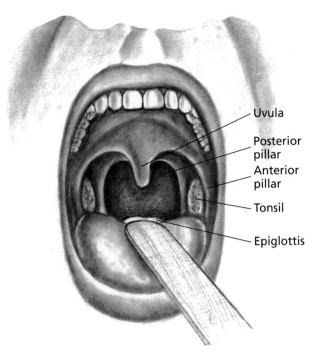

Fig. 11-7 **Structures of the oropharynx.** *(From Thompson et al, 1993.)*

DEVELOPMENTAL CONSIDERATIONS

INFANTS

Although the maxillary and ethmoid sinuses are present at birth, they are very small and not able to be examined until the child is much older; the sphenoid sinus is a tiny cavity at birth that is not fully developed until puberty.

By the time the infant is 3 months old, the infant drools because salivation has increased. The infant continues to drool until he or she learns to swallow the saliva. In the third month of fetal development, deciduous teeth begin to calcify. When each tooth has enough calcification to withstand chewing, it erupts to the surface. The 20 deciduous teeth usually appear between 6 and 24 months of age (Fig. 11-8). The permanent teeth begin forming in the jaw by 6 months of age (Seidel et al, 1995).

🌐 Racial Variation

About 10% of Tlinkit Indian and 2% of Canadian Eskimo infants are born with teeth. The incidence among white infants is quite rare (1:3000). (Jarvis and Gorman, 1972)

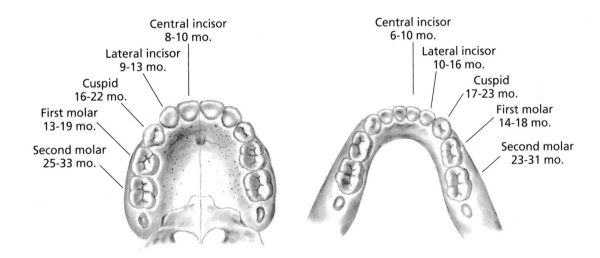

Fig. 11-8 **Dentition of deciduous teeth and their sequence of eruption.** *(From Seidel et al, 1995.)*

CHILDREN

The frontal sinus develops by 7 to 8 years of age.

The roots of the deciduous teeth are reabsorbed by pressure from the permanent teeth until the crown is shed. The permanent teeth begin to erupt when the child reaches about the age of 6 and continue until about age 18, when the third molars, or wisdom teeth, erupt (Seidel et al, 1995).

PREGNANT WOMEN

Elevated levels of estrogen cause increased vascularity of the upper respiratory tract, engorging the capillaries of the nose and pharynx. This leads to symptoms of nasal stuffiness and epistaxis. Connective gum tissue may show increased vascularity and proliferation, which may lead to bleeding gums.

OLDER ADULTS

The nose becomes larger and more prominent because of unabated cartilage formation. The granular lining on the lips and cheeks becomes more prominent, and the gingival tissue is less elastic and more vulnerable to injury. Because of gingival recession, the root surfaces of the teeth are exposed to caries formation. As teeth lose their translucency, they darken and become worn from long use.

The tongue becomes more fissured. The older adult may have altered motor function of the tongue, leading to problems with swallowing. After the age of 45, the papillae on the lateral edges of the tongue gradually atrophy and the number of papillae and taste buds drop in general. As a result, taste perception may be diminished.

HEALTH HISTORY | Nose, Paranasal Sinuses, Mouth, and Oropharynx

The history related to the assessment of the nose, paranasal sinuses, mouth, and oropharynx involves evaluation of any potential underlying disease state or condition and issues related to patterns of care and exposure to risk factors.

QUESTIONS

RATIONALE

NOSE AND PARANASAL SINUSES

NASAL DISCHARGE

- Do you have any nasal discharge or runny nose? Is it only occasionally or constantly? How would you describe the discharge? What color is the discharge? Is it watery, thick, purulent, or bloody? Is it foul-smelling? Is it from only one side or both? Do you have chronic postnasal drip? Does your nose become crusty or painful? Do you use nosedrops or a nasal spray? If so, what kind and how often?
- Do you have allergies? If so, to what and what symptoms do you usually exhibit? Are the allergies seasonal?
- Do you have frequent colds? If so, what is the pattern and what symptoms do you usually exhibit?

◀ *Allergies and colds are the most common causes of nasal discharge. A thin, watery discharge is generally due to excess mucus production resulting from a viral infection or allergy. A thick or purulent green or yellow discharge results most commonly from a bacterial infection. A bloody discharge may result from a neoplasm, trauma, or an opportunistic infection such as a fungal disease. A foul-smelling discharge, especially unilateral discharge, is most commonly associated with a foreign body or chronic sinusitis. A clear, watery discharge from the nose secondary to a head injury may be indicative of cerebrospinal fluid leakage.*

OBSTRUCTION OF NASAL AIR FLOW

- Have you ever had nasal surgery? If so, when and for what? Have you ever had an injury to your nose? If so, what? Was your nose ever broken? Is either side obstructed now, or can you breathe through both sides? If there is obstruction, how long has it been present? Do you have a history of nasal polyps? Describe your sense of smell—is it good? Do you have any allergies or is the obstruction associated with any other symptoms?

◀ *Nasal airway obstruction may be secondary to trauma-induced blockage of nasal passage, allergic response with congestion of the nasal mucosa, or nasal polyps. Nasal polyps may also cause a loss of smell and may be seen in clients with allergic rhinitis or cystic fibrosis.*

SINUS CONGESTION OR PAIN

- Do you have any pain in your sinus areas? Do your sinuses seem congested? If so, do you have pain behind, above, or around your eyes or near your molars? If you have sinus congestion, what do you do to treat it?

◀ *Sinus congestion or infection causes referred pain around the eyes and to the front teeth. Trauma to the face may cause an alteration to the normal facial structures and may cause sinus obstruction, which in turn may promote the growth of organisms leading to infection. Obstruction may also be caused by a deviated septum or foreign body in the nose.*

QUESTIONS

RATIONALE

NOSEBLEED (EPISTAXIS)

- Does your nose bleed? How often? How much? What color is the blood? Is it thin or clotted? Does it come from just one side or both? Is it aggravated by picking your nose or scratching? Is your nose dry? How do you treat your nosebleeds? Are they difficult to stop? Have you ever snorted cocaine?

◀ *Epistaxis may occur secondary to hypertension, trauma, chronic sinusitis, malignancy, or a bleeding disorder. While the most common causes of epistaxis are nose-picking or friable membranes secondary to dryness, it may also result from cocaine abuse.*

- Do you have high blood pressure?

◀ *High blood pressure may precipitate a nose bleed.*

MOUTH AND OROPHARYNX

PAIN

- Do you have pain in your mouth? If so, describe where it is and its severity. How long has the pain been present? What brings it on? What makes it better? Worse? What do you use to treat the pain? Does the pain interfere with eating?

◀ *Mouth pain may be secondary to dental problems or gingival disease. It is important to take a careful dental history.*

MOUTH LESIONS

- Do you have any sores in your mouth or on your lips? If yes, have you ever had a sore like this before? How long has it been present? What have you done to treat it? Have you noticed any odor from your mouth?

◀ *Mouth lesions may be caused by benign causes, such as trauma from a toothbrush or food, or they may be a sign of an infection, immunologic problem, or cancer. It is always important to inquire about a client's smoking history, as well as his or her sexual habits.*

- Are there any other sores anywhere else on your body, such as in the vagina? In the urethra? On the penis? In the anus? Do you have a history of venereal disease? Are the lesions painful?
- Do you smoke? If so, what do you smoke (pipe, cigarettes, or cigars) and how much?
- Do you use smokeless tobacco? If so, how long have you used it?

◀ *Sexually transmitted diseases such as herpes may be transmitted through oral sex.*

DIFFICULTY SWALLOWING (DYSPHAGIA)

- Do you have pain or difficulty when swallowing? If yes, does it occur with liquids, solids, or tablets? Do you have your tonsils? Do you have frequent throat infections? Do you ever have trouble handling secretions?

◀ *Throat pain or difficulty swallowing may be secondary to infection, a foreign body, or an inflammatory process. A sudden onset of drooling or difficulty swallowing is a medical emergency and should be so managed.*

SORE THROAT

- How frequently do you get sore throats? Is your throat sore now? If yes, how long has it felt that way? Describe what it feels like—a lump, burning, scratchy? Does it hurt to swallow? When did it start? Is it associated with fever, cough, fatigue, headache, postnasal drip, or hoarseness? Is it worse when you get up in the morning? Do you notice that you are breathing from your mouth? If so, is it because you are having difficulty breathing through your nose? Are others in your home ill or just recovered from a sore throat or cold? Do you inhale dust or fumes at work? Is the sore throat present constantly, or more often in the morning or evening? Is your home or office dry? Are you hoarse? What have you done for your sore throat?

◀ *A sore throat may be caused by many things from nasal congestion or sinus drainage to an infection or allergy. A careful history will help to determine the etiology of the complaint.*

◀ *Postnasal drip may cause early morning sore throat or a cough on lying down. The maxillary sinuses do not drain when the client is upright, but they do drain when the client lies down.*

QUESTIONS

RATIONALE

HOARSENESS OR VOICE CHANGE

■ Do you use your voice a lot? How long have you had this hoarseness or voice change? Is it constant or does it come and go? Do you smoke? Do you feel like you have to clear your throat a lot? Does the weather affect your voice? Does your voice seem different from what you consider normal (weak, husky, higher, lower)? Do you feel like the hoarseness or voice change is associated with a cold or sore throat?

◀ *Common causes of hoarseness or a voice change are overuse of the voice and laryngeal irritation secondary to smoking. Hoarseness that cannot be traced to an irritation or specific cause should be evaluated for possible neoplastic involvement.*

TEETH, DENTURES, AND DENTAL CARE

■ What are your daily dental care habits? Do you have dentures? Bridges? Other dental appliances? How many times each day do you brush your teeth? Do you use dental floss? Do you use toothpaste?
■ Do you have bad breath frequently? If so, is it just in the morning or does it continue even after you have brushed your teeth?
■ When was your last dental examination? Did you have problems at that time? If so, what?
■ Do you currently have gum or teeth problems? If so, describe them. Are you able to eat/chew all types of foods?
■ (If the client has dentures:) How long have you had this set? Do they fit well? Are they loose or do they rub your gums? Have you noticed any irritation of your gums?

◀ *It is important to determine the client's normal dental care patterns so that health teaching may be developed. If the client had dental or gum problems, a referral to a dentist should be made. If the client wears dentures and reports difficulty with the fitting of the dentures or difficulty with chewing or sore gums, a dental referral should be made.*

 Racial Variation

African Americans have a harder and denser tooth enamel than whites, making their teeth less susceptible to decay.

INFANTS

■ Did the child's mother have a history of maternal infection, alcohol or drug use, irradiation, hypertension, or diabetes during pregnancy?

■ Were any abnormalities present at the child's birth? If so, what were they? Has the infant undergone repair for problems such as cleft lip or cleft palate? Have other members in the family had congenital problems?

◀ *Maternal infection or substance abuse during pregnancy may lead to congenital defects or infection.*
◀ *Identifying problems early can help in providing treatment and proper follow-up.*

QUESTIONS

RATIONALE

CHILDREN

YOUNG CHILD

Questions for the young child should focus on developmental maturation, bottle-feeding or thumb-sucking, infection, and early dental care.

- Are the child's teeth erupting? If so, when did this start and what teeth does he or she have? Does he or she tend to put objects in the mouth or nose? Have you noticed any unilateral nose drainage or odor from the nose? Has the child had frequent colds or sore throats? Does the child have a pacifier?
- Is the child using a bottle? If so, how often? Does he or she go to bed with a bottle? Does the child have any caries? Does the child suck his or her thumb? Does the child have any mouth infections or sores in the mouth such as thrush? If so, how often do they occur? Does the child seem to have sore throats or colds often? How often? How are these treated? Has he or she had strep throat?

- Do you brush your child's teeth? Has the child seen a dentist? If so, how often? Do you use fluoridated water or a fluoride supplement?

◄ *Normal development should be noted with regard to teething and oral behaviors. A delay in tooth eruption may be associated with nutritional deficits or congenital problems such as Down syndrome. Dental problems and caries may be related to the child taking a bottle to bed and the presence of milk on or around the child's teeth overnight. Frequent colds and sore throats may be common but should be evaluated because of risks related to hearing and allergies. Thumb-sucking or using a pacifier should be a concern only if the child's secondary teeth are present.*

◄ *A parent should brush the child's teeth as soon as they are present. Toothpaste may be used. The child should see a dentist by age 3. Good dental hygiene started at a young age serves as a preventative health habit in later life.*

OLDER CHILD

Questions for the older child should include those for the younger child, but should also focus on the characteristics of the teeth as well as dental habits and care.

- How does the child care for his or her teeth each day? Brushing habits? How often does the child see a dentist? Does the child have a habit of grinding his or her teeth (bruxism)? If so, when does this happen (night, day, or both)? Do the child's teeth appear straight? If not, are there plans for correction?

◄ *Parents need to monitor tooth-brushing in the older child to be sure that a complete job of brushing is done.*

OLDER ADULTS

Focus on self-care habits, frequency of visits to the dentist, and client concerns secondary to tooth loss, taking medications, or a change in sense of smell or taste.

- Are you currently taking medications that made your mouth dry (xerostomia)? Is your nose dry? If so, what do you do about the dryness? If you have had a loss of teeth or dentures that do not fit well, does this interfere with your eating or chewing? Are you able to chew the foods that you want to?
- Do you see a dentist on a regular basis? When was your last visit?

◄ *Dry mouth may occur secondary to taking medications (e.g., anticholinergic drugs) or decreased secretion by mouth glands. Tooth loss or malfitting dentures may lead to poor nutrition because the client is unable to chew and may therefore not eat properly.*

EXAMINATION Procedures and Findings

Guidelines While the nose, sinuses, mouth, and oropharynx are all entities that should be considered separately, the sequencing of the examination moves easily from one area to the next, making it appear as a single examination.

EQUIPMENT   Examination gloves
Penlight
Otoscope with broad-tipped nasal speculum or nasal speculum
Transilluminator
Tongue blade
4 × 4 gauze sponges

TECHNIQUES and NORMAL FINDINGS

ABNORMAL FINDINGS

NOSE AND PARANASAL SINUSES

INSPECT and PALPATE the nose for General Appearance and Symmetry. The skin should be smooth and intact, with the color matching the rest of the face. The nose should appear symmetric and midline. The nostrils should be symmetric, dry (no crusting), and not flaring or narrowed.

If nasal discharge is present, describe its character and amount (watery, mucoid, purulent, bloody, etc.)

Apply pressure to one side of the nose to assess for patency; ask the client to close his or her mouth and sniff inward through the opposite side; repeat on the opposite side. There should be noiseless, free exchange of air on each side.

Palpate the external nose to be sure it is firm and not tender.

EVALUATE the olfactory nerve (cranial nerve I) for Intactness. Ask the client to close his or her eyes and mouth. Hold one nostril closed at a time, then hold an aromatic substance (such as coffee or lemon extract) under the nostril. Repeat with the other nostril. The client should be able to identify the smell. (This procedure may be deferred until the neurologic examination.)

INSPECT the internal nasal cavity for Patency. Use a nasal speculum and a good light source. Hold the speculum in the palm of the hand and use your index finger to stabilize the speculum against the side of the nose. Insert the speculum slowly and cautiously about 1 cm and spread the outer naris as much as possible

- Lesions or a warty appearance, redness or discoloration may be signs of a systemic illness.
- Increased vascularity with many small new blood vessels may indicate liver disease.
- Marked asymmetry may be noted secondary to injury.
- Narrowing of the nostrils when the client inhales may be associated with chronic obstruction and mouth breathing.
- Swelling, hypertrophy, nasal discharge, or crusting may all be signs of infection or allergy.
- Watery, unilateral nasal discharge following a history of head injury may be indicative of skull fracture. Likewise, unilateral, purulent, thick nasal drainage may indicate a foreign body.
- Noisy or obstructed breathing may occur secondary to nasal congestion, trauma to the nasal passage, polyps, or allergies.
- Instability or tenderness on palpation.
- Presence of masses.

TECHNIQUES and NORMAL FINDINGS

ABNORMAL FINDINGS

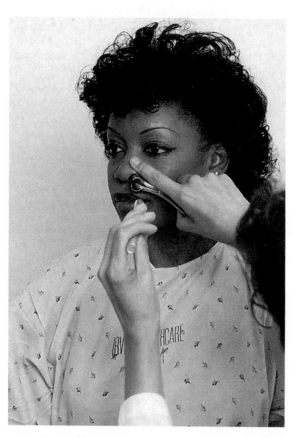

Fig. 11-9 Hold the speculum in the palm of the hand and use your index finger to stabilize the speculum.

without causing pain or discomfort. Use your other hand to adjust the client's head so that the nasal cavity may be visualized (Fig. 11-9). (Alternatively, an otoscope with a nasal speculum attached may be used for the examination.)

The observation of the nares has two focuses. The first is to observe the nasal septum for deviation. Deviation is not an important finding unless the client complains of a decreased air flow through the nares. If breathing through the nares is a problem, then the finding is significant. The second reason for examining the nares is to evaluate the turbinates and nasal mucosa. Observe the following:

(1) With the client's head erect—note floor of the nose, inferior turbinate, nasal hairs, and mucosa, which should be slightly darker red than oral mucosa. Also note the vascular area on the medial side of the septum in the lower third of the nasal cavity (Kiesselbach area). (Most nosebleeds occur from the Kiesselbach area) (Fig. 11-10). The client's nasal septum should be straight and midline. There should be no perforations, bleeding, or crusting.

(2) Client's head back—observe the middle meatus and middle turbinate. The turbinates should be the same color as surrounding tissue, which is a deep pink color.

■ Deviated nasal septum with a decrease in turbulent air flow should be considered abnormal.

■ Rhinitis—indicating that the nasal mucosa is swollen and inflamed-appearing.
■ Sinus drainage or masses.
■ Turbinates may appear pale pink or bluish-gray and swollen, indicating an allergic response. Increased redness may occur secondary to infection, whereas localized redness and swelling in the vestibule may indicate a furuncle or localized infection. A rounded, elongated mass projecting into the nasal cavity may be a polyp.
■ Nasal polyps are benign growths that may occur secondary to chronic allergies or systemic diseases such as cystic fibrosis.

TECHNIQUES and NORMAL FINDINGS

ABNORMAL FINDINGS

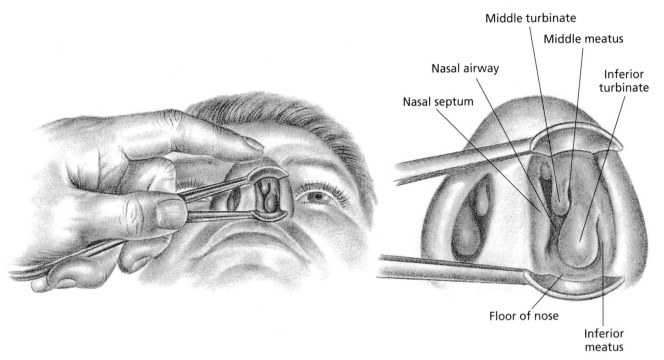

Fig. 11-10 View of the nasal mucosa through the nasal speculum. *(From Seidel et al, 1995.)*

INSPECT the frontal and maxillary sinus area for Swelling (Fig. 11-11). PALPATE the frontal and maxillary paranasal sinus areas for Tenderness or Bogginess. To assess the frontal sinuses, press upward with your thumbs over the sinus areas below the eyebrows. Then to assess the maxillary sinuses, press in the same manner over the sinus areas below the cheekbones. (CAUTION: Do not press directly over the eyeballs.)

■ The appearance of swelling, bogginess, or tenderness on palpation may indicate sinus congestion or infection.

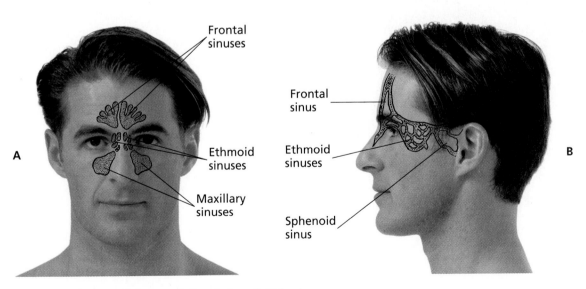

Fig. 11-11 Paranasal sinuses. **A,** Front view. **B,** Side view.

TECHNIQUES and NORMAL FINDINGS

ABNORMAL FINDINGS

If the client complains of sinus pain or shows signs of sinus congestion, perform transillumination of the sinus area. To do this:

1. Darken the room. Use a sinus transilluminator or small bright pen light.
2. Transilluminate the maxillary sinuses by placing the source of light lateral to the nose, just beneath the medial aspect of the eye. Look through the client's open mouth for illumination of the hard palate (Fig. 11-12).
3. Transilluminate the frontal sinuses by placing the light source against the medial aspect of each supraorbital rim. Look for a dim red glow as light is transmitted above the eyebrows (Fig. 11-13).

■ An absence of a glow during transillumination of the sinuses may indicate that the sinus is congested and is filled with secretions or that the sinus has never developed.

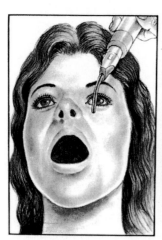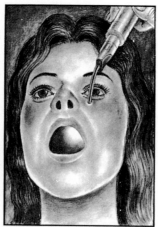

Fig. 11-12   Transillumination of the maxillary sinuses.

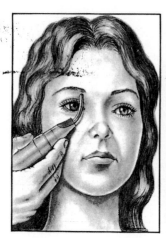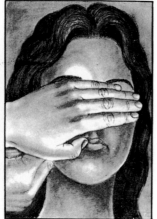

Fig. 11-13   Transillumination of the frontal sinuses.

TECHNIQUES and NORMAL FINDINGS

ABNORMAL FINDINGS

MOUTH AND OROPHARYNX

Examination of the mouth involves inspection and palpation of the temporomandibular joint, lips, gums, teeth, tongue, hard and soft palates, and buccal mucosa.

PALPATE temporomandibular joint for Tenderness or Discomfort.
Place two fingers in front of each ear and ask the client to slowly open and close the mouth and move the lower jaw from side to side (Fig. 11-14). The jaw should move smoothly, opening 1.33 to 1.75 inches (3.5 to 4.5 cm). Note presence of tenderness, crepitus, clicking, or referred pain with jaw movement on either one or both sides.

■ Limited excursion (less than normal). Complaints of tenderness or referred pain, crepitus, or clicking, especially on closure of the jaw.

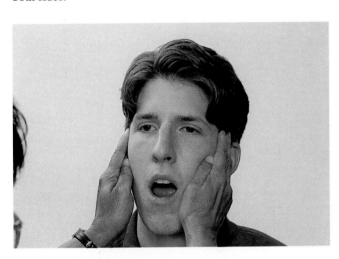

Fig. 11-14 Position fingers in front of each ear in preparation for examination of the TMJ.

General mouth characteristics.
First, as the client opens his or her mouth:

NOTE the Odor of the breath. Normally, mouth odor should be slightly sweet or have no odor at all.
Have the client close his or her mouth.

■ An acetone odor on the breath may indicate diabetic ketoacidosis.
■ A fetid odor may occur secondary to gum disease, caries, poor dental care, or sinusitis.

INSPECT the lips for Color, Symmetry, Moisture, and Texture. Lips should appear pink, symmetric both vertically and laterally. The lips should be smooth and moist and have slight vertical linear markings. There should be a distinct border between the lips and the facial skin (vermillion border) and should not be interrupted by lesions.

■ Pale lips may be indicative of anemia or shock. Cyanotic-colored lips and circumoral cyanosis may indicate lack of adequately oxygenated blood flow related to cardiovascular or respiratory problems or hypothermia. Reddened or cherry-colored lips may indicate carbon monoxide poisoning.

🌐 Racial Variation

Dimpling or lip pits are a normal variation found in the commissure of the lips, occurring in about 20% of African Americans, 12% of whites, and 7% of Asian Americans. Lips may have a natural blue tone in darker-skinned individuals.

TECHNIQUES and NORMAL FINDINGS	ABNORMAL FINDINGS

ABNORMAL FINDINGS

■ Dry, flaking, or cracked lips may be caused by dehydration; chapping may be secondary to dry air or wind or excessive lip-licking or dehydration (Fig. 11-15).

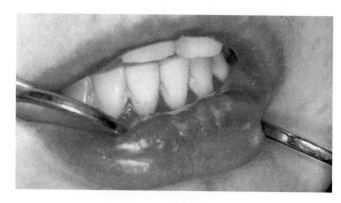

Fig. 11-15   Ulceration of the lower lip.   *(From Tyldesley, 1994.)*

■ Swelling of the lips may be caused by infection or allergy. Lesions, plaques, vesicles, nodules, or ulcerations may be signs of infection, irritation (such as lip biting), or skin cancer.

INSPECT the teeth for Alignment. Ask the client to clench the teeth and smile. (This also partially tests cranial nerve VII—the facial nerve). The upper back teeth should rest directly on the lower back teeth, with the upper incisors slightly overriding the lower ones. The teeth should be evenly spaced.

■ Protrusion of the upper or lower incisors, or upper incisors that do not overlap over the lower ones on closure, are indications of malocclusion (Fig. 11-16).

INSPECT the teeth for Number, Color, and Surface Characteristics. There should be 32 teeth, which should be white, yellow, or gray and have smooth edges. During the examination, note notching, caries, and missing teeth. The characteristics of the teeth may have racial variations.

 Racial Variations

Whites have the smallest teeth.
African Americans have somewhat larger teeth.
Asians and *American Indians* have the largest teeth.

(*Note:* Upper or lower third molars may be congenitally absent.)

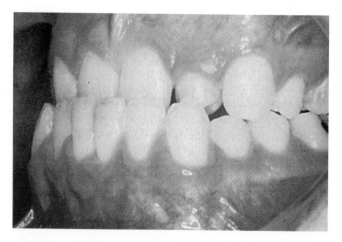

Fig. 11-16   Class III malocclusion.   *(From Scully and Welbury, 1994.)*

TECHNIQUES and NORMAL FINDINGS

ABNORMAL FINDINGS

Classes of Malocclusion

Class I
Molars have customary relationship, but the line of occlusion is incorrect because of malpositioned teeth from rotations or other causes.

Class II
Lower molars are distally positioned in relation to the upper molars; the line of occlusion may or may not be correct.

Class III
Lower molars are medially positioned in relation to the upper molars; the line of occlusion may or may not be correct.

(From Seidel et al, 1995)

■ Missing teeth may occur secondary to tooth extraction or trauma.

■ Darkened or stained teeth may occur secondary to coffee, medications, or poor dental care.

■ Presence of debris, especially at the gum line, usually occurs because of poor dental habits.

■ Excessively exposed tooth neck with receding gums may occur secondary to aging or gingival disease. Gingivitis and edema can develop into advanced periodontal disease, with erosion of gum tissue, destruction of underlying bone, and loosening of the teeth.

PALPATE the teeth for Stability. Wearing examining gloves, attempt to move the teeth with your fingers. The teeth should be firmly anchored and should move little if at all.

■ Marked movement of the teeth or loose teeth may be secondary to either periodontal disease or trauma.

INSPECT and PALPATE inner lips and gums. Ask the client to remove any dental appliances. Have him or her open the mouth slightly so you can inspect and palpate inner lips and upper and lower gingivobuccal fornices.

🌐 Cultural Note

Lower sociocultural populations may have poor dental health secondary to inadequate health insurance and limited access to dental care. Population groups with a higher than average incidence of gingivitis include Mexicans, Cubans, and Puerto Ricans. *(HHANES 1982–1984).*

TECHNIQUES and NORMAL FINDINGS

The gingiva, the gum line around the base of the teeth, should have a pink appearance with a clearly defined margin at each tooth. The gum line beneath dentures should be free of inflammation, swelling, or bleeding.

 Racial Variation

Dark-skinned individuals may have a patchy brown pigmentation of the gums. There may be a dark melanotic line along the gingival margin.

Wearing gloves, palpate the gums for lesions, thickening, tenderness, or masses.

ABNORMAL FINDINGS

- ◼ Color changes of the gums to pale, cyanotic, or red, may indicate systemic problems.
- ◼ Bleeding of the gums may occur secondary to systemic disease or gingival gum disease.
- ◼ Other specific changes of the gums may be indicative of specific problems. For example, a blue-black line along the gum margin may indicate chronic lead or bismuth poisoning.
- ◼ Tenderness on palpation or gum bleeding with brushing, or palpation, thickening, or masses may indicate gingival disease or may occur secondary to Dilantin therapy. (Fig. 11-17).

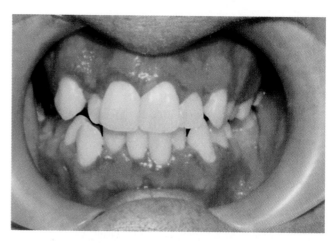

Fig. 11-17   Enlargement of the gums.   *(From Bingham, Hawke and Kwok, 1992.)*

INSPECT buccal mucosa and pillars for Color and Symmetry. Ask the client to open the mouth widely to allow you to inspect buccal mucosa using a penlight and tongue blade. Inspect the anterior and posterior pillars. Note the color of the mucosa and the symmetry of the pillars. The color of the tissue should be pale coral or pink with slight vascularity. Stenson's duct (the parotid duct) should be visualized as a slightly elevated pinpoint red marking. The buccal mucosa should be smooth, with a transverse occlusion line appearing adjacent to where teeth meet. Clear saliva should cover the surface.

 Racial Variation

Darker-skinned individuals often have darker oral pigmentation. This pigmentation increases with age, and may also be seen in older, fair-skinned adults. A gray-white, benign lesion of the buccal mucosa called leukoedema occurs in 70% to 90% of dark-skinned individuals and 40% of fair-skinned individuals. This finding also increases with age.

- ◼ Aphthous ulcers on the buccal mucosa appear as a white, round or oval ulcerative lesion with a red halo.
- ◼ White patches or plaques may indicate infections such as thrush.
- ◼ A dappled brown surface may occur secondary to adrenal insufficiency.
- ◼ Koplik's spots on the buccal mucosa are a classic identification of measles (see p. 243 for further description of Koplik's spots).
- ◼ Excessively dry mouth or excessive salivation may indicate salivary gland blockage or may occur secondary to medications, dehydration, or stress.

TECHNIQUES and NORMAL FINDINGS

ABNORMAL FINDINGS

For clients who wear dentures, observe for any areas where pressure areas or ulcerations occur.

INSPECT the tongue for Movement, Color, Ulceration, and Surface Characteristics. Ask the client to stick out his or her tongue. (This maneuver also tests cranial nerve XII—the hypoglossal nerve). The forward thrust should be smooth and symmetric and the tongue itself should appear symmetric. The tongue should be pink and moist with a glistening covering dorsally and laterally. During the inspection, note any swelling or variation in size, color, coating, or ulceration.

PALPATE the tongue for Irregularities. Following inspection, grasp the tongue with a 4 × 4 inch gauze pad and palpate all sides for texture. Be sure to wear an examination glove (Fig. 11-18). The tongue should feel smooth and even.

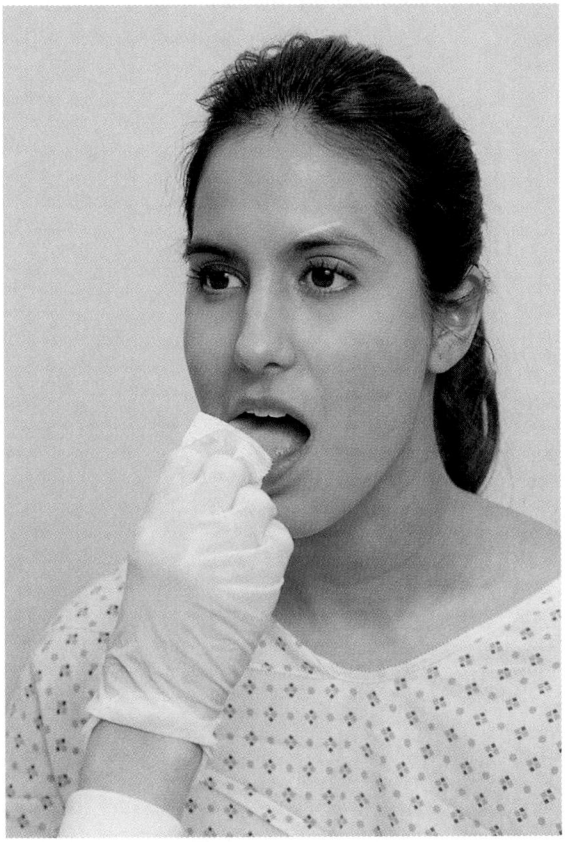

- ■ For clients who wear dentures: gum tenderness, lesions, or thickening may indicate malfitting dentures.

- ■ Atrophy of the tongue on one side or deviation of the tongue may be signs of a neurologic problem.
- ■ A smooth or beefy-colored, red, swollen tongue with a slick appearance may indicate niacin or vitamin B_{12} deficiency.
- ■ A hairy tongue with yellow-brown to black elongated papillae may occur secondary to antibiotic therapy or pipe smoking.
- ■ An enlarged tongue may be seen in clients with mental retardation, hypothyroidism, or acromegaly.
- ■ A small tongue may be seen in clients with malnutrition.

- ■ Lumps, nodules, or masses may indicate local or systemic disease or cancerous lesions.

Fig. 11-18 Grasp the tongue with a 4 × 4 inch gauze pad.

TECHNIQUES and NORMAL FINDINGS

ABNORMAL FINDINGS

During the palpation, note any lumps, nodules, or areas of thickening. Note: After putting on the gloves, wash your hands with water to remove the powder coating before putting your hands in the client's mouth.

Following palpation, pull the tongue to either side.

INSPECT the lateral surfaces of the tongue for Lesions or Ulcerations. If lesions are noted, scrape the area with a tongue blade to differentiate between food particles and actual mouth lesions.

Ask the client to raise the tongue to the roof of the mouth. Inspect and palpate the ventral surface and floor of the mouth. It should be pale, coral, or pink, with the frenulum centered and the submaxillary duct (Wharton's ducts) opening visible.

INSPECT the palate and uvula for Texture, Color, and Surface Characteristics. Instruct the client to tilt his or her head back so that the palate and uvula may be inspected. The hard palate should be smooth, pale, and immovable with irregular transverse rugae. Torus palatinus, a bony protuberance at the midline of the hard palate, is a normal variation and may be seen in approximately 25% of all women (Fig. 11-19). The soft palate and uvula should be smooth and pink, with the uvula in a midline position.

- ■ Leukoplakia is a whitish lesion that may not be scraped off by a tongue blade. Oral candida is similar in appearance.
- ■ Abnormalities include discoloration, ulceration, masses, or other lesions.

- ■ Nodules that are noted on the palate that are not at the midline may indicate a tumor. Other systemic diseases such as HIV infections may show oral lesions, such as Kaposi sarcoma on both the hard and soft palates.
- ■ Opportunistic infections such as candida may occur when an individual has been on antibiotics or is immunosuppressed.
- ■ Failure of the soft palate to rise bilaterally, as well as uvula deviation during vocalization, may indicate a neurologic problem such as paralysis of the vagus nerve.

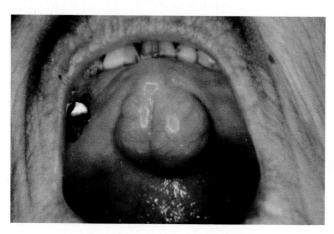

Fig. 11-19   **Torus palatinus of the hard palate.**   *(From Bingham, Hawke and Kwok, 1992.)*

 Racial Variation

Asians and American Indians/Alaskan Natives have a higher prevalence of torus palatinus than African Americans or whites.

INSPECT the Movement of the soft palate. Instruct the client to say "ah." (If necessary, depress the tongue with a tongue blade.) Observe to see if the soft palate rises symmetrically with the uvula remaining in the midline position. (This also tests cranial nerves IX and X—the glossopharyngeal and vagus nerves).

 Racial Variation

A split uvula have been reported as occurring in about 10% of Asians and 18% in some American Indian groups. *(Giger and Davidhizar, 1995).*

TECHNIQUES and NORMAL FINDINGS

ABNORMAL FINDINGS

INSPECT the posterior wall of the pharynx for Color and Surface Characteristics. With the client's mouth wide open and a tongue blade holding the tongue to the side, examine the posterior wall of the pharynx (Fig. 11-20). The tissue should be smooth and have a glistening pink coloration. There may be small irregular spots of lymphatic and some small blood vessels.

■ Exudate or mucoid film on the posterior pharynx may be present secondary to postnasal drip or infection.
■ A grayish tinge to the membrane may occur with allergies or diphtheria.

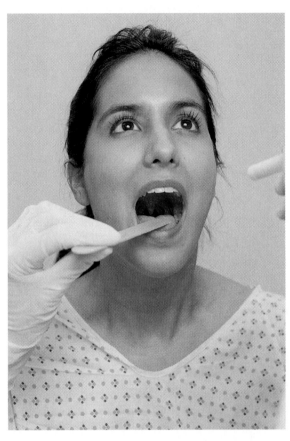

Fig. 11-20 Displace the tongue with a tongue depressor for inspection of the pharynx.

INSPECT the tonsils for Texture and Color. The tonsils extend beyond the posterior pillars. The tonsils should appear slightly pink with an irregular texture.

■ Swollen, reddened tonsils with or without exudate may be indicative of infection. Tonsil swelling ranges from 1+ (slightly swollen) to 4+ (kissing tonsils).

INFANTS/NEWBORNS

■ APPROACH

The physical examination of the nose and mouth is easy and straightforward; the problem arises when the child is uncooperative or unable to hold still. The infant must be carefully and securely restrained by a parent or other adult who acts as a "holder" to ensure the child's safety and to permit the full viewing of the examination area. The restraining is usually done with the infant in a supine position, with the arms extended securely above the child's head (Fig. 11-21). The holder will then be able to secure both the child's arms and head. A second holder or the examiner may need to immobilize the infant's lower extremities.

■ FINDINGS

Nose

The infant's nose is small and difficult to examine. The base of the nose should be appropriate to the size of the face. A wide base nose (greater than 2.5 cm in the term infant) along with widely spaced eyes may be indicative of hypertelorism. The examiner may find milia across the infant's nose.

The infant's nares have only minimal movement with breathing. Slight nasal flaring may be seen if the infant has respiratory distress. The examination of the inside of the nares should be conducted by tilting the infant's head back and shining a light into the nares. Do not attempt to insert a speculum into the nares.

Test the nares' patency by holding one nostril closed and then the other one. Because infants are obligatory nose breathers, any obstruction of the nares secondary to a congenital abnormality such as choanal atresia, foreign body, or nasal secretions will cause the infant to be irritable or distressed. If a newborn has nasal congestion, suction the nares with a bulb syringe or small-lumen catheter.

🌐 Racial Variation

The nasal bridge of African-American, Asian-American, and some American Indian infants may be flat. A cleft lip or cleft palate are most common in Asian and American Indian populations, and rare in African Americans.

Mouth and Oropharynx

The initial examination of the infant's mouth should include an assessment of the integrity of the mouth and the absence of congenital abnormalities such as cleft lip. The examination of the lips may show evidence of a sucking callus. This should disappear after the first few weeks of life.

It is generally possible to examine the infant's mouth while the infant is crying. The buccal mucosa should appear pink, moist, and smooth. If whitish patches are seen along the mucosa, scrape the area with a tongue blade to differentiate between a lesion and milk deposits. Patches that do not scrape clean may indicate candidiasis (thrush). The infant's gums should appear smooth and full. Occasionally, a natal loose tooth may be found. If found, these teeth should be removed to prevent possible aspiration. Other normal findings may include the presence of small white epithelial cells on the palate or gums. These are called Bohn nodules or Epstein pearls (Fig. 11-22).

The infant's tongue should be appropriate to the size of the mouth and should fit well into the floor of the mouth. Macroglossia or aglossia may be signs of Down syndrome or congenital hypothyroidism.

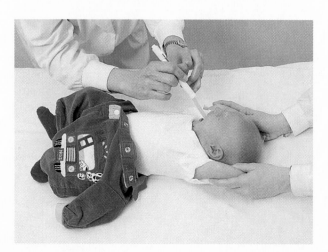

Fig. 11-21　Positioning of infant for examination of nose and mouth.

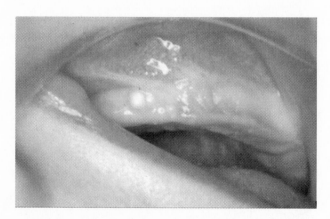

Fig. 11-22　Epstein's pearls (gingival cysts) in an infant. *(From Scully and Welbury, 1994.)*

Finally, the infant's hard and soft palates should be examined. Careful observation of the hard palate should confirm the absence of a cleft palate.

Following inspection, the examiner may use a gloved hand and an examination light to palpate the buccal mucosa and gums. While the examiner's finger is in the infant's mouth, the strength of the infant's suck should also be assessed. The infant should have a strong suck with the tongue pushing upward against the examiner's finger.

CHILDREN

■ APPROACH

Examining the nose and mouth of the toddler and young child presents a cooperative challenge. The very young child will probably tolerate the mouth and nose examination better while sitting on the parent's lap. Have the child sit on the adult's lap with his or her back to the parent. The parent may then immobilize the child's legs by placing them between the adult's legs. The parent then has both hands free. One hand should be used to reach around the child's body to restrain the child's arms and chest. The other hand may be used to assist the examiner by immobilizing the child's head (Fig. 11-23). Once the child becomes too large for the parent's lap, the examination is best performed with the child in a supine position on the examination table. Care must always be taken to prevent the child from making sudden movement during the examination.

Regardless of the immobilization technique used, time should also be taken to try to gain the cooperation of the child. Once the child is old enough to understand and is curious about what is happening, the examiner should also take the time to engage the child. Move slowly and permit the child to handle the equipment, and assure the child that your intent is not to hurt. The actual examination procedure may start by permitting the child to play with the tongue blade and to ask the young child to show you his or her teeth or play smiling and "ahh" games. This is generally nonthreatening and may lead the way to cooperation.

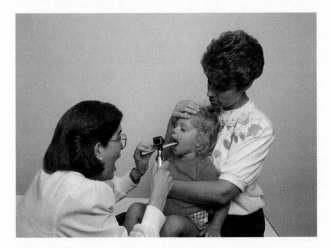

Fig. 11-23 Technique for immobilizing a young child's head before examination.

There is no guarantee that these methods will work with all children. It may be helpful to divide the examination into two phases and work them into the rest of the examination at different points. If all else fails and the child is uncooperative, the child must be immobilized by a "holder" to ensure the child's safety. A sudden move by the child could result in injury.

■ FINDINGS

Nose and Paranasal Sinuses

The young child's nose should be assessed in the same manner as the infant's. The child's external nose should be examined for presence of a transverse crease at the bridge of the nose. This is commonly the result of the "allergic salute," which occurs when a child has a frequent runny nose or allergies and wipes the nose with an upward sweep of the palm of the hand.

The child's head should be tilted backward, and the light should be shone into the nares. The examiner may use his or her thumb on the tip of the nose to make a better visualization. If visualization of a larger area is needed, the examiner may use the otoscope with a large speculum.

If the child has unilateral nasal patency or has an odor from the nose, the examiner should carefully evaluate the nares for a possible foreign body.

The examination of the child's sinuses should become part of the examination after approximately age 8. There is a wide age variation in the development of the sinuses.

Mouth and Oropharynx

Inspect the child's lips for dryness, flaking, or cracking corners of the mouth. If present, these signs may indicate excess licking of the lips, malnutrition, or infection such as impetigo.

Salivation normally increases in children between 3 months and 2 years of age. Note that an excessively dry mouth may indicate dehydration, fever, or drug ingestion such as atropine. Excessive salivation may indicate gingivostomatitis or multiple dental caries. Drooling after 12 months of age may be indicative of a neurologic disorder.

Carefully examine the teeth, noting eruption sequence and timing. Also note the condition and the positioning of the teeth. Flattened edges on the teeth may indicate teeth grinding (bruxism). Also note the health of the teeth and the presence of debris around the teeth or gum line. Darkened, brown, or black teeth may indicate decay or oral iron therapy. Mottled or pitted teeth may result from tetracycline therapy during tooth development.

Note the characteristics and size of the tongue. A strawberry-colored tongue, along with other clinical signs, may be indicative of scarlet fever.

If the mouth has a fetid or musty smell, further investigation should be made regarding hygiene practices, local or systemic infections, or sinusitis.

The child's buccal mucosa should be pink, moist, and without lesions such as Koplik's spots (as seen in measles) or candidiasis (thrush).

The child's tonsils should be dark pink in color and without vertical reddened lines, general redness, swelling, or exudate. The tonsils grow to their maximum size between 2 and 6 years of age and have the maximum potential to obstruct the child's airway during this time. Normally, the child's tonsils should not interfere with swallowing or breathing.

OLDER ADULTS

■ APPROACH

Special considerations for the older client include the physiologic and anatomic changes that occur secondary to aging. The normal bone reabsorption that occurs with aging may be escalated by systemic disease or poor dental care. The older adult's body heals more slowly, thereby leading to a higher risk of infection of the oral cavity. If the client has other physical disabilities, the client may have difficulty performing adequate oral self-care.

Other effects of the aging process include considerations such as dental restorations that may be deteriorating with time; tooth enamel erosion and slow deterioration from years of vigorous brushing; and gum tissue reabsorption that causes the neck of the tooth to become exposed. This in turn makes the tooth vulnerable to decay; the teeth may wear down because of years of chewing; and, finally, the gingival tissue becomes less elastic and more vulnerable to trauma.

In addition to physical changes, older clients may be sensitive to the fact that they are unable to provide the level of dental hygiene that they were capable of when they were younger. Or a client may be aware that the condition of the teeth is poor, and he or she may therefore be sensitive to the examination. Clients with dentures or dental appliances may be sensitive to having their oral cavity examined, especially if the examiner requests that the dentures or appliance be removed. The examiner should be aware of the client's sensitivity, but should reassure the client that a full examination of the gums is necessary to ensure that no problems are present.

■ FINDINGS

The examination of older adults proceeds as for adults. Abnormal findings peculiar to this age group include:

Nose and Paranasal Sinuses

There may be an increase in the amount of nasal hair, especially in men. The hairs are coarse and bristly.

Mouth and Oropharynx

Because of loss of elasticity of joint ligaments, the temporomandibular joint may dislocate when the mouth is opened widely. Care should therefore be taken during the mouth examination to not cause undue stress on the mouth.

The surface of the lips may be marked, with deep wrinkling and fissures at the corner of the mouth (perleche) associated with an inflammatory response to severe overclosure or vitamin deficiency. The older client is at higher risk for squamous cell carcinoma of the lip, especially if the client has been a long-time pipe smoker. The older adult's buccal mucosa may appear thin and less vascular than the younger adult. There may also be a decrease in saliva secondary to medications.

Aging changes cause the gum line to recede secondary to bone degeneration, causing the teeth to appear longer. The gums may become more friable and bleed with slight pressure.

The teeth may become darkened or stained. Many older adults may become edentulous or have caps or bridges. Old dental restorations may be degenerating, especially at margins. Dental occlusion surfaces may be markedly worn down. Malocclusion of the teeth may be common secondary to the migration of the teeth after tooth extraction. Loosening of the teeth is a special hazard associated with periodontal disease and bone reabsorption.

CLIENTS WITH SITUATIONAL VARIATIONS

PREGNANT WOMEN

■ APPROACH

The variations that occur during pregnancy are transitional and will generally disappear after the child's birth.

■ FINDINGS

The nose and mouth of the pregnant woman undergoes several changes related to an increase in vascularization and estrogen levels. The increased systemic vascularization may cause an increase in the redness of the nose, pharynx, and gums; the gums become swollen, spongy, and may bleed during brushing. An increase in the level of systemic estrogen may cause an increase in nasal congestion and sinusitis.

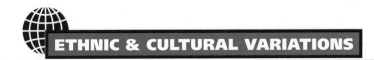

ETHNIC & CULTURAL VARIATIONS

■ FINDINGS

A number of benign physical variations exist in the nasal and oral cavities across racial and ethnic lines. The nose, for example, ranges from flat and broad to prominent and narrow. The nasal bridge is often quite flat in appearance in African-American and Asian-American infants.

Teeth serve as another prime example. Tooth size varies widely between racial groups, with larger teeth often seen in conjunction with a prognathic jaw. A pattern set of either 28 or 32 permanent teeth is typical in adults, with third molar agenesis a common racial variant. Tooth enamel is harder and denser in African Americans, leading to less tooth decay and loss. Congenital tooth formation is seen frequently among some Alaskan Native groups but is quite rare in the general population. Such differences are important to note when using the teeth as an indicator of development, general nutritional status, or hygienic practices.

Coloring of lips, gums, and oral mucosa also vary. Dark-skinned individuals often display darker oral pigmentation, particularly as they age. A dark melanotic line along the gingival margin is a common finding in those with darker skin. Leukoedema is also more common in those with darker pigmentation.

Distinctive findings such as a bifid or split uvula and torus palatinus have definite racial patterns and are seen primarily in American Indian/Alaskan Natives and Asian Americans. While these are benign findings, a split uvula is often a subclinical manifestation of a cleft palate. Cleft lip and cleft palate are abnormal physical findings most commonly seen in American Indian/Alaskan Native and Asian-American infants.

E X A M I N A T I O N S U M M A R Y
Nose, Sinus, Mouth, and Oropharynx

Nose and Paranasal Sinuses *(pp. 223-226)*
- Inspect and Palpate the nose for
  General appearance and symmetry
  Discharge
  Tenderness
- Evaluate the olfactory nerve for
  Intactness
- Inspect the internal nasal cavity for
  Patency
- Inspect and Palpate the paranasal sinuses for
  Swelling
  Tenderness or bogginess

Mouth and Oropharynx *(pp. 227-233)*
- Palpate the temporomandibular joint for
  Tenderness and discomfort

- Note breath for
  Odor
- Inspect the lips, teeth, and gums for
  General appearance
  Teeth alignment and stability
- Inspect the oral cavity and buccal mucosa for
  Color, symmetry, and texture
- Inspect and Palpate the tongue for
  Movement, symmetry, color, ulceration, and
  surface characteristics
- Inspect the hard and soft palates for
  Texture, color, and surface characteristics
- Inspect the posterior pharynx and tonsils for
  Color and surface characteristics

COMMON PROBLEMS/CONDITIONS
associated with the Nose, Sinuses, Mouth, and Oropharynx

NOSE

■ *Nasal polyps:* Smooth, pale gray tissue enlargements in the nasal cavity that occur most commonly in clients with chronic allergic rhinitis (Fig. 11-24). These non-tender growths may become so large that they actually obstruct the nasal passage.

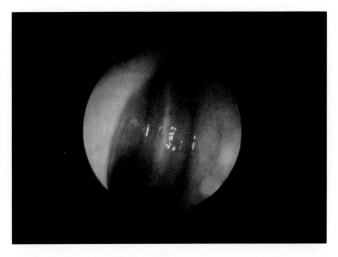

Fig. 11-24 A simple benign nasal polyp (center). It is smooth, semitranslucent and has a gray color. *(From Bingham, Hawke and Kwok, 1992.)*

LIPS, MOUTH, AND OROPHARYNX

LIP LESIONS

■ *Herpes simplex I (cold sore):* A common viral infection of the lip that may occur secondary to fever, colds, allergy, or trauma to the lip (Fig. 11-25). Like other herpes type lesions, the lesion stages progress from a cluster of clear vesicles, to pustules, and finally crusts.

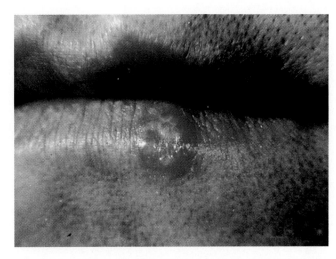

Fig. 11-25 Herpes simplex lesion (cold sore) of lower lip. *(From Grimes and Grimes, 1994.)*

■ *Squamous cell carcinoma of the lip:* Appears as ulcerated sores of the lip (Fig. 11-26). It may also be seen on the floor of the mouth or the lateral border of the tongue. The lesion is usually indurated and has a raised irregular border and an erythematous base.

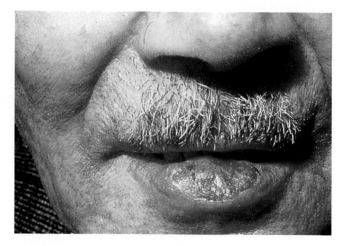

Fig. 11-26   Squamous cell carcinoma.   *(From Hill, 1994.)*

■ *Cleft lip:* This congenital abnormality may occur as a cleft lip only with an intact hard palate, or it may include both the lip and the hard palate (Fig. 11-27).

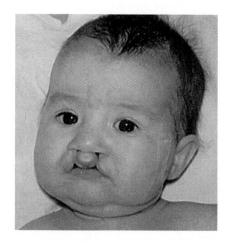

Fig. 11-27   Bilateral cleft lip in an infant.   *(From Scully and Welbury, 1994.)*

TEETH AND GUMS

■ *Advanced pyorrhea:* Gingivitis and edema can develop into advanced pyorrhea with erosion of the gum tissue, destruction of underlying bone, and loosening of the teeth (Fig. 11-28).

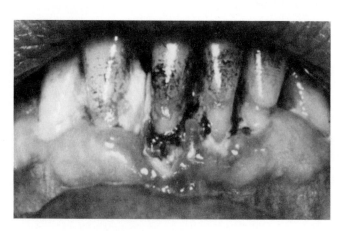

Figure 11-28   Advanced pyorrhea.   *(From DeWeese et al, 1988.)*

TONGUE

■ *Hairy tongue:* Blackish, painful lesions that are felt on top of the tongue (Fig. 11-29). These are reported as feeling like a "hairy" sensation. There is usually a history of excessive antibiotic use, excessive use of mouthwash, smoking, or alcohol consumption.

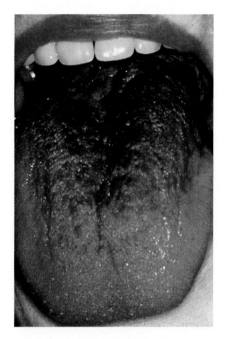

Fig 11-29   Hairy tongue.   *(From Dunlap, Barker, 1991; Colgate-Hoyt/ Gel-Kam.)*

BUCCAL MUCOSA

■ *Candidiasis (thrush) (monilial infection):* Appears on the tongue, buccal mucosa, or posterior pharynx as a whitish, cheesy patch resembling milk curd (Fig. 11-30). If the membrane is peeled off, a raw, bleeding, erythematous area results. Thrush is commonly seen in infants, but in adults is seen primarily in individuals who are chronically debilitated, in clients who are immunosuppressed, persons with HIV/AIDS, or those who have been on antibiotic therapy.

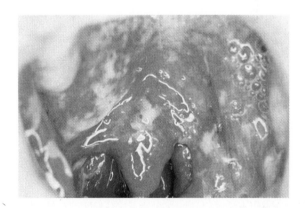

Fig. 11-30   Candidiasis (thrush)   *(From Sigler and Schuring, 1993.)*

■ *Aphthous ulcer (canker sore):* Painful lesions that appear commonly on the buccal mucosa (Fig. 11-31). They may also appear on the lips, tip and side of tongue, or palate. They appear as white, round, or oval ulcerative lesions with a red halo. Ulcers may last up to two weeks; their etiology is unknown.

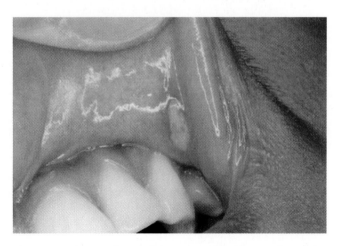

Fig. 11-31   A small aphthous ulcer (canker sore) on the lower lip.   *(From Bingham, Hawke and Kwok, 1992.)*

▪ *Leukoplakia:* Seen as a painless white area on the inside of the cheek, tongue, lower lip, or floor of the mouth (Fig. 11-32). The lesion is hyperkeratinized and cannot be scraped off. Leukoplakia is most frequently seen in older men and may be linked to smoking, AIDS, alcoholism, and chewing tobacco.

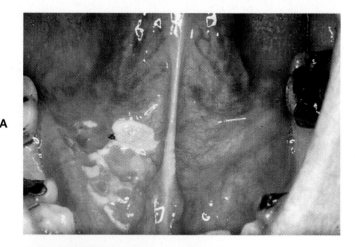

A

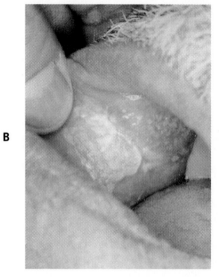

B

Fig. 11-32 **Leukoplakia.** *(A from Dunlap, Barker, 1991; Colgate-Hoyt/Gel-Kam; B from Bingham, Hawke, and Kwok, 1992.)*

■ **Oral Kaposi's sarcoma:** A malignancy seen in persons with AIDS appears as incompletely formed blood vessels in the mouth (Fig. 11-33). These vessels form lesions of various shades and sizes as the blood extravasates in response to the malignant tumor of the membrane.

 Cultural Note

The incidence of oral cavity cancer in the United States is highest among Chinese Americans and African Americans, with African-American men leading the list.

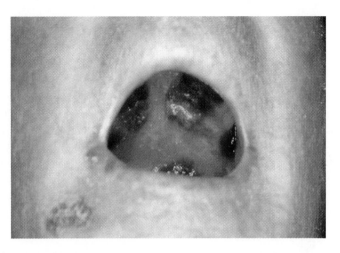

Fig. 11-33 The bluish raised lesion seen on the palate of this patient who has AIDS is Kaposi's sarcoma. *(From Bingham, Hawke, and Kwok, 1992.)*

■ **Koplik's spots:** A classic diagnostic finding of measles (Fig. 11-34). They appear on the buccal mucosa as small bluish white areas with irregular borders.

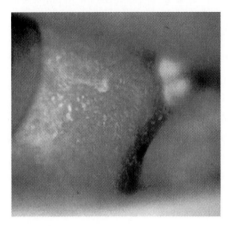

Fig. 11-34 Koplik's spots on the buccal mucosa. *(From Scully and Welbury, 1994.)*

&Nursing Diagnosis

Sample Documentation

CASE 1   42-year-old woman with jaw pain and clicking when she chews.

Subjective

Reports that approximately 2 months ago, when she was chewing food during a routine meal, she felt a "catch and pain" in jaw and was unable to close mouth; during following 30 to 40 minute period, "locking" eased, pain continued, and she was able to close mouth. Since then reports increased jaw pain during chewing, pain radiating to ear; reports "clicking" sensation and sound when attempting to chew.

Since problem began, primarily on liquid diet; reports weight decrease from 130 lb (59 kg) to 115 lb (52.3 kg); last bowel movement 2 days ago, hard texture.

Objective

Height: 5'5" (165 cm). Weight: 115 lbs (52.3 kg). Healthy-appearing female in no acute distress. Able to open and close mouth widely with slight pain on left side, radiating to ear. Teeth align correctly upon closing mouth and clenching teeth; no evidence of malocclusion.

Complains of left-side jaw tenderness with palpation of temporomandibular joint (TMJ); crepitation with clicking felt at left TMJ with opening and closing jaw.

Remaining mouth examination not remarkable.

. . . .

Nursing Diagnosis #1

Pain related to temporomandibular joint dysfunction

Defining Characteristics   Increased jaw pain; clicking sensation when chewing.

Nursing Diagnosis #2

Altered nutrition: less than body requirements related to inadequate food intake secondary to painful chewing.

Defining Characteristics   Too painful to chew; on liquid diet for 2 months; weight loss.

Sample Documentation & Nursing Diagnosis

CASE 2 19-month-old male with nasal discharge and odor about the head.

Subjective

Mother reports 4-day history of yellow nasal discharge. Reports no history of illness, fever, congestion, rash, or nausea or vomiting. Reports slow onset of bilateral nasal stuffiness and discharge, and increasing foul odor about child's head; reports child sits in high chair and feeds self finger food; foods eaten in last week include cheerios, yogurt, raisins, jello squares; reports child is very fussy.

Objective

Tympanic temperature 99.1° F (37.3° C)

Healthy-appearing, playful male child actively exploring examining room.

Nose Bilateral purulent, yellow nasal discharge; internal nasal exam—small, swollen, foul-smelling raisin in left nostril; right nostril clear, no blockage.

Mouth Lips pink, no lesions; 18 primary teeth, all intact, no caries; oral cavity and buccal mucosa pink without lesions; posterior pharynx pink with large tonsils visualized behind posterior pillar; tonsils without exudate or lesions.

Respiratory Bilaterally equal breath sounds; no acute respiratory distress.

••

Nursing Diagnosis #1

Risk for infection related to foreign body in nose.

Defining Characteristics 4-day history of nasal discharge, foul-smelling odor.

Nursing Diagnosis #2

Knowledge deficit related to injury prevention.

Defining Characteristics Raisin found in nostril.

HEALTH PROMOTION

■ **Smoking** Clients who smoke are at risk for mouth and lip cancer. At high risk are clients who smoke a pipe (lip cancer) and who chew smokeless tobacco (mouth cancer and leukoplakia). These individuals should be taught self-examination skills to examine the mouth for sores that won't heal or discolorations in the mouth.

■ **Dental care** All clients, regardless of age, should be encouraged to visit a dentist on a regular basis. Dental visits should begin between 2 and 3 years of age. The American Dental Association (ADA) advises that the frequency of dental examinations be tailored to the individual (ADA, 1985). In addition, clients should be encouraged to use dental floss and regular brushing. Flossing on a regular basis reduces the risk of periodontal disease.

Parents should be taught that young children who take the bottle to bed and suck on the nipple during the night are at higher risk to develop dental caries of the primary teeth. This is especially true if the bottle contains an acidic or cariogenic beverage (fruit juice, milk, or formula). Parents should also be taught that, if their young children have caries of the baby teeth, they should not ignore the problem but should seek dental evaluation. Infection or caries of the primary teeth may affect the secondary teeth.

Parents should be taught to start brushing the child's teeth as soon as they erupt. This not only teaches the child good dental care, but is also a preventative dental practice. It is not necessary for the young child to use toothpaste.

Fluoride is also an important factor in reducing dental caries, especially in children. Clients living in areas where there is no fluoride in the water should be referred for dental evaluation and supplemental fluoride treatments.

■ **Nose sprays** Nose sprays may be very effective in relieving nasal congestion. If used for a long period or routinely, they may indeed cause a "rebound" effect and actually make the nasal congestion problem worse. Clients should therefore be advised to use nose sprays only occasionally. Nose sprays should not be used for more than five consecutive days.

■ **Nasal foreign bodies** Parents should be advised that young children are curious about small objects and may push them up their nose. This may include small objects such as peanuts, corn, beads, or rocks. Children should not be left alone with any small object that may cause them to choke or objects that are smaller than the child's little finger.

??????? STUDY QUESTIONS ???????

1. List three functions of the nose and sinuses.
2. Match the structure to the function.

Septal cartilage	*Drains tears*
Cilia	*Drains paranasal sinus*
Inferior meatus	*Separates the nares*
Middle meatus	*Traps particles*

3. Identify the structures of the mouth and describe their respective functions.
4. What structures make up the oropharynx?
5. Trace the development of deciduous and permanent teeth.
6. List three problems that older adults may face as a result of changes in the structures in the mouth.
7. Match the condition with the correct cause:

Nasal discharge	*Bean lodged in nares*
Nasal obstruction	*Abuse of cocaine*
Epistaxis	*Allergy to ragweed*
Eye pain	*Sinus infection*

8. What historical information would you collect on a client who presents with a mouth ulcer? A sore throat? Difficulty in swallowing?
9. List specific information that is important to gather when taking a history on a young child; an older child; an older adult.
10. What equipment is necessary for performing an examination of the nose, sinuses, mouth, and oropharynx?
11. Describe what you are looking for as you inspect and palpate the nose.
12. Describe nasal signs indicative of allergies; a lodged foreign object; a skull fracture.
13. How is patency of the nose assessed?
14. If an individual complains of sinus congestion, what procedure should you perform? Describe how to perform this procedure. What are you looking for?
15. What characteristics are you looking for when you examine the following structures: (a) lips (b) teeth (c) gums (d) tongue (e) palate.
16. List at least five normal racial variations that may be present on examination of the mouth.
17. Describe how you would differ your approach when examining infants and children of varying ages.
18. List abnormal findings that may be seen primarily in: (a) infants (b) small children (c) older adults.
19. Describe the differences between a cold sore and a squamous cell carcinoma of the lip.
20. Describe the differences in candidiasis and leukoplakia of the buccal mucosa.
21. Describe the appearance of oral Kaposi's sarcoma.
22. List at least three common oral problems that may occur in an individual who is HIV-positive.
23. What behaviors place the young child at risk for developing dental caries? What should parents be taught about dental hygiene for their children?
24. What can occur with prolonged use of nasal sprays?

CHAPTER 12

Ears and Auditory System

ANATOMY AND PHYSIOLOGY

The ear is a sensory organ that functions both in equilibrium and hearing. It is divided into three sections: the outer ear, the middle ear, and the inner ear.

OUTER EAR

The outer ear is made up of the auricle (pinna), which is composed of cartilage and skin, and the auditory ear canal (meatus), which extends for approximately 2 to 3 cm and is covered with cerumen-producing glands (Fig. 12-1).

EXTERNAL EAR CANAL

The adult's external ear canal is configured as an S-shaped pathway leading from the outer ear to the tympanic membrane. The external ear canal in the infant and young child is straighter. This straightness makes the child more prone to ear infections. The canal is covered with sensitive skin and is generally lubricated with cerumen, which is secreted by sebaceous glands in the canal. The underlying structures of the distal half of the external ear and the proximal half of the canal are cartilage and bone, respectively.

TYMPANIC MEMBRANE

The outer ear is separated from the middle ear by the shiny, translucent, pearl-gray tympanic membrane, made up of layers of skin, fibrous tissue, and mucous membrane (Fig. 12-2). This membrane covers the proximal end of the auditory canal. The tympanic membrane is pulled inward at its center by one of the ossicles of the middle ear, called the malleus. Most of the tympanic membrane is taut and is known as the pars tensa; a smaller, less taut part is the pars flaccida, and the dense fibrous ring around the membrane is the annulus. The cone of light may be seen downward and anteriorly. The tympanic membrane is translucent, permitting visualization of the middle ear cavity.

MIDDLE EAR

The middle ear is an air-filled cavity that transmits sound by way of the three tiny bones that make up the ossicle—the malleus, incus, and stapes (Fig. 12-3). The malleus may actually be visualized through the tympanic membrane. The middle ear has a cartilaginous and bony passage, the eustachian tube, between the nasopharynx and the middle ear, which opens briefly during yawning, swallowing, or sneezing to equalize the pressure of the middle ear to the atmosphere.

INNER EAR

The inner ear is a curved cavity inside a bony labyrinth consisting of the vestibule, the semicircular canals, and the cochlea. The vestibule and the semicircular canals make up the organs that coordinate equilibrium. The cochlea is a coiled structure containing the organ of Corti, which transmits sound impulses to the acoustic cranial nerve (VIII).

HEARING

Hearing occurs when sound waves enter the external auditory ear canal and strike the tympanic membrane. The membrane begins to vibrate, which then causes the ossicle behind

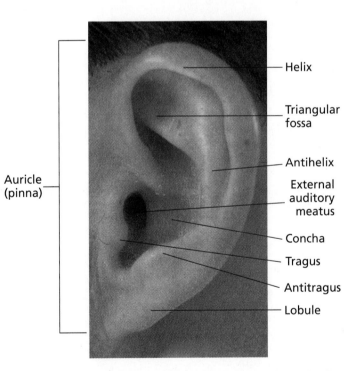

Fig. 12-1 Anatomic structure of the auricle (pinna). The helix is the prominent outer rim, whereas the antihelix is the area parallel and anterior to the helix. The concha is the deep cavity containing the auditory canal meatus. The tragus is the protuberance lying anterior to the auditory canal meatus, and the antitragus is the protuberance on the antihelix opposite the tragus. The lobule is the soft lobe on the bottom of the auricle.

the tympanic membrane to vibrate. The vibrations then travel via the fluid of the cochlea to the hair cells of the organ of Corti. When the delicate hair cells of the organ of Corti are set into motion, cranial nerve VIII is stimulated. The sound wave impulses from the cranial nerve are transmitted to the temporal lobe of the brain for interpretation.

Conductive hearing loss.   This type of hearing loss occurs when a change in the outer or middle ear impairs conduction of sound from the outer to the inner ear. Air conduction is impeded. Common causes of conductive hearing loss include impaction by cerumen (wax in the ear canal), foreign bodies lodged in the ear canal, tumors of the middle ear, and otitis media. Symptoms of conductive hearing loss include diminished hearing and low-volume speaking voice.

Sensorineural hearing loss.   This type of hearing loss is caused by impairment of the organ of Corti. Conditions that commonly cause this type of loss are Meniere's disease and ototoxicity. Presbycusis (a gradual deterioration of hearing secondary to aging) is the most common form of sensorineural hearing loss, and is especially common in the elderly.

DEVELOPMENTAL CONSIDERATIONS

INFANTS

The inner ear develops during the first trimester of pregnancy; an insult to the fetus during that time may impair hearing. The neonate's external auditory canal is shorter than the adult's, with an upward curve. The infant's eustachian tube is wider and, at the same time, shorter and more horizontal than the adult's. Unfortunately, this makes it easier for infection from the pharynx to ascend into the inner ear.

CHILDREN

As the child grows, ear infections usually become less frequent or less likely because the eustachian tube lengthens and its pharyngeal orifice moves inferiorly. However, with the growth of lymphatic tissue, specifically the adenoids, the eustachian tube may become occluded, interfering with aeration of the middle ear.

PREGNANT WOMEN

The capillaries of the eustachian tubes can become engorged with elevated levels of estrogen. This can lead to symptoms of epistaxis, a sense of fullness in the ears, and impaired hearing.

OLDER ADULTS

As the individual ages, the cartilage formation may make the auricle larger and more prominent. A decrease in active sebaceous glands causes the cerumen to become very dry, and this dry cerumen may completely obstruct the external auditory canal. As a result, hearing is diminished. In addition, the tympanic membrane becomes more translucent and sclerotic, causing conductive hearing loss.

As the hair cells in the organ of Corti begin to degenerate, hearing tends to deteriorate, usually after the age of 50. The stria vascularis, a network of capillaries that secrete endolymph and promote sensitization of hair cells in the cochlea, may atrophy with age, contributing to hearing loss. In addition, sensorineural hearing loss first occurs with high-frequency sounds and then progresses to lower-frequency tones.

An excess deposition of bone cells along the ossicle chain can cause fixation of the stapes in the oval window; as a result, hearing further deteriorates.

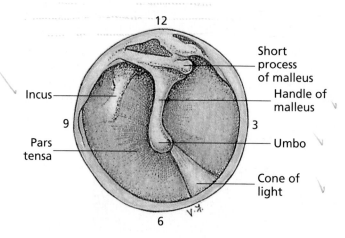

Fig. 12-2   Landmarks of tympanic membrane with "clock" superimposed (right ear).   *(From Wong, 1995.)*

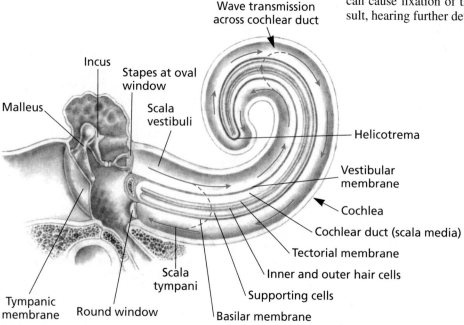

Fig. 12-3   Middle ear, showing relationship of ossicles and cochlea. Communication between scala vestibuli and scala tympani is shown. Arrows indicate displacement of liquid inside bony cochlea and round window from movement of stapedial footplate and displacement of oval window. *(From Thompson et al, 1993.)*

HEALTH HISTORY | Ears and Auditory System

Evaluation of the ear includes not only the physical characteristics of the ear itself but also the assessment of hearing and equilibrium.

● ●

QUESTIONS

RATIONALE

EAR

■ Do you have any problems with your ears, hearing or balance? *If so:* Describe. Have you ever had surgery on your ears to improve your hearing? *If so:* When and for what? Did it help? *If so:* Describe how.

A brief general history about the ears and hearing should provide good information that may then be used during the assessment of specific problems.

■ Have you been struck in the ear or had an injury to your ear? *If so:* Describe when and what happened. *If so:* Was there any type of discharge or bleeding from your ear following the injury?

Ear injuries, either recent or past, may also provide information that may be applied to a client's ear symptoms or complaints. Bleeding or discharge from the ear following an injury may be a sign of basilar skull fracture or a ruptured tympanic membrane.

■ How do you clean your ears? Do you stick anything such as a Q-tip in your ears to clean them?

It is important to assess potential injury to the ear from aggressive cleaning of the ears. Cleaning of the ears with a cotton-tipped applicator may cause cerumen to be impacted against the tympanic membrane. This impaction in turn may cause hearing loss.

■ Have you ever had your hearing tested? *If so:* When was it done and for what reason?

It is important to determine if baseline hearing testing has been performed.

EARACHE OR PAINFUL EAR

■ How long have you had an earache? Does it come and go or is it constant? Does it feel like it is in your ear or deep in your head? Describe what it feels like (sharp, dull, aching, pounding). Does it hurt just when you pull on or touch your ear or does it ache without touching? Does the pain change when you change your position, such as lying down? Is there any discharge from your ear? *If yes:* What does it look like (clear, purulent, bloody)? Does the discharge have an odor?

Determining if the earache or pain is superficial or deep or increases with pulling on the ear may help the examiner to determine if the problem is external to (external otitis) or behind the tympanic membrane (otitis media). External otitis causes pain in the ear canal that may be elicited by pulling on or moving the external ear. Otitis media causes a sensation of pain that is deep in the ear and is not elicited by moving the external ear. A discharge or drainage from the ear may indicate a ruptured tympanic membrane or may be associated with external otitis.

■ Have you recently had or do you now have a cold or any problems or infections in your mouth, teeth, sinuses, or throat?

Ear pain may be referred from a problem in the mouth, sinuses, or throat. Likewise, an infection may migrate from a primary site outside the ears into the middle ear.

■ Have you had ear infections or painful ears in the past or when you were a child? If so, describe type and frequency. How have your earaches been treated in the past?

ITCHING OF THE EARS

■ Describe the sensation, including exactly where it is and how often it occurs. How do you clean your ears? Do you put any cleaning solution in your ears either during bathing or showering? Have you been swimming recently? If so, where and how often?

HEARING

RINGING IN THE EARS

■ Describe the noise that you are hearing. Is it ringing, crackling, or buzzing? When exactly did it start? Does it occur all of the time or just periodically, such as at night?

■ Are you currently taking any medications? *If so:* What are you taking and when did you start taking the medications? Have you taken the same medication in the past? *If so:* Did it cause any similar problems, such as ringing in the ears?

HEARING LOSS

■ How long have you had the feeling that you are having trouble hearing? Has it occurred suddenly or has it become worse gradually?

■ What type of sounds or tones do you have difficulty hearing? Is there a certain pitch you have trouble hearing, such as conversation on the telephone or an alarm clock ringing? Do people tell you that they have to "shout" for you to hear them?

■ Is there a family history of hearing loss? *If so:* Who, and at what age did it start?

■ Where do you work? Do you work or live in an environment where there is a lot of noise, such as a factory or machine shop? *If the client works in one of these environments, ask:* Do you wear a hearing protection device or ear plugs? *If so:* Do you wear it all of the time or just occasionally? Do the earplugs or headset help reduce the environmental noise? *If so:* To what degree? How long have you worked in such an environment? Has your hearing loss become a problem since you have worked there, or did it start before your employment there?

◄ *It is always important to determine a baseline for ear problems. A history of chronic ear infections or problems may shed light on the reason for the client's current problem.*

◄ *Itching in the ears may occur secondary to dry skin in the external canal or an infection in the external canal of the ear, such as swimmer's ear (external otitis). It may also occur if large amounts of soap are allowed in the external canal and not properly rinsed.*

◄ *Ringing is a sensation or sound heard only by the affected individual. It frequently occurs secondary to medications that are ototoxic, such as acetylsalicylic acid (aspirin), quinine, streptomycin, neomycin, gentamicin, furosemide (Lasix), indomethacin (Indocin), or nitrofurantoin. Ringing in the ears may also be a sign of Meniere's disease.*

◄ *It is important to assess if hearing loss has occurred suddenly or over time. A sudden hearing loss in one or both ears that is not associated with an ear infection or upper respiratory infection requires further evaluation.*

◄ *Hearing loss associated with aging (presbycusis) occurs gradually over time and occurs with some pitches or tones more than others.*

> Presbycusis becomes increasingly common after age 50. Hearing impairment is reported by 50% of persons age 65 to 74, 33% of those age 75 to 84, and 48% of persons age 85 and over.

(Guide to Clinical Preventive Services, 1989; Ebersole and Hess, 1994.)

◄ *Repeated and prolonged exposure to loud noise either at work, home, or in the community may lead to hearing loss. Examples of known high-volume noise areas include airports, busy traffic areas, factories, heavy machinery, and construction sites. If any indi-*

QUESTIONS

RATIONALE

🌐 **Cultural Note**

When using communication response patterns to assess hearing or speech status, the examiner is reminded that many American Indians and Alaskan Natives use extended pauses and periods of silence in their speech and that their answers to questions are often discursive and circular.

■ To what degree does your hearing loss bother you? Does it interfere in your activities of daily living, such as causing a problem on the job or during telephone conversations? What do you do to cope with your hearing difficulty? Do you find yourself not going out or being with your friends because you have difficulty hearing?

■ Do you wear a hearing corrective device (e.g., hearing aid)? If so, how long have you worn it? Does it help? Do you wear it all of the time? If not, why not? Do you have any problem with upkeep, cleaning, or changing the batteries?

BALANCE OR EQUILIBRIUM

DIZZINESS OR VERTIGO

■ Describe when the problem started. Does it bother you all of the time or just at certain times, such as when lying down, standing up, or bending over? Describe. Are there any accompanying symptoms such as nausea, vomiting, or visual changes?

■ Describe the sensations you feel: Is it a feeling that you will fall or lose your balance? Is it a sensation that your surroundings are moving or that you are spinning? Does it occur when your eyes are open, closed, or both?

■ Are you currently taking any medications? *If so:* What are you taking and when did you start taking the medications? Have you taken the same medication in the past? *If so:* Did it cause any similar problems, such as ringing in the ears?

■ How much does your dizziness interfere with your daily living? Are you able to function adequately? Are you able to drive or go up and down stairs?

vidual, regardless of age, provides a history of hearing loss and environmental exposure to loud noise, he or she should be referred for further testing.

◀ *Hearing loss that may cause individuals to withdraw or become isolated because they cannot hear or because they are embarrassed has been reported to lead to reduced interpersonal communication, depression, reduced mobility, and exacerbation of coexisting psychiatric conditions.*

◀ *Some clients have hearing devices but do not use them because of the extraneous noise they cause or because the batteries are nonfunctional. If the client has a hearing device but does not wear it, it is very important to determine why.*

◀ *Dizziness may occur secondary to an internal ear problem such as Meniere's disease or medications.*

Vertigo
The sensation of whirling motion when the client feels himself or herself in motion or the room is spinning. It is a dysfunction of the labyrinth.

Dizziness
A sensation of faintness or inability to maintain normal balance in a standing or seated position.

◀ *Some medications are ototoxic and cause a side effect of vertigo or dizziness. If the client reports either dizziness or vertigo and also relays a history of being on an ototoxic medication, the client should be referred for medical reevaluation.*

◀ *If the client reports dizziness or vertigo as a problem, he or she should be advised about the potential hazard of driving or operating machinery.*

QUESTIONS

RATIONALE

BIRTH HISTORY

■ How much did the infant weigh at birth? Were there any congenital infections following birth, such as rubella or meningitis? Were any congenital defects noted at birth, such as cleft palate or malformations of the face or head? Was there any birth trauma or perinatal asphyxia? Was the baby jaundiced? Did he or she have hyperbilirubinemia following birth? Was the baby premature or in the newborn intensive care unit following birth?

◀ *Infants at risk for hearing impairment are those weighing less than 1500 grams or those with congenital infections, perinatal asphyxia, or other high-risk birth problems.*

An estimated 1% to 3% of infants and young children are hearing impaired, and half of these cases are congenital or acquired during infancy. If not identified, hearing impairment at this age may interfere with the development of speech and language skills.

(National Institutes of Health, 1993.)

■ Does the infant jump, startle, or cry when there is a bang or loud noise. Does the older infant turn his or her head toward a noise?

◀ *The parent may be the first to notice that the infant does not respond to noise.*

PRENATAL HISTORY

■ *Ask the mother:* Did you have any viral infections while you were pregnant, such as syphilis or meningitis? Did you have any x-rays while you were pregnant? Did you drink alcohol or smoke tobacco while you were pregnant? *If so:* How much? Do you have diabetes or did you have high blood pressure while you were pregnant?

◀ *A careful prenatal history may also provide information about infants at risk for hearing impairment.*

YOUNG CHILDREN

■ Does the child behave in any way that indicates that there may be a hearing problem, such as not babbling by 6 months or not reacting to loud or strange noises; no attempts of communicative speech by 15 months; not seeming to communicate or be attentive to peers of the same age?

◀ *If a hearing problem is not identified at infancy, it may be identified when the parent notices that the young child is not making noises or talking like other children of a similar age. The Denver Developmental assessment tool, described in Chapter 2, specifically assesses the child's developmental vocabulary and word construction ability.*

■ *If the child is talking:* At what age did the talking begin? How difficult is it for you to understand the child's language?

◀ *If the child has a hearing problem, he or she will not be able to imitate sounds or words.*

■ Does the child ever put objects in the ears?

◀ *Putting objects in the ears is an injury and infection risk.*

■ Does the child have frequent ear infections? If so, how old was the child at the first infection? How many ear infections has the child had during the past 6 months? What has been done to treat these infections? Are the infections increasing in frequency or severity?

◀ *If the child has more than 2 or 3 ear infections (otitis media) each year, the child is said to be "otitis-prone."*

QUESTIONS

■ Does the child seem to pull at the ears or play with the ears? If so, how often?

■ Have you ever had your child's hearing tested? If so, at what age and for what reason? What were the results?

■ Has the child ever had ear surgery, such as having tubes placed in the ears?

OLDER CHILDREN

Questions for the older child should include all of those questions asked of the younger child but should also focus on infections of the ears, hearing problems in school or at home, and exposure to risks, such as loud noise.

■ Do you have frequent ear infections? *If so:* What treatment have you had? Have you ever had to have tubes in your ears?

■ Do you swim? *If so:* Does the water ever bother your ears? Do you wear ear plugs?

■ Do you have any trouble hearing things that you think you should hear? Like the teacher at school?

■ *Ask the parent:* Does the child engage in disruptive behavior in school or does the child act withdrawn?

■ Do you listen to loud music or go places where there is loud noise, such as a concert? *If so:* Does the noise hurt your ears? How often do you listen to loud music?

OLDER ADULT

The major problem with the ears and hearing in the older adult is the gradual loss of hearing due to sensorineural changes of the organ of Corti. The questions already presented in the adult section related to hearing loss, ototoxic medications, and hearing aids should be asked. In addition, a careful history should be taken regarding dizziness and balance, which may have a root cause in the inner ears and put the client at risk for falling and injury.

RATIONALE

◀ *Pulling of the ears is frequently done if the child has an infection of the ear.*

◀ *Children at high risk for hearing problems (see the infant history section) who have not been screened and who have some indication of a possible hearing problem should have screening performed.*

◀ *The placement of tubes in the ears is generally an indication that the child has had numerous ear infections. The tubes are placed as a method to prevent recurrent infections.*

◀ *Because the eustachian tube develops more curvature as the child grows, there should be a decreased frequency of ear infections. If the child continues to have chronic ear infections, a more comprehensive assessment of causation must be made.*

◀ *Frequent swimming may put the susceptible child at greater risk for external ear canal infections.*

◀ *Hearing loss in the school-age child may occur secondary to otitis media with middle ear effusion and is usually self-limiting. A second common cause of hearing difficulty in the child is the build-up of cerumen in the external ear canal. This is especially common if the child routinely cleans the ears with a cotton-tipped applicator.*

◀ *Disruptive behavior may be a result of a sensory deficit.*

◀ *Repeated exposure to loud noise, such as music concerts, starting this early in life places the individual at risk for long-term, nonreversible hearing loss. Risk education may be indicated.*

EXAMINATION Procedures and Findings

Guidelines The examination of the ears actually has three distinct components. First is the examination of the external ear, the ear canal, and the tympanic membrane. Second is the evaluation of hearing. Third is the evaluation of the vestibular apparatus or balance.

EQUIPMENT	Otoscope with clean reusable or disposable speculum (several sizes are helpful)
	Pneumatic bulb attachment for the otoscope (if child is to be examined)
	Tuning forks—500 and 1000 Hz

TECHNIQUES and NORMAL FINDINGS

ABNORMAL FINDINGS

EAR

External Ear: INSPECT the ears for Alignment and Position on the head in relation to the outer canthus of the eyes. The pinna of the ear should align directly with the outer canthus of the eye.

INSPECT both external ears for Size, Shape, Symmetry, Skin Color, Uniformity, and Skin Intactness. The skin should be an even skin tone, with color about the same skin tone as that noted on the face. The color should be uniform throughout. There should be no lesions. A small, painless nodule, called a *darwinian tubercle,* is a normal deviation and may be noted at the helix of the ear (Fig. 12-4).

■ Low-set ears (the pinna is located below the external corner of the eye) or ears that are misaligned (the ear is angled more than 10° from a vertical position) should be considered abnormal (see Fig. 12-15). Low-set ears are seen in persons with congenital diseases such as Down syndrome or renal disorder. Ear size: If the ears are smaller than 4 cm in length, they are referred to as *microtia* ears. Likewise, if the ears are larger than 10 cm in length, they are referred to as *macrotia* ears.

■ Abnormal findings include lesions or deformities of the external ear, such as nodules, tophi (see Common Problems/Conditions, later in this chapter), sebaceous cysts, or cauliflower ear, which may occur secondary to injury.

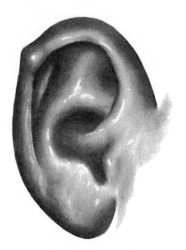

Fig. 12-4   Darwinian tubercle.   *(From Seidel et al, 1995.)*

TECHNIQUES and NORMAL FINDINGS

ABNORMAL FINDINGS

If the ears are pierced, note the skin around the piercing for skin intactness, swelling, discharge, or lesions.

- ■ The color of the ears may change with certain conditions. For example, blueness may indicate cyanosis; redness may indicate flushing, warming after exposure to cold, or vasomotor instability; and pallor may indicate frostbite.
- ■ If areas of redness, swelling, or lesions with discharge are found, then infections such as furuncles should be considered.

INSPECT the external auditory canal for Discharge or Lesions. There should be none.

- ■ Any discharge—clear, purulent, crusty, or bloody—from the ear should be considered abnormal. A bloody or clear discharge from the ear accompanied with a history of head injury should lead to suspicion of possible skull fracture. A purulent or crusty discharge may indicate infection of the external canal, a foreign body, or, if the tympanic membrane has ruptured, infection of the middle ear.

PALPATE both external ears and mastoid areas behind the ears for Tenderness, Swelling, or Nodules. All areas should be firm and without tenderness or swelling. Gently pull on the helix of the ear to determine if there is any discomfort or pain. There should be none. (*Note:* If the client has a painful ear, always examine the unaffected ear first.)

- ■ Tenderness of the mastoid area may indicate mastoiditis.
- ■ Pain when the helix of the ear is pulled may indicate an external ear canal infection.

AUDITORY CANAL AND TYMPANIC MEMBRANE

INSPECT the external auditory canal using an otoscope for Tissue Swelling or Redness, Discharge, and Cerumen. If you have a choice of speculum size, always choose the largest speculum that will comfortably fit into the external auditory meatus. To use the otoscope, grasp the pinna of the client's ear with one hand and gently pull the helix upward and slightly toward the back of the head (Fig. 12-5). This straightens the S-shaped curve of the auditory canal.

With the other hand, gently position the lighted speculum of the otoscope into the client's external auditory canal. Hold the otoscope upside down in the palm of your hand. Rest the back of your hand against the client's temple area to steady the positioning of the otoscope (Fig. 12-6).

(An alternative way to hold the otoscope is to hold the handle downward and immobilize the positioning of the speculum by placing the index finger of the hand holding the handle of the otoscope on the client's face.)

TECHNIQUES and NORMAL FINDINGS

ABNORMAL FINDINGS

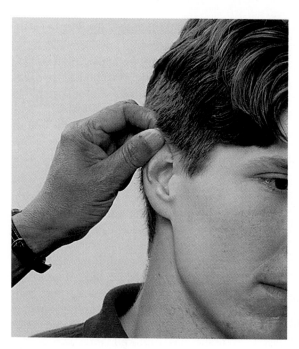

Fig. 12-5   Pull the client's helix upward and slightly toward the back of the head.

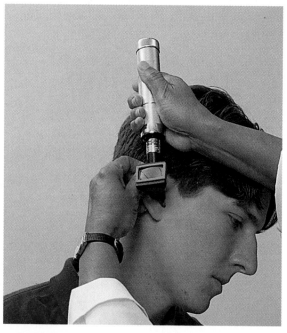

Fig. 12-6   Holding the otoscope "upside down," rest the back of your hand against the client's temple area to steady the otoscope.

Note: If you are unable to visualize the auditory canal because the canal is filled with cerumen, the cerumen must be removed. To do this, the examiner may first fill the canal with a cerumen softening agent such as Aralugan. Block the opening of the canal with a cotton ball and wait 5 to 10 minutes. The cerumen may then be easily removed from the canal by irrigating the canal with warm water. Some examiners prefer to remove the cerumen with a cerumen spoon. This technique requires skill so as not to scrape the walls of the canal or injure the tympanic membrane.

CAUTION: Do not use water irrigation of the canal if any of the following are suspected: otitis externa, tympanic membrane perforation, or myringotomy tubes in place.

Do not release the hand holding the pinna. There must be continuous traction on the pinna throughout the examination of the auditory canal and the tympanic membrane. Watch the insertion of the otoscope as it is placed in the canal, and then look through the lens of the otoscope. Insert the speculum 1.0 to 1.5 cm (0.5 inch). Be careful not to insert the otoscope speculum into the canal too far. If the speculum touches the bony section of the canal (inner ⅔ of the canal), there may be a sensation of pain. If you are unable to see anything but canal walls, reposition the client's head, apply more traction on the pinna, and re-angle the otoscope toward the nose.

Once the otoscope is properly positioned, note any evidence of tissue swelling, redness, or discharge along the walls of the canal. Note the amount, color, and characteristics of cerumen. Some cerumen almost always is in the canal, but it should not occlude the canal or obscure the visualization of the tympanic membrane. Note the characteristics of the cerumen. The color may be black, brown, dark red, creamy, to brown-gray. The texture ranges from moist, to

■ Redness and swelling of the external auditory canal may be an indication of otitis externa. The infection may cause the canal to become swollen and completely closed.

TECHNIQUES and NORMAL FINDINGS	**ABNORMAL FINDINGS**

dry and flaky, to hard. There should be no odor. Finally, note the presence of hair in the canal, as well as any other canal characteristics such as lesions, foreign bodies, or polyps.

🌐 Racial Variations

> *White and dark-skinned races* have cerumen that is moist, sticky, and dark.
> *Asian and American Indian races* have cerumen that is generally sparse, dry, flaky, and lighter.

After the canal has been thoroughly examined, focus your view on the tympanic membrane (TM) (Fig. 12-7).

■ Purulent discharge from the auditory canal may occur secondary to otitis externa or, if the tympanic membrane is ruptured, it may be drainage from behind the eardrum. Clear fluid or frank blood drainage from the auditory canal following a head injury may indicate a basilar skull fracture. To confirm that clear fluid drainage is indeed cerebrospinal fluid, test the drainage with a glucose test strip. Cerebrospinal fluid will test positive for glucose.

■ Other abnormal findings in the auditory canal include the presence of foreign bodies, polyps, exostosis, and furuncles (see photos in Common Problems/Conditions, later in this chapter).

■ Any perforation of the TM or absence or distortion of the landmarks on the TM should be considered abnormal.

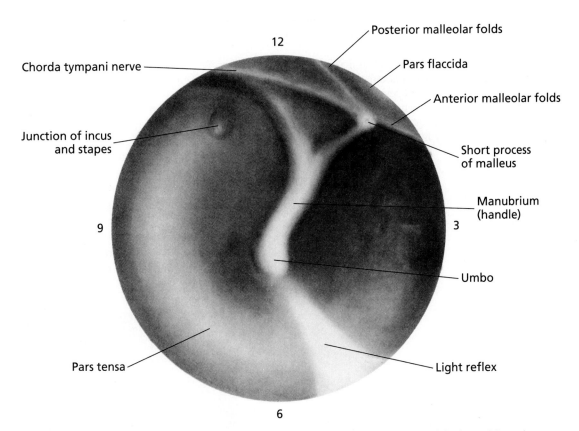

Fig. 12-7 Normal (right) tympanic membrane with usual landmarks noted. (Clock position given as reference.) *(Modified from Barkauskus, 1994.)*

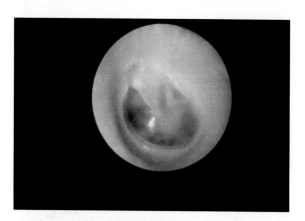

Fig. 12-8   A normal left tympanic membrane with the cone of light visible. *(From Bingham, Hawke, and Kwok, 1992.)*

INSPECT the tympanic membrane for Landmarks, Color, Contour, Translucence, and Fluctuation. First, locate all landmarks (umbo, handle of the malleus, and light reflex).

Next, note the color of the TM, the contour (bulging or retracted), and any indications of perforation. You may need to slightly adjust the light source so that the entire membrane can be evaluated. The TM should be a translucent, pearly gray, be neither bulging nor retracted, and have no perforations (Fig. 12-8). A cone of light reflex should be prominently noted in the lower-anterior quadrant of the drum.

The fluctuation of the TM (which is a further evaluation to determine if the TM is retracted or bulging) may be done by attaching a pneumatic bulb to the otoscope. To perform this procedure, make sure that the speculum is fully inserted into the canal and that the speculum is large enough to completely occlude the canal. *Gently* squeeze the bulb so that puffs of air are transmitted to the TM. A normal response is that the TM itself will slightly fluctuate with the puffs of air.

🌐 Cultural Note

American Indian, Alaska Native, and Pacific Islander children have the highest rates of otitis media in the world. African-American children have the lowest incidence.

■ Variations in the color and characteristics of the TM indicating an abnormality:

■ *Yellow/amber:* Serous fluid in the middle ear, which may indicate serous otitis media or chronic otitis media with air bubbles.

■ *Redness:* Infection in the middle ear, such as acute purulent otitis media.

■ *Chalky white:* Infection in the middle ear, such as otitis media.

■ *Blue or deep red:* Blood behind the TM, which may have occurred secondary to injury.

■ *Red streaks:* Injected/increased vascularization may be due to allergy.

■ *Dullness:* Fibrosis or scarring of the TM secondary to repeated infections.

■ *White flecks/plaques:* Healed inflammation of the TM.

■ *Air bubbles or a fluid level:* Indicates serous fluid in the middle ear (Fig. 12-9).

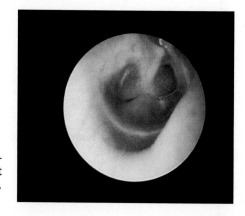

Fig. 12-9   Serous otitis media. An air-fluid level is present behind the right tympanic membrane. *(From Bingham, Hawke, and Kwok, 1992.)*

TECHNIQUES and NORMAL FINDINGS

ABNORMAL FINDINGS

■ Abnormal variations in the mobility of the TM:

■ *Bulging of TM with no mobility:* Indicates pus or fluid behind the TM.

■ *Retraction of TM with no mobility or mobility of the TM with negative pressure only:* Obstruction of the eustachian tube.

■ *Increased mobility of only one part of the TM:* Indicates an area of healed TM perforation (Fig. 12-10).

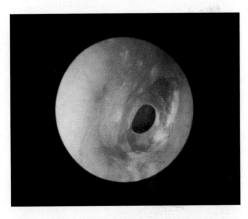

Fig. 12-10 Right tympanic membrane with dry central perforation in the anteroinferior quadrant and scarring. *(From Bingham, Hawke, and Kwok, 1992.)*

HEARING

As you perform the hearing assessment, also watch the client's responses, which may indicate a hearing loss that is not measured by the following testing methods. Subtle indications of hearing loss include such signs as:

■ Asking you to repeat the question.

■ Repeated misunderstanding of the questions you ask.

■ Garbled speech sounds with word distortion.

■ Leaning forward, tilting head, frowning, and seeming to watch your lips as you speak.

■ Speaking in a loud voice that may be monotone.

TEST acoustic cranial nerve (VIII) to evaluate Auditory Function. The following tests are used for screening only and should not be considered diagnostic of hearing problem.

Whispered voice test. Stand 1 to 2 feet in front of or to the side of the client. Instruct the client to cover one ear with his or her hand so that one ear may be tested at a time. Shield your mouth so that the client cannot read your lips. Softly whisper several monosyllabic (e.g., *ball, chair, cat*) and bisyllabic (e.g., *streetcar, baseball, highchair*) words. The client should be able to hear at least 50% of all words whispered. Repeat the procedure with the other ear.

Finger-rubbing test. A gross hearing test may be done by holding your hand 3 to 4 inches from the client's ear and briskly rubbing your index finger against your thumb. The client should be able to hear the noise generated by rubbing the fingers together. Repeat the technique with the other ear.

Tuning fork tests. To activate the tuning fork, hold it by the base stem and softly strike the forked section against the back of your hand. If you strike the fork too hard, the tone is too loud and it will take a long time to fade out.

■ It should be considered abnormal if the client cannot repeat at least 50% of the spoken words. (Each ear must be considered separately.)

■ Clients with a high-frequency hearing loss may not be able to hear the noise generated by your fingers. Consider each ear separately.

TECHNIQUES and NORMAL FINDINGS

Rinne test. This test uses a tuning fork to compare air conduction (AC) to bone conduction (BC). The AC route through the ear canal is a more sensitive route. Strike the tuning fork and place the base of the tuning fork directly on the client's mastoid process (Fig. 12-11, *A*). Begin timing by counting the seconds. The client should be able to hear the tone. Instruct the client to tell you when the tone can no longer be heard. At that time, note the number of seconds counted; quickly remove the fork from the mastoid process, invert the fork, and hold the vibrating section of the tuning fork in front of the client's ear (Fig. 12-11, *B*). Begin counting again. The client should be able to hear the tone again. Instruct the client to tell you when the vibration is no longer heard. Note the time. The tone heard in front of the ear should last twice as long as the tone heard when the fork was on the mastoid process (AC>BC [2:1]). This is the normal, or *positive*, response.

Repeat the test with the other ear.

ABNORMAL FINDINGS

- Consider the test abnormal when the sound is heard longer by bone conduction than air conduction or when AC is not twice as long as BC.
- Clients with *conductive hearing loss* will have bone conduction longer than air conduction in the affected ear.
- Clients with *sensorineural hearing loss* will have air conduction longer than bone conduction in the affected ear, but it will be less than 2:1 ratio.

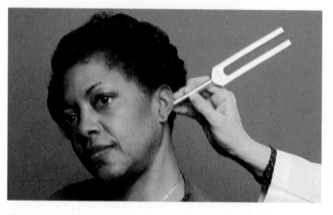 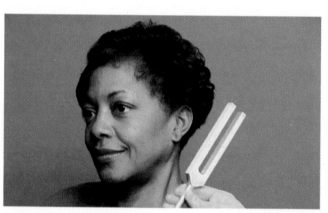

Fig. 12-11 Rinne test. **A,** The tuning fork is placed on the mastoid bone for bone conduction. **B,** The tuning fork is placed in front of the ear for air conduction. *(From Sigler and Schuring, 1993.)*

Weber test. This test assesses bone conduction by testing the lateralization of sounds.

Softly strike the tuning fork and place it in the middle of the client's forehead (Fig. 12-12). The client should hear the tone equally in both ears. If the client reports a lateralization of the sound, ask in which ear the sound was heard loudest and then repeat the test, having the client occlude one ear by placing his or her finger in the ear. The sound should now be heard most loudly in the occluded ear.

- When the sound lateralizes to one side and the client hears the tone better in one ear than the other, the test should be considered abnormal.
- Clients with *conductive hearing loss* will have a lateralization of sound to the deaf ear.
- Clients with *sensorineural hearing loss* will have lateralization of sound to the better ear.

Fig. 12-12 Weber test. The tuning fork is placed on the midline of the skull. *(From Sigler and Schuring, 1993.)*

TECHNIQUES and NORMAL FINDINGS

ABNORMAL FINDINGS

TEST acoustic cranial nerve (VIII) to evaluate Vestibular Function. Romberg test. This test assesses the ability of the vestibular apparatus in the inner ear to help maintain standing balance. To evaluate it, ask the client to stand in front of you and facing you. Instruct the client to stand with his or her feet together, arms at the side, and eyes closed. Wait 20 seconds and watch the client's swaying and ability to maintain balance. The client may sway slightly but should be able to maintain the balance without stepping sideways (Fig. 12-13). *(Stay close to the client to offer balance support if necessary.)*

■ If the client is unable to maintain the position, steps sideways, or widens base support, the test should be considered abnormal, or positive.

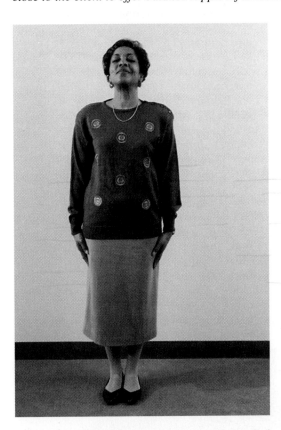

Fig. 12-13 Romberg test evaluates client's balance. Offer balance support to the client if necessary to prevent falls. *(From Sigler and Schuring, 1993.)*

INFANT

■ APPROACH

The infant's ears are often a site where congenital abnormalities are found. It is therefore very important to carefully examine the infant's ears. To ensure safety, the infant must be securely immobilized during the examination. To do this, the infant may be placed in either a supine or prone position. If supine, have a "holder" person secure the infant's arms down at the sides with one hand and turn and immobilize the head to one side with the other (Fig. 12-14, *A*). To examine the infant in a prone position, instruct the "holder" to position the infant's arms down at the side with one hand and turn and hold the infant's head to one side with the other hand (Fig. 12-14, *B*). You will need both hands free to hold the helix of the ear and maneuver the otoscope. It is important to ensure that the infant is securely positioned and that the otoscope is braced against the infant's head to move with the infant if necessary.

To examine the auditory canal and tympanic membrane in the infant, the examiner must alter the method of holding the auricle of the ear. Instead of holding the pinna of the ear and pulling it up and back, for the infant and all children up to age 3 years, grasp the lower portion of the pinna and apply gentle traction down and slightly backward. This is necessary to straighten the canal of the ear.

■ FINDINGS

It is important to carefully assess the formation of the auricles and positioning of the ears on the head. The top of the auricle should form a flat imaginary line to the outer canthus of the eye and the ear should have less than a 10° rotation from a vertical position (Fig. 12-15). Low-set ears or ears with angulation greater than 10° may be an indication of a congenital problem such as Down syndrome. The external ear should be well formed, appear smooth and intact, and have no skin tags or other formations.

The canal and tympanic membrane should be carefully examined as in the adult. The TM of the infant may be difficult to visualize because it is more horizontal. The TM may appear slightly injected (reddened) secondary to crying. Also, because the TM does not become conical for several months, the light reflex may appear diffuse. By age 6 months, the infant's TM takes on an adult-type appearance and is easier to visualize and examine.

It is also important that infants have some type of hearing screening. The screening test to be performed should depend on the risk factors determined during the infant's history. Gross screening of the newborn's ability to hear may be conducted by eliciting a loud noise (e.g., clapping hands or ringing bell) and observing the infant's body movement, startle response, or cry in response to the auditory stimuli. This test, however, is not reliable for actually testing the infant's hearing ability. Two automated devices have been developed to more accurately determine the auditory function of newborns and infants. These tests, the auditory response cradle (ARC) and the crib-o-gram (COG), may be used with high-risk infants

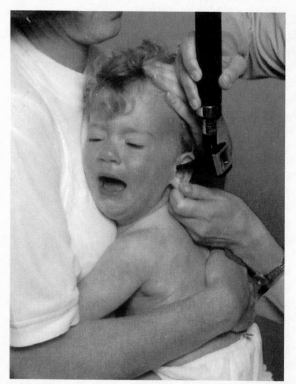

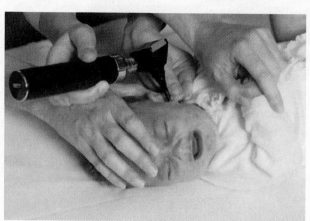

Fig. 12-14 Immobilization of young child or infant. **A,** Prone position. **B,** Supine position. *(From Wong, 1995.)*

to objectively measure the infant's body movements in response to sound.

As the infant becomes older, gross hearing assessment should be conducted and recorded. By age 4 to 6 months, the infant should turn the head toward the source of the sound, should respond to the parent's voice, and should respond to music toys. By 6 to 10 months the child should respond to his or her name and follow sounds.

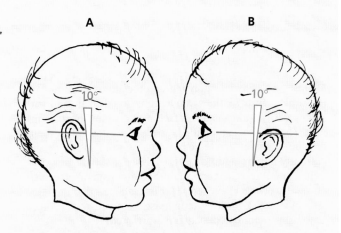

Fig. 12-15 Ear alignment. **A,** Normal alignment. **B,** Low-set alignment. *(From Bowers and Thompson, 1992.)*

CHILDREN

■ APPROACH

The biggest challenge to examining the ears of the young child is immobilization. It is vitally important to immobilize the child in either the supine or prone position and to ensure that the potentially squirmy child will not move during the otoscope examination. If the child moves, it will not only cause pain but also may cause injury to the ear canal itself. Because the otoscope examination may be perceived as traumatic by the child, it may be deferred until the very last procedure of the entire examination. If the child becomes upset during the examination, be sure to quickly return the child to the parent for comforting.

As the child becomes older, the examiner should take the time to elicit the child's cooperation during the examination. If time is taken, and the child is reassured, the examination should not be traumatic. Nevertheless, if the examiner has any question regarding the child's ability to hold perfectly still during the otoscope examination, the parent or adult who is with the child should assist in immobilizing the child to ensure the child's safety.

■ FINDINGS

The findings of the examination do not differ from what has already been presented. If the child is less than 3 years of age, the pinna of the ear should be pulled down during the examination as described for the infant. If the child is older, the pinna should be pulled up and backward as for the adult.

Young children are also at risk for foreign bodies in their ears, and all children presenting with suspect history should be carefully examined. Likewise, when examining the tympanic membrane, note the presence of myringotomy tubes. They are commonly placed in the central section of the TM. The pneumatic bulb is frequently used with young and older children to carefully evaluate the fluctuation of the TM. Review the adult section for the procedure and anticipated findings.

Hearing evaluation of the young child may be necessary if the parent or examiner perceives that the child has some type of lag related to the child's developmental milestones. Behavioral manifestations of the child that may indicate hearing impairment include lag in verbalization skills; speech that is monotone, garbled, or difficult to understand; inattentiveness during conversation; facial expressions that appear strained or puzzled; withdrawal and lack of interaction with others; asking "what" a lot or asking for statements to be repeated; or having frequent earaches.

ADOLESCENTS

■ APPROACH

If the child has had no ear or hearing problems before adolescence, special approach or procedures need not be performed. Instead, the examination should focus on identifying care patterns and risk factors for ear and hearing injury. The adolescent should be carefully questioned about how he or she cleans the ears and any problems he or she currently has. In addition, the adolescent should be questioned about repeated exposure to loud music or excessive noise at work or elsewhere. If it is evaluated that the adolescent is at risk for long-term noise exposure, then protection and prevention education is warranted.

Adolescents participating in contact sports such as wrestling, boxing, football, rugby, or soccer should be carefully assessed and educated about ear protection and injury prevention.

■ FINDINGS

The procedures and findings are the same as those found for the adult. If the adolescent is at risk for hearing injury due to noise or injury and has not had a baseline test, testing may be warranted.

OLDER ADULTS

■ APPROACH

Although there is nothing special with the approach to the older adult, the examiner is reminded to carefully observe the client for subtle symptoms and signs of hearing loss. In addition to a careful history, the examiner should also observe for subtle indications of hearing loss including such signs as asking you to repeat the question; repeatedly misunderstanding the questions you ask; having garbled speech sounds with word distortion; leaning forward, tilting head, frowning and seeming to watch your lips as you speak; or speaking in a loud voice which may be monotone. All of these signs should be considered indications for further evaluation.

■ FINDINGS

The physical characteristics of the older adult are slightly different from those of the younger adult. The ear-lobes may be pendulous and have linear wrinkling. There may be presence of or an increase in wiry hair in the opening of the auditory canal. The tympanic membrane may appear whiter, opaque, and thickened.

As aging progresses, it is normal to have some degree of presbycusis. This is most commonly identified by having difficulty understanding speech, as opposed to having a reduction in the ability to hear sounds of all pitches. The client will have the most difficulty hearing when in a room where there is conversation and competing background noise.

If the client wears a hearing device, the ear should be carefully examined, and assessed for any skin irritation or sores that may be secondary to the molded device. A hearing device may also increase the likelihood of cerumen impaction.

CLIENTS WITH SITUATIONAL VARIATIONS

PREGNANT WOMEN

■ APPROACH

There is no special approach when examining the ears of the pregnant woman.

■ FINDINGS

The examiner may note an increase in vascularization of the ears, the auditory canal, and the tympanic membrane. All other findings are the same as for the adult.

CLIENTS WITH IMPAIRED HEARING

■ APPROACH

It is of first importance to determine to what degree the client can or cannot hear. Hearing loss spans a continuum from diminished auditory acuity to profound deafness. Knowing what type of hearing loss the client has will help to determine your approach. An adult client who has been deaf since birth may have very different coping and communicating skills from a client who suddenly lost hearing secondary to an injury or an older adult who just can no longer hear well. Inquire specifically about reason and type of hearing loss; length of time that the client has had a hearing loss; adaptation to the hearing loss; most common methods of communication; difficulties with communication if any; and knowledge of services and resources for individuals with hearing impairment.

If the client is profoundly deaf and communicates by signing, and you do not sign, it is best to arrange the client's examination so that someone can be with the client who both signs and speaks. If the client reads lips and can speak, then you may be able to communicate just fine. If, on the other hand, the client reads lips but cannot speak, an interpreter is again required. While communication may be done by writing questions and answers back and forth, it is a laborious task and not desirable.

If you are interacting with a client who reads lips or a client who has diminished hearing and you wish to speak to the client, remember to speak slowly and distinctly and to face the client directly so that he or she may see your face.

■ FINDINGS

Hearing loss can occur in low, medium, or high frequencies or in a combination. Hearing is measured in decibels (dB). A decibel is a ratio that compares the relationship between two sound intensities. The American Medical Association's formula for defining hearing loss as impaired is 1.5% for every decibel that the pure tone average exceeds 25 dB. A hearing loss of 40 dB in both ears, or a 22.5% hearing impairment, usually impairs the client's ability to function normally in social situations and usually requires the use of a hearing aid. Profound deafness is defined as 85 to 90 dB below normal.

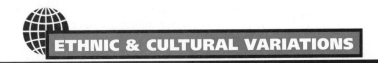

ETHNIC & CULTURAL VARIATIONS

■ APPROACH

It is worth noting that various cultures use a variety of speech and response patterns in communication. When English is a second language or when individuals are actively bilingual, patterns may also vary. These factors need to be considered when using communication response patterns to assist in assessment of hearing.

■ FINDINGS

There are few documented physical variations between races when looking at the ears. The most noted difference is in the consistency and color of cerumen. Most Asian Americans, American Indians, and Alaska Natives have dry cerumen. Most whites and African Americans have wet cerumen. Hispanics may have either type. Cerumen type is genetically determined, with wet cerumen being the result of at least one dominant gene, while dry cerumen results from two recessive genes.

The incidence and severity of otitis media, one of the most common of childhood illnesses, is greatly increased among American Indian, Alaska Native, and Pacific Islander groups. This is important to note, as fluid persisting in the middle ear after treatment can impair hearing and lead to developmental delays in speech and language. Recurrent otitis media may also increase the risk of deafness from other factors such as meningitis, the leading cause of deafness in American Indians and Alaska Natives.

E X A M I N A T I O N S   U   M   M   A   R   Y
Ears and Auditory System

Ear
External Ear (pp. 254-255)
- Inspect both external ears for:
  Alignment, position, shape, and symmetry
  Skin color, uniformity, and intactness
- Inspect external auditory canal for:
  Discharge or lesions
- Palpate both external ears and mastoid areas
  for:
  Tenderness
  Swelling
  Nodules

Auditory Canal and Tympanic Membrane (pp. 255-258)
- Inspect the auditory canal for:
  Tissue swelling or redness
  Discharge
  Cerumen: amount and characteristics

- Inspect the tympanic membrane for:
  Landmarks
  Color
  Contour
  Translucence
  Fluctuation of membrane (if appropriate)

Hearing *(pp. 259-261)*
- Test acoustic cranial nerve (VIII) to evaluate
  auditory function:
  Whispered voice test
  Finger-rubbing test
  Tuning fork tests
  Rinne Test
  Weber Test
- Test acoustic cranial nerve (VIII) to evaluate
  vestibular function:
  Romberg Test

COMMON PROBLEMS/CONDITIONS
associated with the Ear and Auditory System

EXTERNAL EAR

■ **Cauliflower ear:** A thickened, disfigured auricle resulting from repeated injury (Fig. 12-16).

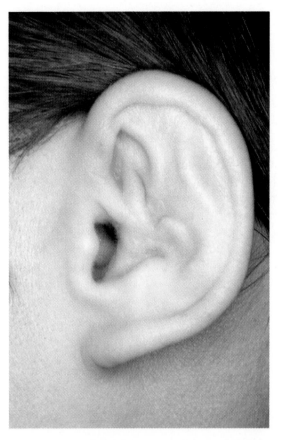

Fig. 12-16 Cauliflower ear. Note loss of definition in the finely sculpted cartilage. *(From Bingham, Hawke, and Kwok, 1992.)*

■ **Darwinian tubercle:** Small, painless congenital nodules found along the helix of the ear (Fig. 12-17).

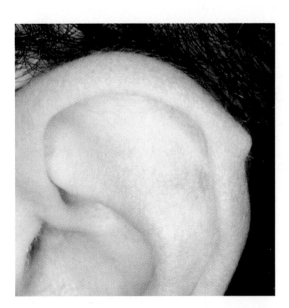

Fig. 12-17 An uncommon darwinian tubercle projecting posteriorly. The common darwinian tubercle projects anteriorly. *(From Bingham, Hawke, and Kwok, 1992.)*

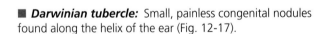

■ **Sebaceous cysts:** Small nodules with a central black punctum (Fig. 12-18). They are most commonly found behind the earlobe in the postauricular fold. If they become infected, they become painful.

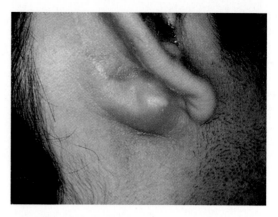

Fig. 12-18　Sebaceous cyst.　*(From Bingham, Hawke, and Kwok, 1992.)*

■ **Tophi:** Small, hard, whitish-yellow, nontender nodules in or near the helix of the ear (Fig. 12-19). They contain uric acid crystals and are a sign of gout.

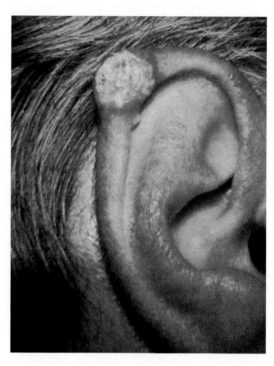

Fig. 12-19　Tophus of the pinna.　*(From Sigler and Schuring, 1993.)*

AUDITORY CANAL

■ **Excessive cerumen:** If the cerumen becomes excessive, it may become impacted and occlude the entire ear canal (Fig. 12-20). If the entire canal is blocked, the client will feel a sense of fullness in the ear and experience decreased hearing.

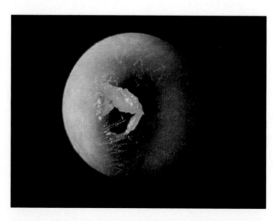

Fig. 12-20　A normal piece of earwax in the outer part of the right external auditory meatus.　*(From Bingham, Hawke, and Kwok, 1992.)*

■ *Foreign body:* Frequently seen in children. If the object is not removed, it may set up a secondary infection (Fig. 12-21). This is especially true if the item is a food substance, such as a raisin or kernel of corn.

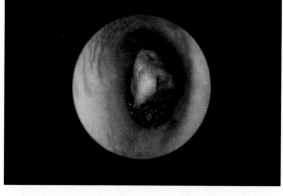

Fig. 12-21 Client inserted a small stone into the deep part of the external ear canal. It is lying against the tympanic membrane. *(From Bingham, Hawke, and Kwok, 1992.)*

■ *Otitis externa (swimmer's ear):* A bacterial or fungal infection of the external ear canal that occurs secondary to tissue injury or a moist environment such as swimming (Fig. 12-22). The tissue appears red and swollen and may obscure the tympanic membrane.

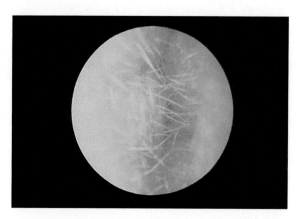

Fig. 12-22 Acute external otitis (swimmer's ear). *(From Cummings, 1993.)*

■ *Polyp:* A sign of possible chronic ear disease that arises from tissue within the auditory canal (Fig. 12-23). The tissue enlarges, becomes reddened, and bleeds easily. There is also an associated purulent discharge.

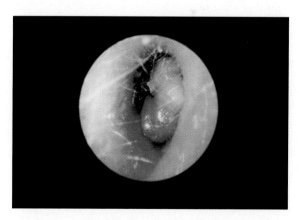

Fig. 12-23 Large solitary osteoma of the external auditory meatus, which is blocking and trapping earwax (to the left and behind the osteoma). *(From Bingham, Hawke, and Kwok, 1992.)*

TYMPANIC MEMBRANE/MIDDLE EAR

■ **Bacterial otitis media:** An infection of the middle ear (Fig. 12-24). The tympanic membrane often appears red, thickened, and bulging. There is accompanying fever and earache. There may be conductive hearing loss and a feeling that the ear is blocked.

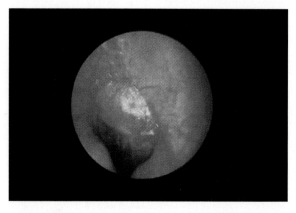

Fig. 12-24   Acute otitis media with redness and edematous swelling of the pars flaccida, shown in the central part of the illustration (left ear).   *(From Bingham, Hawke, and Kwok, 1992.)*

■ **Secretory otitis media (serous otitis media):** The accumulation of serous fluid in the middle ear, secondary to an obstruction or dysfunction of the eustachian tube (Fig. 12-25). The cause ranges from allergies to enlarged lymphoid tissue blocking the eustachian tubes. The tympanic membrane may be retracted, yellow in color, and air bubbles may be seen. The client may complain of a crackling sound when yawning or swallowing.

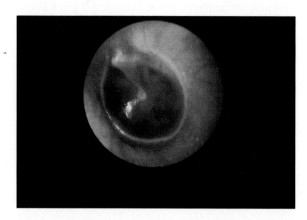

Fig. 12-25   Secretory otitis media. The tympanic membrane is markedly retracted and produces a foreshortened appearance to the handle of the malleus.   *(From Bingham, Hawke, and Kwok, 1992.)*

■ **Perforation of the tympanic membrane:** If the acute otitis media is left untreated, the TM may rupture to release pressure and permit drainage of the substance behind the membrane (Fig. 12-26). Perforation may also occur secondary to a blow to the head or penetration of the ear canal by a foreign body.

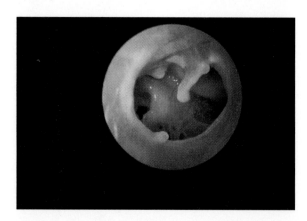

Fig. 12-26   Right tympanic membrane has a total perforation through which can be seen posterosuperiorly the long process of the incus and its articulation with the head of the stapes and stapedius tendon.   *(From Bingham, Hawke, and Kwok, 1992.)*

■ *Tympanotomy or myringotomy tubes:* Small polyethylene tubes that may be surgically placed through the eardrum to relieve middle ear pressure and permit drainage of fluid or material collected behind the TM (Fig. 12-27). They are most commonly put in the ears of young children because of recurrent ear infections. Usually they will spontaneously work their way out of the TM within 6 to 12 months after insertion.

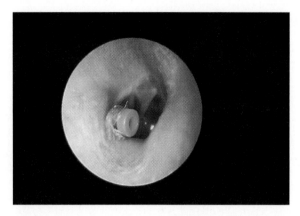

Fig. 12-27 Tympanostomy tube protruding from the right tympanic membrane. *(From Bingham, Hawke, and Kwok, 1992.*

HEARING LOSS

■ *Conductive hearing loss:* Occurs when sound does not reach the inner ear. Thus air conduction is impeded. Common causes of conductive hearing loss include foreign bodies, cerumen build-up, tumors or polyps in the canal, and infection such as otitis media.
■ *Sensorineural hearing loss:* Caused by an impairment of the organ of Corti. Common causes include presbycusis (seen in older adults); Meniere's disease, and ototoxic medications.

VESTIBULAR FUNCTION

■ *Meniere's disease:* A disease affecting the vestibular labyrinth, which, over time, leads to profound sensorineural hearing loss. The disease progresses in steps from a sensation of fullness in the ear with slight hearing loss to ringing in the ears *(tinnitus),* to, finally, disabling vertigo.

Sample Documentation

&Nursing Diagnosis

CASE 1   56-year-old African-American man presents with "funny growths" on his ears.

Subjective

Reports that about 1 month ago noticed small, hard, yellowish-white bumps on top of left ear; 2 weeks later noticed same type of growth on right ear; growths still there and client concerned.

Does not report any recent illness or infection; does not report any serious medical problems, except recent aching and swelling of big toe joints—tested for gout and told uric acid level elevated; reports being given dietary instruction and "some type of medication" for discomfort in toes; since then, aching and swelling of great toe has subsided.

Does not report earaches, ear discharge, hearing loss, tinnitus, vertigo, hearing decrease.

Reports not following special diet received—diet includes foods he does not eat; states will continue to eat what he has always eaten.

Objective

Weight   246 lb (111.8 kg).

Alert male without complaints except for ear lesions. External ears smooth, even color, and without lesions except for multiple small (0.5 cm), whitish-yellow, nontender nodules on helix and antihelix of both ears. No drainage from nodules. Auditory canal clear with small amount of cerumen seen bilaterally. Tympanic membranes pearly gray bilaterally; light reflex and all landmarks clearly visualized. Hearing and vestibular function not tested.

• •

Nursing Diagnosis #1

Anxiety (mild) related to nodules on ears.

Defining Characteristics   Verbalized concern about nodules on ears.

Nursing Diagnosis #2

Noncompliance with diet related to incompatibility of prescribed diet with food preferences.

Defining Characteristics   History of gout, noncompliance with diet, personal eating preferences that do not comply with prescribed diet.

Sample Documentation & Nursing Diagnosis

CASE 2   7-year-old Hispanic female with earache for 1 day.

Subjective

Child, accompanied by mother, complains of "severe" earache in right ear that started yesterday; mother states child swam at camp every day last week. Does not report cold, fever, sore throat, ear congestion, decreased hearing. Reports pain when ear is pulled or touched.

Objective

Temperature   99.2° F (37.3° C).

Weight   42 lb (19.1 kg).

External Ears   Without discoloration, lesions, swelling; small amount of crusted exudate at auditory canal opening on right ear. Left ear without exudate; complains of pain when pinna of right ear is manipulated; no discomfort when left ear manipulated.

Otoscopic Examination   *Left ear:* Canal clear without lesions or swelling; small amount of dry cerumen; tympanic membrane pearly gray—light reflex and landmarks clearly visible; no bulging or retraction of tympanic membrane. *Right ear:* Examination not possible due to increased pain and crying; visualization of canal from outside shows swelling and redness of canal with flaking and crusty, odorless discharge; tympanic membrane not visualized.

Hearing   *Left ear:* Fingers rubbed together at 4 inches clearly heard. *Right ear:* Unable to hear rubbing fingers at 4 inches.

• •

Nursing Diagnosis #1

Acute pain related to inflammation of external auditory canal.

Defining Characteristics   Cries when right ear manipulated; swelling and redness of canal with flaking and crusty discharge.

Nursing Diagnosis #2

High risk for altered growth and development related to growth in 25th percentile.

Defining Characteristics   7-year-old girl, weight 42 lb (19.1 kg).

HEALTH PROMOTION

■ **Protection from Noise** Repeated exposure to excess or constant loud (>80 dB) noise in the work place, home, or during recreational activities is the major cause of permanent hearing loss. See Table 12-1 for a list of common representative sounds and their decibel levels. It has been estimated that over 5 million workers are chronically exposed to hazardous noise levels daily. While most occupational workplaces have noise level thresholds above which earplugs or earphones must be worn, farms and agricultural settings have virtually no regulations. Thus one occupational group that has a high incidence of hearing loss are farmers and agriculture workers who operate farm machinery. Children and adolescents are another group at high risk for repeated hazardous noise exposure. Music and rock concerts are known for loud music in a confined space. Persons living near airports are passively exposed to loud noises every day and even though they may "tune them out," the chronic repeated noise may over time affect their hearing.

TABLE 12-1	Noise Levels

DECIBELS (dB)	REPRESENTATIVE SOUND
0	Softest sound normal ear can hear
10	Heartbeat, rustling of leaves
20	Whisper at 1.8 m (5 feet)
30–45	Normal conversation
60	Noise in average restaurant
70–80	Street noises
80	Loud radio in home
90–100	Train
120	Thunder, rock music
140	Jet airplane during takeoff
>140	Pain threshold

(From Wong, 1995.)

Teach clients and their families first to be aware of hazardous noise levels and then to either limit their exposure to such noise or consistently wear protective earplugs or ear protectors (also called noise defenders). Teach clients to monitor the presence of noise. One way to monitor noise is to listen for a ringing in the ears. If the ears are ringing from noise, ear damage and hearing loss may occur. The best noise defender is one that is comfortable to wear.

Different types of noise defenders are available, made from various materials, including sponge rubber, soft rubber, dense cotton, and molded materials. The client should be advised to try several different types. The one that is most comfortable and blocks the greatest amount of noise will be the one that the client will most likely consistently wear.

If the client is repeatedly exposed to very loud noises, earmuffs are the only defender that will protect the ears. Earmuffs also vary in type. Under rare circumstances, both ear canal noise defenders and ear muffs may be warranted.

■ **Routine Hearing Examinations** Screening for hearing impairment should be routinely performed on all high-risk neonates. Risk factors include family history of childhood hearing impairment; congenital perinatal infection with herpes, syphilis, rubella, cytomegalovirus, or toxoplasmosis; malformations involving the head or neck, including cleft palate; birth weight below 1500 g; bacterial meningitis; hyperbilirubinemia requiring exchange transfusion; or severe perinatal asphyxia. High-risk children not tested at birth should be screened before age 3. Currently there is insufficient evidence to recommend routine otologic testing of all children in this age group. If young children within this age group are tested and have an abnormal test, the results should be confirmed by repeat testing at appropriate intervals. In addition, the child must have careful evaluation of all other aspects of growth and development to determine if he or she is reaching developmental milestones according to the designated time frame.

The National Institutes of Health (NIH) (1993) recommend that all infants who are admitted to the Neonatal Intensive Care Unit (NICU) be screened before discharge and that universal screening be implemented for all infants before 3 months. Other specialists disagree, stating that universal screening can be complex, expensive, and not necessarily justified (Bess and Paradise, 1994).

Hearing screening is not necessary for asymptomatic adolescents and young adults, except those who are exposed regularly to excessive noise. Screening of workers for noise-induced hearing loss should be performed in the context of existing worksite programs and guidelines. Older adults should be periodically evaluated to determine changes in their hearing status.

HEALTH PROMOTION—cont'd

■ **Cleaning of the Ears** Cerumen (earwax) is healthy and serves to actually clean the ears. The sticky nature of the cerumen catches foreign debris in the ear. Most of the time, the ear canals are self-cleaning due to the migration of the wax. If cerumen accumulates and actually blocks the canal, then the ear canal must be cleaned.

There are three methods to clean the cerumen from the ear canal. The first is the careful use of a cotton swab. Only the cotton portion should be placed in the ear. Once it is in place, rotate the swab to clean the distal portion of the canal. Caution is necessary because if the applicator is inserted too far in the canal or if the arm is bumped while the applicator is in the ear, damage to the ear canal and the drum may result. Also, the cotton swab may actually push the cerumen deeper into the canal, causing cerumen impaction.

The second method of cleaning the ear canal is to irrigate the canal with water irrigation using a rubber ear syringe. With this method, use warm water and vigorously but carefully flush the ear. The water will run quickly in and out, so be sure to position the head over a sink or basin. Warn the client that a lot of noise will be generated as water is forced into the ear. If the water is too warm or too cold, temporary dizziness may result. If the irrigation causes pain, stop immediately; the tympanic membrane may be perforated.

The third method of irrigation is to use ear drops that will usually soften and remove the cerumen. Frequently, drops alone are not adequate to clean the wax, especially if there is a large amount of cerumen deep in the canal.

The most effective method of removing cerumen from the ears is to use a combination of softening drops followed by warm water irrigation. To do this, place the softening agent in the ear canal and plug the canal with cotton for 5 to 10 minutes.

Then irrigate the ear with warm water as instructed above. This combination of methods is usually successful.

■ **Foreign Bodies in the Ear** Young children are notorious for putting everything they can find into their mouths, noses, and sometimes ears. Parents must be taught about the hazards of small children having access to objects small enough to be placed in the ear. Parents should also be advised that, if a foreign body in the ear is suspected, they should not attempt to remove it at home by themselves. There are several reasons for this: (1) the object may be pushed further into the ear canal; (2) any object the parent may use to "get the object out of the ear" may actually damage the wall of the ear canal, setting up the possibility of a secondary infection; (3) if the parent does not adequately immobilize the child, the child may jerk during the parent's attempt to remove the object and further injure the ear from the sudden movement; and finally, (4) should the parent believe that the foreign body can be flushed out with water without knowing exactly what the foreign body is, further problems may develop. If the object is a food substance such as a bean or piece of corn, the object may swell in the ear canal. Advise the parent that it is always best to take the child to a health care provider for foreign body removal.

Other foreign bodies that may be a problem for persons of all ages are bugs, spiders, and insects. All persons should be advised about this risk, especially if they spend a lot of time outdoors or camp frequently. If a bug does crawl into the ear, it will make a terrible noise until it is either killed or removed. One safe way to stop the noise and to suffocate the creature until it can be removed is to fill the ear canal with some type of oil, preferably mineral or olive oil. Then, as advised above, care should be sought with a health care provider to actually remove the bug and to ensure that the ear canal is without lesion or damage.

???????? STUDY QUESTIONS ???????

1. List the two primary functions of the ear.
2. List and describe the three sections of the ear.
3. List the five sequential steps that occur so that we can hear.
4. Differentiate between conductive and sensorineural hearing loss.
5. List one developmental problem and describe how it affects the function of the ear in the following groups: infants, children, pregnant women, older adults.
6. Match the condition with the correct cause:

Earache	Soap residue
Itching ears	Infection
Ringing ears	Being a rock musician
Hearing loss	Aspirin overdose

7. What historical information is important to collect for a client who presents with an earache? Ringing in the ears? Progressive hearing loss?
8. Distinguish between dizziness and vertigo. List at least two causes of vertigo or dizziness. What hazard is associated with vertigo?
9. List at least three causes of hearing impairment in infants. Which racial groups are at highest risk for hearing impairment as infants or small children?
10. What questions can you ask when taking a history that will elicit whether a particular infant is at high risk for a hearing impairment?
11. What indicators in young children are suggestive of a hearing loss? Which of these indicators may not be reliable in American Indian and Alaska Native groups? Hispanic groups?
12. List at least two common causes of hearing impairment in older children. What questions would help you elicit whether a particular child is at risk for hearing loss?
13. What is the major problem associated with hearing in the older adult?
14. What equipment is needed for examination of the ear?
15. When inspecting the ear for alignment, what are you looking for? What would be considered abnormal?
16. List four problems that may be indicated if discharge from the external auditory canal is noted.
17. Why is palpation of the external ear important?
18. How is the size of the specula for the otoscope chosen?
19. Describe the steps you would follow to examine the internal ear.

20. What are you looking for as you examine the ear canal? The tympanic membrane?
21. What normal racial variations occur in the characteristics of cerumen?
22. Match the abnormal finding in the color of the TM with the correct cause:

General redness	Allergy
Red streaks	Healed inflammation
Chalky white	Infection in middle ear
White flecks	Purulent otitis media

23. How is movement of the tympanic membrane achieved? What is the purpose of moving the TM? What is the normal response of the TM to puffs of air? List three abnormal responses to air puffs.
24. List and describe four screening tests that you could perform to evaluate auditory function.
25. Define air and bone conduction. What is the normal air-to-bone conduction ratio?
26. What tuning fork results would you expect in someone with a conductive hearing loss? A sensorineural loss?
27. How is vestibular function evaluated? What is a normal result?
28. Describe the specific age-related safety measures that are utilized during examination of the ear.
29. Describe specific techniques that are used in approach if the client is hearing impaired.
30. Describe the following conditions related to the external ear: cauliflower ear; Darwin tubercle; sebaceous cysts; tophi.
31. List four common problems of the external auditory canal and the possible complications that may occur as a result.
32. Discuss two types of otitis media. What can occur if otitis media is not treated? What is the purpose of myringotomy tubes?
33. What are common causes of conductive hearing loss? Sensorineural hearing loss?
34. What would you teach clients about protecting their hearing from repeated noise exposure?
35. List and describe three ways to safely clean cerumen from the ear canal.

CHAPTER 13

Eyes and Visual System

ANATOMY AND PHYSIOLOGY

As one of the sensory organs, the eye transmits visual stimuli to the brain for interpretation via the optic nerve (cranial nerve II). The eye is protected by the bony orbit, which is lined with fatty tissue. Additional protection is provided through the corneal or blink reflex that keeps out foreign objects and spreads tears over the surface of the eyeball. The corneal reflex is mediated by the ophthalmic division of the trigeminal nerve (cranial nerve V) and the facial nerve (cranial nerve VII).

EXTERNAL OCULAR STRUCTURES

The external eyes are composed of the eyebrows, eyelids, eyelashes, conjunctiva, and lacrimal glands. The opening between the eyelids is called the palpebral fissure. The eyelashes curve outward from the lid margins, filtering out dust and dirt. Two different thin, transparent mucous membranes called conjunctivae lie between the eyelids and the eyeball. The bulbar conjunctiva covers the scleral surface of the eyeballs. The palpebral conjunctiva lines the eyelids and contains blood vessels, nerves, hair follicles, and sebaceous glands. One of the sebaceous glands, the *meibomian gland,* secretes an oily lubricating substance that appears as vertical yellow striations in the palpebral conjunctiva. Secretions from these glands lubricate the lids, prevent excessive evaporation of tears, and provide an airtight seal when the lids are closed (Fig. 13-1).

Tears are formed by the lacrimal glands in the anterior lateral fossa of the orbit. They combine with sebaceous secretions to maintain a constant film over the cornea (Fig. 13-1). In the inner (or medial) canthus, small openings called the upper and lower lacrimal puncta drain tears from the eyeball surface into the nasolacrimal ducts.

EYE MOVEMENT

The movement of the eye is provided by six *extraocular muscles* and three cranial nerves. The medial, inferior, and superior rectus muscles, as well as the inferior oblique muscle, control the following eye movement directions: upward outer, lower outer, upward inner, and medial eye movements. These muscles are guided by the oculomotor nerve (cranial nerve III). The superior oblique muscle controls lower medial movement, innervated by the trochlear nerve (cranial nerve IV). The lateral rectus muscle controls lateral eye movement, innervated by the abducens nerve (cranial nerve VI) (Fig. 13-2).

GLOBE OF THE EYE

The globe of the eye is surrounded by three separate layers. The outer layer is the *sclera,* which is the tough, fibrous, layer, sometimes called the "white" of the eye. The sclera merges with the cornea in front of the globe at a junction called the limbus. The cornea covers the iris and the pupil. It is transparent, avascular, and richly innervated with sensory nerves via the trigeminal nerve (cranial nerve V). The constant wash of tears provides the cornea with its oxygen supply and protects its surface from drying. Another corneal function is to allow light transmission through the lens to the retina (Figs. 13-1 and 13-3).

The middle layer, called the uvea, consists of the choroid posteriorly and the ciliary body and iris anteriorly. The choroid layer is highly vascular and supplies the retina with blood. The iris is a circular, muscular membrane that regulates pupil dilation and constriction via the oculomotor nerve

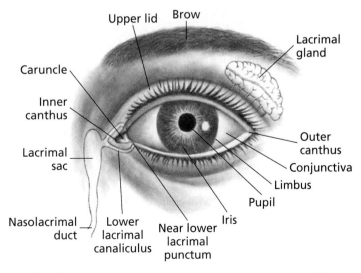

Fig. 13-1 Visible surface of eye. *(From Thompson et al, 1992.)*

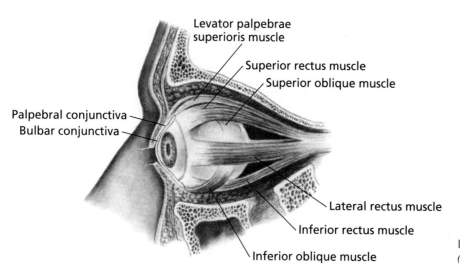

Fig. 13-2 Diagrammatic section of orbit.
(From Thompson et al, 1992.)

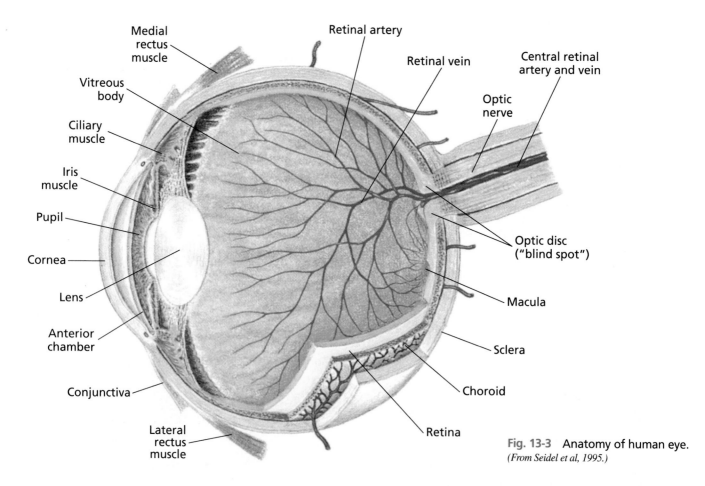

Fig. 13-3 Anatomy of human eye.
(From Seidel et al, 1995.)

(cranial nerve III). The iris' central aperture, the pupil, admits light to the retina. The ciliary body has two functions: its smooth muscle function adjusts the shape of the lens to accommodate vision at varying distances, and its secretory function is the production of aqueous humor (Fig. 13-4). The transparent aqueous humor, which fills the space between the cornea and lens, is secreted by the ciliary epithelium in the posterior chamber. The aqueous humor flows between the lens and the iris and is then reabsorbed by the trabecular meshwork (Fig. 13-5). This meshwork lies at the angle where the iris and cornea merge and encircles the anterior chamber. The trabecular meshwork filters the aqueous humor before it enters the canal of Schlemm and then flows into the anterior ciliary veins. The aqueous humor helps to maintain the in-

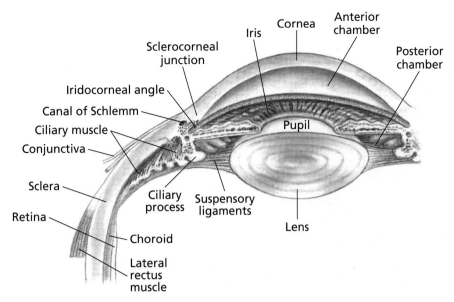

Fig. 13-4　Close-up view of ciliary body, zonules, lens, and anterior and posterior chambers.　*(From Thompson et al, 1992.)*

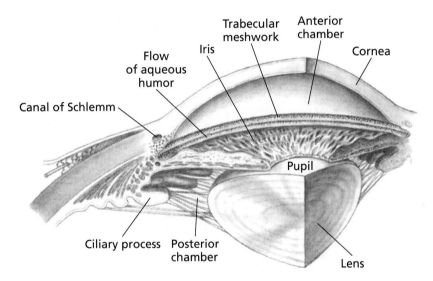

Fig. 13-5　Close-up view of trabecular meshwork and flow of aqueous humor.　*(From Thompson et al, 1992.)*

traocular pressure and metabolism of the lens and posterior cornea. The transparent lens attaches to the ciliary body by suspensory ligaments. The lens alters its shape for visual clarity when the eyes are viewing an object at close range.

Finally, the inner layer of the eyes, the retina, serves as an extension of the central nervous system. This transparent layer has photoreceptor cells, called rods and cones, scattered throughout its surface. As the name photoreceptor suggests, these cells perceive images and colors in response to varying light stimuli. Rods respond to low levels of light, and cones to higher levels of light.

These rods and cones, while scattered throughout the retina, are not at all evenly distributed. The macula lutea, a pigmented area about 4.5 mm in diameter, is densely packed peripherally with rods. At the same time, the fovea centralis, a small depression in the center of the macula lutea on the posterior wall of the retina, contains no rods but is densely packed with cones. Visual acuity is sharpest in this area in higher levels of light.

Perforating the retina is the optic disc, which is the head of the optic nerve (cranial nerve II). It contains no rods or cones, causing a small blind spot located about 15° laterally from the center of vision. The optic disc is where the central retinal artery and central vein bifurcate, emerge, and feed into smaller branches throughout the retinal surface (see Fig. 13-17).

VISION

Rods and cones in the retina perceive images and colors in response to varying light stimuli. The lens is constantly adjusting to stimuli at different distances by accommodation. For example, the normally flat lens becomes thicker and more

LEFT EYE   RIGHT EYE

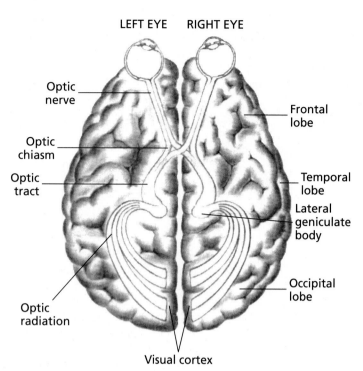

Optic nerve

Optic chiasm

Optic tract

Optic radiation

Visual cortex

Frontal lobe

Temporal lobe

Lateral geniculate body

Occipital lobe

Fig. 13-6   Visual pathway.   *(From Thompson et al, 1992.)*

convex to accommodate near objects. Through lens accommodation, an image is focused on the retina. Nerve impulses then are transmitted along the optic nerve and optic tract, reaching the optic cortex for interpretation. Objects in the visual field stimulate the opposite side of the retina. When nerve fibers pass into the optic nerve, the nasal and temporal fibers are separate within the sheath. The nerves merge at the optic chiasm, and the nasal fibers cross over to the opposite optic tract. Optic tracts emerging from the optic chiasm encircle the hypothalamus and terminate in the lateral geniculate bodies in the temporal lobes. From there, optic impulses are transmitted via visual nerve fibers to the occipital lobe of each cerebral hemisphere (Fig. 13-6).

DEVELOPMENTAL CONSIDERATIONS

INFANTS

Neonates have a visual acuity of 20/200. Peripheral vision is fully developed at birth; however, central vision develops later. The 2- to 3-month-old infant begins to have voluntary control over eye muscles. At around this same time, the lacrimal ducts begin carrying tears into the nasal meatus. By 8 months the infant can distinguish colors, and by 9 months the eyes are able to perceive a single image, reflecting the eye muscles' ability to coordinate.

CHILDREN

Young children's eyes are less spherical than adults', making children's vision myopic. The globe grows gradually until the expected adult visual acuity is achieved around age 6.

PREGNANT WOMEN

During pregnancy, the eye becomes more sensitive and dry, due to a rather insignificant change in lacrimal gland function. This may make it difficult to use contact lenses during pregnancy. During the first 8 weeks of gestation the fetus' eyes are formed, making them particularly sensitive to intrauterine drug exposure or maternal infection, both of which can result in eye malformation.

OLDER ADULTS

Changes in the external structure of the eye, including graying of eyebrows and eyelashes, occur, along with loss of tonus and decreased elasticity of eyelid muscles. Tearing is diminished, resulting in "dry eyes," which causes irritation and discomfort.

Corneal sensitivity often is diminished so that elderly may be unaware of infection or injury. Corneal reflexes are often diminished to absent. As the lens become more rigid, usually by the age of 45, and the ciliary muscle of the iris weakens, the near point of accommodation changes. This loss of lens elasticity is termed *presbyopia*. Increased density of the lens, along with degeneration of cells of the iris, cornea, and lens capsule, cause scattering of light and sensitivity to glare. Color perception is altered, with difficulty seeing blue, violet, and green (Matteson and McConnell, 1988).

HEALTH HISTORY　Eyes and Visual System

The principal areas to be investigated during the history relating to the eyes and visual system are difficulty with vision, pain, redness or swelling, watering or discharge, and ocular problems (strabismus, diplopia, or glaucoma).

QUESTIONS　　　　　　　　　　　　RATIONALE

DIFFICULTY WITH VISION

■ What type of difficulty are you having with vision? When did it begin? Did it begin suddenly or gradually? Does the problem affect one eye or both? Is it constant or does it come and go? How would you describe it—blurring? Cloudiness? Images out of focus? Spots (floaters) in front of your eyes? Many, few, or one?

◀ *The client is the only one who can clearly describe the eye problems he or she is experiencing and you should seek the most accurate representation to aid in identifying any problems. Note that a sudden onset of visual symptoms, which may indicate a detached retina, requires an emergency referral. Floaters in eyes reported by clients usually are not significant.*

■ What have you tried to correct the vision difficulty? Do the problems go away when you blink several times? Do you use any medications for eye problems?

◀ *The methods that relieve the problem often point to its cause.*

■ Have you ever seen a halo or multicolored ring around objects or lights?

◀ *Halos surrounding lights may indicate acute narrow-angle glaucoma or digoxin toxicity.*

■ Have you notice any "blind spot?" Does it move as you shift your gaze? Do you feel your peripheral vision has decreased?

◀ *A blind spot surrounded by an area of normal or decreased vision (a scotoma) occurs in glaucoma and with optic nerve and visual pathway disorders.*

■ Have you noticed any difficulty seeing at night?

◀ *Night blindness can occur in optic atrophy, glaucoma, or vitamin A deficiency.*

■ Do you wear contact lenses or glasses? When were they prescribed? For what problem? How often do you have the lenses checked by a physician or optometrist? Are the contact lenses soft, hard, or extended wear? How long do you wear them each day? Do you ever sleep with contact lenses in place?

◀ *Self-care behaviors should be assessed, particularly in light of any problems the client may be experiencing.*

■ How often do you clean your glasses? Your contact lenses? How do you clean them? Do you remove them (glasses or contacts) for certain activities? How often do you have your eyes checked? Have you had any problems specific to your glasses or contacts?

◀ *Wearing contact lenses too long may lead to infection.*

■ What medications do you take? Do you use eye drops? What kind of drops? How often? For what reason?

■ Have you ever had eye surgery? Have you ever suffered injury or trauma to the eyes?

◀ *Parasympatholytics and sympathomimetics dilate the pupil. Adverse reactions of drugs may cause myopia, blurred vision, or light sensitivity.*

PAIN

■ Do you have pain in your eye(s)? Did it begin suddenly or gradually? Is it sharp? Dull? Throbbing? Burning? Itching? Do you feel that there is a foreign body in your eye? Do you have a headache across the eye area? Are your eyes more sensitive to light than usual?

◀ *Again, the sudden onset of eye pain should be considered an emergency. Although some common eye diseases cause no pain, any complaint of pain should be noted and investigated.*

QUESTIONS	RATIONALE

REDNESS AND/OR SWELLING

■ Have you noticed any redness or swelling in the eye area? Any signs of infection? Have you had eye infections in the past? When do they occur? Are they seasonal? Are they associated with any sport you may be involved in? Do you have allergies? Do any individuals in your family or others in close contact have these same problems?

◀ *Allergies may cause seasonal redness, swelling, or excessive tearing.*
Chlorine from pools may cause redness.

WATERING AND DISCHARGE

■ Do you have watering or excessive tearing? Does this occur constantly or from time to time? Do your eyes feel strained or tired when they water?

◀ *Tearing (lacrimation) and excessive tearing (epiphora) can be caused by irritating substances, allergies, or blocked drainage of tears. Eye strain or fatigue can produce tearing.*

■ Have you noticed a discharge or matter in the eyes? Does it occur only in the morning? Is it hard to open your eyes in the morning because of the discharge? How do you remove the matter?

◀ *Thick yellow or green discharge is abnormal. Crusts can form overnight and make the eyes difficult to open. Hygiene practices and cross-contamination control should be evaluated.*

OCULAR PROBLEMS

■ Have you ever been tested for glaucoma? What were the results? Has glaucoma occurred among members of your family?

◀ *Glaucoma testing is recommended periodically for all persons over age 65 (U.S. Preventive Services Task Force). A tendency for the disease seems to be inherited.*

■ Have you had crossed eyes? Do your eyes cross when they are tired?

◀ *Crossed eyes may indicate strabismus.*

■ Do you have double vision? When does it occur? Does it occur continuously or intermittently? Does it occur when you have one eye or both eyes open?

◀ *Diplopia, the perception of two images of a single object, may indicate extraocular disease.*

■ Have your vision problems interfered with your daily life? Describe how this has happened. Do you have diabetes? Any other diseases that may affect your vision? Do you require books with large print, or those on audiotape, or those in Braille? Are you afraid that you may not be able to see someday?

◀ *Evaluate the adjustments the client has made to lifestyle and routines. Assess the client's attitude and fears concerning blindness.*

■ Does your job involve risks for your vision? For example, are there sparks or flying bits of metal that could injure your eyes? Do you use safety goggles? Are you in front of a computer monitor frequently? Do you read extensively, leading to eye fatigue and strain? When was your last eye examination?

◀ *Ocular diseases or injuries can be related to work.*

INFANTS

Questions that should be asked of the parent or guardian when the client is a newborn or infant include the following:

■ Did the mother have a vaginal infection when she delivered? What was the infection? How was it treated?

◀ *Some vaginal infections, such as gonorrhea and genital herpes, can affect the eyes of newborns.*

■ Has the child achieved all the developmental milestones regarding vision? (See Chapter 22)

◀ *The parent is the most likely person to notice problems with vision.*

QUESTIONS

CHILDREN

In addition to inquiry into the child's achievement of developmental milestones, questions to ask when the client is a child include the following:

- Is the child's vision tested each year at school? Is the child able to see the chalk or markers on the board or overhead transparencies in the classroom without difficulty? Does the child have difficulty reading?
- Are you aware of safety factors when purchasing toys? Do you take measures to protect the child from trauma? Have you taught the child how to handle and use sharp objects?
- Does the child rub eyes excessively? Does the child shut eyes, tilt head, or thrust head forward? Does the child blink more than usual? Does the child hold books close to his or her eyes? Sit close to television? Are the eyes inflamed or watery? Does the child develop frequent sties?

Preventive programs detect problems early.

Safety is of utmost concern in the care of children's vision. Assess the child's compliance with safety precautions. These are additional signs of visual problems in young children.

ADOLESCENTS

In addition to the history taken for adults, adolescents should be asked the following questions:

- Can you see the chalk or markers on the board or overhead transparencies in the classroom?
- Do you sit close to television or have to hold books close to your eyes?
- Do you wear glasses, if prescribed?

They may be self-conscious, influenced by peer pressure not to wear glasses, or concerned about self-esteem.

OLDER ADULTS

The effects of aging on the visual system should be evaluated with the following questions:

- Do you wear glasses? How old are they?
- Do you have any trouble with vision when you are climbing stairs or driving?

- When was your vision examined last? When were you last tested for glaucoma? Do you have glaucoma?
- Have you noticed any pain around the eyes? Do you feel you have lost any peripheral vision? Do you have problems with night vision? Have you noticed a change in recognizing colors?
- Do you have cataracts? Is there a family history of cataracts? Have you had cataracts removed? Have the cataracts progressed, causing decreased vision? Do your eyes feel dry or burn? Do you have increased or decreased tearing? What do you do for these problems?

Loss of depth perception occurs with aging.

Check for the client's self-care behaviors.

Assess the client's health status and ability to cope.

EXAMINATION   Procedures and Findings

Guidelines **The eye examination assesses the function of the eye in three phases: visual acuity, including distant and near vision, peripheral vision, and eye movement, followed by an inspection of the external eye and finally the internal eye.**

> EQUIPMENT   Snellen eye chart or E chart
> Hand-held near-vision screener (Rosenbaum or Jaeger)
> Cover card (opaque)
> Penlight
> Ophthalmoscope

TECHNIQUES and NORMAL FINDINGS

ABNORMAL FINDINGS

VISION

TEST vision for Acuity and observe for any outward cues indicating any difficulty with vision. Measure distant vision using the *Snellen eye chart* (see Fig. 5-13 *A*).

The Snellen eye chart tests the optic nerve (cranial nerve II). Place the Snellen eye chart on the wall in a well-lighted room. The client may sit or stand about 6 meters (20 feet) from the chart. If a client wears contact lenses or glasses, he or she should leave them in place unless they are for reading only.

Have the client cover one eye with an opaque card and read the line of smallest letters possible. Test the other eye using the same procedure. Document the line read completely by the client, using the fraction printed at the end of the line. A finding of 20/30 means the client can read at 20 feet what a person with normal vision can read at 30 feet. If the client can read all the letters in the 20/30 line and two letters in the 20/20 line, document the finding as 20/30 +2.

Also ask the client to use both eyes to name the colors of the two horizontal lines to document red and green color perception. Finally, ask him or her which of the two horizontal lines is longer to assess perception.

Note: Use the Snellen "E" chart for the client who cannot read letters. The client is asked to indicate the direction in which the "E" points (see Fig. 5-7 *B*). Repeat the procedure with the other eye. In all cases, the reading pattern should be smooth and without hesitation. Eyes should remain open without squinting. Record the results using the fraction at the end of the last line that was read successfully. Also record whether the client wore glasses or contact lenses.

Assess near vision for people over 40 years of age or for those who feel they have difficulty reading. Use a Jaeger or Rosenbaum card or a newspaper (Fig. 13-7). NOTE: Myopic (nearsighted) people may be able to read at a normal distance if they remove their glasses. This will be reported as a change in vision because formerly they were able to read while wearing their glasses.

> O.S. = ocular sinister   = left eye
> O.D. = ocular dexter   = right eye
> O.U. = ocular uterque = each eye

■ Note any hesitancy, squinting, leaning forward, or misreading of letters. Blinking or facial expressions indicating that the client is struggling should be noted also. These signal difficulties in perceiving the letters and a possible visual problem.

■ Criterion for legal blindness is 20/200.

■ Note that the larger the denominator, the poorer the vision. If vision is poorer than 20/30, refer the client to an ophthalmologist or optometrist. Impaired vision may be caused by refractive error, opacity of the lens, cornea, or vitreous, or a retinal or optic pathway disorder.

■ With age, there is a tendency for the eyes to lose their ability to perform accommodation; this tendency is known as presbyopia. As a result, the client will need to move the card farther away to see it clearly.

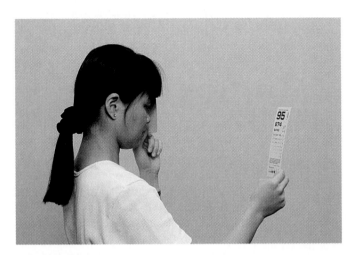

Fig. 13-7 Assessing a client's near vision with the Rosenbaum chart.

ASSESS visual fields for Peripheral Vision. The *confrontation test* assesses the optic nerve (cranial nerve II) function. The examiner faces the client, standing or sitting at a distance of 2 to 3 feet (60 to 90 cm). Have the client cover one eye with an opaque card as you cover your own eye directly opposite the client's covered eye. (NOTE: This test assumes that the examiner has normal peripheral visual fields.) Gaze directly at each other. Hold a pencil or use your finger and extend it to the farthest periphery. Gradually bring the object close to the midline (equal distance between you and the client). Ask the client to report when he or she first sees the object; you should see the object at the same time. Slowly move the object inward from the periphery in four directions: anteriorly (from above the head down into field of vision); inferiorly (from upper chest up toward field of vision); temporally (move in laterally from behind the client's head into field of vision), and nasally (move medially into the field of vision) (Fig. 13-8). Estimate the angle between the anteroposterior axis of the eye and the peripheral axis when the pencil or finger is first seen. Normal values are 50° upward, 90° temporal peripheral, 70° downward, and 60° toward the nose.

■ If the client cannot see the pencil or finger at the same time that you see it, peripheral field loss is suspected. Refer client for more precise testing.

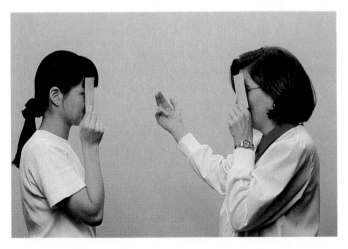

Fig. 13-8 Assessing a client's peripheral vision nasally by moving object medially into the field of vision.

| **TECHNIQUES and NORMAL FINDINGS** | **ABNORMAL FINDINGS** |

INSPECT extraocular muscles for Movement. Inspect eye movement in the *six cardinal fields of gaze* (oculomotor [cranial nerve III], trochlear [cranial nerve IV], and abducens nerves [cranial nerve VI]), as follows (Fig. 13-9):

1. Have client look directly ahead at you.
2. Ask client to keep the head still and use the eyes only to follow your finger or an object in your hand.
3. Move an object from center position to upper outer extreme, hold there, move back to center, to lower inner extreme, and hold there.
4. Move an object to temporal-nasal extremes, holding there momentarily.
5. Move an object to opposite upper outer extreme and back to opposite lower inner extreme.

Normally there will be parallel tracking of the object with both eyes. Mild nystagmus at extreme lateral gaze is also normal. NOTE: An alternative method to steps 3 to 5 above is to move your finger slowly in a circle to each of the six directions. Stop in each position so that client can hold the gaze briefly before moving to the next position.

- Eye movement that is not parallel indicates an extraocular muscle weakness or dysfunction of cranial nerve III, IV, or VI.

- *Exotropia*—outward (temporal) deviation of the eye.

- *Esotropia*—inward (nasal) deviation of the eye. Note any nystagmus other than that considered normal. (Nystagmus is involuntary movement of the eyeball in a horizontal, vertical, rotary, or mixed direction.) Note any lid lag, when the upper eyelid fails to overlap the superior part of the iris and white shows. This may be a sign of hyperthyroidism.

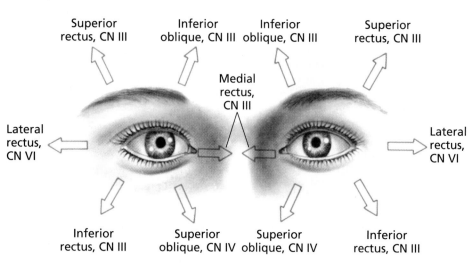

Fig. 13-9 The six cardinal fields of gaze. *(From Seidel et al, 1995.)*

INSPECT the corneal light reflex for Symmetry. (Hirschberg test) Ask the client to stare straight ahead with both eyes open. Shine a penlight toward the bridge of the nose at a distance of 12 to 15 inches (30 to 38 cm). Light reflections should appear symmetrically in both pupils (Fig. 13-10). When an imbalance is found in the corneal light reflex, perform the cover-uncover test.

- If light reflections appear at different spots in each eye (asymmetrically), this may indicate weak extraocular muscles preventing eyes from focusing on an object simultaneously. (Strabismus is the inability of both eyes to focus on an object simultaneously.)

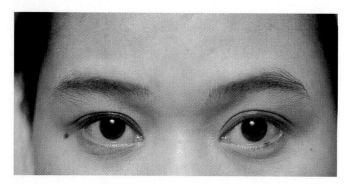

Fig. 13-10 Testing the corneal light reflex. Symmetric light reflections in both corneas is a normal finding.

TECHNIQUES and NORMAL FINDINGS

To perform the *cover-uncover test,* ask the client to stare straight ahead at your nose even though the gaze may be interrupted. Cover one of the client's eyes with the opaque card. Note the uncovered eye, checking for any deviation from a steady, fixed gaze. Then remove the card and observe the just-uncovered eye for movement to focus. It should not move. Repeat with the other eye (Fig. 13-11).

ABNORMAL FINDINGS

■ If the uncovered eye moves to focus, it is the weaker eye.

■ If the just-uncovered eye moves to focus, it is the weak eye because it relaxed while being covered.

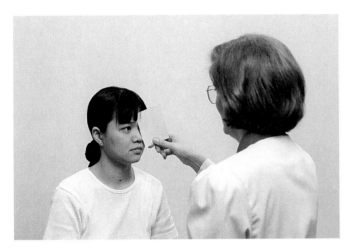 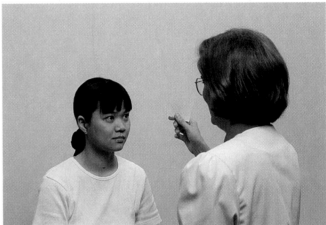

Fig. 13-11　The cover-uncover test is used to evaluate eye fixation.

TECHNIQUES and NORMAL FINDINGS

ABNORMAL FINDINGS

EXTERNAL OCULAR STRUCTURES

INSPECT the eyebrows for Quality, Hair Distribution, Underlying Skin, and Symmetry. Skin should be intact and eyebrows symmetric. Note whether the eyebrow extends over the eye.

■ Flakiness, loss of hair, scaling, and un-equal alignment of movement should not be seen. Loss of the lateral one third of the eyebrow occurs in hypothyroidism.

 Racial Variation

The palpebral fissures are horizontal in nonAsians, whereas Asians nor-mally have an upward slant to the palpebral fissures (Fig. 13-12.)

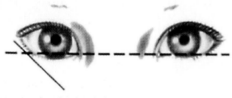

Upward palpebral slant

Fig. 13-12 Narrowed and upwardly slanting palpebral fissures are a normal finding in Asians.   *(From Wong, 1995.)*

INSPECT the eyelids and eyelashes for Symmetry, Position, Closure, Blinking, Discharge, and Color. Palpebral fissures should be bilaterally equal. The upper lid margins should cover part of the iris but not the pupil. The lower lid generally covers to just below the limbus. Lid closure should be complete, with smooth, easy motion. Blinking should generally consist of frequent, bilateral, in-voluntary movements, averaging 15 to 20 blinks per minute. Lid margins should fit flush against the eyeball surfaces, and eyelashes should be equally distributed and curled slightly outward. The color of the lids should correspond to skin color, and margins should be pale pink.

■ Palpebral fissures are asymmetrically po-sitioned. Sclera is visible between the upper lid and iris in hyperthyroid exoph-thalmos. The lid of either eye covers part of pupil, causing ptosis, which may be congenital or acquired. Closure of the lid that is incomplete or accomplished only with pain or difficulty may occur with in-fections. Edema of the lid may occur with trauma or infection. The presence of lesions, nodules, redness, flaking, crusting, excessive tearing, or discharge is noted. Note lid deformity and whether lashes are absent or turned in. Red, swollen eyelids may indicate infec-tion, e.g., sty (hordeolum), or inflamma-tion, e.g., meibomian cyst (chalazion).

 Racial Variation

For white clients, the eyeball does not protrude beyond the supraorbital ridge of the frontal bone. For African-American clients, the eyeball may protrude slightly beyond the supraorbital ridge.

INSPECT and PALPATE the globe in the bony socket for Position and Indentation. Ask the client to look down with lids closed so that you will not pal-pate the cornea. Gently palpate the eyeball; it should indent with slight pressure. Palpate the lower orbital rim near the inner canthus. This pressure slightly everts the lower lid.

■ Asymmetric placement of the globe should be noted. Note whether the placement is too far forward (exoph-thalmos) or backward (enophthalmos). An eyeball that is rigid may occur in glaucoma.

TECHNIQUES and NORMAL FINDINGS

ABNORMAL FINDINGS

INSPECT the lacrimal puncta for Color, Moisture, Discharge, Tenderness, and Nodules. Puncta are seen as small elevations on the nasal side of the upper and lower lid margins. Mucosa should be pink and intact despite pressure. Eyes should be moist, without excessive tears. Gently palpate the upper and lower lids for tenderness or nodules.

INSPECT the bulbar conjunctiva for Color and Clarity. Ask client to look up. Gently separate the lids widely with the thumb and index finger, exerting pressure over the bony orbit surrounding the eye. Have client look up, down, and to each side. The bulbar conjunctiva should be clear, possibly with tiny red vessels.

Pull down and evert the lower lid; ask the client to look up. The palpebral conjunctiva should be opaque, pink, and vascular (Fig. 13-13).

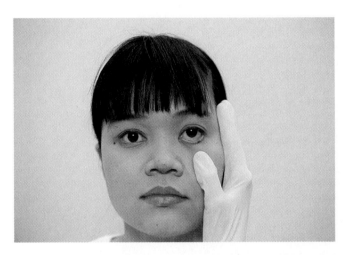

Fig. 13-13   To inspect the palpebral conjunctiva, gently pull down and evert the lower eyelid.

■ Lacrimal puncta that are clogged with mucus or dirt cause inflammation (dacryocystitis). Fluid or purulent material may be discharged from the puncta in response to pressure. Excessive tearing (epiphora) may be caused by blockage of nasolacrimal duct.

■ Tenderness, nodules, or irregularities should be noted.

■ Blood vessels should not be dilated. Conjunctiva appear red and congested in conjunctivitis. A sharply defined area of blood adjacent to normal-appearing conjunctiva may indicate subconjunctival hemorrhage. Lesions, nodules, or foreign bodies should be noted. Pale conjunctiva occurs in anemia. Observe for discharge and crusting. Note any tissue growth of bulbar conjunctiva from the periphery toward the corneal center (pterygium).

TECHNIQUES and NORMAL FINDINGS

ABNORMAL FINDINGS

Eversion of the upper lid. Although not a part of routine screening, this maneuver is used when you must inspect the conjunctiva of the upper lid, such as when clients complain of eye pain or a foreign body is suspected. To ensure the client's cooperation, explain the procedure before performing it (Fig. 13-14).

- Ask client to look down but keep eyes slightly open; this relaxes the levator muscle of the eyelid.
- Gently grasp the upper eyelashes and pull gently downward. Do not pull the lashes outward or upward, causing muscle contraction.
- Place a cotton-tipped applicator stick about 1 cm above the upper lid margin and push gently down with the applicator while still holding the lashes to evert the lid.
- Hold the lashes of the everted lid against the upper ridge of the bony orbit, just below the eyebrow but not pushing against the eyeball.
- Examine the lid for swelling, infection, or foreign bodies.
- Return the lid to normal by moving the lashes slightly forward and asking clients to look up and then blink. The lid returns easily to normal.

- Swelling, presence of a foreign body, and redness should be noted, with the client referred for further examination.

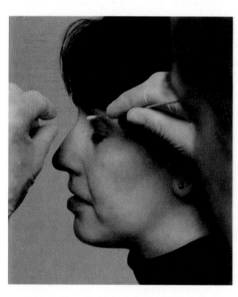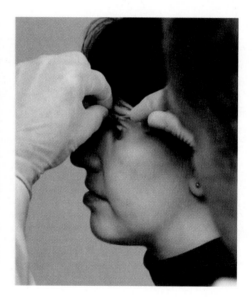

Fig. 13-14   Everting upper eyelid.   *(From Seidel et al, 1995.)*

GLOBE OF THE EYE

INSPECT the sclera for Color and Clarity. Sclera should be white and moist.

- Yellow sclera may indicate jaundice.

 Racial Variation

The sclera appears white except in darker-skinned clients, in whom it is normally a darker shade. Tiny black dots of pigmentation may be present near the limbus in dark-skinned individuals. In light-skinned individuals, there may be a slight yellow cast.

TECHNIQUES and NORMAL FINDINGS

INSPECT the cornea for Transparency and Surface Characteristics. Use oblique lighting and slowly move the light reflection over the corneal surface. Observe for transparent quality and a smooth surface that is clear and shiny.

Test the corneal reflex only in selected cases, such as unconscious clients. Lightly touch the cornea with cotton. The lids of both eyes close when either cornea is touched. This reflex tests the sensory reception of the ophthalmic branch of the trigeminal nerve (cranial nerve V) and the motor branch of the facial nerve (cranial nerve VII) which creates a blink.

INSPECT the anterior chamber for Transparency, Iris Surface, and Chamber Depth by using a penlight or ophthalmoscope. Shine light from the side across the iris to note transparency, a flat iris, and adequate chamber depth (enough clearance between the cornea and iris) (Fig. 13-15).

ABNORMAL FINDINGS

■ Note opacities, irregularities in light reflections, lesions, abrasions, or foreign bodies. Especially note any white opaque ring encircling the limbus, called *corneal arcus*. The arc is composed of lipids deposited at the periphery. It is seen in many clients over 60 and is associated with type II hyperlipidemia when seen in clients younger than age 40.

■ Edema of the brainstem might impair the function of cranial nerve V and cranial nerve VII and may occur after head injury or with hemorrhage or tumor.

■ Cloudiness or visible material or blood should be noted. The iris should not bulge toward the cornea, and the chamber should not be shallow. Also note iris or pupil shapes other than round, inconsistent iris coloration, and unequal pupil sizes. About 5% of the population normally have unequal pupils (anisocoria), but it may occur due to past eye surgery, trauma, or congenital anomalies.

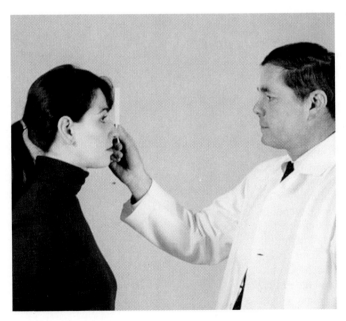

A

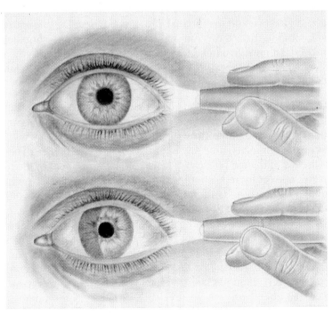

B

Fig. 13-15 Evaluation of depth of anterior chambers. **A,** Normal anterior chamber. **B,** Shallow anterior chamber. *(From Seidel et al, 1995.)*

TECHNIQUES and NORMAL FINDINGS

ABNORMAL FINDINGS

INSPECT the iris for Shape and Color. It should be round with consistent coloration.

INSPECT the pupils for Size, Shape, and Reaction to Light. Pupils should be round and equal in size. Next, dim the room lights if possible. Ask the client to hold the eyes open and fix gaze straight ahead. Approach with a penlight beam from the side and shine it directly on the pupil. The illuminated iris should constrict (direct response) (oculomotor cranial nerve III) and the other iris constricts simultaneously (consensual response). The optic nerve (cranial nerve II) senses the light and cranial nerve III creates the constriction of the iris, which makes the pupil appear smaller. Repeat with the other eye.

- ■ Failure of either one or both eyes to constrict to light in speed or magnitude indicates dysfunction of the oculomotor nerve (cranial nerve III). *Mydriasis* is pupil size greater than 6 mm that fails to constrict; it may occur with diabetes, epilepsy, head trauma, or high blood alcohol level.
- ■ *Miosis* is constriction to less than 2 mm caused by drugs such as morphine.

INSPECT pupils for Accommodation. Ask the client to fix the gaze at a distant object across the room. The pupils should dilate when visualizing a distant object. Then ask the client to shift gaze to your finger, placed about 6 inches from the client's nose. The usual response is bilateral constriction and convergence of the eyes.

- ■ Failure of pupil to converge or constrict may occur in diabetes or syphilis.

OPHTHALMOSCOPIC EXAMINATION (INTERNAL EYE)

Darken the room to help dilate the pupils. Have client remove glasses; contact lenses may be left in. The examiner may leave his or her own glasses or contact lenses in place. Ask client to fixate on a distant point. Turn on the ophthalmoscope light by pressing the on/off switch and turning the rheostat control clockwise. Set the diopter wheel to 0. To examine the client's right eye, hold the ophthalmoscope in your right hand and use your right eye. Place your right index finger on the selection wheel so that you can change the diopter settings as needed to focus on the internal structures. Direct the client to continuously gaze at a point across the room and slightly above your shoulder. Begin about 10 inches (25 mm) from client's eye at a 15° angle lateral to the client's line of vision. Shine the light of the ophthalmoscope on the pupil while looking through the viewing lens.

- ■ Decreased or irregular red reflex, dark spots, and opacities should be noted.

OBSERVE the red reflex. Observe a red glow over the client's pupil; this is the red reflex (Fig. 13-16, *A*) created by light illuminating the retina. Keep this red reflex in sight and move closer to the eye, adjusting the lens with the diopter wheel as needed to focus; note any interruption in the red reflex. There should be none. Absence of the red reflex may be caused by movement of the light away from the pupil; correct by repositioning the light (Fig. 13-16, *B*). Continue to move closer until you nearly touch foreheads with the client. Placing your middle finger on the client's cheek will stabilize the ophthalmoscope. Focusing varies depending on the refractive state of both the examiner and the client. Remember that the myopic (near-sighted) client has longer eyeballs so that light rays focus in front of the retina. To see the retina of this client, you use the minus (red) numbers by moving the diopter wheel up, or counterclockwise. By contrast, the hyperopic (far-sighted) client has shorter eyeballs, so that light rays focus behind the retina. For this client, use the positive (black) numbers by moving the diopter wheel down, or clockwise. When you locate a blood vessel, follow it inward toward the nose until you see the optic disc.

- ■ Dark shadows or black dots may indicate opacities that occur with cataracts or may be due to hemorrhage in the vitreous humor.

INSPECT the optic disc for Discrete Margin, Shape, Size, Color, and Physiologic Cup. The margin should be regular and have a distinct, sharp outline. Scattered or dense pigment deposits may be seen at the border. A gray crescent may appear at the temporal border.

- ■ Blurred margin may indicate papilledema, which is caused by increased intracranial pressure relayed along the optic nerve.

A 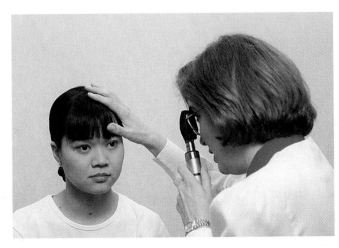 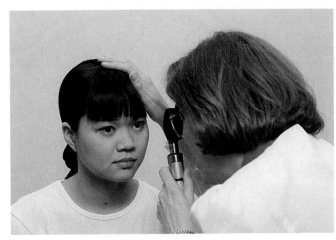 B

Fig. 13-16 Examining the retina. **A,** The red reflex is created by light illuminating the retina. **B,** Move close to the client until you nearly touch foreheads.

The optic disc should be round or slightly vertically oval. Its size measures about 1.5 mm (it is magnified 15 times through the ophthalmoscope). Marked myopic refractive errors may make the disc appear larger, and hyperopic errors may make it appear smaller. The optic disc's color should be creamy yellow to pink, lighter than the retina, possibly with tiny blood vessels visible on the surface. The physiologic cup is a small depression just temporal to the disc center that does not extend to the border. It usually appears lighter than the rest of the disc and occupies less than ½ of the disc's diameter. Vessels entering the disc may drop abruptly into the cup or appear to fade gradually.

Follow each of the four sets of retinal vessels from the disc to the periphery.

INSPECT the retinal vessels for Color, Arteriolar Light Reflex, Artery to Vein (A:V) Ratio, and Arteriovenous Crossing Changes. Arteries are on average ¼ narrower than veins; artery-to-vein width should be 2:3 to 4:5. Arteries are light red in color and may have a narrow band of light in the center. By contrast, veins are larger than arteries and have no light reflex. They are darker in color, and venous pulsations may be visible (Fig. 13-17).

Overall, the caliber of both arteries and veins should be regular and uniformly decreasing in size as they branch and move toward the periphery. Artery and vein crossing should give no evidence of constricting either vessel.

■ Irregular disc or discs that differ in size or shape between the two eyes should be noted.

■ Note diffuse or pallor sectional of the disc, which always extends from the center of the disc to the border. Hyperemic discs with engorged or tortuous vessels on the surface are abnormal. The depression of the physiologic cup should not extend to the border of the disc and should not occupy more than ½ of the diameter of the disc. The physiologic cup's appearance (size or placement) should not differ between eyes.

■ Extremely narrow arteries are abnormal. The width of the light reflex should not cover more than ⅓ of the artery. They should not be pale or opaque.

■ Irregularities of caliber, either dilation or constriction, should be noted. Compact areas of tortuous, narrow vessels should be investigated. Indentations or pinched appearances where veins and arteries cross occur with hypertension and are called A-V nicking.

TECHNIQUES and NORMAL FINDINGS

ABNORMAL FINDINGS

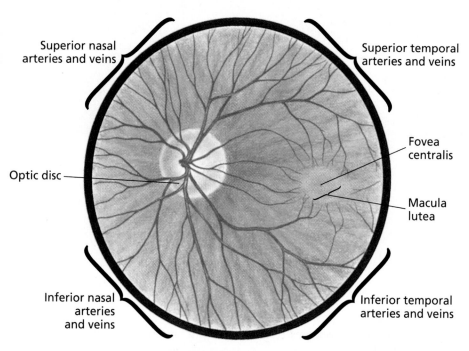

Superior nasal arteries and veins

Superior temporal arteries and veins

Fovea centralis

Optic disc

Macula lutea

Inferior nasal arteries and veins

Inferior temporal arteries and veins

Fig. 13-17   Retinal structures of the left eye.   *(From Seidel et al, 1995.)*

🌐 Racial Variation

The fundi of black persons may be heavily pigmented and uniformly dark.

INSPECT the retinal background for Color, Presence of Microaneurysms, Hemorrhages, and Exudates. The color is uniform throughout and may be pink, red, or orange; it varies with skin color (Fig. 13-18, *A-C*).

The retinal surface should be finely granular, with choroidal vessels possibly visible. Movable light reflections may appear on the surface, usually in young persons.

■ Pale fundus, either in general or in localized areas, or hemorrhages (linear, flame-shaped, round, dark red, large, small) must be noted.

■ Note microaneurysms, which appear as fine red dots, and any exudates, soft, hard, fuzzy, or well-defined.

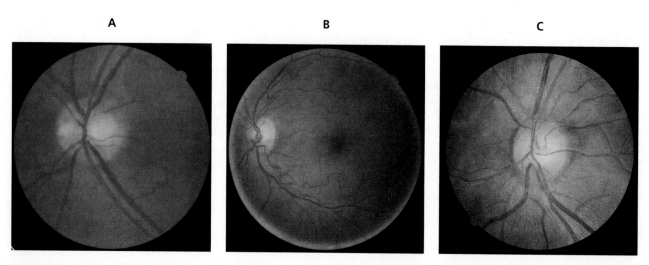

A   B   C

Fig. 13-18   Fundus of **A**, white client, **B**, black client, and **C**, Asian client.   *(Courtesy Dr. Frances C. Gaskin.)*

TECHNIQUES and NORMAL FINDINGS

ABNORMAL FINDINGS

INSPECT the macula for Color and Surface by asking the client to look directly into the ophthalmoscope light. The macula is about one disc diameter (DD) in size and lies about two DDs temporal to the optic disc. The macula and its center, the *fovea centralis,* should be slightly darker than the rest of the retina. The fovea may appear as a tiny bright light. Tiny vessels may appear on the surface. Fine pigmentation and granular appearance may be visible. The macula may be difficult to see if the client's pupil has not been chemically dilated.

Repeat the same examination on the other eye, holding the ophthalmoscope in the left hand and using your left eye to assess the client's left eye.

■ Note any abnormalities or lesions, as already outlined.

AGE-RELATED VARIATIONS

INFANTS

■ APPROACH

Newborns frequently have edema of the lids, either from the trauma of birth or in response to eye drops or ointments such as prophylactic instillation of silver nitrate. The edema may delay the examination for a few days. To begin the assessment, hold or rock the infant into an upright position to elicit eye opening. An alternative strategy is to hold the infant supine with the head gently lowered.

Examination of the infant can be a challenge to collect necessary data during the short time period that the infant is willing to cooperate. Being patient and creating a game out of the exam is helpful.

■ FINDINGS

Visual Acuity

Blink a penlight on and off several times, then move it around slightly about 10 inches (25 cm) from the baby's face. The infant should indicate some degree of recognition of the light and follow it momentarily. Visual acuity at birth ranges from 20/100 to 20/400 (Wong, 1995).

Specific age-related responses may be observed that indicate the infant's attention to visual stimuli.

- 0–2 weeks: Eyes do not reopen after exposure to bright light; there is increasing alertness to objects.
- 2–4 weeks: Infant is capable of fixating on object.
- 1 month: Infant can fixate and follow a bright toy or light.
- 3–4 months: Infant can fixate, follow, and reach for a toy, since binocular vision is normally achieved at this age.
- 6–10 months: Infant can fixate and follow toy in all directions.

Absence of these attending behaviors indicates a problem that may be visual or neurologic.

Extraocular Muscles

Perform corneal light reflex test as described for adults followed by the cover-uncover test. Transient strabismus is common during the first few months of life due to lack of binocular vision. If it continues beyond 6 months of age, however, a referral to an ophthalmologist is needed because early recognition and treatment can restore binocular vision.

Position and Alignment of Eyes

The eyes are symmetric and the outer canthus of the eye aligns with the pinna of the ear. Asymmetry of eyes or the presence of epicanthal folds should be noted, as should wide-set eyes (hypertelorism) or those that are close together (hypotelorism). A pronounced slant may indicate a chromosomal abnormality.

Eyebrows, Eyelids, and Eyelashes

Eyes of newborns usually are closed; often no eyebrows are present. Their eyes are symmetric, and eyelashes may be long. Eyelids may have edema, as mentioned previously, due to instillation of medications. Birth trauma can cause eyelid capillary hemangiomas.

Lacrimal Apparatus

A purulent discharge from eyes shortly after birth is abnormal. It may indicate ophthalmia neonatorum and should be reported. There are no tears until about 4 weeks of age. Excessive tearing before the third month or no tearing by the second month are deviations from normal.

Sclera and Bulbar Conjunctiva Characteristics

Infant sclera may have a blue tinge caused by thinness; otherwise sclera are white. Tiny black dots (pigmentation) or a slight yellow cast may appear near the limbus of dark-skinned infants. Note any discolorations of the sclera, such as dark blue sclera, or any dilated blood vessels. Hyperbilirubinemia may cause jaundiced (yellow) sclera in newborns.

Palpebral conjunctiva are pink and intact without discharge. Observe for abnormalities such as redness, lesions, nodules, discharge, or crusting of the conjunctiva. Birth trauma may cause conjunctivitis or conjunctival hemorrhage.

Pupil Reaction, Shape, and Size

Pupils should constrict in response to bright light. The blink reflex also is present in normal newborns and infants. Absence of these reflexes (no blinking or constriction) should be noted. If the pupillary response is not present after 3 weeks, the infant may be blind. A dilated, fixed, or constricted pupil may indicate anoxia or brain damage.

Pupils are round, about 2 to 4 mm in diameter, and equal in size. Dilated, constricted, or unequal pupils may indicate brain damage. A white pupil may occur in retinoblastoma, a relatively rare congenital malignant tumor arising from the retina (Wong, 1995). A white pupil in conjunction with a cloudy cornea or anterior chamber may indicate congenital cataracts.

Presence of Red Reflex

Using an ophthalmoscopic light, you should note a bilateral red reflex, which is a bright, round, red-orange glow seen through the pupil. It may be pale in dark-skinned newborns. Presence of the red reflex rules out most serious defects of the cornea, aqueous chamber, lens, and vitreous chamber. Absence of the red reflex may indicate the presence of retinal hemorrhage or congenital cataracts (Wong, 1995).

■ APPROACH

Most of the examination of children is the same as that for adults. Vision can be assessed when performing developmental tests such as the Denver II, e.g., noting the child's ability to stack blocks or identify animals. The assessment of vision and eyes should be appropriate for the developmental stage and age of the child. Prepare children for the ophthalmoscope exam by showing them the light, explaining how it shines in the eye and why the room must be darkened.

■ FINDINGS

Visual Acuity

Visual acuity of 20/20 is achieved during toddler years, although 20/40 is considered acceptable (Wong, 1995.) Use the *Allen test* to screen children 2½ to 3 years of age. Show the large cards with pictures to the child up close to be sure the child can identify them. Then present each picture at a distance of 15 feet from the child. Normally the child will be able to name 3 of the 7 cards within three to five trials.

Use the *Snellen "E" test* for children 3 to 6 years of age. Have children point their fingers in the direction of the "arms" of the E. By 7 to 8 years of age, begin to use the standard Snellen chart, as described for adults. Test each eye separately with and without glasses as is appropriate. If the child cannot cooperate for this test, wait. Be sure to screen children two separate times before referring them.

Color Vision

Test for color vision once between the ages of 4 and 8. use *Ishihara's test,* which consists of a series of polychromatic cards that have numbers and patterns embedded in different colors. Ask the child to identify each pattern. A child with normal color vision will see the number or pattern. A color-blind person will not be able to see the pattern against the background. Color blindness or deficiency may affect the child's school performance.

Extraocular Muscles

Perform corneal light reflex test as described for adults, followed by the cover-uncover test if necessary.

Screening for *strabismus* is important because early recognition and treatment can restore binocular vision; diagnosis after age 6 has a poor prognosis. Strabismus can lead to amblyopia, a type of blindness. Children who are found to have strabismus need to be referred to an ophthalmologist.

Screen for *nystagmus* by inspecting the movement of the eyes to the six cardinal fields of gaze. It may be necessary to stabilize the child's chin with your hand to prevent the entire head from moving. Both eyes should exhibit coordinated parallel movements in all directions. End-point nystagmus may occur if the eye is held in extreme gaze, and is seen as mild rhythmic twitching with quick movement in the direction of gaze with slow drift in the other direction. Eye movements that are not coordinated or parallel indicate the need for further testing. If one or both eyes fail to follow your hand in any direction or if there are sporadic or nonpurposeful movements, a referral may be needed. Note any pathologic nystagmus, that is, quick movement always in the same direction regardless of the direction of gaze.

Alignment of Eyes

Note whether the outer canthus of the eyes align with the pinna of the ear (Fig. 13-19). If the canthus is higher or lower than the pinna, report as an abnormal finding.

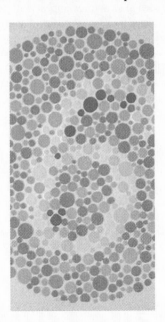

Ishihara's test. *(From Epstein, 1992.)*

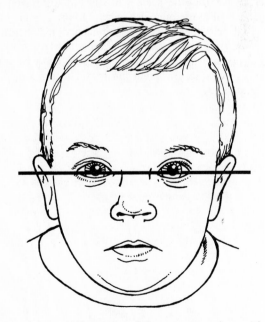

Fig. 13-19 Alignment of the outer canthus with the pinna of the ear is a normal finding.

ADOLESCENTS

■ APPROACH

Overall the examination should be conducted in the same manner as for adults. If client is accompanied by an adult (parent or guardian), allow client to decide whether the adult waits in or outside the exam room during the physical examination.

■ FINDINGS

Eye Strain

Muscle imbalances are common findings of adolescents, as well as eye strain from not wearing prescribed eye glasses for self-esteem or image reasons.

Competitive Sports

Whether an adolescent who has absent or loss of function of one eye can participate in competitive sports should be judged on an individual basis. The American Society for Testing and Materials (ASTM) has approved eye guards for use in competitive sports (Neinstein, 1991.)

OLDER ADULTS

■ APPROACH

Overall the examination should be conducted in the same manner as for younger adults.

■ FINDINGS

Visual Acuity

Central and peripheral vision may be decreased after age 70. Acuity of 20/20 or 20/30 with corrective lenses is common. Accommodation takes longer. Color perception of blue, violet, and green may be impaired.

Eyebrows and Eyelids

Eyebrows may be thin along the outer edge and the remaining brow hair may appear coarse. There may be wrinkles or crow's feet in the skin around the eyes, because the elastic tissues have atrophied. Pseudoptosis, or relaxed upper eyelid, may be seen, with the lid resting on the lashes. Actual ptosis may also occur. Orbital fat may have decreased, so that the eyes appear sunken, or may herniate, causing bulging on the lower lid or inner third of the upper lid. Ectropion, wherein the lower lid drops away from the globe, or entropion, wherein the lower lid turns inward, may be present.

Lacrimal Apparatus

The lacrimal apparatus may function poorly, giving the eye a lack of luster; the client may report a burning sensation or dry eyes.

Sclera and Bulbar Conjunctiva

Sclera are white. Brown spots may appear near the limbus as a normal variation. Bulbar conjunctiva may appear dry, clear, and light pink without discharge or lesions.

Cornea

The cornea is transparent, clear, often yellow; arcus senilis (a gray-white circle around the limbus) is common. Soft, raised yellow plaques (xanthelasma) may be noted on the lids at the inner canthus, but these are of no clinical significance.

Internal Structures of the Eye

Usually the retinal structures appear dull, with pale, attenuated blood vessels. The arterioles display a narrower light reflex and are straighter. More crossing defects are also seen. Benign degenerative hyaline deposits may be noted on the retinal surface (drusen); these do not interfere with vision.

CLIENTS WITH SITUATIONAL VARIATIONS

PREGNANT WOMEN

■ APPROACH

Although the examination should proceed as for other adults, some of the findings of an eye examination in a pregnant woman will differ.

■ FINDINGS

Eyelids darken from melanin pigment. Pale conjunctivae may indicate anemia.

Contact lenses may be uncomfortable to wear due to increased dryness. Both eyesight and the corrective prescription may change as corneal fluid shifts during pregnancy or as the pituitary gland enlarges, compromising visual fields.

Toxemia may cause blurred vision. Chromatopsia may be noted, characterized by unusual color perception, seeing spots, blindness in the lateral eye halves, retinal arteriole constriction, sheen, disk edema, or retinal detachment, which is an emergency.

After delivery, the eyelids lighten and the cornea curves change as fluid levels or the pituitary gland returns to the prepregnant state. Failure to return to the prepregnant state following delivery should be reported.

CLIENTS WITH DECREASED OR ABSENT VISION

■ APPROACH

When performing a physical assessment on a blind person, you must remember to alert the client to all actions *before* you perform them.

■ FINDINGS

The history questions will be revised to delete all those relating to vision and ocular problems. However, questions dealing with pain, swelling, watering, and discharge still are appropriate. Additional questions are needed concerning how the individual has adapted to the loss of sight. The physical examination includes only inspection of the external eye structures as described for the adult.

CLIENTS WITH PROSTHETIC EYE

■ APPROACH

Clients who have had an enucleation of an eye replaced by a prosthesis appear to have binocular vision. The examiner, however, must remember that the clients have no sight on the affected side and must be approached from the sighted side.

■ FINDINGS

Some artificial eyes are permanently implanted. Others are removed for daily cleaning.

CLIENTS WITH SUSPECTED DRUG INTOXICATION

■ APPROACH

The examination should be conducted in the same manner as for adults. Include questions about recent drug use, which drugs, and what dosage.

◼ FINDINGS

When assessing a client whom you suspect is intoxicated, use the Rapid Eye Test in Table 13-1 to collect data to confirm or refute your suspicion. Data from Table 13-2 may help you identify from the client's eye signs which drug(s) may have been abused.

TABLE 13-1	Rapid Eye Test to Detect Current Drug Intoxication

General Observation

Look for redness of sclera, ptosis, retracted upper lid (white sclera visible above iris, causing blank stare), glazing, excessive tearing of eyes, and swelling of eyelids.

Pupil Size

Dilated (>6.5 mm) or constricted (<3.0 mm).

Pupil Reaction to Light

Slow, sluggish, or absent response

Nystagmus

Hold finger in vertical position and have the client follow finger as it is moves to the side, in a circle, and up and down. Positive test is failure to hold gaze or jerkiness of eye movements.

Convergence

Inability to hold the cross-eyed position after an examining finger is moved from one foot away from client's nose and held there for 5 seconds.

Corneal Reflex

Decreased rate of blinking after touching cornea with cotton.

TABLE 13-2	Common Eye Signs Detected after Abuse of Selected Drugs

	MARIJUANA	**HEROIN**	**ALCOHOL**	**COCAINE**	**PCP**
Pupil size	normal	constricted	normal	dilated	normal
Slow or no reaction of pupil to light	yes		yes	yes	yes
Nonconvergence	yes				
Redness of sclera	yes		yes		
Glazing of cornea	yes	yes	yes		
Nystagmus	yes		yes		yes
Swollen eyelids	yes	yes			yes
Watering eyes	yes				
Ptosis		yes			
Decreased corneal reflex		yes		yes	yes

Data from Tennant F: Is your patient abusing drugs? Postgrad Med 84:108–114, 1988.
PCP, Phencyclidine.

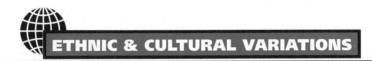

ETHNIC & CULTURAL VARIATIONS

■ **FINDINGS**

The most distinctive ethnic physical variation of the eye is the upward slant and narrowing of the palpebral fissures seen in Asian Americans. This normal feature in Asian Americans is usually indicative of Down syndrome in those of nonAsian descent. Other physical variations include a slight protrusion of the eyeball beyond the supraorbital ridge in African Americans. This should not be mistaken for exophthalmos. Asian American, American Indian and Alaskan Native infants often display a pseudostrabismus as the result of a flattened nasal bridge. This must be distinguished from true strabismus in the assessment process. Skin color also dictates variations in the eye. The sclera is darker in dark-skinned individuals, as are the iris and the fundus of the retina.

It is important to note that many of the minority populations in the United States have a disproportionate incidence of diseases, such as diabetes and hypertension, that place them at increased risk for ocular retinopathies and other complications of the eye. Many of these groups also have a higher incidence of cataract formation.

EXAMINATION SUMMARY
Eyes and Visual System

Test Visual Acuity *(pp. 284-285)*
- Test distant vision using Snellen eye chart or Snellen E chart
- Assess near vision using Jaeger or Rosenbaum card or newspaper
- Assess peripheral visual fields using confrontation test

Inspect Extraocular Muscles *(pp. 286-287)* for movement using:
- Six cardinal fields of gaze
- Corneal light reflex
- Cover-uncover test

Inspect the External Ocular Structures *(pp. 288-292)*
- Inspect eyebrows for:
  Quality
  Hair distribution
  Underlying skin
  Symmetry
- Inspect eyelids and eyelashes for:
  Position
  Symmetry
  Closure
  Blinking patterns
  Discharge
  Color
- Inspect and palpate orbital area for:
  Position
  Indentation
- Inspect lacrimal puncta for:
  Color
  Moisture
  Discharge
  Tenderness
  Nodules
- Inspect conjunctiva and sclera for:
  Color and clarity
  Discharge
  Tenderness
  Pterygium

Crusting
Lesions
Nodules
Foreign bodies
- Inspect cornea for:
  Transparency
  Surface characteristics
- Inspect anterior chamber for:
  Transparency
  Iris surface
  Chamber depth
- Inspect iris for:
  Shape
  Color
- Inspect pupil for:
  Size
  Shape
  Reaction to light and accommodation

Inspect the Internal Ocular Structures *(pp. 292-295)*
- Observe the red reflex
- Inspect optic disc for:
  Margins
  Size and shape
  Color
  Physiologic cup
- Inspect retinal vessels for:
  Color
  Arteriolar light reflex
  Artery-to-vein ratio
  Arteriovenous crossing characteristics
- Inspect retinal background for:
  Color
  Presence of microaneurysms, hemorrhages, exudates
- Inspect macula and fovea centralis for:
  Color
  Surface

COMMON PROBLEMS/CONDITIONS
associated with Eyes and the Visual System

EXTERNAL EYE

■ ***Ectropion:*** An eversion of the lower lid caused by decreased muscle tone (Fig. 13-20). The palpebral conjunctiva is exposed, increasing the risk of conjunctivitis.

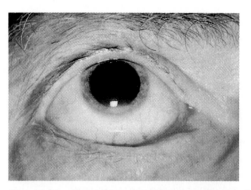

Fig. 13-20   Ectropion. In older persons the lower lid loses its tone and drops away from the globe, particularly on the medial side.   *(From Bedford, 1986.)*

■ ***Exotropion:*** An eversion of the lid and lashes caused by muscle spasms of the eyelid (Fig. 13-21). Friction from lashes may cause corneal irritation.

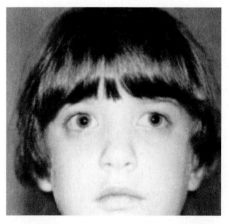

Fig. 13-21   Exotropion. Client has a 30 prism diopter exotropia at distance.   *(From Helveston, 1993.)*

■ ***Enophthalmos:*** Sunken eyes occurring with chronic wasting illnesses such as cachexia (Fig. 13-22).

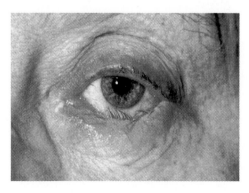

Fig. 13-22   Enophthalmos. The eyelid and lashes are rolled in.   *(From Bedford, 1986.)*

■ **Exophthalmos:** A forward bulging of the eyes associated with hyperthyroidism and caused by deposits of fat and fluid in the retroorbital tissues, forcing the eyeballs forward (Fig. 13-23). Upper eyelids usually are retracted so that when the eye is open, the sclera above the iris is visible. Lids may not close completely.

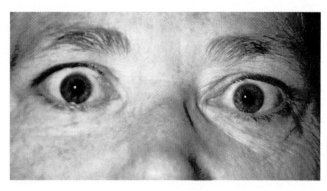

Fig. 13-23 Exophthalmos. Thyrotoxicosis with bilateral symmetric lid retraction, with sclera showing above the iris. *(From Bedford, 1986.)*

■ **Blepharitis:** An inflammation of the lash follicles and meibomian glands cause red, scaly, and crusted lid margins. Chronic blepharitis may be associated with seborrhea or dandruff or may be caused by bacterial infection (Fig. 13-24).

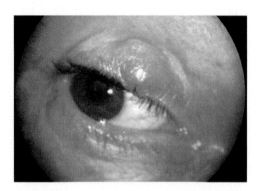

Fig. 13-24 Blepharitis. Swelling of the meibomian glands caused by eruption of sebum outside the walls of the gland. *(From Bedford, 1986.)*

■ **Chalazion:** A firm, nontender nodule of a meibomian gland in the eyelid; often follows hordeolum or chronic inflammation such as conjunctivitis, blepharitis, or meibomian cyst (Fig. 13-25).

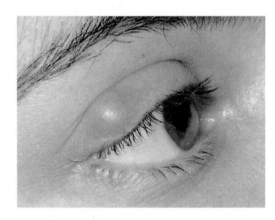

Fig. 13-25 Chalazion (right upper eyelid). *(From Newell, 1992.)*

■ **Hordeolum (sty):** An acute infection of hair follicles of the eyelid, usually caused by *Staphylococcus aureus* (Fig. 13-26). The affected area usually is very painful, red, and edematous.

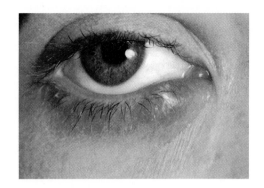

Fig. 13-26 Hordeolum (sty). *(From Bedford, 1986.)*

■ **Ptosis:** Drooping of the eyelid due to paralysis of oculomotor nerve (cranial nerve III) or systemic neuromuscular weakness such as myasthenia gravis (Fig. 13-27).

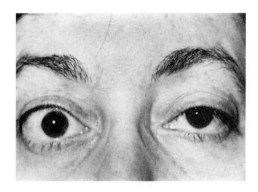

Fig. 13-27 Ptosis. Client with left ptosis and right upper lid retraction. *(From Rocca, Nesi, and Lisman, 1987.)*

■ **Pterygium:** Growth of bulbar conjunctiva toward the center of the cornea (Fig. 13-28). Usually it invades from the nasal side and obstructs vision as it covers the pupil. Occurs usually from chronic exposure to hot, dry, sandy climate.

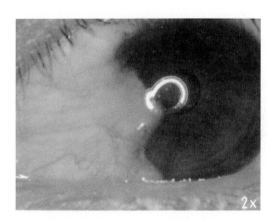

Fig. 13-28 Pterygium. *(From Newell, 1992.)*

■ *Conjunctivitis:* Inflammation of the palpebral or bulbar conjunctiva caused by bacteria, virus, chlamydia, allergic reaction, systemic infections, or chemical irritation (Fig. 13-29).

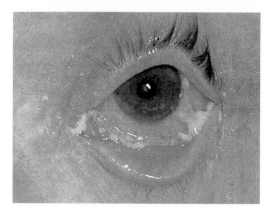

Fig. 13-29 Conjunctivitis (acute). *(From Newell, 1992.)*

■ *Corneal abrasion or ulcer:* Disruptions of the corneal epithelium and stroma caused by viral or bacterial infections or desiccation because of incomplete lid closure or poor lacrimal gland function (Fig. 13-30). Commonly caused by scratches, foreign bodies, or poorly fitted, overworn contact lenses. Client feels intense pain, has a foreign body sensation, and reports photophobia. Tearing and redness are observed.

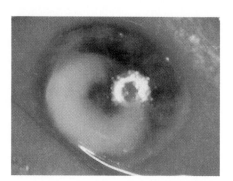

Fig. 13-30 Fungus corneal ulcer. *(From Newell, 1992.)*

■ *Dacryocystitis:* Inflammation of the lacrimal sac; is an infection and blockage of the sac and duct (Fig. 13-31). Pain, warmth, redness, and swelling occur in the inner canthus. Tearing is present and may occur in newborns through older adults. Pressure on the sacs produces purulent discharge from the puncta.

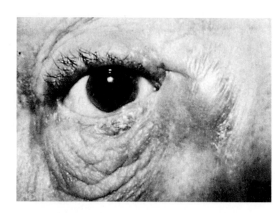

Fig. 13-31 Dacryocystitis. Acute dacryocystitis in right eye of 71-year-old man. *(From Newell, 1992.)*

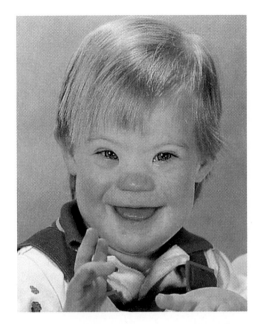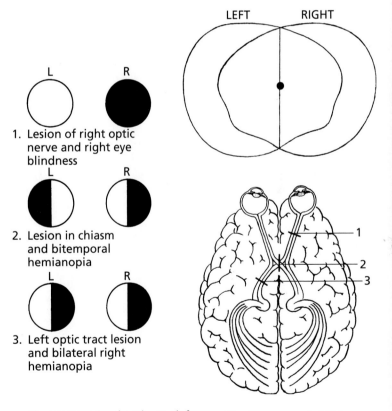

■ *Upper palpebral slant of the eyes:* Seen in children with Down's syndrome, along with epicanthal folds and hypertelorism (Fig. 13-32).

Fig. 13-32 Note upslanting palpebral fissures in child with Down syndrome. *(From Zitelli and Davis, 1992.)*

PERIPHERAL VISUAL DEFECTS

Visual field defects can often be traced to disorders in specific anatomic locations because of the arrangement of nerve fibers (Fig. 13-33). A left or right optic nerve lesion could cause a defect in the corresponding left or right eye. A common chiasm defect is bitemporal hemianopia, which results from a pituitary tumor. A left optic tract lesion would result in a bilateral right visual field defect.

1. Lesion of right optic nerve and right eye blindness

2. Lesion in chiasm and bitemporal hemianopia

3. Left optic tract lesion and bilateral right hemianopia

Fig. 13-33 Visual pathway defects. *(From Thompson et al, 1992.)*

EXTRAOCULAR MUSCLES

■ **Strabismus:** An abnormal ocular alignment in which the visual axes do not meet at the desired point (Fig. 13-34). Nonparalytic strabismus is due to muscle weakness, focusing difficulties, unilateral refractive error, nonfusion, or anatomic differences in eyes. Paralytic strabismus is a motor imbalance caused by paresis or paralysis of an extraocular muscle. Two of the most common types of strabismus are esotropia and exotropia. *Esotropia* is an inward-turning eye and is the most common type of strabismus in infants. *Exotropia* is an outward-turning eye.

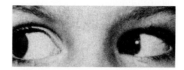
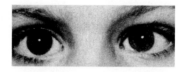
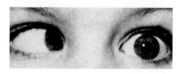

Fig. 13-34 Paralytic strabismus involving left lateral rectus muscle innervated by cranial nerve VI (abducens nerve). *(From von Noorden, 1990.)*

INTERNAL EYE

■ **Pupil abnormalities:** See Table 13-3.

■ **Cataract:** An opacity of the crystalline lens, most commonly from denaturation of lens protein caused by aging (Fig. 13-35). Cataracts due to aging usually are central, but peripheral cataracts are seen in hypoparathyroidism. Congenital cataracts can result from maternal rubella or other fetal insults during the first trimester of pregnancy.

A

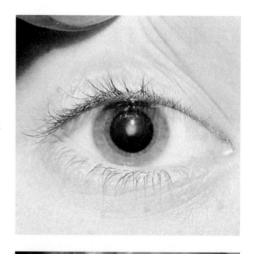

B

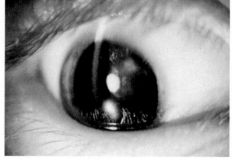

Fig. 13-35 **A,** Anterior polar cataract, a developmental abnormality, which in most cases remains stable and rarely affects vision. **B,** Cataract of galactosemia. Early lens changes in galactosemia are reversible. *(From Zitelli and Davis, 1992.)*

TABLE 13-3	Pupil Abnormalities	

ABNORMALITY	CONTRIBUTING FACTORS	APPEARANCE
Bilateral		
Miosis (pupillary constriction; usually less than 2 mm in diameter)	Iridocyclitis; miotic eye drops (such as pilocarpine given for glaucoma)	
Mydriasis (pupillary dilation; usually more than 6 mm in diameter)	Iridocyclitis; mydriatic or cycloplegic drops (such as atropine); midbrain (reflex arc) lesions or hypoxia; oculomotor (CN III) damage; acute-angle glaucoma (slight dilation)	
Failure to respond (constrict) with increased light stimulus	Iridocyclitis; corneal or lens opacity (light does not reach retina); retinal degeneration; optic nerve (CN II) destruction; midbrain synapses involving afferent pupillary fibers or oculomotor nerve (CN III)(consensual response is also lost); impairment of efferent fibers (parasympathetic) that innervate sphincter pupillae muscle	
Argyll Robertson pupil	Bilateral, miotic, irregular-shaped pupils that fail to constrict with light but retain constriction with convergence; pupils may or may not be equal in size; commonly caused by neurosyphilis or lesions in midbrain where afferent pupillary fibers synapse	
Oval pupil	Sometimes occurs with head injury or intracranial hemorrhage; transitional stage between normal pupil and dilated, fixed pupil with increased intracranial pressure (ICP); in most instances returns to normal when ICP is returned to normal	
Unilateral		
Anisocoria (unequal size of pupils)	Congenital (approximately 20% of normal people have minor or noticeable differences in pupil size, but reflexes are normal) or caused by local eye medications (constrictors or dilators), amblyopia, or unilateral sympathetic or parasympathetic pupillary pathway destruction (NOTE: Examiner should test whether pupils react equally to light; if response is unequal, examiner should note whether larger or smaller pupil reacts more slowly [or not at all], since either pupil could be abnormal size)	Normal eye Affected eye
Iritis constrictive response	Acute uveitis is frequently unilateral; constriction of pupil accompanied by pain and circumcorneal flush (redness)	Normal eye Affected eye

Continued

TABLE 13-3   Pupil Abnormalities—*cont'd*

ABNORMALITY	CONTRIBUTING FACTORS	APPEARANCE
Oculomotor nerve (CN III) damage	Pupil dilated and fixed; eye deviated laterally and downward; ptosis	Normal eye Affected eye
Horner's syndrome	Miotic pupil; ptosis; interruption of sympathetic nerve supply to dilator pupillae muscle; may be caused by goiter, cervical lymph enlargement, apical bronchogenic carcinoma, or surgical injury to neck	Normal eye Affected eye
Adie's pupil (tonic pupil)	Affected pupil dilated and reacts slowly or fails to react to light; response to convergence normal; caused by impairment of postganglionic parasympathetic innervation to sphincter pupillae muscle or ciliary malfunction; often accompanied by diminished tendon reflexes (as with diabetic neuropathy or alcoholism)	

Other Irregularities

Iridectomy	Sector iridectomy	
	Peripheral iridectomy Surgical excision of portion of iris usually done in superior area so upper lid will cover additional exposure	
Coloboma (localized absence of portion of iris)	Congenital absence of area of iris; remaining iris shows normal light response	
Iridodialysis (circumferential tearing of iris from scleral spur)	Blunt trauma; more than one "pupil" in eye can cause diplopia	

From Thompson JM, McFarland GK, Hirsch JE, Tucker SM: Mosby's clinical nursing, *ed 3, St. Louis, 1992, Mosby.*

■ *Diabetic retinopathy:* Visual alterations occurring in diabetics caused by changes in the retinal capillaries (Fig. 13-36). Diabetic retinopathy is divided into background and proliferative. Background retinopathy is marked by dot hemorrhages or microaneurysms and the presence of hard and soft exudates. Hard exudates are thought to result from lipid transudation through incompetent capillaries, have sharply defined borders, and tend to be bright yellow. Soft exudates are caused by infarctions of the nerve layer and appear as dull yellow spots with poorly defined margins.

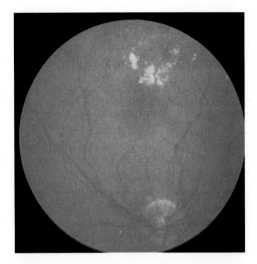

Fig. 13-36 Diabetic retinopathy. The retinal changes are predominantly at the posterior pole with microaneurysms and "dot and blot" hemorrhages, together with hard exudates in the macular area. *(From Bedford, 1986.)*

■ *Diabetic retinopathy (proliferative):* Development of new vessels as a result of anoxic stimulation (Fig. 13-37). New vessels lack support structures of healthy vessels and are more likely to hemorrhage. Bleeding from these vessels is a major cause of blindness in clients with diabetes.

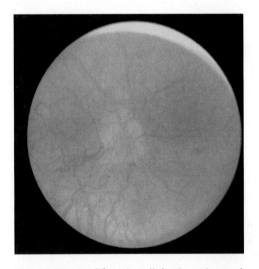

Fig. 13-37 Proliferative diabetic retinopathy. *(From Seidel et al, 1995; courtesy John W. Payne, MD, The Wilmer Ophthalmological Institute, The Johns Hopkins University and Hospital, Baltimore.)*

■ *Cytomegalovirus (CMV) infection:* An increasingly common cause of blindness as the human immunodeficiency virus (HIV) epidemic spreads (Fig. 13-38). It is characterized by hemorrhage, exudates, and necrosis of the retina. CMV infection is said to create a "pizza pie" appearance in the retina.

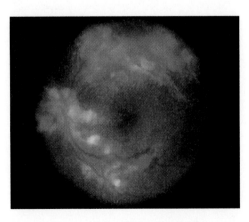

Fig. 13-38 Cytomegalovirus infection. *(From Seidel et al, 1995; courtesy Douglas A. Jabs, MD, The Wilmer Ophthalmological Institute, The Johns Hopkins University and Hospital, Baltimore.)*

■ *Glaucoma:* a condition of increased intraocular pressure caused by obstruction of the outflow of aqueous humor. The increased pressure damages the retina and may cause atrophy of the optic nerve. Vision loss is gradual and painless, with loss of peripheral vision occurring first.

■ *Hypertensive retinopathy:* changes in the retina are classified using the Keith-Wagner-Barker (KWB) system, which evaluates changes in the vascular supply, the retina itself, and the optic disc. These changes occur bilaterally. The normal artery-to-vein ratio (2:3 or 4:5) decreases due to the vascular smooth muscle contraction, hyperplasia, or fibrosis (Fig. 13-39).

- Group I of the KWB classification has arterioles with an increased light reflex. There is moderate arteriolar constriction, but no changes in the arteriovenous crossings.
- Group II has changes in the arteriovenous crossing. Arterioles are reduced to half the usual size, and areas of local vasoconstriction may be noted.
- Group III has shining retina and yellow areas with poorly defined margins (cotton wool spots) that result from ischemic infarcts of the retina.
- Group IV has papilledema, edema of the optic disc (Seidel et al, 1995).

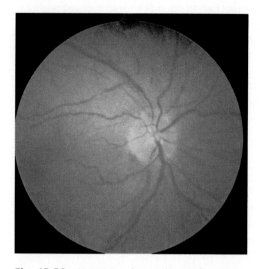

Fig. 13-39 Hypertensive retinopathy. Narrowing of the caliber of the arterioles, and crossing of these arterioles over the veins and a few hemorrhages, can be seen. *(From Bedford, 1986.)*

Sample Documentation & Nursing Diagnosis

Nursing Diagnosis

CASE 1   Mother brings 15-month-old girl to clinic for well-child check-up, immunizations, and "lazy eye."

Subjective

Mother reports, "I brought my daughter for shots and for you to look at her lazy eye." Reports concern about "lazy eye" that drifts when child looks at mother—noticed several months ago; reports no excessive blinking, watering, or discharge from eyes, redness or swelling of eyes, or impaired vision. Reports child is walking, feeding self, scribbling without difficulty. Last physical examination 3 months ago.

Objective

Weight   24 lb (11 kg).

Height   30" (76.2 cm).

Active, alert 15-month-old girl. Extraocular muscles parallel except for inward deviation of left eye (esotropia); no nystagmus; corneal light reflex asymmetric; cover-uncover test revealed left eye moves when uncovered; eyelids and eyelashes symmetric; conjunctiva clear bilaterally; sclera white; corneas clear; lacrimal structures without tearing or redness; pupils equal, round, and react to light (PERRL); red reflex noted bilaterally.

Denver II appropriate for age.

· ·

Nursing Diagnosis #1

Sensory/perceptual alteration (visual) related to lazy eye

Defining Characteristics   Esotropia; asymmetric corneal light reflex; left eye deviation when uncovered.

Nursing Diagnosis #2

Health-seeking behaviors related to expressed desire to ensure health of child

Defining Characteristics   Mother brought child for immunizations.

Sample Documentation

&Nursing Diagnosis

CASE 2   66-year-old man with blurred vision states, "I can't see as well as I used to."

Subjective

Reports gradual changes in vision over past 6 months. Wears glasses for reading; stopped driving at night due to halo around street light blurring vision. Reports no eye pain, discharge, watering from eyes, excessive blinking, redness or swelling of eyes, or trauma to eyes. Last eye exam 3 years ago. Walks dog around block daily for exercise. Usual food intake: breakfast—eggs, bacon, toast, jelly, coffee with milk, juice; lunch—sandwich, chips, soft drink; dinner—at local cafeteria. Lives alone; concerned about who will help him at home. One married daughter in area who just had baby.

Objective

Height   5'11" (180 cm).

Weight   225 lbs (102 kg).

Visual acuity   O.D. 20/40; O.S. 20/40.

Obese, cooperative, reliable.

Brows, lids, lashes evenly distributed; extraocular muscles intact; no lid lag; no nystagmus; visual fields equal to examiner's; no tearing; conjunctiva pink without discharge; pupils round, react to light, and accommodation. Unable to assess red reflex or perform ophthalmic examination due to opacities of lens.

• •

Nursing Diagnosis #1

Sensory/perceptual alteration (visual) related to cataract formation

Defining Characteristics   Halo around lights, blurred vision, decrease in vision, corneal opacities.

Nursing Diagnosis #2

Anxiety related to anticipated need for help with failing vision

Defining Characteristics   Reported concern about caring for self with blurred vision; lives alone.

Nursing Diagnosis #3

Altered nutrition: more than body requirements related to lack of knowledge about nutrition

Defining Characteristics   Diet inconsistent with food pyramid; walks around block for exercise; height 5'11" (180 cm), weight 225 lbs (102 kg).

HEALTH PROMOTION

■ **Children** Vision screening is recommended for all children before entering school, preferably at age 3 or 4 (U.S. Preventive Services Task Force, 1989). Every toddler should be screened for strabismus as part of the routine eye examination during well-child visits (Edelman and Mandle, 1994). After age 8, vision should be fully integrated. Routine vision testing is *not* recommended as a component of the periodic health examination of asymptomatic school children. Secondary visual problems may be the basis for behavioral problems.

■ **Adolescents** Routine vision testing is *not* recommended as a component of the periodic health examination of asymptomatic clients.

Teens who participate in school shop or science labs or in certain sports (racquetball, squash) should wear safety lenses and safety frames approved by the American National Standards Institute. Teens with good vision in only one eye should wear safety lenses and frames to protect the good eye, even if they do not otherwise need to wear glasses (USDHHS, 1994).

■ **Adults** A comprehensive eye examination, including screening for visual acuity and glaucoma, should be performed every 2 years beginning at age 40 in African Americans and at age 60 in all other individuals. Diabetic clients, at any age, should have an annual eye examination by an ophthalmologist (USDHHS, 1994).

Clients who work outside should protect their conjunctiva from excessive exposure to sunlight by wearing sunglasses.

■ **Older adults** The American Ophthalmologist Association recommends that adults over 40 years of age be screened for glaucoma. The U.S. Preventive Services Task Force, however, reports that there is no evidence to suggest a need for a specific testing schedule. The Task Force recommends that clients over 65 years of age be tested periodically for glaucoma by an eye specialist.

??????? STUDY QUESTIONS ???????

1. List and describe the five structures of the external eye.
2. Identify two structures of the eye that serve as protection. How do they perform this function?
3. Describe how eye movement is controlled.
4. Describe how the oculomotor nerve controls pupil constriction and dilation.
5. Discuss how images are received and transformed into vision.
6. Define accommodation.
7. Describe at least one visual characteristic that is different in infants, children, pregnant women, and older adults.
8. What questions would you ask to assess reported eye pain? Redness? Swelling?
9. What are the recommendations for glaucoma testing for adults?
10. List one concern that needs to be addressed when recording history information specific to newborns, children, adolescents, and older adults.
11. What are the three phases of the eye exam?
12. What equipment is needed for an eye examination?
13. Describe the steps in using the Snellen eye chart.
14. What equipment should be used for individuals who cannot read?
15. How should visual fields be tested for near vision? Peripheral vision?
16. What process is used to inspect eye movement in six gaze fields?
17. How is the corneal light test performed? Cover-uncover test?
18. List the findings for which each of the following external ocular structures should be inspected: eyebrows, eyelids, globe, lacrimal puncta, bulbar conjunctiva.
19. List three normal physical variations of the eye that are seen in different ethnic groups.
20. What does the acronym PERRLA mean?
21. How is the test for accommodation completed?
22. Describe the steps in performing an ophthalmoscopic examination.
23. What is the normal color of the optic disc?
24. What is the relationship between the sizes of the arteries and veins of the retina?
25. How would you approach an infant for an eye examination?
26. List the specific age-related responses to visual stimuli that are expected to be seen in infants from birth to 10 months of age.
27. What is the process for testing color vision?
28. Describe specific eye problems that may be present in adolescents.
29. Discuss the specific changes in vision that occur with aging.

30. Match the eye condition with the correct description.

Exotropia	*Eversion of the lower lid*
Exophthalmos	*Inversion of the eyelid*
Ectropion	*Sinking of the orbit*
Enophthalmus	*Bulging of the globe*
Ptosis	*Droopy eyelid*

31. Match the eye condition with the correct description.

Chalazia	*Inflamed lid margins*
Hordeolum	*Nodule of meibomian gland*
Pterygium	*Infection of eyelash follicles*
Blepharitis	*Growth of bulbar conjunctiva*

32. What are the differences and similarities between conjunctivitis and a corneal abrasion?

33. Distinguish between diabetic and hypertensive retinopathy.

34. Discuss the health promotion activities for children, adolescents, adults, and older adults.

35. Describe how to conduct a rapid eye test. What signs would you expect to see in an individual who is intoxicated by alcohol? Cocaine? PCP?

Lungs and Respiratory System

ANATOMY AND PHYSIOLOGY

INTERNAL RESPIRATORY STRUCTURES

The primary purpose of the respiratory system is to supply oxygen to the body cells and rid the cells of excess carbon dioxide. Respiratory functions include the following: ventilation (distribution of air), diffusion and perfusion (movement of oxygen and carbon dioxide across the alveolar-capillary membrane to the blood in the pulmonary capillaries), blood flow (in particular, the transportation of respiratory gases), and the control of breathing.

The actual transfer of oxygen and carbon dioxide between environmental gases and the blood occurs in the alveoli. While these are not directly available for clinical examination, respiratory efficiency is assessable by appraising other structures that support alveolar function, primarily those most directly involved in ventilation. Ventilation is the process that moves air from the outside of the body to the gas-exchange units of the lungs. This process involves both primary and accessory muscles and the lungs, housed in the right and left pleural cavities of the thorax. These two cavities are separated by the mediastinum, containing the heart and other structures that connect the head to the abdomen. The pleural cavities are lined with two types of serous membranes: the parietal and visceral pleurae. The chest wall and diaphragm are protected by the parietal pleura; the outside of the lungs is protected by the visceral pleura. A small amount of lubricating fluid coats the space between the pleurae.

The lungs are not symmetric; the right lung has three lobes, and the left has two. Each lobe has a major, oblique fissure dividing the upper and lower portion; however, the right lung has a lesser horizontal fissure dividing the upper lung into upper and middle lobes. The entire lung parenchyma is encased by an elastic subpleural tissue. Each lung extends anteriorly about 4 cm above the first rib into the base of the adult neck. Posteriorly, the lungs' apices rise to about the level of T1, while the lower borders, on deep inspiration, reach to about T12 and, on expiration, rise to about T9 (Fig. 14-1).

The primary muscles of inspiration are the diaphragm and external intercostal muscles. During inspiration, as the diaphragm contracts and pushes the abdominal contents down, the external intercostal muscles aid in increasing the intrathoracic space. The decrease in intrathoracic pressure causes the lungs to expand and the ribs to flare. Then, with expiration, a relatively passive action, the diaphragm relaxes, expelling the air. The accessory muscles—specifically, the internal intercostals and scalene muscles—are used to facilitate both inspiration and expiration.

During inspiration, as the diaphragm and primary muscles increase the thoracic space, pressure changes cause air to enter the body through a system of connecting flexible tubular structures, beginning with its entrance through the mouth or nose, passing through the respiratory portion of the larynx to reach the trachea, a flexible tube approximately 10 or 11 cm long in the adult. These structures—the nose, pharynx, larynx, and intrathoracic trachea—constitute what is referred to as the *upper airway*. The upper airway has three functions in respiration: to conduct air to the lower airway; to protect the lower airway from foreign matter; and to warm, filter, and humidify this inspired air.

The *lower airway* consists of the trachea proper, the mainstem and segmental bronchi, the subsegmental and terminal bronchioles, and the gas exchange units (alveoli). This lower airway has three functions: to conduct air to the alveoli, to clear the mucociliary structures, and to produce pulmonary surfactant via the type II cells of the alveoli (Fig. 14-2).

The trachea splits into a left and right bronchus at about the level of T4 and T5. This division occurs posteriorly and slightly below the manubriosternal junction anteriorly; the right bronchus is shorter, wider, and more upright than the left one. The bronchi serve two functions: to transport air in and out of the lungs and to filter that air by entrapping foreign particles in mucus, which is swept into the throat by ciliary movement and then expectorated.

The bronchi are further subdivided into increasingly small bronchioles. Each bronchiole opens into an alveolar duct and terminates in multiple alveoli, where the actual gas exchanges occur.

EXTERNAL CHEST

The bulk of the respiratory system is protected by a thoracic cage consisting of, in addition to the muscles just discussed, 12 thoracic vertebrae, 12 pairs of ribs, and the sternum. All the ribs are connected to the thoracic vertebrae posteriorly. The first seven ribs are also connected to the sternum by the costal cartilages. The costal cartilages of the

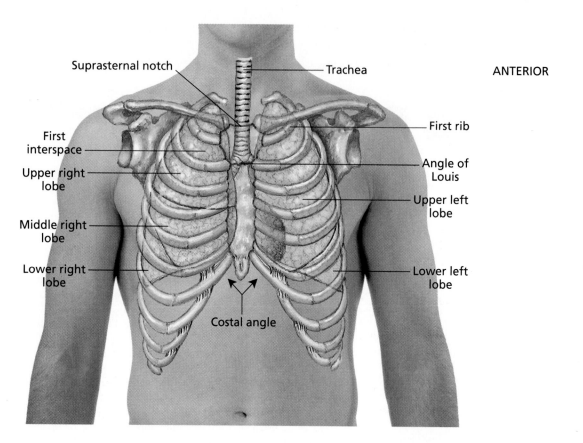

Suprasternal notch

Trachea

ANTERIOR

First rib

First interspace

Upper right lobe

Angle of Louis

Upper left lobe

Middle right lobe

Lower right lobe

Lower left lobe

Costal angle

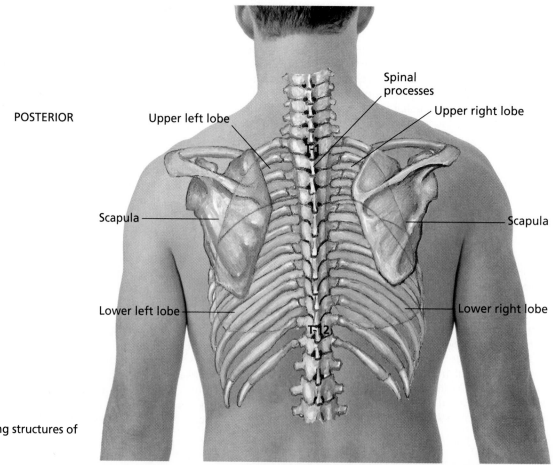

POSTERIOR

Spinal processes

Upper left lobe

Upper right lobe

Scapula

Scapula

Lower left lobe

Lower right lobe

Fig. 14-1   Underlying structures of the thorax.

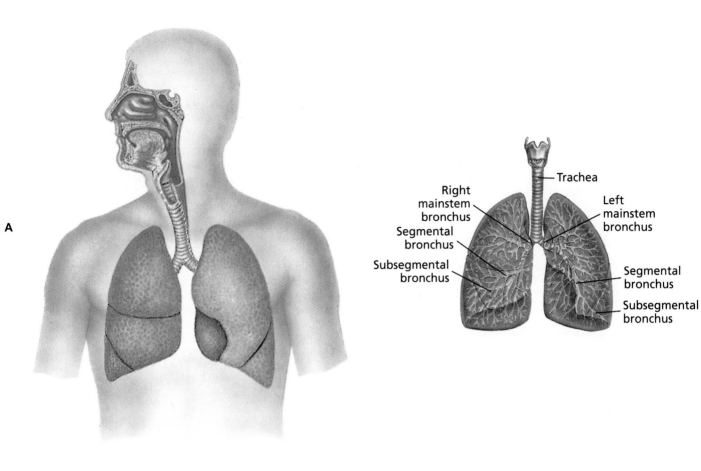

A

B

Trachea

Right
mainstem
bronchus

Left
mainstem
bronchus

Segmental
bronchus

Subsegmental
bronchus

Segmental
bronchus

Subsegmental
bronchus

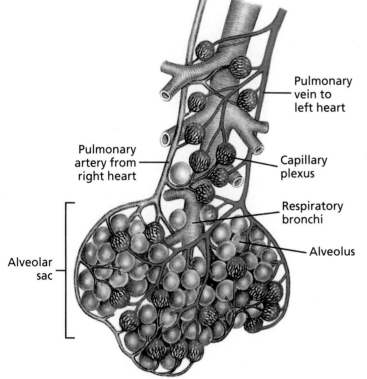

C

Pulmonary
vein to
left heart

Pulmonary
artery from
right heart

Capillary
plexus

Respiratory
bronchi

Alveolus

Alveolar
sac

Fig. 14-2   Airway structures. **A,** Upper and lower airways. **B,** Trachea and lungs. **C,** Structure of an acinus.

eighth to tenth ribs are connected immediately superior to the ribs. The eleventh and twelfth ribs are unattached anteriorly; hence their name, the "floating ribs." The tips of the eleventh ribs are located in the lateral thorax, and those of the twelfth in the posterior thorax (Fig. 14-3, *A* and *B*).

The adult sternum is about 17 cm long and has three components: the manubrium, the body, and the xiphoid process. The first two components articulate with the first seven ribs; the manubrium also supports the clavicle. Only the xiphoid does not articulate with any of these. The intercostal spaces (ICS)—the spaces between the ribs—are each named according to the rib immediately superior to it.

Racial Variation

The size of the thoracic cavity varies by ethnic group. Whites have the largest chest capacity, followed by African Americans, Hispanics, Asian Americans, and American Indians/Alaska Natives. Size has an influence on pulmonary functioning. Those with larger cavities generally have larger air-exchange capacities.

Topographic markers.   The following surface landmarks are helpful in locating underlying structures and in describing the exact location of physical findings (Fig. 14-4).

Anterior chest wall.
- *Nipples.*
- *Manubriosternal junction* (angle of Louis). The junction between the manubrium and sternum; useful for rib identification.
- *Suprasternal notch.* The depression at the ventral aspect of the neck, just above the manubrium.
- *Costal angle.* Intersection of the costal margins, usually no more than 90 degrees.
- *Midsternal line.* Imaginary vertical line through the middle of the sternum.
- *Clavicles.* Bones extending out both sides of the manubrium to the shoulder. They cover the first ribs.
- *Midclavicular lines.* Right and left imaginary lines through the clavicle midpoints, parallel to the midsternal line.

Lateral chest wall.
- *Anterior axillary lines.* Left and right imaginary vertical lines from anterior axillary folds through the anterolateral chest, parallel to midsternal line.

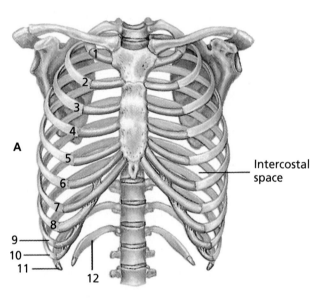

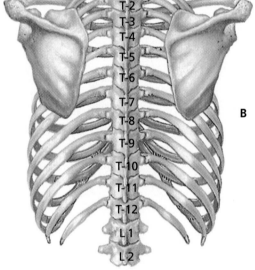

Fig. 14-3   Rib cage. **A,** Anterior view. **B,** Posterior view.

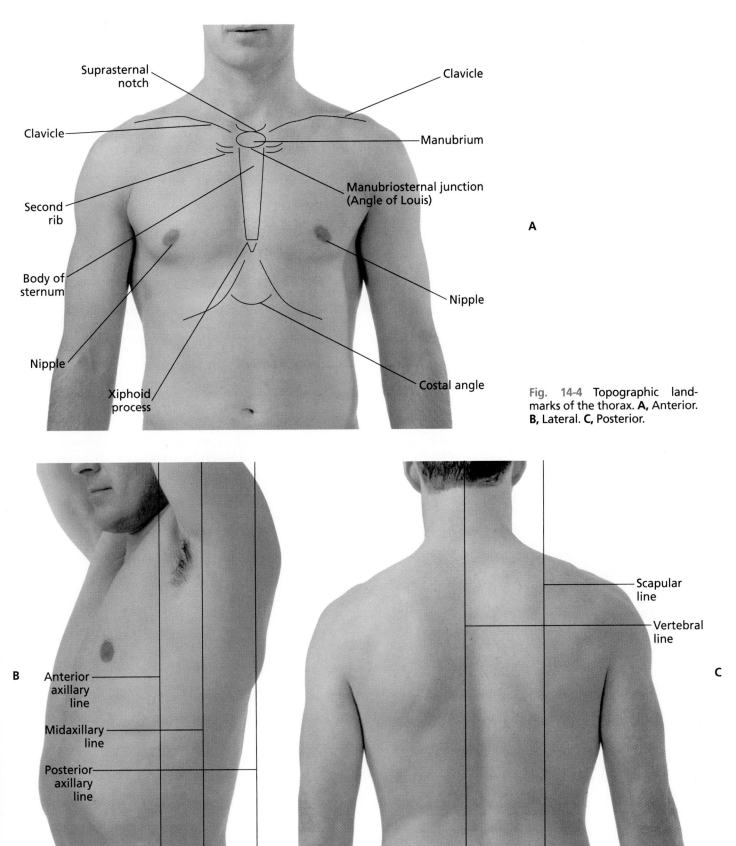

Fig. 14-4 Topographic landmarks of the thorax. **A**, Anterior. **B**, Lateral. **C**, Posterior.

- *Posterior axillary lines.* Left and right vertical imaginary lines from the posterior axillary folds along the posterolateral thoracic wall with abducted lateral arm.
- *Midaxillary lines.* Left and right vertical imaginary lines from axillary apices; midway between and parallel to anterior and posterior axillary lines.

Posterior chest wall.

- *Vertebra prominens.* Spinous process of C7; visible and palpable with the head bent forward; if two palpable prominences are felt, the upper is the spinous process of C7 and the lower is that of T1.
- *Midspinal line.* Imaginary vertical line along the posterior vertebral spinous processes.
- *Scapular lines.* Left and right vertical imaginary lines, parallel to midspinal line; they pass through inferior angles of the scapulae in the upright patient with arms at sides.

DEVELOPMENTAL CONSIDERATIONS

INFANTS

Prenatal. In the fetus, even when the lungs are fully evolved, the alveoli are collapsed, and the lungs contain no air. Throughout gestation, passive respiratory motions do not contribute to respiration; fetal gas exchange is supplied by the placenta. Instead, these passive movements prepare the lungs to respond to chemical and neurologic stimuli during and after the birth process.

Infancy. After birth, once the umbilical cord is cut, the lungs fill with air with a great deal of effort. More changes occur as a result of this first breath; blood flows through the lungs more vigorously, expanding and relaxing pulmonary arteries. The resultant decrease in pulmonary pressure closes the foramen ovale within minutes, increasing oxygen tension in the arterial blood, and thus stimulating the ductus arteriosus to contract and close. These actions help both the pulmonary and systemic circulations to mature and the lungs to become fully integrated and functioning.

CHILDREN

In children, the respiratory rate is much faster than it is in adults. Children use the abdominal muscles to assist with breathing until ages 7 to 8. The chest's bony structure tends to be more prominent as well, largely due to the relatively thinner chest wall. The more cartilaginous structure is more yielding, and the xiphoid process is not only more movable but also often more prominent. By the time the child reaches 8 to 10 years of age, the respiratory rate drops to that of an adult.

PREGNANT WOMEN

Changes in the pregnant woman's respiratory function are due to both mechanical and chemical alterations. First, of course, the enlarged uterus pushes the diaphragm upward, putting pressure on the lungs and causing, in some cases, shortness of breath. As a result, breathing frequently becomes more thoracic than abdominal, and the thoracic cage widens. An increase in the level of progesterone may stimulate an increased tidal volume (deeper inspiration) without necessarily changing respiratory frequency, although many pregnant women experience an increased breathing rate for oxygenation and compensation for structural changes. Pregnant women normally exhibit increased respiratory tract vascularity.

After delivery, the chest wall may remain wider, not returning to its prepregnancy state, although all respiratory characteristics should return to their prepregnancy states.

OLDER ADULTS

With aging, the vital capacity is altered. A loss of muscle strength (particularly tensile muscle) in the thorax and diaphragm, as well as skeletal changes, contribute to the development of a broadened thoracic cavity in many older adults. If an individual has chronic lung disease or emphysema, he or she may develop what is called a "barrel chest." This refers to a condition in which the anterior-posterior (AP) diameter increases demonstrably, emphasizing the dorsal curve of the thoracic spine. Sometimes the chest wall may also exhibit a stiffening and may have decreased expansion. This may be due to calcification at rib articulation points.

As the alveoli become less elastic and more fibrous, there is some loss of interalveolar folds, decreasing the amount of alveolar surface available for gas exchange. As a result, breathing on exertion becomes more difficult; exceeding a tolerant level of exertion may result in dyspnea. Also, with age, mucous membranes become drier and less able to clear retained mucus; this predisposes the older adult to bacterial growth and respiratory infection.

HEALTH HISTORY Lungs and Respiratory System

The history related to the lungs and respiratory system focuses on the problems of coughing, shortness of breath, other breathing problems, chest pain, substance use such as cigarette or pipe smoking, and possible environmental exposure to harmful agents. Assessment of self-care behaviors should also be determined at this time.

QUESTIONS

RATIONALE

BREATHING AND RESPIRATORY PROBLEMS

COUGH

■ Do you have a cough? If so, how long have you had it? Did it begin suddenly or gradually? When do you cough the most? Does the cough awaken you at night?

Some conditions are characterized by a specific onset of coughing or are associated with a specific time during the day or night. Coughs associated with acute illnesses usually continue throughout the day; those caused by environmental exposures to irritants usually occur at times in relation to the exposure to the irritant; and post-nasal drip or sinusitis coughing occurs at night when the individual lies down.

■ How would you describe your cough—Dry? Moist? Wet? Hacking? Hoarse? Barking? Whooping? Bubbling? Productive? Nonproductive?

Certain types of coughs are associated more commonly with certain conditions; for example, mycoplasma pneumonia causes a hacking cough; croup causes a barking cough; colds, pneumonia, and bronchitis cause a congested cough; and early congestive heart failure causes a dry cough.

■ Do you cough up phlegm or sputum? If so, what color is it? Does it have a foul odor? Do you cough up blood? Does it look like streaks or just blood? If so, is it bright red or a dark red-purple color? If you are coughing up sputum, is it all of the time or just periodically? How long has this been going on? Is it related to any activity or exposure that you are aware of? If so, what? Has it changed over time? If so, how?

Some conditions have characteristic sputum production, such as the following:
White or clear mucus—*colds, viral infections, or bronchitis*
Yellow or green material—*bacterial infections*
Rust-colored material—*tuberculosis, pneumococcal pneumonia, or perhaps blood*
Bright red or dark purple—*blood (hemoptysis)*
Pink frothy sputum associated with dyspnea—*pulmonary edema; some medications may cause the sputum to be a pink-tinged color.*

QUESTIONS

- Have you noticed any other symptoms along with the cough, such as shortness of breath, chest pain or tightness with breathing, fever, stuffy nose, noisy respiration, hoarseness, gagging, or stress? Does activity make it worse? Does the cough tire you out? Does it keep you awake at night?

- Do you have allergies? If so, what type? For how long? What are your symptoms usually like? Is there a history of allergies in your family? Do you smoke tobacco, or are you often exposed to the smoke of others who smoke in your home or environment?

- How do you treat the cough? Over-the-counter medications? Vaporizer? Prescribed medications? How effective are these measures?

SHORTNESS OF BREATH

- Have you ever noticed shortness of breath or times when it was hard to breathe? Does anything seem to trigger these episodes? Do you become short of breath with activity or exercise? If so, how long has this been going on? How severe is the shortness of breath? How long does it last?

- Do you experience shortness of breath at a certain time of day or night? How does changing your position affect the problem? Does the shortness of breath interfere with your activities? Is it harder to inhale or exhale or are both equally affected? Do the episodes appear to be related to certain foods, pollen or dust, animals, seasons, or emotions?

- Do you experience any other problems when you are short of breath? Night sweats? Cough? Chest pain? Bluish color around the lips or nails? Do your ankles swell?

RATIONALE

Associated signs and symptoms are important factors to assess when trying to determine the underlying cause of the cough. For example, a cough associated with a fever, shortness of breath, and noisy breath sounds may be indicative of a lung infection, whereas tightness of the chest associated with shortness of breath and a nonproductive cough is more likely to be associated with a problem such as asthma or bronchitis.

Allergies are sensitivities to certain substances or types of substances. Their presence may produce irritated tissues that are more prone to cough. Some allergies tend to be inherited. It is useful to have an index of how the client views the cough, with anxiety a possible contributing factor to cough.

It is important to determine the current treatment and the effectiveness of such treatments.

The exact causative factors should be determined, meaning exactly how much exercise brings on the episode (number of steps climbed, blocks walked, etc.).

Knowing the exact timing and places where shortness of breath occurs helps in determining cause and, hopefully, preventive strategies.

- *Paroxysmal nocturnal dyspnea is shortness of breath that awakens the individual in the middle of the night. Comfort is usually achieved by sitting up.*

- *Asthma attacks are triggered by a specific allergen. This may be external to the individual (extrinsic), such as a pet, or internal (intrinsic), such as stress or emotions.*

Shortness of breath may be simply a problem of the respiratory system, or it may be a symptom associated with the cardiovascular system, such as congestive heart failure or a severe heart murmur.

<table>
<tr><td>

QUESTIONS

■ What do you do when you experience shortness of breath? What relieves the symptoms?
- Special positioning, using multiple pillows? If so, how many pillows do you use, or what position do you sleep in? Do you sleep in a recliner?
- Taking medication? Using oxygen or an inhaler? Describe what, how much, and how often.

■ Do you think the shortness of breath is getting better or worse?

CHEST PAIN WITH BREATHING

■ Have you had pain in your chest when you breathe? If so, indicate the exact area where you feel the pain. What does the pain feel like? Viselike, tight, sharp, burning, etc? How long have you had pain? Did it start suddenly or gradually? Is the pain constant or does it come and go? When it started, was it associated with an injury or a respiratory infection (cold, virus, or otherwise)? Is your pain worse with deep inspiration?

■ Does the pain interfere with you getting enough breath? Does the pain radiate to other areas, such as the neck or arms?

■ Have you had a recent fall or injury to your ribs? If so, describe.

■ What have you done to treat the pain? Heat? Splinting? Pain medication? Do these things help?

DIAGNOSED RESPIRATORY CONDITIONS

■ Have you been diagnosed as having a respiratory disease such as asthma, bronchitis, bronchiectasis, emphysema, cystic fibrosis, lung cancer, or tuberculosis? If so, please describe. Is there a family history of any of these conditions?

■ Have you ever had a lung or breathing evaluation, such as pulmonary function tests, TB tests, fungal skin tests, chest x-ray, and allergy testing? If so, when were they and what were the results?

■ Have you ever had injury to your chest wall? Broken ribs? A collapsed lung? Lung or thoracic surgery? If yes to any of these, please describe why and when. Also, please describe any breathing problems you have had.

PERSONAL AND ENVIRONMENTAL EXPOSURE TO RESPIRATORY IRRITANTS

SMOKING/TOBACCO

■ Do you smoke? Do you smoke cigarettes, pipe, or cigars? Do you use smokeless tobacco? How many packs or how much tobacco do you use each day? How long have you been smoking or using tobacco this much each day? When did you start smoking or using tobacco? How old were you?

</td><td>

RATILONALE

◀ *Orthopnea is difficulty breathing when the individual is lying down. Clients may describe using several pillows to "prop" themselves up in bed so that they can sleep. If 2 pillows are used, it is called "2-pillow orthopnea," if 3 pillows it is "3-pillow orthopnea," etc.*

◀ *Assess the efficacy of treatment and any progression the client has noted.*

◀ *Pain with deep breathing may be an indication of pleural lining irritation.*

◀ *Even though the pain is associated with breathing, it is important to evaluate the possibility of the pain being related to a cardiovascular problem.*

◀ *Injured ribs will not only cause pain when the individual breaths but also, because of the pain, the client is likely to breathe more shallowly, which may lead to respiratory congestion.*

◀ *Assess self-care behaviors and successful relief of pain.*

◀ *Other respiratory tract problems should be evaluated. Family history may be used to determine risk for the client.*

◀ *All are objective evaluation measures that may be used as baseline information or used to confirm a diagnosis.*

◀ *The incidence of surgery or injury may provide additional information about a possible respiratory or lung problem.*

◀ *Tobacco, both smoked and smokeless, is a known respiratory irritant that may lead to respiratory compromise and disease, including such problems as chronic bronchitis, emphysema, chronic obstructive lung disease, and cancer.*

</td></tr>
</table>

QUESTIONS

RATIONALE

 Cultural Note

Cultural differences have been identified in smoking habits of individuals in the United States. For example, a greater number of African-American and Hispanic males smoke than white males. Other ethnic groups generally smoke less than whites and women smoke less than men.

■ Have you ever tried to quit smoking or using tobacco? What helped you? Why do you think your attempt was not successful? What activities do you normally associate with smoking?

Assess self-care behaviors and level of awareness or risk. Evaluate patterns of smoking behavior to form the basis for a smoking cessation program should the client desire to quit.

HOME ENVIRONMENT

■ Are you exposed to the smoke of others in your home? If so, does their smoke seem to be an irritant to you?
■ The following items may cause respiratory irritation. Describe how each of these affect you and your breathing:
  • House location.
  • Possible allergens in home, such as pets.
  • Type of heating and or air conditioning, including filtering system, humidification, and ventilation.
  • Hobbies: woodworking, plants, animals, metal work.

OCCUPATIONAL ENVIRONMENT

■ Are there environmental conditions that may affect your breathing where you work? What are they? Where do you work? In a factory? Outdoors? In a mine? In a chemical plant? On a farm? In heavy traffic?
■ Are you frequently exposed to dust? Vapors? Chemicals? Paint fumes? Irritants such as asbestos? Known allergens?
■ If you are exposed to respiratory irritants, do you wear a mask or a respirator mask? Does your work area have a special ventilatory system to clear out pollutants? Do you wear a monitor to evaluate exposure? Do you have periodic health examinations, pulmonary function tests, or x-ray examinations?

Both the home and the work environment are common places for exposure to respiratory irritants that may cause temporary or permanent lung damage. The client may not be able to alter the presence of environmental irritants that are in the work environment. Instead, he or she must use masks, respirators, ventilation hoods, etc. to reduce the amount of exposure to respiratory irritants. Regulatory agencies such as the Occupational Safety Health Administration (OSHA) have developed guidelines and regulations to reduce the amount of occupational exposure to respiratory irritants.

TRAVEL

■ Have you recently traveled to countries or areas of the United States where you may have been exposed to uncommon respiratory diseases (e.g., histoplasmosis in the southeast and midwest United States; schistosomiasis in Southwest Asia, the Caribbean, and Asia)?

Often, travel to areas of the country or world where the individual is exposed to unusual infections that he or she has little or no resistance to will increase that person's susceptibility to infection.

INFANTS

The major areas to be evaluated with infants are prematurity, low birth weight, coughing or difficulty breathing, frequent colds, difficulty feeding, and apnea. Questions that should be asked include the following:

■ Was the infant premature? What was his or her birth weight? Was the infant ever in the newborn intensive care unit? Was ventilation assistance needed? If so, for how long? Were you ever told that the baby had a breathing problem or respiratory distress syndrome?

Low birth weight and prematurity are risk factors for respiratory difficulties.

QUESTIONS

RATIONALE

 Racial Variation

African-American fetuses reach lung maturity about 1 week sooner (34 weeks) than white fetuses (35 weeks), thus decreasing the incidence of respiratory distress syndrome in premature African-American infants.

■ Does the child have a cough? Does he or she seem congested? Is the breathing noisy, or is there any wheezing or obvious breathing difficulty?

It is important to determine baseline and screening information about the child's current breathing difficulties and the possibility of a respiratory problem. It may be considered normal for young children to have four to six upper respiratory infections (URIs) a year.

■ Does the baby ever have spells when he or she breathes and then does not breathe for a while? Do you use an apnea monitor?

Periods of apnea are most likely to occur if the infant is premature. Newborn apnea is usually identified while the infant is in the nursery, but if it is not, it is important to continue to assess if the child is having apnea now. Unidentified apnea can lead to infant death.

■ Is the baby being breast-fed or bottle-fed? Have you noticed any breathing difficulty with feeding, such as increased perspiration, cyanosis, tiring quickly, or disinterest in feeding?

■ Does the baby ever have choking spells or seem to spit up a lot? Has the child had recurrent episodes of lung infections such as pneumonia?

Recurrent choking or infection may be an indication of possible gastroesophageal reflux.

■ How have you child-proofed your house and yard against things that the child could choke on?

Assess safety and emergency first aid knowledge. Determine whether the parent protects the child by keeping small items out of reach. Suffocation is the leading cause of unintentional childhood death under the age of one year.

■ Do you know what emergency measures to take if the infant inhales or chokes on a toy, food product, or other household object? Have you ever been taught rescue breathing or the Heimlich maneuver?

Evaluate the awareness of the parent or caregiver with regard to rescue breathing and first aid measures.

CHILDREN AND ADOLESCENTS

YOUNG CHILD

In addition to the questions and areas addressed above, young children are at great risk of unintentional drowning, aspiration, or poisoning; thus safety is an important concern. Questions that address this area include:

■ Does the child frequently eat foods such as peanuts, popcorn, hot dogs, raw carrots, and peas? If so, does he or she eat them when sitting to eat or when playing? If hot dogs are eaten, are they cut into very small pieces? Has the child ever choked on any food?

Choking is a common problem with food substances, especially when the child is permitted to be up and playing while also eating.

QUESTIONS

■ Does the child know how to swim? Do you have a swimming pool? Does the child ever play unsupervised around or near water (including the bathtub)?

■ Does the child have recurrent respiratory infections, allergies, or breathing problems? If so, how often do the problems occur? How long does it usually last? What are the precipitating factors? Current medications? Effects of activities, including outdoor playing and sports?

■ *Ask child:* What do you understand about your breathing problem? How do you feel about having to take the treatments or medications that you have to take? How does all of this affect your ability to do what you want to do with your friends?

OLDER CHILD AND ADOLESCENT

In addition to all previously discussed areas of health history questioning, it is important to specifically inquire about risk-taking behaviors that have direct effects on the respiratory system. Specifically, this behavior includes smoking and inhaling toxic substances such as glue, hair spray, spray paint, or lighter fluid fumes.

■ Have you ever smoked a cigarette or chewed tobacco? If so, have you done it in the past week? How often and how much do you smoke or chew? How old were you when you started smoking or using tobacco? Have you tried to quit? Do you want to quit? What makes it difficult for you to quit?

■ Do you sniff glue or inhale any other volatile substances? If so, have you done it in the past week? How often and how much do you inhale the substance? Does it make you sick? How old were you when you started inhaling? Have you tried to quit? Do you want to quit? What makes it difficult for you to quit?

OLDER ADULTS

The general health of older adults should be noted, as well as any lifestyle changes made in response to respiratory symptoms. Questions that should be asked in addition to those for adults include the following:

■ Do you have frequent respiratory infections? Do you get a flu shot every year? Do you get a shot to prevent you from getting pneumonia? Do you notice any breathing problems related to the effects of weather?

■ How much activity do you usually engage in each day or each week? Have you noticed any fatigue or shortness of breath while following your daily routine?

RATIONALE

◀ *Water and swimming pools are hazardous for all unsupervised children whether they can swim or not. Drowning is the third leading cause of unintentional childhood death (Children's Safety Network, 1994).*

◀ *Children with asthma, bronchitis, or other chronic conditions such as cystic fibrosis should be questioned about the overall progress of their disease and how they are coping with it.*

◀ *Many times how the child feels about the breathing problem determines the actual sequelae of the respiratory problem.*

◀ *Public health authorities report that childhood and adolescent smoking is on the rise and that, for those children who do smoke, many smoked their first cigarette before 10 years of age.*

◀ *Likewise, the prevalence of toxic fume inhalation by school-age children and adolescents is also a common, serious, and sometimes deadly problem.*

◀ *Assess the client's level of self-care, as well as his or her exposure to respiratory pathogens.*

◀ *Older adults may have a reduced ability to exercise because pulmonary function tends to decrease with age. Specific changes that may occur include reduced vital capacity and diminished surface area for gas exchange. Sedentary or bedridden clients are at increased risk for respiratory dysfunction.*

QUESTIONS

■ Have you been diagnosed as having any type of respiratory problem, including asthma, chronic obstructive pulmonary disease, lung cancer, or tuberculosis? If you have, has the disease been bothering you lately? Have you gained or lost weight over the last few months? If so, how much?

■ Does it seem to be harder to breathe than it used to be? Do you feel that you cannot breathe as deeply as you used to?

■ Have you noticed sweating at night? Have you had a low-grade fever periodically? Do you feel any sensations in the chest other than pain—perhaps a feeling of heaviness?

RATIONALE

◄ *Baseline information and coping skills are important to assess.*

◄ *A decrease in weight without an adjustment of caloric intake may be a sign of cancer. An increase in weight may be a sign of congestive heart failure.*

◄ *Decreased elastic lung recoil, increased residual volume, and decreased vital capacity are common among older adults.*

◄ *The incidence of chronic respiratory disease is higher in older adults, and these questions make note of symptoms of respiratory disorders.*

EXAMINATION Procedures and Findings

Guidelines **To adequately assess the lungs and respiratory status, the client should be either undressed to the waist or wearing a gown that opens in the back. If the client is undressed to the waist, which is desirable, provide the client with a drape to use as a cover when full exposure is not necessary. Position the client in a sitting position on the side of the examination table.**

EQUIPMENT   **Stethoscope (for infants and young children, use a stethoscope that has a small diaphragm)**
Ruler and tape measure, marked in centimeters
Marking pen

TECHNIQUES and NORMAL FINDINGS

ABNORMAL FINDINGS

Examination of the lungs and respiratory system include the four techniques of inspection, palpation, percussion, and auscultation.

GENERAL PRESENTATION

With the client sitting on the edge of the examination table, perform a general inspection of the anterior and posterior chest.

■ An appearance of apprehension with restlessness, a forward-leaning posture, possible nasal flaring, supraclavicular or intercostal retractions or bulging with expiration, or use of accessory muscles during breathing are all signs of respiratory compromise and distress.

INSPECT the client for General Appearance, Posturing, Breathing Effort, and Trachea Position. The client's general appearance and posturing should be relaxed. The posturing should be upright. Breathing should occur with no effort and at a rate that is appropriate for the client's age.

Inspect the trachea for position. It should be midline in the neck.

■ Tracheal deviation to one side or the other may indicate atelectasis, partial or complete pneumothorax, or pulmonary fibrosis.

CHEST WALL CONFIGURATION

INSPECT the chest wall for Form and Symmetry, Muscle Development, Anterior:Posterior (AP) Diameter, and Costal Angle. The thorax should be symmetric, in an elliptical form, with ribs sloping down at about 45 degrees relative to the spine. Muscle development should be equal. The spinous processes should appear in a straight line. The scapulae should be symmetric in each hemithorax. Anteriorly the costal angle should be less than 90 degrees. Note the underlying fat and relative prominence of the ribs (Fig. 14-5).

■ Asymmetry or unequal muscle development is abnormal. Skeletal deformities such as scoliosis or kyphosis may limit the expansion of the chest.

TECHNIQUES and NORMAL FINDINGS

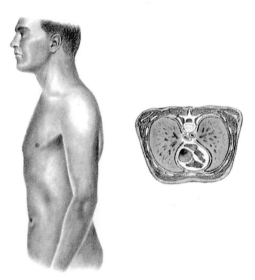

Fig. 14-5   Normal chest of healthy man. Note AP-to-transverse ratio.

ABNORMAL FINDINGS

■ In chronic lung hyperinflation conditions such as chronic emphysema, the chest wall may have a *barrel chest* appearance (Fig. 14-6). In this situation, the ribs are more horizontal and the chest looks like it is held in constant inspiration. The costal angle is greater than 90 degrees.

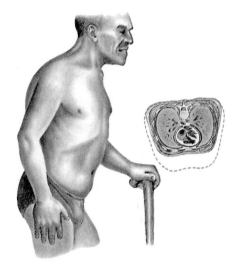

Fig. 14-6   Barrel chest with increased AP diameter.

■ Other chest wall skeletal deformities include pectus carinatum (Fig. 14-7) and pectus excavatum (Fig. 14-8).

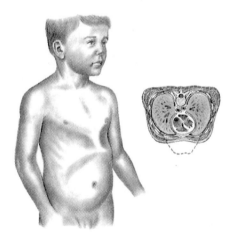

Fig. 14-7   Pectus carinatum, or pigeon chest. Note prominent sternum.

TECHNIQUES and NORMAL FINDINGS

ABNORMAL FINDINGS

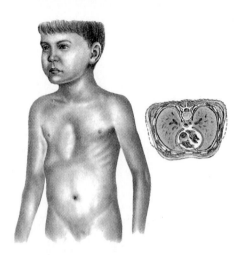

Fig. 14-8 Pectus excavatum, or funnel chest. Note sternum is indented above xiphoid.

GENERAL OXYGENATION

To evaluate client's oxygenation:

INSPECT the client's nails, skin, and lips for Color. Note any cyanosis or pallor (see Chapters 8 and 15 for details). If there is any question about adequate oxygenation, measure the client's oxygen saturation level using pulse oximetry (see Chapter 5).

■ Cyanosis or pallor of the nails, skin, or lips may be a sign of an underlying respiratory or cardiovascular condition.

RESPIRATORY EFFORT

OBSERVE and EVALUATE respirations for Rate and Quality, Breathing Pattern, and Chest Expansion. Note the respiratory rate. In men this is generally more diaphragmatic or abdominal, and in women more thoracic. Breathing should be smooth and even. In the adult, passive breathing should occur at a rate of 12 to 20 breaths per minute. The ratio of respirations to pulse rate should be 1:4.

Evaluate the rhythm or pattern of breathing. The chest wall should symmetrically rise and expand and then relax. It should appear easy and without effort. There should be no bulging or retractions observed (Fig. 14-9).

■ Abnormal breathing rates include:
  ■ *Tachypnea:* A persistent respiratory rate greater than 20 breaths per minute.
  ■ *Bradypnea:* A persistent respiratory rate slower than 12 breaths per minute.
■ Abnormal breathing patterns include:
  ■ *Hyperventilation:* Breathing is rapid and shallow. This may occur secondary to anxiety or exercise or a metabolic disease.
  ■ *Kussmaul Breathing:* Breathing appears very deep, rapid, and laborious. This type of breathing may be associated with metabolic acidosis.
  ■ *Hypoventilation:* Breathing is very shallow. This may be seen in clients with broken ribs or pleuritic pain where inspiration is painful.

| **TECHNIQUES and NORMAL FINDINGS** | **ABNORMAL FINDINGS** |

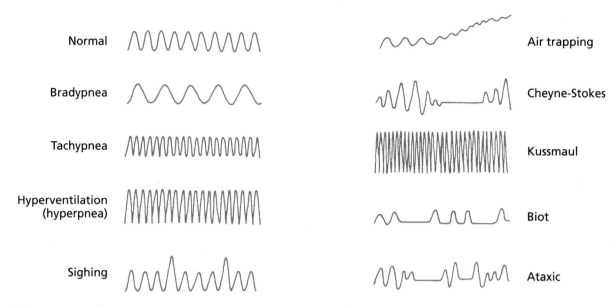

Normal

Bradypnea

Tachypnea

Hyperventilation (hyperpnea)

Sighing

Air trapping

Cheyne-Stokes

Kussmaul

Biot

Ataxic

Fig. 14-9 Patterns of respiration. In certain circumstances, some of these patterns may be abnormal.

Evaluate for symmetric expansion of the chest. Warm your hands and place them on the posterolateral chest wall with your thumbs at the level of T9 or T10. Slide your hands toward the midline, pushing up a small fold of skin between your thumbs. Have the client take a deep breath. As he or she inhales deeply, your thumbs should move apart symmetrically.

ANTERIOR AND POSTERIOR CHEST ASSESSMENT

PALPATE the trachea for Position. It should be palpable just below the thyroid. The trachea should be midline and slightly moveable (Fig. 14-10).

■ If the trachea is not midline, it may be an indication of some degree of lung collapse.

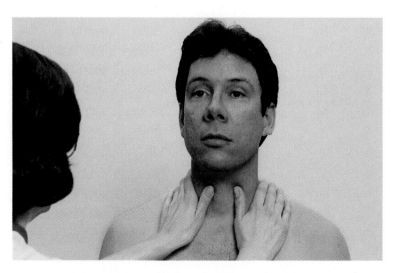

Fig. 14-10 Palpating to evaluate midline position of trachea.

TECHNIQUES and NORMAL FINDINGS

ABNORMAL FINDINGS

PALPATE the chest wall for Symmetry. With the palmar surface of your fingers, use both hands simultaneously to compare the two sides of the posterior chest wall. The skin should be smooth and warm and the spine should be straight and nontender from C7 through T12.

The scapulae should be symmetric and the surrounding musculature well developed. The posterior ribs should be stable and nontender.

Repeat the palpation techniques on the anterior chest. The skin should be smooth, and the rib cage should be symmetric and firm. The sternum and xiphoid should be relatively inflexible.

PALPATE the chest wall for Thoracic Expansion. During respiration place both thumbs at about the tenth rib along the spinal process. While maintaining the thumb position, extend the fingers of both hands outward over the posterior chest wall (Fig. 14-11). Instruct the client to take a deep breath. Observe for bilateral outward movement of your thumbs during the client's inspiration. Both thumbs should move symmetrically. A unilateral or unequal movement of your thumbs should be considered abnormal.

■ Note any *crepitus,* which feels like a crinkly or crackly sensation under your fingers. This abnormal finding indicates air in the subcutaneous tissue. The air has escaped from somewhere in the respiratory tree.

■ *Pleural friction rub* may be felt as a coarse grating sensation during inspiration. It occurs secondary to inflammation of the pleural surface.

■ Note any curvature of the spine, scoliosis, or kyphosis (see Chapter 21 for details of assessment).

■ Muscular development that is asymmetric or an unstable chest wall may indicate a thoracic disorder. Note areas that are tender, where there are masses, or where you note crepitus. These should be evaluated further.

■ Asymmetry of expansion is abnormal. Note if there is any lag between the movement of your thumbs. Unequal chest expansion can accompany atelectasis, pneumonia, traumatic injury such as fractured ribs, or pneumothorax. Pain is noted when there is inflammation of the pleurae.

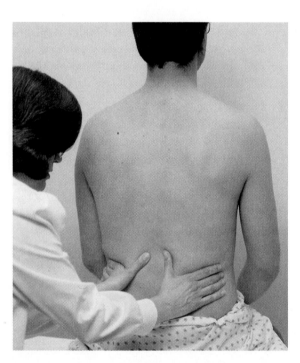

Fig. 14-11   Assessment of posterior thoracic expansion.

TECHNIQUES and NORMAL FINDINGS

PALPATE the chest wall for Vocal (Tactile) Fremitus. (Fremitus is a palpable vibration.) Using the palmar or ulnar surface of your hands, systematically position your hands over both sides of the right and left lung fields and instruct the client to recite "*One, two, three*" or "*99*" while you systematically palpate the chest wall from apices to bases (Fig. 14-12).

Although the quality of the vibrations may vary from person to person because of chest wall density and relative location of the bronchi to the chest wall, the fremitus should feel bilaterally equal.

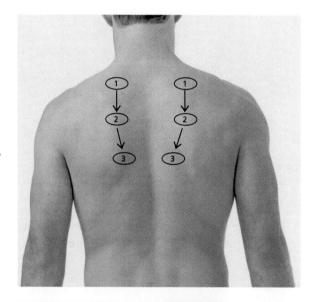

A

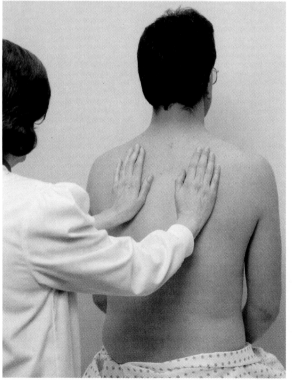

B

Fig. 14-12 Assessing for vocal (tactile) fremitus. **A,** Hand positions for assessment. **B,** Position hands over both lung fields.

ABNORMAL FINDINGS

- *Decreased* or *absent fremitus* occurs any time there is an obstruction to the transmission of vibrations. It often occurs with emphysema, pleural thickening or effusion, massive pulmonary edema, or bronchial obstruction.
- *Increased fremitus* occurs when lung tissue is compressed or consolidated, as in lobar pneumonia.
- *Rhonchal fremitus* is palpable when bronchial secretions are thick.
- *Pleural friction fremitus* or *palpable friction rub* occurs when there is inflammation of either the parietal or visceral pleurae, causing a decrease in normal lubrication. Thus a grating feeling may be palpated. (Although pleural friction rub is most easily identified by auscultation if it is severe enough, it may be identified through palpation.)

PERCUSS the thorax for Tone and Respiratory Excursion. *Percussion* is the tapping of an object to set the underlying structures in motion and thus produce a sound. If performed correctly, it will penetrate to a depth of 5 to 7 cm into the chest. If necessary, review the techniques of performing percussion in Chapter 6. **Tone.** Systematically percuss first the posterior and then the anterior chest wall. Start posteriorly above the scapula and end at the bottom of the rib area (Fig. 14-13). Percuss down the posterior chest from side to side, comparing the two sides. Do not percuss over bone surfaces (Fig. 14-14). The sound should be resonance, which is loud in intensity, low in pitch, long in duration, and hollow in quality (Table 14-1). Move to the anterior chest, instruct the client to pull the shoulders back, and repeat the percussion techniques.

■ *Hyperresonance* is heard when there is overinflation of the lungs. It has a very loud resonance of low pitch that lasts longer than normal and seems "booming." This may be found in individuals with emphysema. *Dull tones* may be heard in clients with pneumonia, pleural effusion, or atelectasis.

> **Clinical Notes**
>
> Anterior chest percussion is not done often because of breast tissue and the position of the heart.

Diaphragmatic (respiratory) excursion. The diaphragm is normally located at approximately the level of the tenth rib posteriorly. The diaphragm is usually slightly higher on the right side because of the location of the liver.

If the client has shallow or painful breathing, respiratory excursion should be assessed. To do this, instruct the client to sit upright, exhale, and hold. (Note: Hold your breath at the same time you ask your client to do so. When you run out of air, you have probably reached the client's limit also, especially if he or she has a breathing problem.) Quickly percuss down the posterior chest wall along the midscapular line until the sound changes in tone from resonant to dull. Use a marking pen to make a small line at that spot. Then instruct the client to take another deep breath and hold. Repeat the midscapular percussion down the posterior chest and again note and mark the point along the chest wall where the sound changes from

■ Note any unusually high or unequal level of the diaphragm. This may be seen in clients with pleural effusion or atelectasis.

TABLE 14-1	Percussion Tones over the Lungs		
	DESCRIPTION	**ADULT PERIPHERAL LUNG**	**CHILD LUNG**
Tone	Description of tone	Resonance	Hyperresonance
Intensity	Loudness or softness of the tone heard	Loud	Very loud
Pitch	Number of vibrations per second: Fast vibrations— high pitch Slow vibrations— low pitch	Low	Very low
Duration	Length of time a vibration note is sustained	Long	Long
Quality	Subjective assessment of characteristics of tone	Hollow	Booming

TECHNIQUES and NORMAL FINDINGS

ABNORMAL FINDINGS

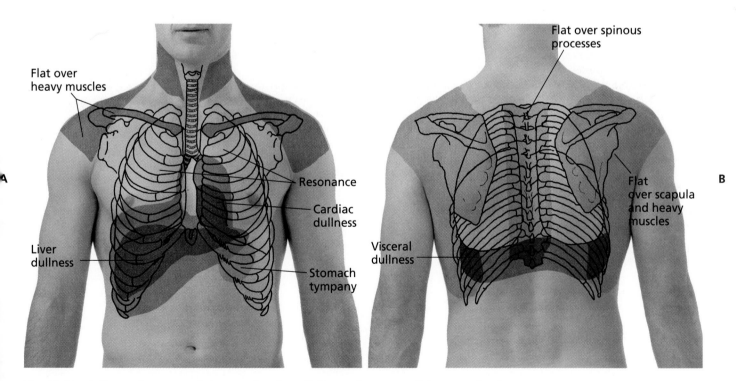

A
B
C

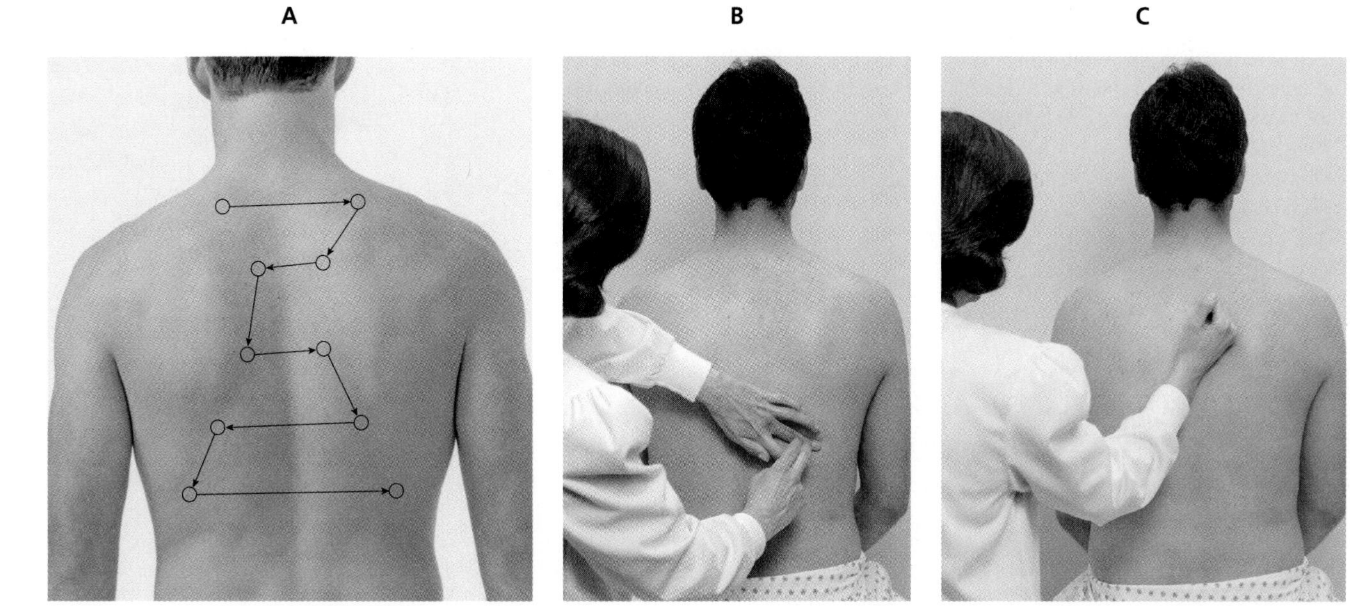

Fig. 14-13 The positioning and pattern for systematic assessment of the posterior chest is the same for percussion and auscultation. **A,** Landmarks for percussion and auscultation. **B,** Indirect percussion. **C,** Direct percussion.

A
Flat over heavy muscles
Resonance
Cardiac dullness
Liver dullness
Stomach tympany
Flat over spinous processes
Flat over scapula and heavy muscles
Visceral dullness
B

Fig. 14-14 **A,** Percussion tones of the anterior chest. **B,** Percussion tones of the posterior chest.

resonant to dull at the bottom of the lungs. The difference between the two marks on each side is called the amount of respiratory excursion (Fig. 14-15). It should be equal on both sides and measure at least 3 to 5 cm; in well-conditioned individuals it may measure as much as 7 to 8 cm.

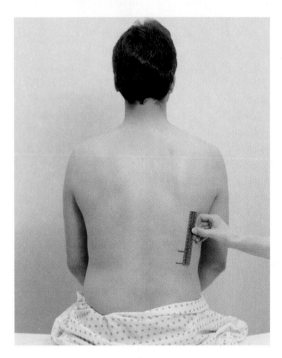

Fig. 14-15 Measuring amount of respiratory excursion.

AUSCULTATE breath sounds for Location. Evaluate the client's breath sounds over the posterior, anterior, and lateral chest walls. Instruct the client to sit upright and breathe deeply and slowly through the mouth. Using the diaphragm of the stethoscope, start *posteriorly* and then more *laterally* to auscultate the chest from apex to base. Follow the same auscultation pattern that was used for percussion (see Figure 14-13). Always listen during both inspiration and expiration and compare one side to the other side (Table 14-2). Listen for the following sounds over the posterior and lateral chest wall:

Vesicular breath sounds should be heard over almost all of the posterior lung fields and all of the lateral surfaces.

■ *Bronchial breath sounds* are abnormal anywhere over the posterior or lateral chest. If heard, there is evidence of consolidation of the lung, as may be seen in clients with pneumonia. (The sound heard will be loud and high-pitched. It sounds as if the air source is just under the stethoscope).

TECHNIQUES and NORMAL FINDINGS

ABNORMAL FINDINGS

TABLE 14-2 Characteristics of Breath Sounds

	BRONCHIAL	BRONCHOVESICULAR	VESICULAR
Pitch	High	Moderate	Low
Intensity	Loud	Medium	Soft
Duration: Inspiration	Insp < Exp	Insp = Exp	Insp > Exp
& Expiration	1:2	1:1	2.5:1
Normal Location	Over trachea	First & second intercostal spaces at sternal border anteriorly; posteriorly at T4 medial to scapula	Peripheral lung fields
Abnormal Location	Over peripheral lung fields	Over peripheral lung fields	Not applicable

Bronchovesicular breath sounds are normally heard over the upper center area of the back on either side of the spine (Fig. 14-16).

Following posterior and lateral chest auscultation, move to the front of the client and use the same techniques to auscultate the anterior chest breath sounds. Listen for the following normal sounds:

Bronchial breath sounds are normally heard over the trachea and the area immediately above the manubrium.

Bronchovesicular breath sounds are normally heard over the central area of the anterior chest around the sternal border.

■ *Bronchovesicular breath sounds* should be considered abnormal when heard over the peripheral lung areas.

■ As with the abnormal sounds heard on the posterior lung fields, *bronchial* or *bronchovesicular* sounds heard in areas where they are not normally heard should be considered abnormal.

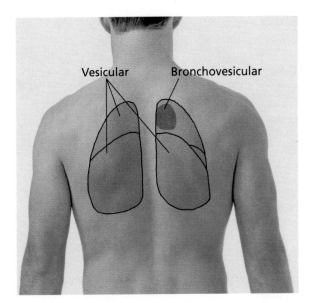
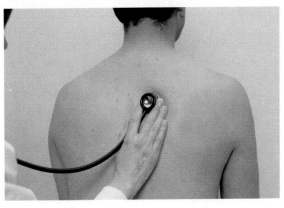

Fig. 14-16 Auscultatory sounds of the posterior chest.

TECHNIQUES and NORMAL FINDINGS

ABNORMAL FINDINGS

Vesicular breath sounds are heard throughout the periphery of the lungs, including the apex of the lungs above the clavicles (Fig. 14-17).

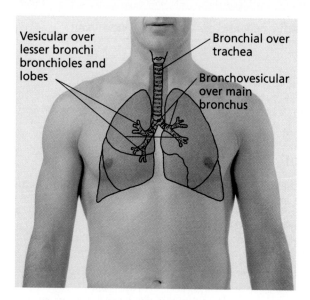

Vesicular over
lesser bronchi
bronchioles and
lobes

Bronchial over
trachea

Bronchovesicular
over main
bronchus

Fig. 14-17   Auscultatory sounds of the anterior chest.

AUSCULTATE chest for Adventitious Breath Sounds. While auscultating the anterior, lateral, and posterior chest, also listen for adventitious sounds. These are extraneous sounds that are superimposed on the breath sounds. Adventitious sounds are not considered normal.

If an adventitious sound is heard, have the client cough; then repeat the examination to see if the sound has changed or disappeared.

■ Adventitious sounds are abnormal (Table 14-3).

Clinical Notes

Before you firmly decide that the client has an adventitious sound, remember that the following may also be causes of sound distortion:

■ If you bump the stethoscope tubing against something or if the client touches the tubing, the sound will be distorted.

■ If the client is cold and is shivering, the sound will be distorted.

■ The stethoscope placed and unintentionally moved on a client's excess chest hair may give a false finding of crackles or pleural friction rub.

■ Extraneous environmental noises such as the rustling of a paper gown or drape may sound like crackles or pleural friction rub.

AUSCULTATE chest for Vocal Sounds (Vocal Resonance). When there is an indication of consolidation of the lung, or if there was an abnormal finding when tactile fremitus was performed, evaluate for vocal resonance. This includes three techniques testing for bronchophony, whispered pectoriloquy, and egophony.

The spoken voice vibrates and transmits sounds through the lung fields. These sounds are normally muffled and cannot be clearly understood. The sound is loudest medially and softer at the periphery of the lung. If there is consolidation of the lung caused by disease, *bronchophony,* which is an increase in loudness and clarity of vocal resonance, will be present.

TECHNIQUES and NORMAL FINDINGS

ABNORMAL FINDINGS

TABLE 14-3 Characteristics of Adventitious Sounds

ADVENTITIOUS SOUNDS	CHARACTERISTICS	CLINICAL EXAMPLES
Crackles (previously called *rales*)		
Fine Crackles 	Fine, high-pitched crackling and popping noises (discontinuous sound) heard during the end of inspiration. Not cleared by cough.	May be heard in pneumonia, congestive heart failure, chronic bronchitis, asthma, and other restrictive and obstructive diseases.
Medium Crackles 	Medium-pitched, moist sound heard about halfway through inspiration. Not cleared by cough.	Same as above, but condition is worse.
Coarse Crackles 	Low-pitched, bubbling or gurgling sounds that start early in inspiration and extend into the first part of expiration.	Same as above, but condition is worse or in terminally ill clients with diminished gag reflex. Also heard in pulmonary edema and pulmonary fibrosis.
Rhonchi		
Sibilant Rhonchi (also called *sibilant wheezes*) 	High-pitched, musical sound similar to a squeak. Heard most commonly during expiration, but may also be heard during inspiration. Occurs in small airways.	Heard in obstructive lung diseases such as asthma or emphysema.
Sonorous Rhonchi (also called *sonorous wheezes*) 	Low-pitched, coarse, loud, low snoring or moaning tone. Actually sounds like snoring. Heard primarily during expiration, but may also be heard during inspiration. Coughing may clear	Heard in problems causing obstruction of the trachea or bronchus, such as bronchitis.
Pleural Friction Rub 	A superficial, low-pitched, coarse rubbing or grating sound. Sounds like two surfaces rubbing together. Heard throughout inspiration and expiration. Loudest over the lower anterolateral surface. Not cleared by cough.	Heard in individuals with pleurisy (inflammation of the pleural surfaces).

TECHNIQUES and NORMAL FINDINGS

ABNORMAL FINDINGS

First, instruct the client to repeat one of the following phrases as you auscultate the posterior chest to assess vocal resonance:

"Ninety-nine," "e-e-e," or "one-two-three."

Bronchophony. Using the diaphragm of the stethoscope, systematically auscultate the posterior chest. As the client repeats either "ninety-nine" or "one-two-three," listen for the response. A normal response is a muffled tone like "nin-nin" or muffled "one-two-three."

- It is abnormal if the sound is louder and clearer. if there is consolidation or compression of the lung, the sound will actually sound like "ninety-nine" or "one-two-three."

Whispered pectoriloquy. Perform when there is a positive finding of bronchophony. It is used to more clearly specify the problem and is referred to as an *exaggerated bronchophony*. To perform whispered pectoriloquy, ask the client to *whisper* "one-two-three." Again, systematically auscultate the posterior chest, listening for the quality of the whispered tones. A normal response is a muffled "one-two-three."

- Again, an abnormal finding is increased clarity and loudness of the sounds, which may be found in consolidation or compression of the lung.

Egophony. Egophony is the final test for vocal resonance. It evaluates the intensity of the spoken voice. Instruct the client to say "e-e-e" as you auscultate the posterior chest. If normal, the sound should be a muffled "e-e-e."

- Changes in intensity and pitch so that the sound appears to be an "a-a-a" occur if there is consolidation of the lung.

AGE-RELATED VARIATIONS

INFANTS

■ APPROACH

Assessing the respiratory status of a newborn or infant is usually straightforward and follows the same sequence as for an adult. Six things are of utmost importance. First, the infant must be undressed at least to the diaper to perform an adequate assessment of the thorax and lungs. Be sure to provide covering for the infant when you are not performing the examination to prevent exposure and cooling. Second, try to inspect the chest configuration and breathing of the child without disturbing him or her. Third, if the child is crying or starts to cry, it is almost impossible to adequately address the respiratory status. Take time to comfort the child, allow the parent to hold the child, or, if all else fails, offer a pacifier or bottle. One of these techniques will help, hopefully, so that you can perform a full assessment. Fourth, consider the size of the diaphragm of your stethoscope before you begin the examination. If the child is very young or small, an adult-size stethoscope diaphragm head will cover at least half of the infant's chest. While this may be adequate for a quick assessment of respiratory rate, it is inappropriate for an accurate assessment of the infant's respiratory status. You should use a stethoscope diaphragm that is appropriate for the size of the child. Fifth, percussion is not routinely performed during infant assessment. Finally, when counting the respiratory rate in the infant, count for an entire minute to obtain a true estimate of breathing.

■ FINDINGS

Inspection of the infant's thoracic cage should show a smooth, rounded, and symmetric appearance The "Harrison's groove" may be seen on the chest wall. This normal anatomic deviation is a horizontal groove in the rib cage at the level of the diaphragm. It extends from the sternum to the midaxillary line. The average chest circumference at the level of the nipples ranges from 30 to 36 cm. This measurement should be 2 to 3 cm smaller than the child's head circumference. Room temperature may greatly affect the child's peripheral skin color. If the infant becomes cold, mottling of the hands and feet may be noted. Once the child is warmed up, the mottling should disappear. If it remains, a more in-depth assessment is needed.

Observe the rate, pattern, and quality of respirations. Infants are obligate nose breathers. Should their nasal passages become occluded, they may have difficulty breathing. The respiratory pattern in the newborn may be irregular, having a Cheyne-Stokes type pattern. Premature newborns may have periods of apnea for as long as 10 to 15 seconds. Stimulation by the adult caregiver can generally produce a quick breath. The respiratory rate in the newborn and infant ranges from 30 to 60 times per minute (Table 14-4). It is important to note that if the child is ill and has a rapid respiratory rate for a prolonged period of time, he or she will tire and may subsequently become physiologically distressed.

Auscultation of the infant's breath sounds is performed in the same manner as for the older child and adult. Because of the thin chest wall of the infant, breath sounds are difficult to localize. They are commonly transmitted from one auscultatory area to another. Because of this, the predominant breath sound you will hear while auscultating the peripheral lung fields is bronchovesicular. This is the predominant sound heard until the child reaches age 5 or 6 years.

Several respiratory sounds and findings, heard or seen, indicate that the infant or young child is in respiratory trouble. These are *stridor, grunting, sternal* or *supraclavicular retractions,* and *nasal flaring.* All are indications of respiratory distress and warrant immediate medical attention. *Stridor* is a high-pitched, piercing sound that is primarily heard in a distressed infant during inspiration. It occurs secondary to upper airway obstruction. The obstruction may cause the infant's inspiratory cycle to be 3 or 4 times longer than expiration. *Respiratory grunting* is a mechanism by which the infant tries to force trapped air out of the lungs while still trying to maintain adequate air in the lungs. *Sternal and supraclavicular retractions* and *nasal flaring* are indications of respiratory distress. Clinically, this may be observed as "see-saw" type breathing with alternating movements of the chest and abdomen. If any of these are observed, the infant is working very hard to try to maintain adequate breathing.

TABLE 14-4	**Respiratory Rates in Children**
AGE	**RATE PER MINUTE**
Newborn	30-60
Less than 1 year	30-50
1-2 years	30-40
3-5 years	20-30
6-10 years	16-20
Over 10 years	12-20

CHILDREN

■ APPROACH

By age 2 or 3 years, the child is usually very cooperative during the respiratory examination. Even before that age, if the examiner takes the time to develop a relationship with the child, cooperation can usually be obtained. Tricks that may help to gain cooperation are such things as letting the child play with the stethoscope before beginning the examination; pretending that your finger is a candle and asking the child to blow it out; or having the child blow out the light of the otoscope or penlight both before and during the examination.

■ FINDINGS

The techniques for examining the lungs and respiratory system of the child are the same as for the adult. Differences in findings include the following. By age 5 or 6, the rounded thorax of the infant approximates the 1:2 or 5:7 (anterior-posterior:lateral) proportional measurements of the adult. If the child's chest proportion remains rounded, it may be an outward indication of a significant problem such as asthma or cystic fibrosis. By age 6 or 7, the child's breathing pattern should change from primarily nasal and abdominal to mostly thoracic in girls and abdominal in boys. As noted in Table 14-4, the child's respiratory rate should gradually slow as the child becomes older. The depth of respirations may be quickly determined by holding your hand at varying distances in front of the child's

nose. Breathing distance responses that are a quick screen of normal respiration depth are as follows:

- 2 years old—6 inches
- 3 to 4 years old—8 inches
- 5 to 6 years old—9 inches
- 8 to 10 years old—10 inches

Palpation findings for the child are the same as for the adult. The examiner should adjust the number of fingers used to palpate the chest wall to be appropriate for the size of the chest. For example, if the child is small you may use only two or three fingers. On the other hand, if the child is large, you may use three fingers or all four.

Percussion may continue to be unreliable until the child is older, at least 8 to 10 years of age. At that time, the techniques are the same as for the adult. If percussion is performed, the examiner should note that young children will have a normal hyperresonance tone.

Auscultation findings for the child range between the findings of the infant and the findings of the adult. Again, depending upon the size of the child and the musculature of the chest, the examiner may find slight variations. Findings for a small or young child with undeveloped chest musculature may include more bronchovesicular breath sounds in the peripheral lung areas, whereas if the child is larger and has started to develop more, the breath sounds will be equivalent to those of the adult (vesicular in the peripheral lung fields).

ADOLESCENTS

■ APPROACH

Examination techniques for the adolescent are the same as for the adult. As with all clients, no matter what age, it is important to have the client disrobe to the waist. The examiner should be sensitive to the possible modesty of the adolescent and provide a drape for the breasts when the anterior chest is not being assessed.

Although smoking and toxic fume inhalation have already been covered in the history section, the examiner may again take time during the examination period to inquire about tobacco and inhalation (sniffing) practices.

■ FINDINGS

The techniques and findings for the adolescent's lung and respiratory assessment are the same as for the adult.

OLDER ADULTS

■ APPROACH

The approach and techniques of examining the lungs and respiration of an older person are the same as for the younger adult. It is important to correlate the client's history with the physical findings. For example, if the client has been a 35-year smoker and now has adventitious sounds present on auscultation, it may have a different meaning and significance from a client who has never smoked and now has shortness of breath and presence of adventitious sounds.

Also, be alert to client fatigue or dizziness during auscultation. If you ask the client to breathe deeply while you

auscultate the chest and you take a long time, the client may become fatigued or dizzy.

■ FINDINGS

The findings of the assessment of the lungs and respiration in the older person are basically the same as for the adult, but several structural and functional differences may be seen. Posterior thoracic stooping or bending or kyphosis may alter the chest wall configuration and make adequate lung expansion more difficult. This in turn may result in decreased tidal volume and thus more shallow breathing. The older adult may also have decreased expansion of the lungs secondary to a sedentary lifestyle or general physical health disability or weakness.

Clients with chronic lung diseases frequently also have an increased anterior:posterior chest wall diameter. The chest wall may actually take on a "barrel" appearance. Clients with chronic obstructive lung problems, such as COPD, usually also have hyperresonance of the lung to palpation.

CLIENTS WITH SITUATIONAL VARIATIONS

PREGNANT WOMEN

◼ APPROACH

During early pregnancy, the client will feel the same and may be examined in the same way as all other adults. As the pregnancy progresses, however, the fetus grows and crowds the abdominal cavity. Increased pressure on the diaphragm occurs secondarily. This in turn may cause decreased lung expansion and may result in an increased respiratory rate and shortness of breath, especially when exercising and lying flat. If the client is near term or has difficulty breathing when lying down, be sure to perform the respiratory assessment when the client is in a sitting position. In addition, the client may need education and reassurance that the shortness of breath she is experiencing is situational and will disappear following delivery.

◼ FINDINGS

The breathing pattern may show shallow, rapid breathing. The thoracic cage usually widens and the costal angle increases from 68° to 103°. Shortness of breath can result from upward movement of the diaphragm and pressure on the lungs from the enlarged uterus. The rate of breathing may increase as much as 15%. This is necessary to compensate for the increase in oxygen demand and the thoracic space structural changes. Diaphragmatic excursion may also decrease secondary to the growing fetus.

CLIENTS WITH OBSTRUCTIVE LUNG DISEASES

◼ APPROACH

Clients with obstructive lung diseases include clients with chronic obstructive pulmonary disease (COPD), emphysema, asthma, and chronic bronchitis. Clients with severe disease may require continuous oxygen therapy. If the client being examined is using oxygen, it is important to inquire about the number of hours per day that oxygen is required, the oxygen concentration required, and the limitation of activity because of either the disease or the oxygen use. Because these clients are also usually on multiple medications, obtaining a careful medication history is important.

◼ FINDINGS

It is difficult to generalize the degree of findings of an individual with an obstructive lung disease. If the disease is not severe, the client may have only symptoms that are exacerbated by illness or stress. On the other hand, if the obstructive disease is severe, the client may have significant respiratory compromise. Possible clinical findings of an individual with an obstructive lung disease include the following. If the client is in distress, he or she may have forward posturing of the upper trunk, or sit in a tripod position with arms forward and supported on knees or on an overbed table. This is known as "the position of air hunger." The nurse may first note dyspnea, cough, and an audible expiratory wheeze. The chest wall may have an increased A:P diameter or appear "barrel-shaped." Percussion of the chest may indicate hyperresonance secondary to chronic hyperinflation of the lungs. Auscultation of breath sounds may indicate prolonged expiration and diminished breath sounds over the diseased area.

CLIENTS WITH CYSTIC FIBROSIS

■ APPROACH

No generalizations should be made about assessing the client with cystic fibrosis other than to note that it is a systemic exocrine gland disease that causes respiratory system dysfunction due to heavy, thick mucus production. This in turn can lead to respiratory system dysfunction. Cystic fibrosis is a multisystem disease, affecting almost all body systems. The primary glands affected by the disease are the pancreas and the sweat glands. Inquire about whether the client has ever been considered for lung transplant. If so, has it been done? What is the current status for consideration?

■ FINDINGS

The thick mucus secretions may cause bronchial obstruction. This primarily leads to areas of atelectasis and hyperinflation. Clinical signs of this sequelae include coughing, congestion, tachypnea, retractions, dyspnea, decreased chest wall movement, and labored breathing. The chest wall may have an increased A:P diameter or a "barrel-shaped" appearance. There may be dullness of percussion tones over areas of consolidation or atelectasis. Breath sounds may have moist crackles or wheezes. If the client's breathing is compromised, there may be unequal or decreased breath sounds.

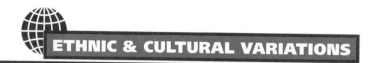

ETHNIC & CULTURAL VARIATIONS

■ FINDINGS

Some variations have been noted in chest capacity and pulmonary function across racial groups. Whites have the largest thoracic cavities and American Indians the smallest. These normal variations affect the amount of air exchange and are reflected in pulmonary function studies of tidal volume and forced expiratory capacity. Lung maturity also differs in fetuses of various racial groups. African-American infants have a much decreased incidence of respiratory distress syndrome because of an earlier lung maturation rate.

Common diseases of the lung strike different cultural groups disproportionately. Tuberculosis and pneumonia pose a much more serious health threat to American Indians than to the general population. Lung cancer is a serious health threat to most Americans. However, it poses a particular risk for African-American men and Pacific Islanders. American Indians and Alaska Natives have an extremely low incidence of lung cancer. Smoking patterns of the various cultural and gender groups explain most, although not all, of the group differences.

E X A M I N A T I O N   S U M M A R Y
Lungs and Respiratory System

General Presentation *(p. 330)*
- Inspect the client for:
  General appearance
  Posturing
  Breathing effort
  Position of trachea

Chest Wall Configuration *(p. 330-332)*
- Inspect the chest wall for:
  Form and symmetry
  Muscle development
  Anterior:posterior diameter
  Costal angle

General Oxygenation *(p. 332)*
- Inspect skin, nails, and lips for:
  Color

Respiratory Rate *(pp. 332-333)*
- Observe and evaluate respirations for:
  Rate and quality
  Breathing pattern
  Chest expansion

Anterior and Posterior Chest Assessment *(pp. 333-342)*
- Palpate the trachea for:
  Position
- Palpate chest wall for:
  Symmetry
  Thoracic expansion
  Vocal (tactile) fremitus
- Percuss the thorax for:
  Tone
  Diaphragmatic (respiratory) excursion
- Auscultate breath sounds for:
  Location of the various sounds
  Presence of adventitious breath sounds
  Vocal sounds (vocal resonance)

COMMON PROBLEMS/CONDITIONS
associated with the Lungs and Respiratory System

■ **Asthma:** A disease marked by increased responsiveness of the trachea and bronchi to various stimuli (Fig. 14-18). It results in widespread narrowing of the airways and bronchospasm with increased mucous secretions that improve either spontaneously or as a result of therapy.

Clinical Findings

Inspection: Increased respiratory rate with prolonged expiration, audible wheeze, shortness of breath, anxious appearance, possible use of accessory muscles, cough.

Palpation: Decreased tactile fremitus, tachycardia.

Percussion: Occasional hyperresonance, decreased diaphragmatic excursion.

Auscultation: Prolonged expiration, expiratory and occasionally inspiratory wheeze, diminished breath sounds.

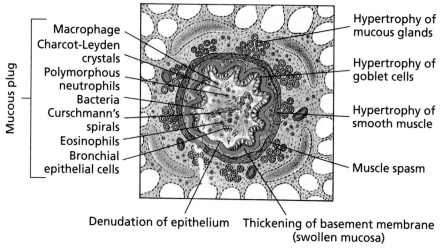

Macrophage
Charcot-Leyden crystals
Polymorphous neutrophils
Bacteria
Curschmann's spirals
Eosinophils
Bronchial epithelial cells

Mucous plug

Hypertrophy of mucous glands
Hypertrophy of goblet cells
Hypertrophy of smooth muscle
Muscle spasm

Denudation of epithelium   Thickening of basement membrane (swollen mucosa)

Fig. 14-18   Asthma.

■ **Atelectasis:** A failure of a portion of the lung to expand (Fig. 14-19). This may be the collapse of a previously expanded lung or an acquired condition secondary to a disease process.

Clinical Findings

Inspection: Cough, tachypnea, tachycardia, decreased chest wall movement on the affected side, and possible tracheal deviation if a large portion of the lung is involved.

Palpation: Diminished fremitus, possible tracheal deviation, decreased chest wall expansion on affected side.

Percussion: Dull over affected area.

Auscultation: Upper lobe above affected area—bronchial breathing, egophony, whispered pectoriloquy. Lobe below affected area—diminished or absent breath sounds. If there is an incomplete blockage, possible wheezing and crackles.

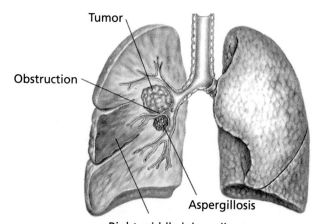

Tumor
Obstruction
Aspergillosis
Right middle lobe collapse

Fig. 14-19   Atelectasis.

■ *Bronchiectasis: (Most common in the older adult.)*
Chronic dilation of the bronchi or bronchioles caused by repeated respiratory infections (Fig. 14-20).
Clinical Findings
Inspection: Respiratory distress, tachypnea, possible rounded chest wall.
Palpation: Normal findings.
Percussion: Normal findings.
Auscultation: Crackles and wheezing that may clear after cough.

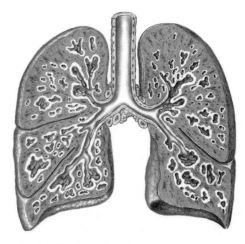

Fig. 14-20 Bronchiectasis.

■ *Bronchitis:* Inflammation of the mucous membranes of the bronchial tree (Fig. 14-21). May be episodic or chronic. If chronic and severe, it is sometimes classified as emphysema.
Clinical Findings
Inspection: Cough, occasional tachypnea, sometimes sputum production.
Palpation: Normal findings.
Percussion: Resonance.
Auscultation: Possible crackles and expiratory wheezing, occasional prolonged expiration.

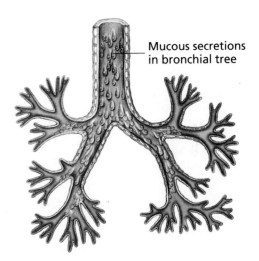

Mucous secretions in bronchial tree

Fig. 14-21 Bronchitis. Irritation of the bronchi causes inflammation.

■ *Chronic obstructive pulmonary disease (COPD):* Nonspecific designation given to a cluster of respiratory problems in which chronic cough and frequently excessive sputum production and dyspnea are prominent (Fig. 14-22). Most commonly seen in older clients who have a history of smoking.
Clinical Findings
Inspection: Possible signs of respiratory distress, wheezing, and other signs associated with emphysema, asthma, and chronic bronchitis.
Palpation: Possible decreased vocal fremitus.
Percussion: Hyperresonance may be present.
Auscultation: Both sonorous and sibilant wheezing may be present, diminished breath sounds.

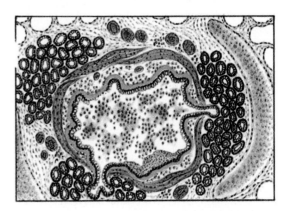

Fig. 14-22 Chronic obstructive pulmonary disease (COPD), a group of diseases including chronic bronchitis.

■ *Cystic fibrosis:* Autosomal recessive disorder of the exocrine glands affecting the lungs, pancreas, and sweat glands (Fig. 14-23). Salt water loss is significant.

Clinical Findings

Inspection: Thick mucous secretion, cough, congestion, tachypnea, retractions, decreased chest movement, labored breathing, dyspnea, barrel chest.

Palpation: Decreased fremitus.

Percussion: Tympanic percussion tones over consolidation or areas of atelectasis.

Auscultation: Moist breath sounds with crackles and wheezes; breath sounds may be unequal or decreased.

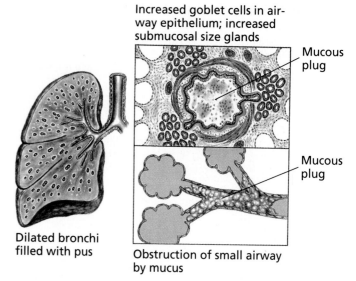

Increased goblet cells in airway epithelium; increased submucosal size glands

Mucous plug

Mucous plug

Dilated bronchi filled with pus

Obstruction of small airway by mucus

Fig. 14-23   Cystic fibrosis.

■ *Croup: (Seen almost exclusively in young children under the age of 3 years.)* Croup is a syndrome that usually results from a viral infection.

Clinical Findings

Inspection: Anxious-appearing child, "bark"-type cough, usually fever, labored breathing, possible inspiratory stridor.

Palpation: No specific findings.

Percussion: Not usually performed.

Auscultation: Crackles may be present, breath sounds are usually clear.

■ *Emphysema: (Most common in the older adult)* Chronic obstructive pulmonary disease in which there is an anatomic alteration of the air spaces distal to the conducting airways (Fig. 14-24). There is a permanent abnormal enlargement of the air spaces. This results in destruction of the alveolar walls and, finally, increased airway resistance.

Clinical Findings

Inspection: Tachypnea, barrel chest, obvious difficulty breathing with forward posturing; may be thin and underweight.

Palpation: Diminished fremitus.

Percussion: Hyperresonance, decreased diaphragmatic excursion.

Auscultation: Diminished breath and voice sounds, possible wheezing or crackles.

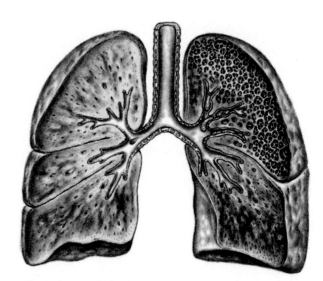

Fig. 14-24   Lobar emphysema.

■ *Pneumonia with lobar consolidation:* Inflammatory process of the respiratory bronchioles and the alveolar spaces that is caused by infection (Fig 14-25).

Clinical Findings

Inspection: Tachypnea, restlessness, retractions in children, labored breathing, hypoventilation.

Palpation: Increased fremitus, if there is also consolidation of the lung tissue.

Percussion: Dull tone over area of consolidation.

Auscultation: Possible crackles and wheezes, change of vesicular breath sounds to bronchovesicular and bronchial, egophony, bronchophony, and whispered pectoriloquy may be present.

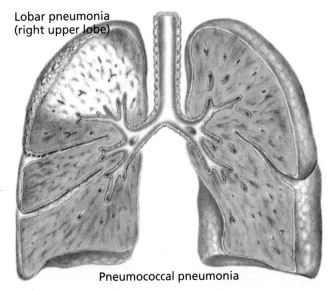

Lobar pneumonia (right upper lobe)

Pneumococcal pneumonia

Fig. 14-25   Pneumonia with lobar consolidation.

 Cultural Note

Pneumonia and tuberculosis are serious health threats for American Indians and Alaska Natives. Death from tuberculosis is over 500% greater for these groups than for the general population, while pneumonia-related deaths are 40% greater than the general population.

■ *Tuberculosis:* Chronic pulmonary and extrapulmonary infectious disease acquired by inhalation of a dried-droplet nucleus containing a tubercle bacillus (Fig. 14-26). The patient is usually asymptomatic during the early stages of the disease. The first signs may be regional lymph node enlargement, night sweats, chronic cough, blood-streaked sputum, weight loss, fatigue, fever, and a positive TB test or chest x-ray.

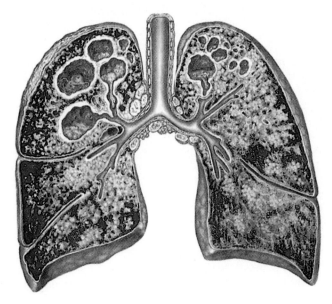

Fig. 14-26   Tuberculosis.

■ *Lung cancer:* Uncontrolled growth of anaplastic cells in the lung (Fig. 14-27). Etiologic factors include such agents as tobacco smoke, asbestos, ionizing radiation, and other noxious inhalants. Cancer develops when the genes responsible for sequential cell division, called *proto-oncogenes,* change to a type of cell called *oncogenes.* Adenocarcinoma appears to be increasing in frequency and is probably the most common type, accounting for 40% of all cases. Adenocarcinoma arises in peripheral lung tissue or in areas scarred from pulmonary infarction, infection, or idiopathic fibrosis. Squamous cell carcinoma accounts for about 30% of all lung cancers.

Clinical Findings

Inspection: Depending on stage, client may appear healthy, or client may have weight loss, cough, congestion, wheezing, hemoptysis, labored breathing, or dyspnea.

Palpation: No specific findings for cancer itself.

Percussion: Depending on the presentation, the percussion tones may be the same as for clients with emphysema, atelectasis, and pneumonia.

Auscultation: Depending on the presentation, the breath sounds heard on auscultation may be the same as for clients with emphysema, atelectasis, and pneumonia.

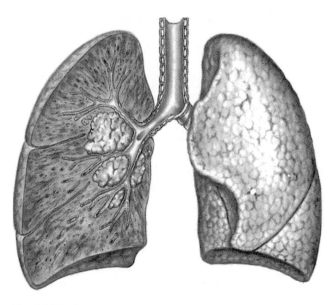

Fig. 14-27   Lung cancer.

 ## Cultural Note

Lung cancer rates vary by gender and cultural grouping. Men have a higher incidence of and mortality from lung cancer across all groups. African Americans have the highest lung cancer rates (1 in 1500), closely followed by Pacific Islanders. White incidence rates are roughly those of the general population (1 in 2000). Rates for other minority groups are below that of the general population, and rates for American Indians/Alaska Natives are extremely low (1 in 16,000).

■ *Pleural effusion:* Pleurisy with effusion (Fig. 14-28). It develops when excess nonpurulent fluid accumulates in the pleural space between the visceral and parietal pleurae. Normally, less than 10 ml of fluid is in the space between the two pleurae. When more fluid accumulates, it is called pleural effusion. The accumulation of excess fluid usually occurs secondary to another problem, such as infection, cancer, or injury. The degree of clinical symptoms depends greatly on the amount of fluid accumulation and the position of the client. The fluid will gravitate to the most dependent position in the lung.

Clinical Findings

Inspection: The degree of respiratory distress depends on the amount of fluid accumulation. If the effusion has occurred rapidly and if it is large, there may be dyspnea, intercostal bulging, or decreased chest wall movement.

Palpation: Fremitus ranges from normal to absent, depending on the amount of fluid that has accumulated. If present, it will be decreased over the affected area.

Percussion: Dull to flat over the affected area, depending on the amount of fluid accumulation. The tone may change as the client changes position.

Auscultation: Breath sounds will be muted or decreased over the affected area. Egophony above effusion site.

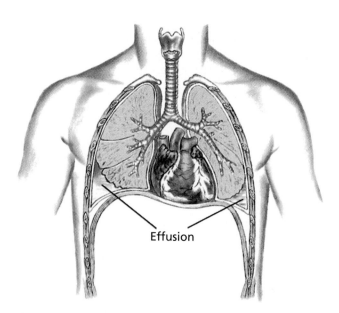

Fig. 14-28   Pleural effusion.

■ *Pneumothorax:* Three types exist: (1) *closed,* which may be spontaneous, traumatic, or iatrogenic; (2) *open,* which occurs following penetration of the chest by either injury or surgical procedure; and (3) *tension,* which develops when air leaks into the pleura and cannot escape (Fig. 14-29). While all types cause respiratory compromise, the tension pneumothorax is life-threatening and requires immediate intervention.

Clinical Findings

Inspection: The clinical signs vary depending on the amount of lung collapse. If there is very minor collapse, the client may be slightly short of breath, anxious, and have chest pain. If there is a large amount of lung collapse, the client will be in severe respiratory distress, including dyspnea, tachypnea, and cyanosis. The client may also have paradoxic chest wall movement.

Palpation: Decreased chest wall movement on the affected side. If severe, there may be tracheal displacement toward the unaffected side with a mediastinal shift.

Percussion: Booming quality percussion tone over affected area.

Auscultation: Distant and hyperresonant breath sounds over the affected area.

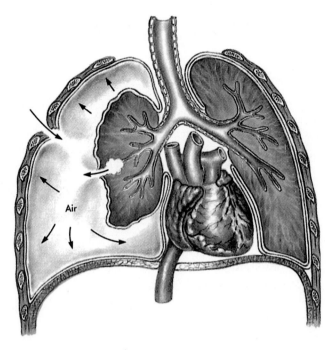

Fig. 14-29   Pneumothorax.

■ *Hemothorax:* The presence of blood in the pleural space (Fig. 14-30). It occurs most frequently following either blunt or penetrating injury to the chest wall.

Clinical Findings

Inspection: Same findings as for pneumothorax. Expect to see chest wall injury.

Palpation: Same as for pneumothorax. May also feel chest wall injury such as broken ribs.

Percussion: Dullness on percussion.

Auscultation: Distant and muffled breath sounds.

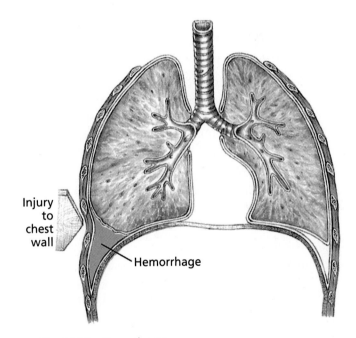

Fig. 14-30   Hemothorax.

Sample Documentation &Nursing Diagnosis

CASE 1   9-year-old Hispanic male with 2-hour history of wheezing.

Subjective

Frightened, anxious-appearing boy states that he has asthma. Earlier today he was outdoors playing soccer with his friends. Reported that he normally takes Proventil inhaler but forgot it today. Did not want to stop playing to get care—until he couldn't breathe well and got scared. Mother present and appears both frightened and frustrated. Reports history of asthma since 5 years old. Usually responds well to Proventil inhaler. Had two puffs just before coming to clinic, approximately 30 minutes ago—no noted relief. No previous hospitalizations for asthma. States no other health problems.

Objective

Pulse   122.

Respiratory rate   42.

Oxygen saturation on room air   91%.

9-year-old boy appears anxious, sitting in tripod position, leaning forward, attempting to breathe with mouth open.

Inspection   Chest wall smooth and normal configuration; no retractions or bulges noted.

Palpation   Deferred because of client's anxious state.

Percussion   Deferred because of client's anxious state.

Auscultation   Noted expiratory wheezes bilaterally; prolonged expiration; diminished breath sounds throughout.

• •

Nursing Diagnosis #1

Ineffective breathing pattern related to bronchospasm and anxiety.

Defining characteristics   Stated difficulty with breathing, history of asthma, reported use of albuterol (Proventil) inhaler before incident; client anxious, tripod position, leaning forward, respiratory rate 42, SaO_2 91%, expiratory wheezes, diminished breath sounds.

Nursing Diagnosis #2

Ineffective coping related to anxiety.

Defining characteristics   Client and mother reported feeling frightened and anxious; client appeared anxious, respiratory rate 42, heart rate 122.

Nursing Diagnosis #3

Noncompliance related to prevention of exercise-induced bronchospasm.

Defining characteristics   Client forgot inhaler, did not want to stop playing soccer to get care; has Proventil inhaler, which, when used appropriately, can usually prevent exercise-induced bronchospasm.

&Nursing Diagnosis

CASE 2   61-year-old white woman with weight loss and a dry, hacking cough.

Subjective

Small-framed, ambulatory woman states that she has had a "dry hacky cough" for the past 3 months, and it just won't go away. Also states 12-pound weight loss during same period. Denies other symptoms or other problems. Reports 41-year history of cigarette smoking. Amount has decreased during past 6 months from 1½ packs of nonfiltered cigarettes to ½ pack per day. She also reports that cough is worse in the morning when she awakens. On two unrelated occasions during the past week she has coughed up "specks of bright red blood." Reports dyspnea on exertion of going up and down stairs but denies other symptoms. Toward end of interview client started crying and stated fear of having cancer.

Objective

Weight   104 lb (47.3 kg).

Temperature   98.4° F (36.9° C).

Pulse   96.

Respiration rate   22.

Inspection   Small-framed, white woman sitting erect on examination table; no noted respiratory distress; A:P chest diameter without noted enlargement; slight kyphosis noted; thoracic expansion symmetric; respirations even and without noted distress.

Palpation   No friction rubs or rib tenderness noted; tactile fremitus increased over most of posterior left lung.

Percussion   Resonance over right lung fields; dullness over most of left lung.

Auscultation   Breath sounds present bilaterally; (R) vesicular breath sounds heard throughout; without adventitious sounds; (L) combination of bronchovesicular and vesicular breath sounds heard; slightly diminished breath sounds on (L) when compared to (R); egophony and whispered pectoriloquy present on (L).

• •

Nursing Diagnosis #1

Impaired gas exchange related to left lung consolidation.

Defining characteristics   Dyspnea on exertion, smoking history, hemoptysis, left lung dull to percussion, diminished breath sounds on left; egophony and whispered pectoriloquy on left.

Nursing Diagnosis #2

Altered breathing patterns related to bronchial irritation and inflammation.

Defining characteristics   41-year history of smoking, now decreased to ½ pack per day; dry hacking cough.

Nursing Diagnosis #3

Fear related to diagnosis of lung cancer.

Defining characteristics   Smoking history, weight loss, fear of cancer, crying; left lung dull to percussion, egophony and whispered pectoriloquy on left.

HEALTH PROMOTION

■ **Smoking** In one year a heavy smoker can spend as much as $1000 on cigarettes. In addition to lung cancer and chronic lung disease being a major continuing problem in the United States, the number of young people who are smoking is increasing each year. The American Cancer Society and most large health care facilities now have a variety of "stop smoking" programs that use a variety of strategies. Factors that seem to contribute to the success of a stop-smoking program are client readiness, finding a program that works for that individual client, and ongoing support by the client's health care provider. Giving the client only written materials about the hazards of smoking and ways to quit smoking is generally thought to have minimal impact on the client's success in actually quitting smoking. The use of nicotine patches or gum may gradually wean the client's dependence.

■ **Smokeless Tobacco** Tobacco chewing and the use of smokeless tobacco have many of the same harmful effects on the body as does smoking cigarettes. In addition, individuals with this behavior are at increased risk for mouth cancer and leukoplakia. The same strategies apply to stopping smokeless tobacco use as for smoking. The American Cancer Society has programs and related materials.

■ **Inhalants** Inhalants such as gasoline, glue, hair spray, deodorant sprays, liquid paper, and liquid cement are used, mainly by young persons, to "get high." These are often the first mood-altering substance used by children. Inhalants may be attractive to the child and adolescent because of their rapid onset of action, low cost, and easy availability. They are typically used by inhaling from a plastic bag containing the substance or by inhaling a cloth saturated with the substance. The initial effect is usually stimulation and excitation, but may lead to death or cause permanent lung, liver, kidney, or brain damage. It is vitally important to determine if the client is now using or has ever used an inhaled agent—even on a single occasion. If you assess that the client is either at risk for using inhalants or is currently a user of inhalants, the client should be clearly informed of the risks associated with their continued use and ultimately referred to a clinical

resource that can provide adequate counseling. Your local public health office or teen clinic will most likely have materials and resources that may be helpful.

■ **Occupational or Home Exposure to Irritants and Carcinogens** All individuals who work in areas where there are fumes are at risk for lung damage and subsequent respiratory problems. The exposure could be to a known harmful agent such as asbestos, or it could be to less obvious toxins such as hair spray, paint fumes, pesticides, herbicides, coal dust, secondary cigarette smoke, wood-burning fireplace fumes, or even dust. Regardless of the toxin or irritant, individuals should be cautioned either to avoid areas where the toxins are present or to wear a filtering mask or respirator to keep from inhaling the fumes. An ounce of prevention is worth a pound of cure.

■ **Preventing Respiratory Infections** Respiratory infections are most serious for the elderly and any individual with chronic lung disease. The following guidelines may be helpful for those clients at high risk for infection:
1. Follow all guidelines from health care providers, such as taking prescribed medications or using supplemental oxygen if ordered.
2. Take care of yourself: drink at least 6 glasses of water each day (unless advised otherwise), eat nutritious meals, get adequate sleep each night (7 to 8 hours), take several short rest periods during the day, learn to conserve your energy so as not to get too tired.
3. Stay away from people who have colds and the flu. If this is not possible, wear a disposable mask when around ill people.
4. Avoid air pollution, including tobacco smoke, wood or oil smoke, car exhaust, and industrial fumes.
5. If you are older or in a group at high risk for infection, consult your health care provider about receiving a pneumovax every 5 years or a flu vaccine every fall.
6. Take special precautions with personal hygiene and always wash hands.
7. If you should become ill, seek medical attention.

??????? STUDY QUESTIONS ???????

1. What is the purpose of the respiratory system? List and describe the four functions that assist in fulfilling this purpose.

2. Describe the process of inspiration and expiration.

3. Draw a picture of the anterior chest wall. Identify and locate the seven topographic markers on your drawing. Repeat the process for the posterior and lateral chest walls.

4. Describe what occurs to an infant's lung after delivery.

5. What is the average respiratory rate for a newborn? A 3-year-old? A 10-year-old? A 16-year-old?

6. Describe changes that occur in a woman's respiratory function as a result of pregnancy.

7. What is a "barrel chest"? Who develops a barrel chest?

8. List the changes in the lungs that occur as a result of aging.

9. An individual reports that he has been coughing up "yellow stuff." What else do you want to know about the expectorated substance?

10. An individual reports trouble breathing when he lies down. What else do you want to know?

11. While taking a history, you discover that the individual is a smoker. What do you need to know about his smoking habits?

12. When a person is experiencing respiratory symptoms, why is it important to know about where they work and what type of job they do?

13. What areas of assessment are important when taking a history for an infant?

14. What kinds of questions might you direct to a 5-year-old with asthma?

15. As a school nurse in a high school, what two topics warrant specific exploration when assessing the respiratory system?

16. What do you expect to find when inspecting a normal chest wall?

17. Describe how you would evaluate whether an individual had adequate oxygenation.

18. How do you know whether inspiratory effort is normal? List and describe two abnormal breathing patterns.

19. What are you looking for as you palpate the anterior chest?

20. Describe the steps you would take in percussing the posterior chest.

21. Describe the procedure you would use to auscultate breath sounds. What are you listening for?

22. Where should you hear bronchial breath sounds? Bronchovesicular sounds? Vesicular sounds? When are these sounds considered abnormal?

23. Match the adventitious sound with the appropriate description:

Rales　　　　　　*Continuous grating sound*
Sibilant rhonchi　*Snoring sound*
Sonorous rhonchi　*Crackling on inspiration*
Pleural friction rub　*Wheezy squeak*

24. What is the purpose of auscultating vocal sounds? What test should you perform first? If the results are positive, what do you do next?

25. List six things that you need to consider in preparing to do a respiratory exam of an infant.

26. List normal variations in the respiratory pattern that you might expect in a newborn. What respiratory sounds are indicative of respiratory distress in an infant?

27. When performing a respiratory exam on a child, list two normal findings that differ from those expected in an adult.

28. List three normal physical findings that occur as a result of pregnancy.

29. Which cultural group has the highest rate of smoking? Which group has the highest incidence of lung cancer? Which group has the lowest lung cancer rate?

30. Match the lung disease to the appropriate physical finding:

Asthma　　　*Barking cough, labored breathing*
Bronchitis　*Prolonged expiration, wheezing*
Croup　　　*Resonance, crackles, cough*
Pneumonia　*Increased fremitus, hypoventilation*

31. List six guidelines that you might use in teaching an at-risk individual about preventing respiratory infections.

CHAPTER 15

Heart and Peripheral Vascular System

ANATOMY AND PHYSIOLOGY

The cardiovascular system transports oxygen, nutrients, and other substances to all the body's tissues, and disposes of metabolic waste products through the kidneys and the lungs. This is accomplished largely by the heart and a system of blood vessels. The heart is about the size of a fist and beats 60 to 100 times a minute without rest, responding to both external and internal demands such as exercise, temperature changes, and stress. Many of these stimuli are communicated to the cardiovascular system through the endocrine and nervous systems. In turn, the cardiovascular system adjusts to these stimuli by constricting or dilating blood vessels, altering the rate of cardiac output, and redistributing blood flow.

THE HEART AND GREAT VESSELS

The heart is a pump divided into right and left sides. Each side of the heart has two chambers, an atrium and a ventricle. The right side receives blood from the superior and inferior vena cava and pumps it through the pulmonary arteries to the pulmonary circulation; the left side receives blood from the pulmonary veins and pumps it through the aorta into the systemic circulation. The upper part of the heart is the base, and the lower left ventricle is called the apex. The heart lies behind the sternum and above the diaphragm in the mediastinum at an angle so that the right ventricle makes up most of the anterior surface and the left ventricle lies to the left and posteriorly. The right atrium forms the right border of the heart and the left atrium lies posteriorly. The aorta curves upward out of the left ventricle and bends posteriorly and downward just above the sternal angle. The pulmonary arteries emerge from the superior aspect of the right ventricle near the third intercostal space (Fig. 15-1).

PERICARDIUM AND CARDIAC MUSCLE

The heart is encased in the pericardium, a double-walled fibrous sac of elastic connective tissue that shields the heart from trauma and infection. The pericardium contains fluid within its layer to reduce friction of cardiac movement. Beneath the pericardium lie three layers of the heart. The epicardium covers the heart surface and extends to the great vessels with a visceral layer of serous pericardium; the middle layer, or myocardium, is thick muscular tissue that controls the

pumping action; and the endocardium lines the inner chambers and valves (Fig. 15-2). Blood is supplied to the myocardium by the coronary arteries, which are the first branches off the aorta. The right coronary artery supplies the sinoatrial and atrioventricular nodes and most of the right side of the heart with a small volume of blood sent to the left ventricle. The left coronary artery supplies blood to the left side of the heart with a small volume of blood sent to the right ventricle.

BLOOD FLOW THROUGH THE HEART: THE CARDIAC CYCLE

Four valves govern blood flow through the four chambers. The tricuspid valve on the right and mitral valve on the left are called the atrioventricular (AV) valves because they separate the atria from the ventricles. The aortic valve emerges from the left ventricle into the aorta, and the pulmonic valve opens from the right ventricle into the pulmonary artery (Fig. 15-3). The aortic and pulmonic valves are called semilunar valves because of their half-moon shape.

Diastole. The valves open and close in response to pressure gradients that maintain the forward flow of blood. Blood flow into the atria from the systemic and pulmonic circulation creates positive pressure. When the pressure in the

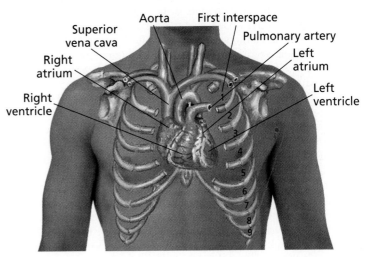

Fig. 15-1 Position of the heart chambers and great vessels.

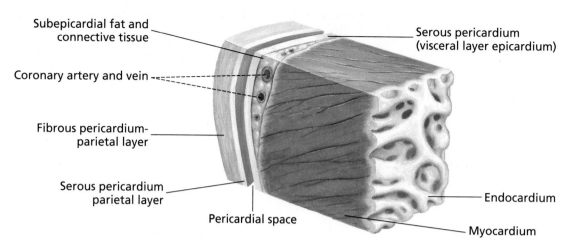

Fig. 15-2 Cross section of cardiac muscle. *(From Canobbio, 1990.)*

Subepicardial fat and connective tissue

Coronary artery and vein

Fibrous pericardium-parietal layer

Serous pericardium parietal layer

Pericardial space

Serous pericardium (visceral layer epicardium)

Endocardium

Myocardium

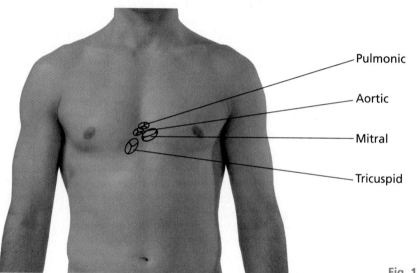

Pulmonic

Aortic

Mitral

Tricuspid

Fig. 15-3 Anatomic location of the heart valves.

atria is higher than the pressure in the ventricles, the atria contract, the AV valves open, and the ventricles fill with blood. About 80% of the blood from the atria flows into relaxed ventricles. Then atrial contraction forces the remaining 20% of the blood into the ventricles. This added atrial thrust is referred to as the "atrial kick." The phase in the cardiac cycle when the ventricles are relaxed and filling with blood is called diastole (Fig. 15-4).

Systole.   When the pressure of blood in the ventricles becomes higher than the pressure in the atria, the AV valves close, preventing the backflow or regurgitation of blood into the atria. The force of blood filling the ventricles stretches the myocardium. When the pressure in the ventricles exceeds the diastolic pressure in the great vessels, the semilunar valves open, pumping blood into the pulmonary arteries and aorta. The ejection of blood out of the ventricles lowers the pressure in the ventricles causing the semilunar valves to close. This phase in the cardiac cycle when the ventricles are contracting is called systole (Fig. 15-5).

ELECTRIC CONDUCTION

The heart is stimulated by an electric discharge that originates in the sinoatrial (SA) node in the superior aspect of the right atrium. The node, called the cardiac pacemaker, discharges about 60 to 100 impulses per minute. The electric discharge stimulates contraction of both atria and then flows to the AV node in the inferior aspect of the right atrium. The impulses are then transmitted through a series of branches (bundle of His) and Purkinje's fibers in the myocardium, which results in ventricular contraction (Fig. 15-6). The AV node prevents excessive atrial impulses from reaching the ventricles. If the SA node fails, the remaining electrical system can generate ventricular contraction at a slower rate, 40 to 60 impulses per minute. If both SA and AV nodes are ineffective, the bundle branches may take over contraction, but at a very slow rate of 20 to 40 impulses per minute. The sequence of electric impulses slightly precedes cardiac cycle events. The electric discharges are measured in an electrocardiogram (ECG).

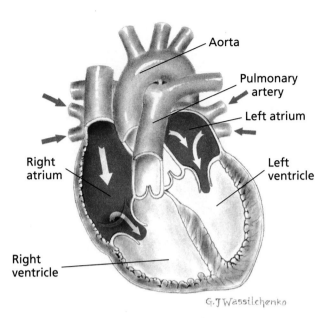

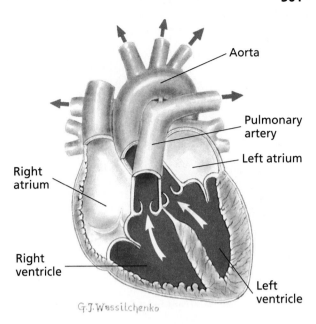

Fig. 15-4 Blood flow during diastole. *(From Canobbio, 1990.)*

Fig. 15-5 Blood flow during systole. *(From Canobbio, 1990.)*

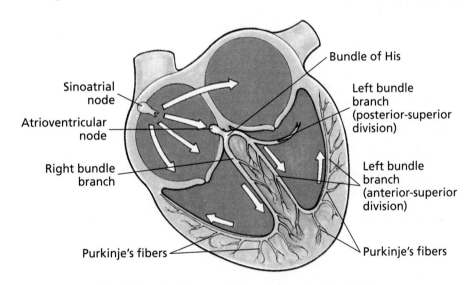

Fig. 15-6 Cardiac conduction. *(From Canobbio, 1990.)*

BLOOD CIRCULATION

The heart and systemic circulatory system work together with the pulmonary system to deliver oxygen to the body, responding not only to electrical stimuli but also to mechanical stimuli. For example, during exercise, blood is redistributed to muscles instead of to other systems, such as the gastrointestinal system.

The circulatory system is composed of arteries, capillaries, and veins. The tough and tensile arteries (Fig. 15-7) and their smaller branches, the arterioles, are subjected to remarkable pressures. They constrict and dilate in response to parasympathetic, sympathetic, endocrine, and temperature stimuli and are responsible for maintaining blood pressure. The more passive veins (Fig. 15-8, *A*) and their smaller branches, the venules, are less sturdy but more expansible, enabling them to act as a repository for extra blood, if needed, to decrease the workload on the heart. Veins are a low-pressure system, compared with arterial circulation. The valves in each vein keep blood flowing in a forward direction toward the heart (Fig. 15-8, *B*).

🌐 Racial Variation

African Americans have more venous valves in the lower legs than whites.

Blood leaving the heart in the aorta is oxygen-rich. It flows from the aorta to arteries to arterioles and into capillaries. Capillaries deliver oxygen and nutrients to cells and collect waste products. The capillary blood flows into the venules, through the veins, and delivers the deoxygenated blood to the right side of the heart. The blood is then pumped into the pulmonary circulation where the carbon dioxide diffuses across the alveolar-capillary membranes to be exhaled. Oxygen diffuses in the opposite direction from alveoli into pulmonary capillaries. Other waste products are eliminated as the blood flows through the glomeruli of the kidneys.

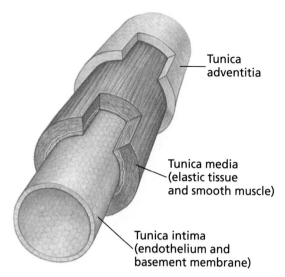

Fig. 15-7   **Arteries.**   *(From Seeley, Stephens, Tate, 1995.)*

DEVELOPMENTAL CONSIDERATIONS

NEWBORNS

The newborn's heart is developmentally similar to the adult's, even before birth, with one notable exception: oxygenation occurs through the placenta to compensate for the nonfunctional fetal lungs. Arterial blood is returned via the umbilicus to the right side of the heart. The foramen ovale is an opening between the left and right atria that allows blood to flow into the left side of the heart, where about two thirds is pumped into the aorta. The remaining third is pumped from the right ventricle directly into the aorta through the patent ductus arteriosus. After birth, as the pressure in the left atrium rises, the foramen ovale closes usually within the first hour. The ductus arteriosus usually closes within 10 to 15 hours. The usual newborn heart rate is between 120 and 160 beats per minute.

PREGNANT WOMEN

During pregnancy, the heart must work harder to accommodate a total plasma volume increase. The degree of blood volume varies considerably, with a range of about 25% to 45%. The left ventricle thickens and increases its mass; similarly, the heart valve orifices increase in size to a maximum of 13% to 14% over their nonpregnant states. Thus cardiac output increases approximately 40% to 50%, returning to normal in about 2 to 3 weeks after delivery. Audible murmurs, increased first heart sound (S_1) split, and heart palpitations may occur. The heart's position shifts up and to the left, rotating so that the apex moves laterally as the uterus and diaphragm shift.

Palmar erythema and spider telangiectases are common changes noted on the skin at this time due to increased vascular resistance and peripheral vasodilation. Blood pressure decreases in the second trimester and may rise in the third, but the change should not exceed 30 mm systolic or 15 mm diastolic over the prepregnant condition.

Edema of the lower extremities, varicosities in the legs, and hemorrhoids are frequently reported signs of blood stagnation in the lower extremities due to occlusion of pelvic veins and inferior vena cava from pressure created by the enlarged uterus.

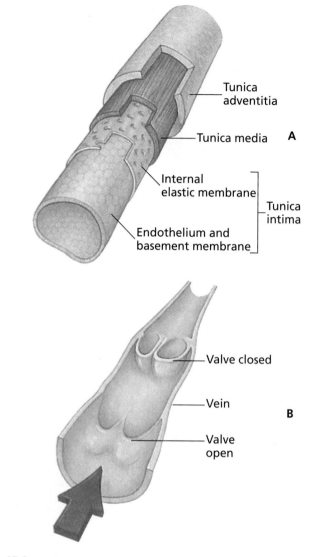

Fig. 15-8   **Veins.**   *(From Seeley, Stephens, Tate, 1995.)*

During delivery, as the uterus empties, pressure is removed from the vena cava. After delivery, the heart will shift back in place and the prepregnant state will return within days.

OLDER ADULTS

With increased age the heart size tends to decrease. The cardiac output declines 30% to 40% due to decreased heart rate and myocardial contractility. Sudden or prolonged stress and tachycardia are poorly tolerated. Response to stress or increased oxygen demand is less efficient, and the return to baseline heart rate takes longer. Physiologic changes, such as thickening of the endocardium and decreased elasticity of the myocardium, contribute to delayed recovery from myocardial contractility and irritability.

Arterial walls and some superficial vessels become less efficient in complying with changing needs as they become more dilated, prominent, tortuous, and calcified. Increased blood pressure, both systolic and diastolic, occurs in response to increased peripheral vascular resistance. In addition, the older adult's cardiac function is affected by fibrosis and sclerosis involving the SA node and mitral and aortic valves.

HEALTH HISTORY | Heart and Peripheral Vascular System

The focus of the history includes personal habits contributing to or preventing disease, chest pain, shortness of breath, nocturia, cough, fatigue, syncope, dependent edema, leg pain, and past history or family history of cardiovascular problems.

QUESTIONS

RATIONALE

PERSONAL HABITS

■ Do you work in an area where there are factors that may affect your cardio-vascular system? For example, are there extensive physical demands? Emotional stress?

■ Do you exercise? What kind of exercise? How often? How long?

■ Do you smoke? Do you use tobacco in any form, such as smokeless or chewing tobacco? How long have you done this? How much?

■ Have you ever quit smoking? *If so:* How and for what length of time? Are you interested in quitting smoking? Do you know how smoking affects the cardiovascular system?

■ Describe your usual eating habits. How often do you eat red meat? Do you monitor your fat or salt intake? Have you dieted recently, or do you diet often? Have you lost or gained weight lately? How much? Do you drink alcoholic beverages? How much? How often? Have you been diagnosed as having high levels of cholesterol or elevated triglycerides? Do you have high blood pressure?

■ How would you describe yourself? Are you intense? Often angry? Able to relax? How do you deal with stress? (Observe the client as he or she responds, and throughout the examination, to evaluate the accuracy of the client's answers.)

■ What do you do to relax? Hobbies? Sports? Meditation? Yoga?

■ Do you take any medicine for your heart or high blood pressure? *If so:* What drugs are they? How much do you take? How often? Do you take them as prescribed? Do you take aspirin on a regular basis as an anticoagulant? What over-the-counter drugs do you use? How frequently? Do you use cocaine? Other street drugs? What drugs do you use?

◀ *These may increase the workload on the heart.*

◀ *Nicotine in tobacco causes vasoconstriction, which may decrease bloodflow to extremities or increase blood pressure.*

◀ *Determine the client's knowledge level and desire for lifestyle change.*

◀ *Modifiable risk factors for heart disease include hypercholesterolemia, obesity, and high blood pressure.*

◀ *Stress and persistent intensity are risk factors for heart disease.*

◀ *Over-the-counter decongestants may be contraindicated for clients with hypertension.*

◀ *Cocaine use has been associated with myocardial infarction and strokes.*

CHEST PAIN

■ Have you ever had any pain in your chest? *If so:* When did it start? Are you currently having this problem? For how long? How often do you have this pain?

■ Where do you feel the pain? Does it radiate? Describe the pain. Is it crushing? Stabbing? Burning? Viselike? (*Note:* Allow the patient to describe it in his or her own words before suggesting any of these descriptors.)

◀ *Angina is an important symptom of coronary artery disease. It indicates that the heart cannot supply the body's demand for oxygen.*

◀ *The origin of chest pain may be cardiac, pulmonary, musculoskeletal, or gastrointestinal. If the patient uses a clenched fist placed on the sternum (Levine's sign) to describe the pain, angina is extremely likely. Pain may radiate to jaw and left arm.*

QUESTIONS

- What factors seem to precede the pain? Exercise? Rest? Highly emotional situations? Eating? Sexual intercourse? Cold?
- What symptoms have you noticed along with the pain? Sweating? Turning pale or gray? Heart skipping beats or racing? Shortness of breath? Nausea or vomiting? Dizziness? Anxiety? Swelling or edema?
- What makes it worse? Moving the arms or neck? Breathing? Lying flat? Exercise?
- What relieves the pain? Rest? Nitroglycerin? How many nitroglycerin tablets does it take to relieve chest pain?

SHORTNESS OF BREATH (DYSPNEA, ORTHOPNEA)

- What types of activities bring on the shortness of breath? How much activity? Does the shortness of breath occur more frequently or with less exertion than it did 6 months ago? Does the shortness of breath come on gradually or suddenly? Is it constant or does it come and go? Does your position affect it? Do you awaken from sleep at night because of shortness of breath?

- Does the shortness of breath interfere with your daily activities? How many level blocks can you walk before you become short of breath? How many blocks could you walk 6 months ago? Do you become short of breath walking up stairs?
- How many pillows do you require when you lie down to sleep?

NOCTURIA

- Have you been awakened at night with an urgent need to urinate? How long has this been happening? Have there been any recent changes?

COUGH

- Do you have a cough? *If so:* When did it start? How often do you cough? How would you describe the cough? Hacking? Dry? Barking? Congested? Hoarse? Do you cough up anything? What does it look like? Does the mucus have an unusual smell? Is there blood mixed with the mucus?
- Is your cough associated with position (more coughing when lying down), with anxiety, or with talking or activity? What makes it worse? Is the cough relieved by rest or medications?

RATIONALE

◄ *These questions help distinguish angina from other causes of chest pain.*

◄ *Determine the extent of the problem to help diagnose the possible cause, which may be cardiac or pulmonary in origin. Shortness of breath that awakens the client from sleep (paroxysmal nocturnal dyspnea) occurs in congestive heart failure. The supine position increases intrathoracic blood volume. A weak heart may not be able to handle the increased workload.*

◄ *These data provide a rough indication of the severity of dyspnea.*

◄ *In orthopnea, a person needs a more upright position to breathe. It is important to note exactly how many pillows the client uses.*

◄ *Nocturia occurs with heart failure in individuals who are ambulatory during the day. Lying down at night promotes the reabsorption of fluid and its excretion.*

◄ *Coughing up blood (hemoptysis) is a symptom of mitral stenosis, as well as of pulmonary disorders. Coughing up frothy sputum occurs in congestive heart failure.*

QUESTIONS

RATIONALE

FATIGUE

■ Have you noticed any unusual or persistent fatigue? Is the fatigue worse in the morning or evening? Is it worse at work or home? Do you have trouble keeping up with your friends? Are you too tired to take part in normal activities? Does rest reduce the fatigue? Do you go to bed earlier because you are too tired to stay awake? Do you take vitamin or iron pills? Do you eat foods with iron, such as green leafy vegetables and liver? *For women:* Do you have a heavy menstrual flow?

◄ *When cardiac output is decreased, fatigue results. It is generally worse in the evening. Fatigue due to other causes, for example, psychogenic (depression or anxiety), occurs all day or is worse in the morning and varies by location.*

■ When did you first notice the fatigue? Was the onset sudden or gradual? Have you noted any recent changes in your activity level?

◄ *Note any progression of the fatigue syndrome.*

SYNCOPE

■ What were you doing just before you fainted? Did you feel dizzy? Has this happened to you before? How often? Was there an abrupt onset of fainting? Did you lose consciousness? Was fainting preceded by any other symptom? Nausea? Chest pain? Diaphoresis? Palpitation? Confusion? Numbness? Hunger? Did you have black, tarry bowel movements after fainting?

◄ *These questions attempt to determine whether the cause of fainting is a cardiovascular problem or a neurologic, metabolic, or bleeding problem.*

DEPENDENT LEG EDEMA

■ When did you first notice the swelling in your legs? Are both legs affected equally?

◄ *Localized edema of one leg may be caused by venous insufficiency from varicosities or thrombophlebitis. Edema of both legs may be caused by systemic disease (e.g., heart failure, renal failure, or liver disease).*

■ Does the swelling disappear after a night's sleep?
■ Does elevating your feet reduce the swelling? Do you wear support stockings?

◄ *Edema that increases during day and decreases at night or with elevation may be related to stasis (e.g., heart failure).*

■ Do you have kidney, heart, or liver disease?

◄ *Kidney, heart, or liver disease may be origins of the dependent edema.*

■ Are you short of breath?

◄ *Shortness of breath may be caused by pulmonary edema from excess fluid.*

■ Do you have pain in your legs?

◄ *Edema of the legs can cause pain on palpation.*

■ Do you have sores on your legs?

◄ *Venous insufficiency can produce ulcers.*

■ *For women:* Are you taking oral contraceptives?

◄ *Oral contraceptives may be associated with thrombophlebitis, which may cause localized edema.*

■ Is the swelling associated with your menstrual period?

◄ *Changes in estrogen and progesterone levels can contribute to fluid retention, resulting in dependent edema.*

QUESTIONS

LEG CRAMPS OR PAIN

■ Are you having leg cramps or leg pain? Do your legs feel heavier than usual? *If so:* When did it start? Does it occur more with activity or with rest? Do you notice pain when you elevate your legs or when you lower your legs? Have you recently been injured or had an extensive period of immobility?

■ Describe the leg pain. Is it a burning in the toes? Pain when pointing the toes? Pain in the thighs or buttocks? Charley horses? Aching? Pain over a specific location? Have you noticed any changes in the skin of your legs, such as coldness, pallor, hair loss, sores, redness or warmth over the veins, or visible veins? Have you had any swelling of your feet or legs? *If so:* When did you first notice this? Has it grown worse or better over the last 6 months? When does the swelling occur? Does it persist or go away with rest or elevation? Are both legs equally swollen?

PAST HISTORY

■ Have you had any hypertension? Elevated blood cholesterol or triglyceride levels? Heart murmur? Congenital heart disease or heart defect? Coronary artery disease? Rheumatic fever? Unexplained joint pains as a child or youth? Swollen joints? Inflammatory rheumatism? St. Vitus' dance (Sydenham chorea)? Recurrent tonsillitis? Anemia? Bleeding disease? Diabetes? Other heart disease? Was this treated by surgery or medication? How long ago? When did you last have an ECG, stress ECG, or other heart test?

■ In the last few weeks, have you had dental work or an invasive procedure (e.g., endoscopy)? *If so:* When?

■ In your family, is there a history of diabetes, heart disease, hyperlipidemia, or hypertension? Is there any family history of congenital heart defects? Sudden death, especially among young and middle-aged relatives?

NEWBORNS/INFANTS

■ What was the mother's health status during pregnancy? Did she have rubella during the first trimester? Unexplained fever? Any infections? Did she use drugs (over-the-counter, prescribed, or illicit)? Did she have hypertension?

RATIONALE

◄ *Arterial insufficiency produces pain that worsens with activity, especially prolonged walking. Leg pain is worse when legs are elevated, improved when legs are lowered. The pain is usually relieved quickly (within 2 minutes) when movement ceases. Determine exactly how much activity brings on the pain. Venous insufficiency pain intensifies with prolonged standing or sitting in one position. Pain is worse when legs are lowered, relieved when legs are elevated. Discomfort increases through the day, being worse at the end of the day.*

◄ *Signs that indicate a severe disorder include reddened areas, ulcers, or taut, shiny skin and pain that is not relieved by rest.*

◄ *These data help identify factors contributing to the symptoms previously reported. Innocent or functional murmurs may be asymptomatic and unrelated to structural heart defects. Murmurs caused by heart defects (e.g., valvular stenosis) require further evaluation. Recurrent tonsillitis is associated with scarlet fever, which may lead to rheumatic heart disease.*

◄ *Invasive procedures may allow entry of bacteria (*Streptococcus, *pneumococcus,* or *Staphylococcus) that may cause infective endocarditis.*

◄ *This history identifies nonmodifiable risk factors for heart disease that may contribute to the client's health status.*

◄ *Congenital rubella, fever, and drug use may cause congenital heart defects (e.g., patent ductus arteriosus).*

◄ *Maternal hypertension may contribute to premature birth.*

QUESTIONS

- Have you noticed any breathing changes in the infant? Does the infant breathe more heavily or rapidly than expected while feeding or defecating? Does the infant seem to tire easily while eating? Does the infant take breaks from feeding to catch his or her breath? Does the infant turn blue around his or her mouth while feeding? Is there more widespread or persistent cyanosis (turning blue)? Does this seem related to crying?

- Is the infant gaining weight appropriately? Is he or she growing well? Is he or she achieving developmental milestones as expected? Does the infant tire easily while playing? How many naps does the infant take each day? How long does a nap last? What position does the infant favor for resting? On his or her back? In the knee-chest position?

CHILDREN

- Has the child achieved developmental milestones (physical and cognitive) as expected? Has the child gained weight and height as appropriate? Does he or she tire easily during play? How long does the child play before becoming tired? What activities are tiring? Can he or she keep up with other children? Is he or she reluctant to go out to play because of an inability to keep up? Does the child turn "blue" or become short of breath during activities?
- Does the child take longer-than-usual (for his or her age) naps? Does the child squat instead of sit while at play or watching television? Does the child complain of leg pains during exercise? Headaches? Nosebleeds? Unexplained joint pain?

- Has the child had any unexplained fever? Does the child have frequent respiratory infections? How many per year? How are these treated? Have any been streptococcal infections?
- Is there a brother or sister in the family with a heart defect? Does anyone in the family have a chromosomal anomaly, such as Down syndrome?

PREGNANT WOMEN

- How does your prepregnant blood pressure compare with your current blood pressure? Have you had any associated symptoms of high blood pressure: protein in urine, visual changes, headaches, rapid onset of facial or abdominal edema, or pitting edema in feet and legs after a night of rest? Do you have varicose veins? Are they worse with this pregnancy?

OLDER ADULTS

- Do you have any known heart or lung disease, such as emphysema, hypertension, coronary artery disease, or chronic bronchitis? What medications do you take for this disease?

- Does the heart disease interfere with your normal activities? Have you or your family had to make changes in lifestyle to accommodate the effects of heart disease? Have you noticed any progression of symptoms or changes recently? Are there stairs at home? How many times do you need to climb them each day? Have you experienced any confusion, dizziness, blackouts, or fainting? Have you noticed any palpitations? Do you cough and wheeze often?

RATIONALE

◄ *An infant with congestive heart failure takes only a few ounces during each feeding, becomes short of breath during sucking, may be diaphoretic or cyanotic, falls asleep as if exhausted, and then awakens a short time later, hungry again.*

◄ *Infants with cardiovascular problems have poor weight gain in addition to the poor sleeping pattern noted with feeding disorders.*

◄ *It is important to record the limitations observed during the child's activities. Note any poor weight gain or cyanosis.*

◄ *Squatting relieves dyspnea.*

◄ *Answers to these questions may suggest congenital heart disease.*

◄ *Streptococcal infections may cause rheumatic fever, which is associated with rheumatic heart disease.*

◄ *Early in pregnancy vasodilation may cause decrease in blood pressure and syncope, especially when changing positions. Later in pregnancy the blood volume of the mother increases. Women who have hypertension before pregnancy must be managed closely during their pregnancies.*

◄ *These diseases of the cardiovascular and respiratory systems may contribute to altered perfusion or ventilation.*

◄ *Cardiorespiratory diseases may interfere with activities of daily living.*

◄ *Decreased perfusion of the brain can cause confusion, dizziness, or fainting.*

EXAMINATION Procedures and Findings

Guidelines Assessing the cardiovascular system involves collecting data about arteries (blood pressure, pulses, and bruits), veins, precordium, and heart sounds. In this chapter these assessment techniques are discussed in this order; however, when integrating them into a physical examination, the examiner probably will not perform these techniques in the order presented here. For example, the temporal pulses will be palpated during the examination of the head, and the popliteal, posterior tibial, and dorsalis pedis pulses will be palpated when examining the legs and feet. When assessing the heart, use the techniques of inspection, palpation, and auscultation. (Percussion of the heart is an optional technique.)

EQUIPMENT   Stethoscope, with a bell and diaphragm (*Note:* For children, the diaphragm and bell may be smaller.)
Sphygmomanometer with appropriately sized cuff
Tape measure (paper or cloth; for circumference of limbs when edema occurs)
Marking pen or pencil and centimeter ruler (optional; used if cardiac percussion performed)

TECHNIQUES and NORMAL FINDINGS

ABNORMAL FINDINGS

EVALUATE the client's General Condition. Observe the client while he or she is lying supine or at an elevation of 30° to 45°. The client should achieve a relaxed, comfortable posture and have deep, even respirations.

■ Abnormal findings include the sensation of pain, coughing, choking, or smothering, with an inability to lie flat for an extended period of time; uneven, shallow, or gasping respirations with inadequate exchange of gases; cyanosis or gray pallor to the skin; mottling; or abnormal color around the lips, neck, or upper chest.

ARTERIAL ASSESSMENT: BLOOD PRESSURE

PALPATE, then AUSCULTATE the brachial artery to Evaluate Arterial Blood Pressure in both arms. (See Chapter 6 for procedure). Blood pressure will vary with sex, body weight, and time of day, but the upper limits for adults are 140 mmHg systolic, 90 mmHg diastolic, and 30 to 40 mmHg pulse pressure. The pressure should not vary more than 5 to 10 mmHg systolic between the two arms (Fig. 15-9).

■ Note elevated systolic or diastolic pressures; widened or narrowed pulse pressures; and lowered systolic or diastolic pressures. Also note significant discrepancies in measurements between the two arms.

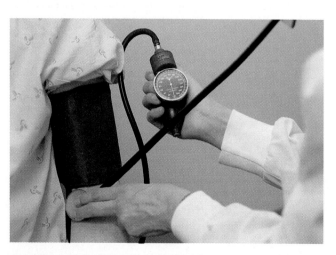

Fig. 15-9   Assessing blood pressure.

TECHNIQUES and NORMAL FINDINGS

ABNORMAL FINDINGS

 Racial Variation

African Americans have generally higher blood pressure readings than whites. These higher readings are thought to be related to differences in renin activity and the regulation of angiotensin II, which acts as a vasoconstrictor. African Americans also retain sodium and chloride better in heat-related situations than do whites.

If the client offers a history of syncope or dizziness or is taking antihypertensive medications, measure the client's blood pressure and heart rate while he or she is sitting, standing, and lying. On standing, pressure may drop 10 to 15 mmHg systolic and 5 mmHg diastolic.

If the pedal, popliteal, and femoral pulses are weak or absent, measure blood pressure in both legs. The systolic pressure in the popliteal artery should be 5 to 15 mmHg higher than that in the brachial artery. The diastolic readings should be the same or similar.

- A decrease in systolic blood pressure greater than 20 mmHg and symptoms such as dizziness indicate orthostatic (postural) hypotension. Diastolic pressure may decrease also. This may be due to fluid volume deficiency, drugs (e.g., antihypertensives), or prolonged bed rest.
- Note any systolic pressure that is lower in the leg(s) than the arm(s). Arterial occlusion of the aorta or femoral or popliteal arteries may decrease perfusion to the lower extremities.

ARTERIAL ASSESSMENT: PULSES

— outline or shape

PALPATE each of the nine arterial pulses for Rate, Rhythm, Amplitude, and Contour. *p. 28* | strength 0 – 4+ / 2+ = normal

Rate: 60 to 100 beats per minute (bpm) (conditioned athletes may be as low as 50 bpm). *temporal, carotid, radial, brachial, femoral, popliteal, posterior tibial, dorsalis pedis, apical*

Rhythm: Regular, that is, equal spacing between beats.

Amplitude: Easily palpable, smooth upstroke. Compare the strength of upper extremity pulses with lower extremity and the left with the right (see box below).

Pulse Amplitude Ratings	
0+	Absent
1+	Diminished, barely palpable
2+	Normal
3+	Full volume
4+	Full volume, bounding hyperkinetic

- Rates above 100 bpm (tachycardia) or below 60 bpm (bradycardia) are abnormal, although recent exertion, smoking, or anxiety will elevate the pulse.
- Irregular rhythms without any pattern should be noted. Coupled beats (two beats that occur close together) are abnormal.
- Note any exaggerated or bounding upstroke or, conversely, pulses that are weak, small, or thready, or where the peak is prolonged. Upstrokes should not vary (seen in pulsus alternans). The force of the beat should not be reduced during inspiration (known as paradoxical pulse) (Table 15-1).

TABLE 15-1	Arterial Pulse Abnormalities	

TYPE	DESCRIPTION	POSSIBLE CAUSES
Diminished, weak, hypokinetic	Pulse is difficult to feel, easily obliterated by the fingers, and may fade out Pulse is slow to rise, has a sustained summit, and falls slowly If both weak and variable in amplitude, pulse is termed "thready"	Hypovolemia Depressed left ventricular function (low ejection fraction) Aortic stenosis
Increased, strong, bounding, hyperkinetic	Pulse is readily palpable, not easily obliterated by fingers, and does not fade Pulse is felt as a brisk impact; can occur with or without increased pulse pressure	Exercise Fever Rigid arterial walls and systolic hypertension Hyperthyroidism (in combination with normal pulse pressure) Chronic severe mitral regurgitation
Water-hammer, collapsing	Pulse has greater amplitude than normal pulse Pulse marked by rapid rise to a narrow summit followed by a sudden descent	Chronic aortic regurgitation Patent ductus arteriosus
Pulsus bisferiens (double-peaked)	Best felt by palpating carotid artery Two systolic peaks can occur in disorders that cause rapid left ventricular ejection of large stroke volume with wide pulse pressure	Aortic regurgitation Large left-to-right shunt Patent ductus arteriosus Hypertrophic obstructive cardiomyopathy
Pulsus alternans	Pulses have large amplitude beats followed by pulses of small amplitude Rhythm remains normal	Depressed left ventricular function
Bigeminal pulse	Normal pulses are followed by premature contractions Amplitude of premature contraction is less than that of normal pulse Rhythm is irregular	Dysrhythmias Premature ventricular contraction
Pulsus paradoxus	Pattern is exaggerated (>10 mmHg) during inspiration, and amplitude is increased during expiration Heart rate and rhythm are unchanged	Cardiac tamponade Constrictive pericarditis Pulmonary emphysema (noncardiac)

Modified from Canobbio MM: Cardiovascular disorders, *St Louis, 1990, Mosby.*

TECHNIQUES and NORMAL FINDINGS

Contour: Smooth and rounded, a series of pulse strokes unvaried, symmetric responses. (*Note:* There may be a slight transient increase in rate during inspiration, especially in clients younger than 40.)

Palpate arteries using the finger pads of the first two fingers. Simultaneous palpation for comparison is customary unless contraindicated.

Temporal: Palpate over the temporal bone on each side of the head lateral to each eyebrow (Fig. 15-10).

Carotid: Palpate along medial edge of sternocleidomastoid muscle in lower third of the neck. Palpate one carotid pulse at a time to avoid reducing bloodflow to the brain (Fig. 15-11).

Auscultate the carotid artery for bruits using the bell of the stethoscope. Ask client to hold breath while you listen. Normally you hear no sound over these arteries (Fig. 15-12).

Apical: Palpate over the apex of the heart at the fourth or fifth intercostal space, left midclavicular line (Fig. 15-13).

The pulse can be assessed as part of the palpation of the heart.

ABNORMAL FINDINGS

■ Note any asymmetry in force or pulse contour, as well as any increased resistance to compression.

■ Bruits are low-pitched blowing sounds usually heard during systole that indicate a narrowing of the vessel by arteriosclerosis. Other arteries to listen to are the temporal, abdominal, aortic, renal, and femoral arteries.

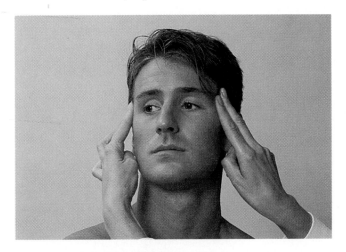

Fig. 15-10 Palpating temporal pulse.

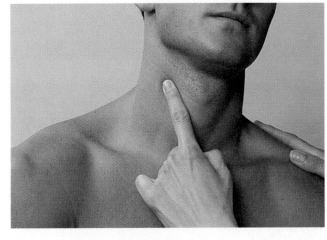

Fig. 15-11 Palpating carotid pulse.

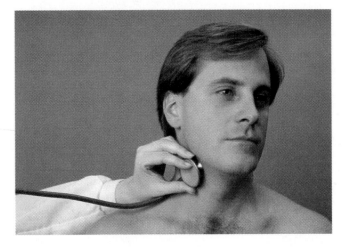

Fig. 15-12 Auscultating carotid pulse. *(From Canobbio, 1990.)*

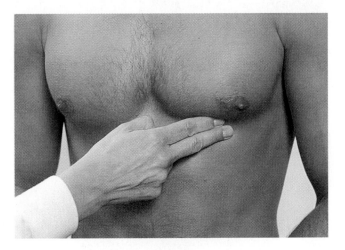

Fig. 15-13 Palpating apical pulse.

Brachial: Palpate in the groove between the biceps and triceps muscle just medial to the biceps tendon at the antecubital fossa (in the bend of the elbow) (Fig. 15-14).

Radial: Palpate at the radial or thumb side of the forearm at the wrist (Fig. 15-15).

Femoral: Palpate below the inguinal ligament, midway between the symphysis pubis and anterior superior iliac. Firm compression may be needed for obese clients (Fig. 15-16).

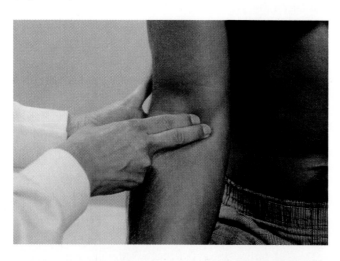

Fig. 15-14   Palpating brachial pulse.

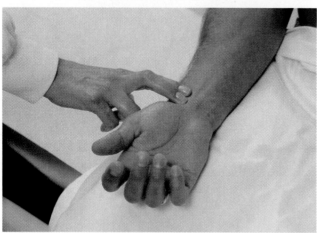

Fig. 15-15   Palpating radial pulse.

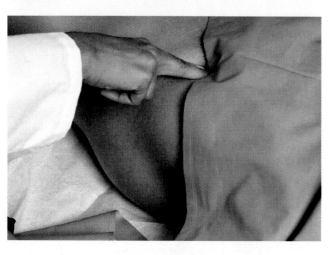

Fig. 15-16   Palpating femoral pulse.   *(From Canobbio, 1990.)*

Popliteal: Palpate behind the knee in the popliteal fossa (Fig. 15-17). This pulse may be difficult to find.

Posterior tibial: Palpate on the inner aspect of the ankle behind and slightly below the medial malleolus (ankle bone) (Fig. 15-18).

Dorsalis pedis: Palpate lightly over the dorsum of the foot between the extension tendons of the first and second toe (Fig. 15-19). (This pulse may be difficult to find or absent in normal persons.)

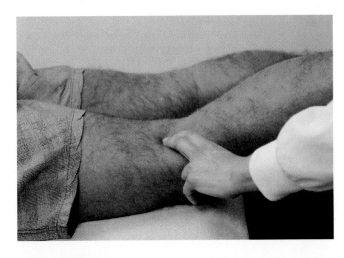

Fig. 15-17   Palpating popliteal pulse.

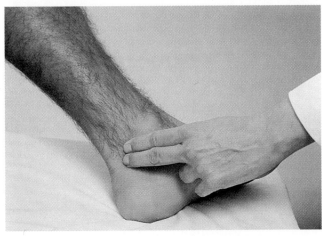

Fig. 15-18   Palpating posterior tibial pulse.

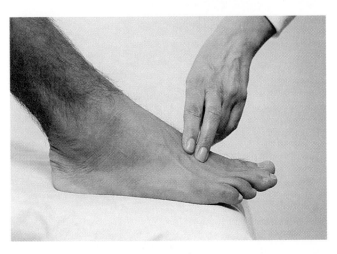

Fig. 15-19   Palpating dorsalis pedis pulse.

TECHNIQUES and NORMAL FINDINGS

ARTERIAL ASSESSMENT: SKIN, HAIR, AND NAILS

INSPECT and PALPATE the extremities for Appearance, Color, Temperature, Hair Distribution, and Capillary Refill. There may normally be no hair over the digits or dorsum of the hands and feet. The skin should be pink or brown (as appropriate) and warm with no evidence of edema. Gently squeeze pads of fingers and toes until they blanche. Release pressure and observe capillary refill, i.e., how many seconds it takes for original color to appear; should be less than 4 seconds.

Nails should be pink, with an angle of 160° at the nail bed.

If arterial insufficiency is suspected, have the client lie down. Elevate his or her legs 12 inches (30 cm) above the level of the heart. Then ask the client to move his or her feet up and down at the ankles for 60 seconds. The feet should exhibit mild pallor. Next have the client sit up and dangle the legs. Original color should return in about 10 seconds, with the foot veins filling up in about 15 seconds. (*Note:* This can also be done with the arms and hands.)

ABNORMAL FINDINGS

■ Note an obviously reduced amount or lack of hair peripherally or skin that appears thin, shiny, and taut. Cold extremities in a warm environment and mild edema are also abnormal. Note marked pallor or mottling when the extremity is elevated or any ulcerated digit tips. There should not be tenderness on palpation or the sensation of "stocking anesthesia," wherein the legs feel numb in a pattern resembling the area covered by a sock.

■ Clubbing of nails (angle disappears, becoming >160°) indicates chronic cyanosis (Fig. 15-20).

■ Note any marked pallor in one or both feet, any delayed return of color or mottled appearance, delay in filling of the veins, or marked redness in the dependent foot (or hand).

Clubbing—early

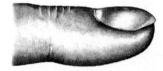

Clubbing—middle

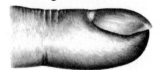

Clubbing—severe

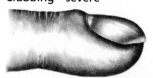

Fig. 15-20 Clubbing of fingers.
(From Canobbio, 1990.)

TECHNIQUES and NORMAL FINDINGS	ABNORMAL FINDINGS

VENOUS ASSESSMENT

INSPECT jugular vein for Pulsations. Inspect both sides of the client's neck for venous pressure as he or she lies at a 30° to 45° angle. Elevate the client's chin slightly and tilt the head away from the side being examined. <u>Illuminate the jugular veins for pulsations</u> with a tangential light source, such as a penlight (Fig. 15-21).

■ Note any fluttering or oscillating of the pulsations. Note irregular rhythms or unusually prominent waves. These may indicate right-sided heart failure.

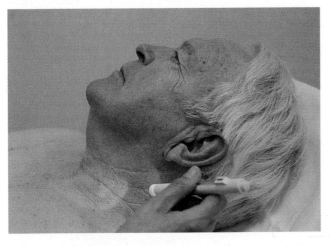

Fig. 15-21 Tangential light to view jugular veins and pulsations.

ESTIMATE Jugular Venous Pressure. <u>Identify the highest point at which the jugular vein blood level or pulsations can be seen.</u> Use the sternal angle as a reference point ("zero") to estimate jugular venous pressure in centimeters. This pressure should not rise more than 1 inch (2 cm) above the sternal angle. (*Note:* If you cannot find the jugular vein, have the client lie down flat for a few minutes so that it will distend) (Fig. 15-22).

■ Note if the jugular venous pressure exceeds 1 inch (2 cm) above the level of the manubrium. (*Note:* If venous pressure is elevated, meaning that the vein is distended up to the neck, the client's head is raised until the highest jugular pulsation can be detected. The distance in inches above the sternal angle and the angle at which the client is reclining should be recorded.) Also note if other veins in the neck, shoulder, or upper chest are distended.

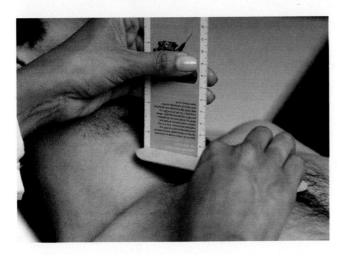

Fig. 15-22 Measuring jugular venous pressure. *(From Canobbio, 1990.)*

TECHNIQUES and NORMAL FINDINGS

Pulsations should be regular, soft, and of an undulating quality. The level of pulsation decreases with inspiration, and the pulsation increases in recumbent position.

Inspect and palpate the legs for the presence or appearance of superficial veins. There should be distention in the dependent position, and the venous valves may appear as nodular bulges. The veins collapse with elevation of the limbs.

Inspect and palpate the thigh and calf for surface characteristics. The legs should be symmetric, nontender, and without excess warmth.

Sharply dorsiflex the client's foot (with the knee slightly flexed) to assess the calf pain response. No pain should be reported.

INSPECT and PALPATE the extremities for evidence of Skin Turgor, Color, and Skin Integrity. Skin turgor should be elastic without tenting or edema. Color is as appropriate for race. Skin integrity is intact without lesions.

ABNORMAL FINDINGS

- Note any fluttering or oscillating of the pulsation. Note irregular rhythms or unusually prominent waves.
- Note if there are distended veins in the anteromedial aspect of the thigh and lower leg or on the posterolateral aspect of the calf from the knee to the ankle.
- Note any swelling of one or both legs (especially if one calf appears larger than the other), tenderness on palpation, warmth, or redness. Measure any apparent swelling of the thighs and calves with a tape measure to ensure accuracy. Measure at the widest point; measure the other leg in the same location.
- If pain results, this is known as <u>Homan's sign</u> and may indicate thrombophlebitis.

- Peripheral cyanosis, edema (bilaterally or unilaterally; see Table 15-2 for interpretation), pigmentation around the ankles, thickening skin, or ulceration, especially around the ankles, are abnormal findings. Varicose veins appear as dilated, often tortuous, veins when legs are in a dependent position.

TABLE 15-2	Pitting Edema Scale	
SCALE	**DEGREE**	**RESPONSE**
1+ Trace	Slight	Rapid
2+ Mild	0-0.6 cm (0-0.25 inch)	10-15 seconds
3+ Moderate	0.6-1.3 cm (0.25-0.5 inch)	1-2 minutes
4+ Severe	1.3-2.5 cm (0.5-1 inch)	2-5 minutes

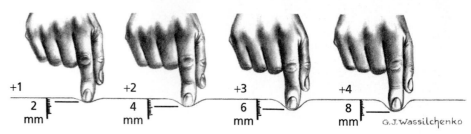

From Canobbio MM: Cardiovascular disorders, *St Louis, 1990, Mosby.*

TECHNIQUES and NORMAL FINDINGS	ABNORMAL FINDINGS

Perform the Trendelenburg test to evaluate venous competence. With client in supine position, lift one leg above the level of the heart until the leg veins are empty. Lower the leg quickly.

- ■ If the veins fill slowly, the veins are competent; rapid filling indicates incompetent veins.

🌐 Racial Variation

African Americans have fewer varicosities than whites. This finding is probably related to the greater number of venous valves present in most African Americans.

CARDIAC ASSESSMENT

INSPECT the anterior chest wall for Contour, Pulsations, Lifts, Heaves, or Retractions. Provide modesty and privacy while inspecting the client's unclothed chest. Movement may be subtle. Use tangential light to inspect client's chest at eye level. Chest should be rounded and symmetric. Slight retraction medial to the left midclavicular line at the fourth or fifth intercostal space is normal; this is the apical impulse.

- ■ Note any kyphosis, sternal depression, or asymmetry.
- ■ Marked retraction of apical space may indicate pericardial disease or right ventricular hypertrophy.

INSPECT the apical impulse for Visible Pulsations. Pulse may be visible only when client sits up and leans forward, bringing the heart closer to the anterior chest. It may be obscured by obesity, large breasts, and muscularity.

- ■ Apical pulsation may be observed after exertion, in hyperthyroidism, or in left ventricular hypertrophy. Pulsations may be displaced left, right, or downward due to cardiac anomalies or change in heart size.

PALPATE the precordium for Pulsations, Thrills, Lifts, and Heaves using the palmar surface of the hand and finger pads. Supine is the preferred position for cardiac palpation; however, the sitting position may be necessary to feel impulses. Use a gentle touch, allowing the movements of the chest to lift the hands. Respiratory movements should be even.

Palpate systematically from the base to the apex or from apex to base. The former sequence is described on the next page.

- ■ Note whether the entire chest seems to lift or heave with the heartbeat. A *thrill* is a palpable vibration over the precordium or artery; it feels like touching a purring cat's stomach. A thrill is a palpable manifestation of a murmur. A *lift* feels like a more sustained thrust than an expected apical pulse. A *heave* feels like an excessive thrust of the heart against the chest wall during systole. A lift or heave may indicate left ventricular enlargement.

Abbreviations	
ICS	intercostal space
RICS	right intercostal space
LICS	left intercostal space
SB	sternal border
RSB	right sternal border
LSB	left sternal border
MCL	midclavicular line
RMCL	right midclavicular line
LMCL	left midclavicular line

TECHNIQUES and NORMAL FINDINGS

Palpate the aortic valve area over second intercostal space (ICS), right sternal border (RSB) for pulsations.

Palpate the pulmonic valve area (base) over second ICS, left sternal border (LSB) for pulsations (Fig. 15-23, *A*).

Palpate the LSB (Fig. 15-23, *B*) to assess right ventricle (RV) function. The RV is best felt with the heel of the hand between the third, fourth, and fifth left ICS.

Palpate the apical pulse (mitral valve area) for rate, rhythm, lift, and heave, using finger pads of right hand. Palpate over the apex at the fifth ICS midclavicular line (MCL) (Fig. 15-23, *C*). This is the point of maximum impulse (PMI). Apical pulse has small amplitude, brief duration, and is no larger than 2 to 3 cm in diameter.

ABNORMAL FINDINGS

■ Pulsations may indicate an aortic aneurysm. A thrill may be associated with aortic valve stenosis.

■ Sustained lifts or palpations may indicate RV hypertrophy; pulsations may indicate pulmonary hypertension. A thrill is associated with pulmonic valve stenosis.

■ Forceful pulsation, displaced laterally or downward associated with increased cardiac output or left ventricular hypertrophy. *Presence of a thrill indicates a murmur.*

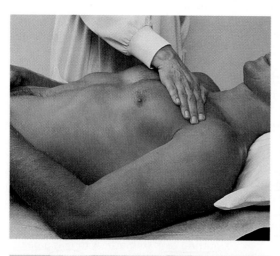

A

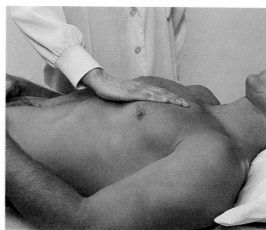

B

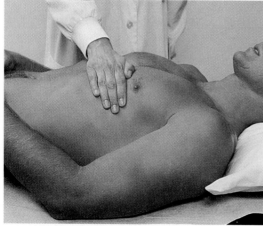

C

Fig. 15-23 Palpation of precordium. **A,** Palpating base. **B,** Palpating left sternal border. **C,** Palpating apex.

Palpate the epigastric area for pulsations. There should be an aortic pulsation with forward thrust and right ventricular pulsation with downward thrust.

■ Bounding pulsations may indicate abdominal aortic aneurysm or aortic valve regurgitation.

TECHNIQUES and NORMAL FINDINGS

ABNORMAL FINDINGS

PERCUSS the heart borders for the Heart Size. (This is an *optional* assessment technique, because chest x-rays provide more precise information.) Percussion is performed at the third, fourth, and fifth ICS from the left anterior axillary line to the right anterior axillary line. The expected finding is a change from resonance to dullness about 6 cm lateral to the left of the sternum. The areas of dullness are marked with a pencil and the distance from the sternum measured with a ruler. Percussion of the heart may be difficult with obese or large-breasted clients.

- ■ Deviation of the left border further to the left is associated with dilated LV, right pneumothorax, or pericardial effusion. Deviation of the left border to the right is associated with dextrocardia or left pneumothorax.

AUSCULTATION

AUSCULTATE S₁ and S₂ heart sounds for Rate, Rhythm, Pitch, and Splitting. (See box for technique for auscultation of the heart). Use the diaphragm and bell to listen at each of the five auscultatory areas. The sounds generated by valve closure are best heard where blood flows away from the valve instead of directly over the valve area (Fig. 15-24). Heart sounds are low-pitched, making them difficult to hear. When first learning heart sounds, the examiner may want to close her or his eyes to concentrate on each specific sound. Begin with the client sitting upright. A systematic approach is used to listen in the five auscultatory areas, with the client breathing normally and then holding the breath in expiration. This allows you to hear the heart sounds better. Begin with the aortic valve area (second ICS, RSB) (Fig. 15-25, *A*), then the pulmonic valve area (second ICS, LSB) (Fig. 15-25, *B*), then Erb's point (third ICS, LSB) (Fig. 15-25, *C*), tricuspid valve area (fourth ICS, LSB) (Fig. 15-25, *D*), and finally the mitral valve area/apical pulse (fifth ICS, left MCL) (Fig. 15-25, *E*).

Rate: Count the apical heart rate. Normal range is 60 to 90 beats per minute; conditioned athletes or joggers may have slower rates normally.

Rhythm: Heart rate is regular.

- ■ Note rates that are over 100 or under 60 beats per minute.
- ■ Irregular, nonpatterned rhythm or sporadic extra beats or pauses between beats should be noted.

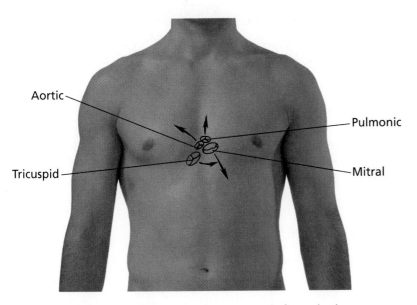

Fig. 15-24   Transmission of closure sounds from the heart valves.

A

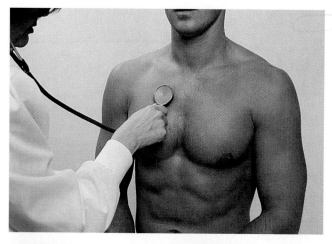

B

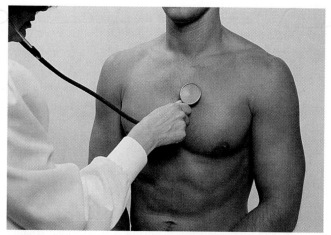

C

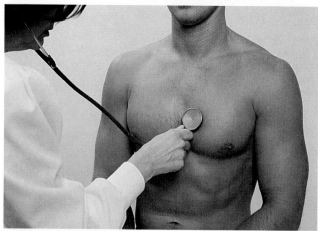

D

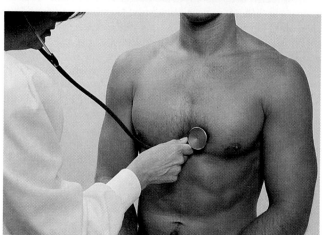

E

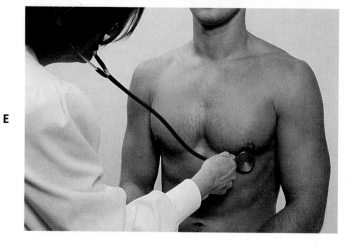

Fig. 15-25 Position for cardiac auscultation. **A,** Aortic area. **B,** Pulmonic area. **C,** Erb's point. **D,** Tricuspid area. **E,** Mitral area.

TECHNIQUES and NORMAL FINDINGS

ABNORMAL FINDINGS

Technique for Locating Intercostal Spaces for Auscultation of the Heart

A systematic approach is needed for this assessment. Some examiners begin at the apex and proceed upward toward the base of the heart, while others begin at the base and proceed downward toward the apex. The sequence is irrelevant as long as the assessment is systematic. Listen first with the diaphragm to hear high-pitched sounds, then with the bell to hear low-pitched sounds.

■ When auscultating from base to apex, begin at the second intercostal space (ICS). Locate this ICS by palpating the right sternoclavicular joint (where the left clavicle joins the sternum.)

■ Palpate the first rib and then move down to palpate the space between the first and second ribs; this is the first ICS.

■ Continue palpating downward to the space between the second and third ribs. This is the second ICS at the right sternal border (RSB), the auscultatory site for the aortic value area. This is not the anatomic site of the aortic valve, but the site on the chest wall where sounds produced by the valves are heard best.

■ Moving to the left side of the sternum at the second ICS, the area for auscultating the pulmonic valve area is found.

■ Remaining at the LSB, move the stethoscope down to the third ICS, which is called Erb's point, an area to which pulmonic or aortic sound frequently radiate. The fourth ICS, LSB is over the tricuspid valve area.

■ At the fifth ICS, move the stethoscope laterally to the left midclavicular line, where the mitral valve area is located.

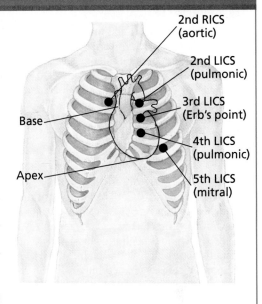

2nd RICS (aortic)
2nd LICS (pulmonic)
3rd LICS (Erb's point)
Base
4th LICS (pulmonic)
Apex
5th LICS (mitral)

First heart sound (S$_1$) is made by the closing of the mitral (M$_1$) and tricuspid (T$_1$) valves. (When the heart sounds are described as "lubb-dubb", the "lubb" represents S$_1$.) This heart sound should be heard at all sites; often louder at the apex; usually lower in pitch than the second heart sound; almost synchronous with the carotid impulse; splitting heard occasionally in the tricuspid area with deep inspiration and varies from beat to beat, occasionally heard as a narrow split.

■ Note if the first heart sound appears accented, diminished or muffled, or varying in intensity with different beats. Observe whether the frequency (pitch) becomes higher with accented intensity. Note that the fourth heart sound is sometimes mistaken for the splitting of the first heart sound.

Second heart sound (S$_2$) is made by the closing of the aortic (A$_2$) and pulmonic (P$_2$) valves. (S$_2$ is the "dubb" of the "lubb-dubb" heart sound.) This heart sound usually heard at all sites; often louder at the base where the aortic and pulmonic sites are auscultated; usually higher in pitch than the first heart sound; duration shorter than with the first heart sound; splitting (physiologic splitting) is commonly heard in the pulmonic area on inspiration in young adults and usually disappears on expiration.

■ Note any increased intensity, especially in the aortic or pulmonary areas, or any decreased intensity. Wide, fixed, or paradoxic splitting are abnormal.

■ One form of pathologic splitting is *paradoxic* or *reversed* splitting that appears on expiration and disappears on inspiration. The most common cause is a left bundle branch block.

Palpation and auscultation may be repeated with the patient lying in the left decubitus position and sitting.

■ See box on page 387 for discussion of abnormal heart sounds.

NEWBORNS/INFANTS

■ APPROACH

Examine the heart within the first 24 hours of birth and again at 2 to 3 days to assess changes from fetal to systemic and pulmonic circulation. Auscultation of the heart must be done when the client is quiet. Thus it may be performed out of sequence when the examiner can take advantage of a happy, quiet infant. The stethoscope used must have a small diaphragm and bell to detect specific cardiac sounds of the newborn or infant.

■ FINDINGS

Skin and Mucous Membranes

Pallor suggests shock, and purplish skin tone may indicate polycythemia. While central cyanosis may indicate congenital heart defects, acrocyanosis (cyanosis of hands and feet) without central cyanosis is of little concern and usually disappears within hours to days of birth. Note if cyanosis increases with crying or sucking. Severe cyanosis that appears shortly after birth may indicate transposition of great vessels, tetralogy of Fallot, a severe septal defect, or severe pulmonic stenosis. Cyanosis that appears after the first month of life suggests pulmonic stenosis, tetralogy of Fallot, or large septal defects.

Heart

The apical impulse of the newborn normally is felt in the fourth or fifth ICS just medial to the midclavicular line. Note any enlargement of the heart and the position of the heart if the infant is having dyspnea. A pneumothorax shifts the apical impulse away from the area of the chest where the pneumothorax is located. The infant's heart may be shifted to the right by a diaphragmatic hernia commonly found on the left. Dextrocardia causes the apical impulse to be on the right.

Weak or thin pulses may be due to decreased cardiac output or peripheral vasoconstriction. Bounding pulses may indicate a patent ductus arteriosus creating a left-to-right shunt. Coarctation of the heart is suspected when the femoral pulses are absent or there is a difference in pulse amplitude between upper extremities or between femoral and radial pulses. Blood pressure measurement is difficult to obtain for newborns and young infants. Electronic sphygmomanometers with a Doppler technique are relatively sensitive and useful for this age group. Capillary refill in infants is very rapid—less than 1 second. Prolonged refill times (more than 2 seconds) may indicate dehydration or hypovolemic shock.

Splitting of heart sounds is common in infants until about 48 hours after birth due to the transition from fetal circulation to systemic and pulmonic circulation. Innocent murmurs, Grade I or II, accompanied by no other signs or symptoms frequently disappear within 2 to 3 days. Murmurs that persist after 3 days or radiate must be referred for further evaluation. If the examiner pushes on the infant's liver, the pressure to the right atria is increased. Murmur with a left-to-right shunt through a septal opening or patent ductus will disappear briefly with pressure to the liver, while murmurs of right-to-left shunt will increase. Auscultate the infant's head and abdomen for bruits to detect arteriovenous malformations.

CHILDREN

■ APPROACH

Auscultation can be difficult and requires a quiet, extremely cooperative child. Although the child's chest is auscultated in the same areas as the adult's, it may take a considerably longer time to be sure of the sounds, which may be upsetting to the parents. Explanations should be given in advance. All of the techniques used require that the child wear only underwear and sit on the table or the caregiver's lap. Cooperative children may recline at a 45° angle. If this is not possible, the child may lie supine to allow the examiner to hear more cardiovascular "sounds."

■ FINDINGS

Position. Squatting may be a compensatory position for a child with a heart defect.

Skin. Cyanosis or pallor may indicate poor perfusion due to congenital heart defects. Note if there is more cyanosis with crying, facial edema, or pedal edema. Note signs of poor feeding, which may indicate a heart problem.

Respirations. Labored respirations could indicate a cardiovascular problem.

Blood pressure. Coarctation of the aorta may be indicated by a systolic pressure in the thigh lower than that in the arm.

Pulse. If an irregular rhythm is noted, have the child hold his or her breath while you continue to feel the pulse; it should become regular. A child's pulse may normally increase on inspiration and decrease on expiration. If the child has suggestive symptomatology, palpate the radial artery, popliteal, dorsalis pedis, posterior tibial, and femoral pulses. Note differences between pulses, particularly the radial and femoral. Weak or absent femoral pulses may indicate coarctation of the aorta.

Venous hum (vibration heard over the jugular vein) is caused by turbulent blood flow in the jugular vein and is an expected finding in children. Auscultate with the bell of the stethoscope over the right supraclavicular space at the medial end of the clavicle along the anterior border of the sternocleidomastoid muscle (Fig. 15-26). Hum is a continuous, low-pitched sound louder during diastole. It may be stopped by gentle pressure between the trachea and the sternocleidomastoid muscle at the level of the thyroid cartilage.

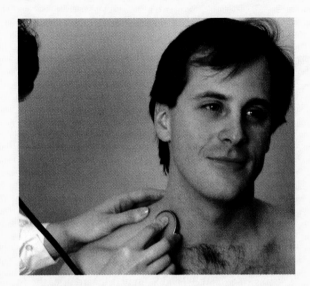

Fig. 15-26 Auscultation for venous hum. *(From Canobbio, 1990.)*

OLDER ADULTS

■ APPROACH

Some expected physiologic changes of aging alter the cardiovascular system and must be distinguished from pathologic findings. The heart of healthy older clients often becomes smaller, with enlargement due to hypertension or other diseases of the heart or vessels. Cardiac output decreases 30% to 40% by 65 to 70 years of age, but the body's general atrophy and reduced exertion also reduce the need for greater output. In general, the aging heart functions well under normal conditions, but may be unable to compensate for extremes of stress, blood loss, tachycardia, unusual exertion, or fever.

■ FINDINGS

Older adults may have variations in heart rate. It may be slower due to increased vagal tone or more rapid, with a range from the low 40s to greater than 100 per minute. Occasional ectopic beats are common and may or may not be significant. The S_4 heart sound is common in older adults and may be associated with decreased left ventricular compliance.

Systemic blood pressure increases with age due to stiffness of the aorta. Check the pressure in both arms when the client is lying down and when standing up. A maximum of 160 mmHg systolic may be within normal limits if it remains stable over time and the client has no symptoms or evidence of end-organ damage. Pressures in both arms should not vary more than 5 to 10 mmHg systolic. Systolic pressure that drops more than 20 mmHg may result in postural or orthostatic hypotension.

Systolic murmurs: Soft, early systolic murmurs may be "functional" in elderly clients. They are often found and represent the effects of aortic lengthening, tortuosity, and sclerotic changes. Note loud aortic (ejection) murmurs that radiate into the neck, which can indicate obstructive aortic disease. Systolic murmurs heard at the apex may indicate mitral calcification.

CLIENTS WITH SITUATIONAL VARIATIONS

PREGNANT WOMEN

■ APPROACH

For the pregnant client there are two heart rates to assess: maternal and fetal. The fetal heart can be heard by Doppler at 12 weeks and by fetoscope at 16 weeks. The procedure for fetal heart tones is in Chapter 6. Blood pressure should be measured throughout pregnancy because pregnancy-induced hypertension may occur.

■ FINDINGS

Dyspnea, orthopnea, fatigue, and palpitations may be attributed to the pregnancy, but should be evaluated for other causes.

Heart rate increases 10 to 15 beats per minute in adjusting to the increased blood volume. The heart itself shifts transversely in response to the positions of the uterus and diaphragm. Audible murmurs, splitting of S_1 and S_2, and S_3 may be heard after the twentieth week of gestation.

Preexisting cardiac conditions may have pronounced symptoms due to the pregnancy-induced increased volume.

Blood pressure may decrease in the second trimester and then return to the usual level during the third trimester. Report blood pressure exceeding 140/90 mmHg (pregnancy-induced hypertension) or hypertension that occurs before the twentieth week and worsens, especially during the third trimester (risk of cerebral hemorrhage).

Vascular changes causing faintness, palpatations, sweating, or pallor when lying on the back are due to pressure from the uterus on the vessels (supine hypotension syndrome).

Edema of the legs and increased varicosities may occur due to increased blood volume, decreased venous tone, or pressure on the inferior vena cava.

After delivery, cardiac function should return to normal. The heart should shift back toward normal position; supine hypotension ceases; pressure by the uterus is relieved from the vena cava; and bradycardia (40 to 50 beats per minute) may occur early in the postpartum period.

Note any signs of heart failure (cardiac patients are at most risk 1 to 3 days after delivery). Note low blood pressure or tachycardia occurring during this period.

CLIENTS WITH DIABETES MELLITUS

■ FINDINGS

Clients who have insulin-dependent diabetes mellitus (IDDM) are at risk for cardiovascular diseases. Diabetes mellitus causes an increase in the basement membrane of capillaries, which makes these vessels more narrow. This narrowing contributes to hypertension, as well as impaired perfusion to the lower extremities. Additionally, diabetes causes increases in platelet adhesion, blood clot size, and clotting factors, which increases the risk of thrombus formation. To minimize the effects of these changes, clients with diabetes must keep their blood glucose levels within normal range with diet, exercise, and insulin therapy. Fluid intake of at least 3 liters daily will help reduce blood viscosity, thereby minimizing blood clotting. These clients may have decreased sensation of chest pain. Any complaints of chest pain must be thoroughly evaluated.

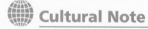 Cultural Note

Diabetes is ranked as the seventh leading cause of death in the United States. The incidence of diabetes mellitus varies greatly among various cultural groups. American Indians and Alaskan Natives have an incidence 10 times that of the general population. Pima Indians over age 35 have a 1:2 incidence rate. Hispanics have a rate 3 times that of the general population, and African Americans have a rate 33% higher than whites. Asian Americans have a fairly low incidence of diabetes, but the incidence is higher than their native-born counterparts and is rising.

ETHNIC & CULTURAL VARIATIONS

■ FINDINGS

Racial variations in the cardiovascular system are not widely described in the literature, but higher blood pressure readings from an increase in renin activity and salt retention in African Americans have been documented, as well as the finding that they possess greater numbers of venous valves in the lower legs than whites, which probably contribute to a lower incidence of varicosities.

Disease incidences are greatly affected by cultural variations. American Indians and Alaskan Natives have higher incidences of diabetes and cardiac disease and lower incidences of hypertension. Hispanics have higher rates of diabetes and hypertension. African Americans have higher incidences of diabetes, hypertension, strokes, and coronary artery disease. Asian Americans have a lower rate of diabetes and hypertension.

EXAMINATION SUMMARY
Heart and Peripheral Vascular System

- Evaluate client's general condition

Arterial Assessment (pp. 368-374)

Blood pressure
- Palpate, then auscultate arterial blood pressure in both arms

Pulses
- Palpate each pulse for:
  Rate
  Rhythm
  Amplitude
  Contour
- Auscultate carotid artery for:
  Bruits

Skin, hair, and nails
- Inspect and palpate extremities for:
  Appearance
  Color
  Temperature
  Hair distribution
  Capillary refill

Venous Assessment (pp. 375-376)
- Inspect jugular veins for:
  Pulsations
- Estimate jugular venous pressure
- Inspect and palpate lower extremities for:
  Skin turgor
  Color
  Skin integrity

Cardiac Assessment (pp. 377-381)
- Inspect anterior chest for:
  Contour
  Pulsations
  Lifts
  Heaves
  Retractions
- Palpate precordium for:
  Pulsations
  Thrills
  Lifts
  Heaves
- Percuss heart borders for heart size (optional)
- Auscultate heart sounds over aortic area, pulmonic area, tricuspid area, mitral area, and apical areas for:
  Rate
  Rhythm
  Pitch
  Splitting
  Murmurs
  Extra sounds

COMMON PROBLEMS/CONDITIONS
associated with the Heart and Peripheral Vascular System

CARDIAC DISORDERS

■ **Murmurs:** A series of prolonged sounds heard either during systole or diastole. They are produced by vibrations created by blood flow that becomes agitated as it flows through structural changes or defects in the heart itself, valves, or great vessels. Murmurs are best heard over the auscultatory areas, rather than over the actual heart defect. Table 15-3 shows the classification of cardiac murmurs.

■ **Systolic murmurs:** Murmurs occurring during the ventricular ejection phase of the cardiac cycle. Most systolic murmurs are caused by obstruction of the outflow of semilunar valves or by incompetent AV valves. The vibration is heard during all or part of systole. Other causes of systolic murmurs are structural deformities of the aorta or pulmonary arteries. A ventricular septal defect (discussed below) results in a murmur classified as pansystolic or holosytolic because it occupies all of systole.

TABLE 15-3 Characterization of Heart Murmurs

	CLASSIFICATION	DESCRIPTION
Timing and duration*	Early systolic	Begins with S_1, decrescendoes, ends well before S_2
	Midsystolic (ejection)	Begins after S_1, ends before S_2; crescendo-decrescendo quality sometimes difficult to discern
	Late systolic	Begins mid to late systole, crescendoes, ends at S_2; often introduced by mid to late systolic clicks
	Early diastolic	Begins with S_2
	Middiastolic	Begins at clear interval after S_2
	Late diastolic (presystolic)	Begins immediately before S_1
	Holosystolic (pansystolic)	Begins with S_1, occupies all of systole, ends at S_2
	Holodiastolic (pandiastolic)	Begins with S_2, occupies all of diastole, ends at S_1
	Continuous	Starts in systole, continues without interruption through S_2, into all or part of diastole; does not necessarily persist throughout entire cardiac cycle
Pitch	High, medium, low	Depends on pressure and rate of blood flow; low pitch is heard best with the bell
Intensity†	Grade I	Barely audible in quiet room
	Grade II	Quiet but clearly audible
	Grade III	Moderately loud
	Grade IV	Loud, associated with thrill
	Grade V	Very loud, thrill easily palpable
	Grade VI	Very loud, audible with stethoscope not in contact with chest, thrill palpable and visible
Pattern	Crescendo	Increasing intensity caused by increased blood velocity
	Decrescendo	Decreasing intensity caused by decreased blood velocity
Quality	Harsh, raspy, machine-like, vibratory, musical, blowing	Quality depends on several factors, including degree of valve compromise, force of contractions, blood volume
Location	Anatomic landmarks (e.g., second left intercostal space on sternal border)	Area of greatest intensity, usually area to which valve sounds are normally transmitted
Radiation	Anatomic landmarks (e.g., to axilla)	Site farthest from location of greatest intensity at which sound is still heard; sound usually transmitted in direction of blood flow
Respiratory phase variations	Intensity, quality, and timing may vary	Venous return increases on inspiration and decreases on expiration

*Systolic murmurs are best described according to time of onset and termination; diastolic murmurs are best classified according to time of onset only.
†Discrimination among the six grades is more difficult for the diastolic murmur than for the systolic.
From Seidel HM et al: Mosby's guide to physical examination, ed 3, St Louis, 1995, Mosby.

Abnormal Heart Sounds

Abnormal heart sounds and murmurs are described by where they occur in the cardiac cycle. The normal sequence of events in the cardiac cycle can be diagrammed as shown below:

$$S_1 \rightarrow \text{systole} \rightarrow S_2 \rightarrow \text{diastole} \rightarrow S_1 \rightarrow \text{etc.}$$

To determine if an abnormal sound occurs in systole or diastole, determine if the sound occurs after S_1 or after S_2.

- During diastole, when 80% of the blood in the atria rapidly fills the ventricles, a third heart sound may be heard (S_3). It is often heard at the apex. An S_3 occurs just after the S_2 and lasts about the same time as it takes to say "me too." The "me" is the S_2 and the "too" is the S_3. An S_3 is normal in children and young adults. However, when an S_3 is heard in adults over 30 years of age, it signifies fluid volume overload to the ventricle that may be due to congestive heart failure or mitral or tricuspid regurgitation (Swartz, 1994).

- At the end of diastole, when atrial contraction completes the filling of the ventricle, a fourth heart sound may be heard (S_4). An S_4 occurs just before the S_1 and lasts about the same time as it takes to say "middle." The "mi" is the S_4 and the "ddle" the S_1. An S_4 is normal in children and young adults. However, when an S_4 is heard in adults over 30 years of age, it signifies a noncompliant or "stiff" ventricle. Hypertrophy of the ventricle precedes a noncompliant ventricle. Also, coronary artery disease is a major cause of a stiff ventricle (Swartz, 1994). Useful mnemonics for remembering the cadence and pathophysiology of the third and fourth heart sounds (Swartz, 1994) are as follows.

SLOSH'-ing-in	SLOSH'-ing-in	SLOSH'-ing-in
S_1 S_2 S_3	S_1 S_2 S_3	S_1 S_2 S_3

a-STIFF'-wall	a-STIFF'-wall	a-STIFF'-wall
S_4 S_1 S_2	S_4 S_1 S_2	S_4 S_1 S_2

Another way to remember the cadence of the S_3 and S_4 heart sounds is using the words "Kentucky" and "Tennessee."

Ken-tuck-y	Ken-tuck-y	Ken-tuck-y
S_1 S_2 S_3	S_1 S_2 S_3	S_1 S_2 S_3

Ten-ness-ee	Ten-ness-ee	Ten-ness-ee
S_4 S_1 S_2	S_4 S_1 S_2	S_4 S_1 S_2

Thus the third and fourth heart sounds can be abnormal when they occur in adults over 30. Both sounds occur in diastole.

The opening *snap* caused by the opening of the mitral or tricuspid valves is another abnormal sound heard in diastole when either valve is thickened, stenotic, or deformed. The sounds are high-pitched and occur early in diastole.

- In systole, *ejection clicks* may be heard if either the aortic or pulmonic valve is stenotic or deformed. The aortic valve ejection click is heard at either apex or base of the heart and does not change with respiration. The less common pulmonic valve ejection click is heard over the second or third left ICS. It increases with expiration and decreases with inspiration.

- *Pericardial friction rubs* are caused by inflammation of the layers of the pericardial sac. A rubbing sound is usually present in both diastole and systole and is best heard over the apical area.

■ **Diastolic murmurs:** Murmurs occurring in the filling phase of the cardiac cycle. Incompetent semilunar valves or stenotic AV valves create diastolic murmurs. These murmurs almost always indicate heart disease. Early diastolic murmurs usually result from insufficiency of a semilunar valve or dilation of the valvular ring. Mid- and late-diastolic murmurs are generally caused by narrowed, stenosed mitral and tricuspid valves that obstruct blood flow (Table 15-4).

A loud murmur that is accompanied by a thrill usually indicates a pathologic condition.

TABLE 15-4	Murmurs due to Valvular Defects		
TYPE	**DETECTION**	**QUALITY/PITCH**	**VARIABLES**
Systolic Ejection Murmur	Systole Diastole ... S_1 S_2 S_1 S_2 S_1 S_2		
Aortic Stenosis	Heard over aortic valve area; ejection sound at second right intercostal border. Radiates to neck, down left sternal border.	Medium pitch, coarse, with crescendo-decrescendo pattern. Pitch low.	May radiate as far as apex and to carotid with thrill; S_1 may be followed by ejection click; S_2 soft or absent; S_4 palpable.
Pulmonic Stenosis	Heard over pulmonic valve; radiates left to neck; thrill at second and third left intercostal spaces.	Same as for aortic stenosis. Pitch medium.	S_1 usually followed by quick ejection click; S_2 often diminished with wide split; P_2 may be soft or absent; S_4 common if right ventricular hypertrophy present.
Diastolic Regurgitant Murmur	Systole Diastole ... S_1 S_2 S_1 S_2 S_1 S_2		
Aortic Regurgitation	Diaphragm, client sitting and leaning forward. Second right intercostal space radiates to left sternal border.	Blowing in early diastole. Pitch high.	Decrescendo midsystolic murmur common; early ejection click may be present; S_1 soft; S2 split may have tambour-like quality; summation gallop common. Wide pulse pressure; bisferiens pulse common in carotid, brachial, and femoral arteries.
Pulmonic Regurgitation	Diaphragm, client sitting or leaning forward. Third and fourth left intercostal spaces.	Blowing. Pitch high or low.	Difficult to distinguish from aortic regurgitation on physical examination

■ *Valvular heart disease (VHD):* An acquired or congenital disorder of the cardiac valve characterized by stenosis and obstruction or by valvular degeneration and regurgitation of blood. A stenotic valve is one that does not open completely so that bloodflow through the valve is reduced and a back flow is created. Conversely, regurgitation is caused by valves that do not close completely, so that blood leaks through the valve during ventricular contraction. Rheumatic fever and endocarditis account for most cases of acquired VHD (see Table 15-4). A common cause of endocarditis is intravenous drug use.

TABLE 15-4 Murmurs due to Valvular Defects—*cont'd*

TYPE	DETECTION	QUALITY/PITCH	VARIABLES
Diastolic Murmur	Systole Diastole S_1 S_2 S_1 S_2 S_1 S_2		
Mitral Stenosis	Bell at apex with patient in left lateral decubitus position	Low rumble more intense in early and late diastole. Pitch low.	Thrill at apex in late diastole common; S_1 increased and often palpable at left sternal border; accentuated P_2 common, followed closely by opening snap. Decreased arterial pulse amplitude.
Tricuspid Stenosis	Bell over tricuspid area.	Similar to mitral stenosis but louder on inspiration. Pitch low.	Thrill over right ventricle; S_2 may split during inspiration. Decreased arterial pulse amplitude. Jugular pulse prominent.
Holosystolic Murmur	Systole Diastole S_1 S_2 S_1 S_2 S_1 S_2		
Mitral Regurgitation	Diaphragm at apex, radiates to left axilla or base.	Harsh blowing quality. Pitch high.	Thrill may be palpable at base; S_1 decreased; S_2 increased, with P_2 often accentuated; S_3 often present. If mild, late systolic crescendo present; if severe, early systolic decrescendo and summation gallop present.
Tricuspid Regurgitation	Fifth intercostal space, left lower sternal border.	Blowing. Pitch high.	Murmur increases during inspiration, decreases during expiration.

🌐 Cultural Note

Heart disease and stroke are major killers of individuals in the United States, and minority cultural groups have disproportionately high losses. American Indians and Alaskan Natives have a cardiac disease mortality rate twice the rate of the general population. African Americans have a higher morbidity and mortality rate from coronary artery disease and stroke than the general population.

■ *Left ventricular hypertrophy:* An increase in the size of the myocardial cells of the left ventricle caused by overwork. Aortic stenosis or hypertension increases the resistance that the left ventricle must work against to maintain adequate cardiac output. The hypertrophy creates a lift palpable during systole and displaces the apical pulse laterally.

■ *Right ventricular hypertrophy:* An increase in the size of the myocardial cells of the right ventricle caused by overwork. Pulmonary hypertension increases the resistance that the right ventricle must work against to maintain adequate bloodflow to the lungs. Pulmonary capillaries compensate for chronic hypoxia by constricting, which can cause pulmonary hypertension resulting in right ventricular hypertrophy. Chronic obstructive pulmonary disease is a cause of chronic hypoxia. Right ventricular hypertrophy can cause a lift along the left sternal border in the third and fourth left intercostal spaces.

■ *Angina pectoris:* Chest pain due to ischemia of the myocardium as a result of atherosclerosis of the coronary arteries. Angina can occur during activity, stress, or expose to intense cold due to an increase demand on the heart or during rest due to spasms of the coronary arteries. Descriptions of pain are that it is squeezing, suffocating, or constricting; it is a steady pain, lasting less than 5 minutes; it may radiate to the left shoulder, jaw, arm, or other areas of the chest; and it is relieved by rest or vasodilating drugs, e.g., nitroglycerin (see Table 15-4).

■ *Myocardial infarction:* Ischemic myocardial necrosis with destruction of myocardial cells. The left ventricle is more commonly affected, but the right ventricle may be affected. Description of pain is that it is the worst chest pain ever experienced, a crushing pain that lasts longer than 5 minutes and is not relieved by rest or nitroglycerin. Dysrhythmias are common. Heart sounds may be distant with a thready pulse.

■ *Heart failure:* A syndrome in which the ventricle fails to pump blood efficiently into the aorta or pulmonary arteries. The left ventricle may fail for two reasons: (1) due to increased resistance that occurs with aortic stenosis or hypertension when the ventricle can no longer compensate effectively for the increased work load, or (2) due to weakening of the left ventricle that occurs after a myocardial infarction when myocardial cells are necrosed, rendering the ventricle ineffective. Since the left ventricle cannot pump sufficient blood forward, some of the blood backs up into the left ventricle and eventually into the pulmonary capillaries, causing pulmonary edema. Assessment finds precordial movement, displaced apical pulse and palpable thrill, S_3, and systolic murmur at apex. In the acute phase the client usually has crackles bilaterally in the lungs from pulmonary edema.

The right ventricle may fail due to hypertrophy from pulmonary hypertension or from necrosis from a myocardial infarction. The failure of the right ventricle to pump blood into the pulmonary arteries causes a back flow of blood into the vena cava. Assessment findings are precordial movement at xiphoid or left sternal border, heptojugular reflex and elevated jugular venous pressure, S_3 at lower left sternal border, and systolic murmur.

■ *Cor pulmonale:* Right-sided heart failure due to pulmonary disease such as chronic obstructive disease or cystic fibrosis. The mechanism of altered blood flow is the same as that in right-sided congestive heart failure, but the cause is different. The pulmonary capillaries compensate for chronic hypoxia by constricting, which increases the workload on the right ventricle. After continual stress on the right ventricle, it fails to pump blood effectively. A back flow of blood occurs into the vena cava.

■ **Bacterial endocarditis:** A bacterial or, infrequently, fungal infection of the endothelial layer of the heart, including the cardiac valves. This commonly occurs from intravenous drug use. Bacteria are attracted to damaged cardiac structures, particularly in areas of turbulent bloodflow (Fig. 15-27). A sterile vegetation, or thrombus, forms on the valves where endocardial tissue is damaged. Vegetations break apart and become emboli, producing infarctions or abscesses in heart, lungs, brain, kidneys, spleen, or extremities. Heart sounds are normal during the early infection. In late infection, murmur heard if valve damage occurs. Ventricular gallop (S$_3$) indicates ventricular failure.

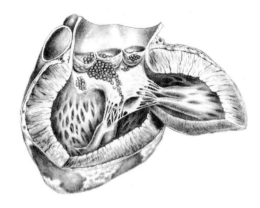

Fig. 15-27 Bacterial endocarditis.

■ **Pericarditis:** An inflammatory process involving the parietal and visceral layers of the pericardium and outer myocardium (Fig. 15-28). Pericarditis may be a consequence of numerous inflammatory or infectious processes, since the pericardium lies in close proximity to the pleura, lungs, sternum, diaphragm, and myocardium. Exudates are formed that may be serous, fibrinous, or purulent. A pericardial friction rub is best heard with client leaning forward; listen in the second, third, or fourth intercostal spaces to left sternal border or at the apex; it is louder during inspiration.

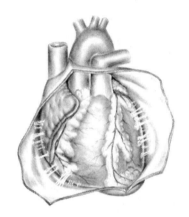

Fig. 15-28 Pericarditis. *(From Canobbio, 1990.)*

Congenital heart defects

■ **Patent ductus arteriosus (PDA):** Ductus arteriosus is a vascular connection that, during fetal life, permits blood to flow from the pulmonary artery to the aorta, bypassing the lungs (Fig. 15-29). Functional closure usually occurs shortly after birth. If the ductus remains open or patent, blood is shunted from the high systemic pressure in the aorta through the ductus to the pulmonary artery, raising the pressure in the pulmonary circulation and increasing the workload of the right ventricle.

Children's growth and development are normal. Blood pressure has wide pulse pressure and bounding pulses. Thrill may be palpable at left upper sternal border. Continuous murmur heard in systole and diastole is called a machinery murmur.

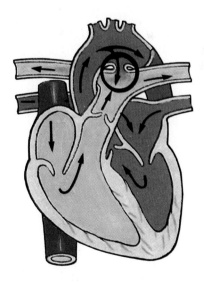

Fig. 15-29 Patent ductus arteriosus. *(From Wong, 1995.)*

■ *Atrial septal defect (ASD):* A defect in the septum that allows blood flow between the left and right atria (Fig. 15-30). With increasing age this defect increases pressure on the right ventricle, causing fatigue and dyspnea in children or young adults. S_2 has splits, with P_2 often louder than A_2. The murmur is due to increased blood flow through the pulmonic valve. It is heard at the base in the second left interspace and is called a systolic ejection murmur of medium pitch.

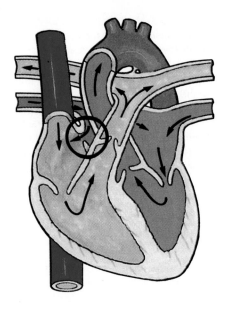

Fig. 15-30   Atrial septal defects.   *(From Wong, 1995.)*

■ *Ventricular septal defect (VSD):* A defect in the septum between the ventricles (Fig. 15-31). The side of the defect determines the extent of the shunting of blood and clinical findings. Infants with large defects have slow weight gain, dyspnea, feeding problems. A loud, harsh, holosytolic murmur is best heard at the left lower sternal border, and may be accompanied by a thrill.

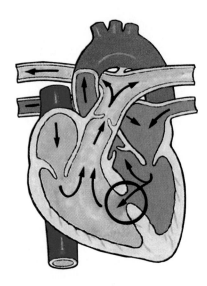

Fig. 15-31   Ventricular septal defects.   *(From Wong, 1995.)*

■ *Tetralogy of Fallot:* Involves four cardiac defects, comprising ventricular septal defect, pulmonic stenosis, dextroposition of the aorta (aorta overrides ventricular septum), and right ventricular hypertrophy (Fig. 15-32). The right ventricular outflow is obstructed, resulting in right ventricular hypertrophy and shunting of venous blood directly into the aorta away from the pulmonary artery, preventing blood from being oxygenated. Infants have severe cyanosis as they grow, and the pulmonic stenosis becomes worse. Infants have dyspnea and use squatting position when walking begins. A palpable thrill is felt at the left sternal border: S_1 is normal, S_2 has a loud A_2 and diminished P_2; the murmur is systolic, loud, crescendo-decrescendo.

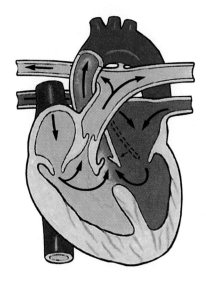

Fig. 15-32 Tetrology of Fallot. *(From Wong, 1995.)*

■ *Coarctation of the aorta:* A narrowing or partial obstruction of a section of the aorta (Fig. 15-33). The narrowing increases pressure in the proximal aorta and diminishes output distal to the narrowing, which decreases bloodflow to the kidneys. The increased pressure in the aorta increases the work load on the left ventricle. Symptoms are usually not present in childhood. Blood pressure on the arms may be 10 to 15 mmHg higher than the legs. Most important finding is absent to diminished femoral pulses.

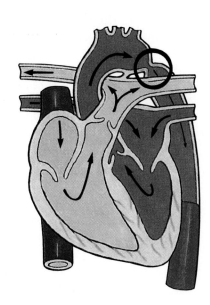

Fig. 15-33 Coarctation of the aorta. *(From Wong, 1995.)*

VESSEL DISORDERS

■ *Hypertension:* Sustained elevation in systolic blood pressure on two or more occasions above 140 or diastolic blood pressure above 90 (Fifth Report, 1993). The elevated blood pressure results from an increase in peripheral resistance due to vasoconstriction of arterial vessel or excess fluid volume in the vascular space. The exact cause of hypertension is unknown. There are no specific symptoms of hypertension, which is why periodic screening is important. Hypertension increases the workload of the heart by increasing the resistance against which the left ventricle must pump to maintain cardiac output. Some factors that contribute to hypertension are obesity; high fat, cholesterol, and salt intake; race; and genetic factors.

■ *Venous thrombosis/thrombophlebitis:* Venous thrombosis is an abnormal condition in which a *thrombus* (clot) develops within a vein. In contrast, thrombophlebitis is inflammation of a vein that may or may not be accompanied by a clot. The triad of stasis, damage to the inner layer of veins (intima), and hypercoagulability usually is responsible for both venous thrombosis and thrombophlebitis. Either may occur in the lower extremity (Fig. 15-34), usually in deep veins, and are recognized by calf pain and tenderness when the foot is dorsiflexed (Homan's sign), dilated superficial veins, edema of the involved extremity, and increased circumference of the involved leg. In the upper extremity, either may occur in superficial veins and are recognized by redness, warmth, and tenderness over the affected area. Veins may be visible and palpable.

■ *Peripheral atherosclerosis disease (arteriosclerosis obliterans):* Chronic arterial insufficiency that occurs when atherosclerotic plaques occlude the blood supply to the legs. A primary symptom is intermittent claudication, which produces leg pain, cramping, and aching during exercise that is relieved by rest period. Progressive occlusion results in severe ischemia, in which the leg or foot becomes cold and numb and skin appears dry and scaly with poor hair and nail growth.

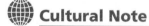

Cultural Note

Hypertension is generally more prevalent in minority cultural groups in the United States than in whites. Higher incidences have been reported in African Americans, Hispanics, and Pacific Islanders. Asian Americans and American Indians and Alaskan Natives have lower prevalence of hypertension than the general population.

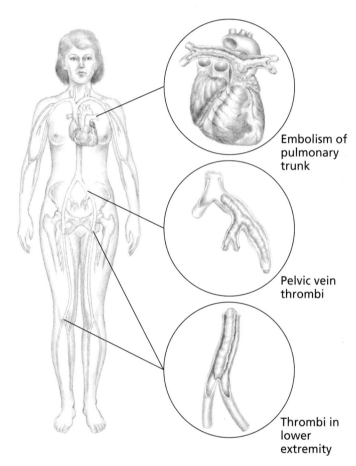

Embolism of pulmonary trunk

Pelvic vein thrombi

Thrombi in lower extremity

Fig. 15-34   Sites of venous thrombosis.   *(From Canobbio, 1990.)*

■ *Raynaud's phenomenon and disease:* An idiopathic intermittent spasm of arterioles of the digits, nose, and ears. Vasospasms may last minutes to hours and may occur bilaterally. They are secondary to connective tissue diseases such as scleroderma, rheumatoid arthritis, and systemic lupus ethythematosis, as well as drug intoxication, myxedema, and primary pulmonary hypertension. Signs and symptoms include blanching of the extremities followed by cyanosis, then redness along with numbness, tingling, burning, and pain. Ulcers may form on the tips of the digits. The diagnosis of Raynaud's disease is applied when there is a history of symptoms for at least 2 years with no progression of symptoms and no evidence of underlying cause.

■ *Arterial aneurysm:* Localized dilation of an artery caused by weakness in the arterial wall (Fig. 15-35). Aneurysms occur anywhere along the aorta and iliac vessels; abdominal aortic aneurysm is most common. A thrill or bruit may be noted over the aneurysm.

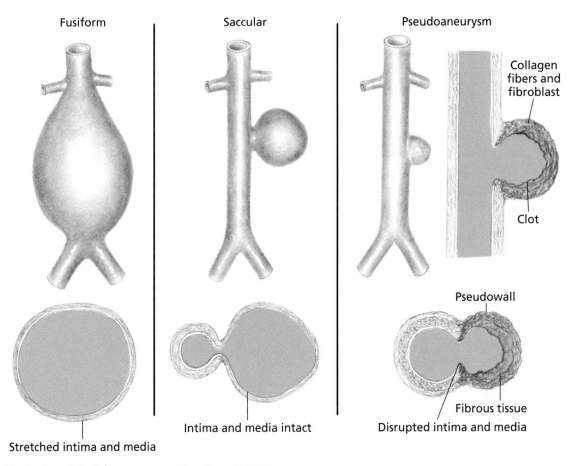

Fig. 15-35 Arterial aneurysm. *(From Canobbio, 1990.)*

Sample Documentation & Nursing Diagnosis

CASE 1   45-year-old black man

Subjective

Client here for annual physical examination as required by his company. He has no complaints.

Past medical history   Appendectomy, age 15; vasectomy, age 44.

Last exam   Medical, does not remember; dental, 2 years ago.

Family history   Paternal grandfather died of heart attack, age 65; paternal grandmother died of breast cancer, age 50.

Social history   Married with two teenage sons, employed full time as engineer. Worked for this company for 1 year, likes his job, but becomes stressed when there are deadlines to meet, every 2 to 3 months. Rarely exercises, smokes ½ pack of cigarettes per day. Interested in stopping smoking since there are "so few places I can smoke anymore." Takes no medications regularly, does not drink alcohol, and does not use street drugs.

Objective

Alert, cooperative, healthy-appearing man.

Height   6'1" (185 cm).

Weight   190 lbs (86 kg).

Temperature   98.4° F (37° C).

Pulse   88.

Resp   16.

BP   150/95 right arm—sitting, 148/97 left arm—sitting.

Serum cholesterol   230 mg/dl.

Heart   No lifts, heaves, or pulsations on inspection or palpation. PMI palpable at fifth ICS, MCL, S_1 loudest at apex, and S_2 loudest at base; normal, with regular rate and rhythm without murmur or S_3 or S_4.

Pulses   Temporal, carotid, brachial, radial, femoral, posterior tibial, dorsalis pedis 2+, symmetric. No carotid bruits.

Extremities   Warm, dry without pallor, cyanosis, or edema; elastic skin turgor, usual hair distribution.

• •

Nursing Diagnosis #1

Altered health maintenance related to inadequate information about exercise, healthy diet, stress reduction, and lowering blood pressure.

Defining characteristics   Rarely exercises, eats whatever he desires, smokes ½ PPD, family history of heart disease, stressful job; cholesterol 230 mg, weight 190 lb (86 kg), BP 150/95.

Nursing Diagnosis #2

Knowledge deficit related to stopping smoking.

Defining characteristics   Smokes ½ PPD × 25 years, desires to stop smoking.

Sample Documentation & Nursing Diagnosis

CASE 2   89-year-old African-American man with complaints of cold feet and hair loss on legs.

Subjective

Reports changes in his feet over the last 6 months. Stopped walking when he got pain in his calf when walking, but the pain went away when he would stop. Toes have started burning. Elevates his feet in his recliner; they hurt more. Reports no other problems or illnesses.

Lives with wife in apartment with small garden, which he cares for when he is not volunteering at the church. Smokes 1½ packs of cigarettes per day.

Objective

Alert, cooperative man with a slow gait.

Temperature   97.8° F (36.5° C).

Pulse   88.

Resp   20.

BP   140/88.

Lower extremities   Glossy, cool, smooth skin; pallor that increases with elevation of extremity; hair loss of lower leg bilaterally.

Ulceration (1 cm) over lateral malleolus with clear exudate. Numbness in tips of toes bilaterally.

Pulses, pressure   Temporal, carotid, brachial, radial strong and symmetric. Femoral, posterior tibial and dorsalis pedis palpable by Doppler. Capillary refill >5 sec. Bruits over abdominal and femoral arteries.

• •

Nursing Diagnosis #1

Altered peripheral tissue perfusion related to arterial insufficiency.

Defining characteristics   Glossy, cool, smooth skin; pallor that increases with elevation of extremity; hair loss of lower leg bilaterally, bruits over abdominal and femoral pulses, increased capillary refill.

Nursing Diagnosis #2

Altered skin integrity related to impaired circulation.

Defining characteristics   Ulceration over lateral malleolus (1 cm) with clear exudate; bruits over abdominal aorta and femoral pulses, decreased capillary refill.

HEALTH PROMOTION

■ **Risk Factors** Factors that increase the risk of heart disease have been identified and separated by modifiable and nonmodifiable risk factors. Risk factors that cannot be modified include heredity (a tendency toward heart disease runs in families), race (African Americans have a higher incidence of hypertension), sex (men have more myocardial infarctions [MI] than women), and age (over half the MIs occur in people over the age of 65).

Health promotion activities are aimed at modifying those risk factors that can be changed. These factors include smoking, hypertension, obesity, hypercholesteremia, stress, and alcohol intake.

■ **Smoking** The nicotine in tobacco vasoconstricts blood vessels, which increases the workload on the heart, increases blood pressure, and decreases peripheral perfusion. Smokers have more than twice as many heart attacks as nonsmokers. Peripheral vascular disease is almost exclusively a disease of smokers. When people stop smoking, their risk of heart disease drops rapidly and 10 years after quitting their risk of death from heart disease is about the same as for people who never smoked. Stop-smoking programs are available through the American Lung Association, American Cancer Society, and American Heart Association.

■ **Hypertension** Elevated blood pressure—over 140 systolic or 90 mmHg diastolic on more than one measurement—indicates hypertension. In addition to smoking, obesity and hyperlipidemia contribute to hypertension. Hypertension increases the workload on the heart and can lead to stroke, myocardial infarction, kidney failure, and congestive heart failure. The first line of management for hypertension is changing lifestyle, for example, eating a low-fat diet, exercising regularly (a minimum of 20 minutes three times a week), reducing salt intake, stopping smoking, limiting alcohol intake, and using stress-reduction techniques. When these techniques do not lower the blood pressure sufficiently, medications can be used.

Blood pressure screening is recommended every 2 years for clients with a diastolic pressure below 85 mmHg and systolic below 140 mmHg. Screening is recommended annually for clients with a diastolic between 85 and 89. Persons with higher blood pressures require more frequent measurements (Report of the U.S. Preventive Services Task Force, 1989, p. 25).

■ **Obesity and Hypercholesteremia** Cholesterol levels between 200 and 240 mg/dl increase the risk of heart disease. Obesity increases the workload on the heart, and excessive lipids, cholesterol, and triglycerides increase the fatty plaque that forms on blood vessels, making them narrow. Exercise and a low-fat diet are recommended to maintain an ideal body weight and a cholesterol level under 200 mg/dl. A progressive walking program, beginning with 5 minutes of brisk walking and progressing to 30 minutes daily, is recommended. A low-fat diet can be accomplished by eating more chicken, turkey, fresh fruits and vegetables, and less beef and yellow cheese. Preparing food by baking or broiling is preferred over frying.

■ **Stress** Psychologic stress increases the heart rate and can increase the workload on the heart. Relaxation techniques are useful in reducing stress. Techniques such as relaxation, yoga, music therapy, and mental imagery are some of the techniques proven to reduce stress.

 Cultural Note

When viewing risk factors for cardiovascular disease, cultural variations need to be considered. For example, more African-American and Hispanic men smoke than whites. Other ethnic groups generally smoke less than whites. Hispanics have generally higher levels of cholesterol than whites, while Asian Americans and American Indians and Alaskan Natives have lower levels. Levels of African Americans and whites are about the same. Obesity is most prevalent in African-American women. Cultural variations in the incidence of hypertension was covered earlier in this chapter.

??????? STUDY QUESTIONS ???????

1. Trace the blood flow through the heart and the changes that occur during systole and diastole. When are the valves of the heart open and closed?
2. Describe the electric conduction through the heart and how each area affects the heart rate.
3. Trace the blood flow as it leaves the heart and circulates through the body.
4. List the changes that occur in the heart when a baby is born.
5. List the normal changes that occur in the heart of a pregnant woman. What changes may be visible on physical exam?
6. Identify the physiologic changes that occur in the cardiovascular system as the client ages.
7. What is the general focus of history-taking of the client's cardiovascular system?
8. Identify lifestyle factors that have a negative effect on the cardiovascular system. What is the reason for the negative effect?
9. When an individual has chest pain, what information do you need to collect to distinguish between angina and pain associated with a myocardial infarction?
10. How are the following related to the cardiovascular system: shortness of breath, swelling of the extremities, nocturia, cough, fatigue?
11. What information would you want to elicit from an individual complaining of leg cramps?
12. List two maternal factors that need investigation when taking an infant history. List infant habits that may change if cardiovascular problems are present.
13. Why would you want to know whether a child squats or sits while at play?
14. What tools are needed for examination of the cardiovascular system?
15. What criteria are used for the classification of pulses?
16. Identify the location of the following pulses; temporal, carotid, apical, brachial, femoral, popliteal, posterior tibial, and dorsal pedis. Describe how to palpate each.
17. Identify the differences in the assessment of the arterial and venous systems.
18. When inspecting the chest wall, what are you looking for?
19. Describe the process of palpation of the precordium. What is a thrill? What is a lift?
20. Describe the technique for percussion of the heart.
21. Describe the sequence for auscultation of the heart. How should the client be positioned?
22. What occurs during the first and second heart sounds? When are the third and fourth heart sounds considered abnormal?
23. How is the technique for assessment of an infant different than that of an adult?
24. A venous hum is heard over the jugular vein on a child. What would this indicate?
25. What are the expected physiologic changes in the cardiovascular system of the older adult? How do these changes relate to vital signs changes?
26. What normal cardiovascular changes are expected during pregnancy?
27. Describe the specific changes that occur in the cardiovascular system of an individual with diabetes mellitus.
28. How are heart murmurs classified?
29. Differentiate between right and left ventricular hypertrophy.
30. Distinguish the pain caused by angina from that caused by myocardial infarction.
31. How is cor pulmonale different from right-sided heart failure?
32. Describe what occurs to the heart in heart failure.
33. Differentiate between bacterial endocarditis and pericarditis.
34. Match the congenital defect with the appropriate characteristic.

PDA	*Narrowing of descending aorta*
ASD	*Hole from pulmonary artery to aorta*
VSD	*Hole between the atria*
Coarctation	*Hole between ventricles*

35. How does hypertension affect the heart?
36. Differentiate between thrombophlebitis and peripheral atherosclerosis.
37. What are common physical findings of Raynaud's syndrome?
38. How do the risk factors associated with heart disease vary across cultural groups?

CHAPTER 16

Breasts and Axillae

ANATOMY AND PHYSIOLOGY

The breasts are paired mammary glands located on the ventral surface of the thorax, within the superficial fascia of the anterior chest wall. They extend vertically from the second or third rib to the sixth or seventh intercostal space and laterally from the sternal margin to the midaxillary line.

The female breast is composed of glandular and fibrous tissue and subcutaneous and retromammary fat (Fig. 16-1). The breasts' functional components include the acini (milk-producing glands), ductal system, and nipple. The glandular tissue is arranged into 15 to 20 lobes per breast, radiating around the nipple in a circular, spokelike pattern. Each lobe is composed of 20 to 40 lobules, or alveoli, containing the milk-producing acini cells that empty into the lactiferous ducts. A lactiferous duct drains milk from the lobes to the surface of the nipple.

Centrally located on the breast, the nipple is surrounded by the pigmented areola. The nipples are composed of epithelium intertwined with circular and longitudinal smooth muscle fibers. These muscles contract in response to sensory, tactile, or autonomic stimuli, producing erection of the nipple and causing the lactiferous ducts to empty. A number of sebaceous glands, called Montgomery's glands, are located within the areolar surface, aiding in lubrication of the nipple during lactation.

The subcutaneous and retromammary fat that surrounds the glandular tissue composes most of the bulk of the breast. The breast is supported by a layer of subcutaneous fibrous tissue and by multiple fibrous bands called Cooper's ligaments. These sensory ligaments extend from the connective tissue layer and run through the breast, attaching to the underlying muscle fascia.

The largest amount of glandular tissue lies in the upper outer quadrant of each breast. From this quadrant, the breast tissue extends into the axilla, forming the axillary tail of Spence. The majority of breast tumors are located in the upper outer breast quadrant and in the tail of Spence (Fig. 16-2).

Each breast contains a lymphatic network that drains the breast radially and deeply into the underlying lymphatics. Lymphatic drainage of the breast occurs largely through axillary nodes. The three types of lymphatic drainage of the breast follow:

- *Cutaneous lymphatic drainage* occurs from the skin of the breast, excluding the areolar and nipple area. This lymph flows into the ipsilateral axillary nodes. Fluid from the medial cutaneous breast area may flow to the opposite breast. It is possible for lymph from the inferior portion of the breast to reach the lymphatic plexus of the epigastric region and subsequently extend to the liver and other abdominal regions and organs.
- *Areolar lymphatic drainage* involves lymph formed in the areolar and nipple areas and flowing into the anterior axillary group of nodes (the mammary or pectoral nodes).
- *Deep lymphatic drainage* originates from the deep mammary tissues; this lymph flows into the anterior axillary nodes. Some of this fluid also flows into the apical, subclavian, infraclavicular, and supraclavicular nodes. Lymph from the retroareolar areas and the medial and lower glandular breast tissue areas communicates with lymphatic systems draining into the thorax and abdomen.

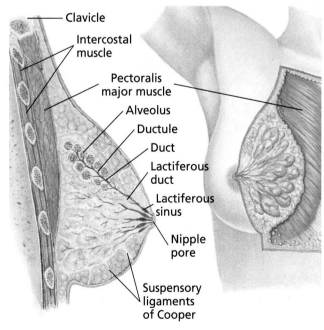

Fig. 16-1 Anatomy of the breast, showing position and major structures. *(From Seidel et al, 1995.)*

Labels: Clavicle; Intercostal muscle; Pectoralis major muscle; Alveolus; Ductule; Duct; Lactiferous duct; Lactiferous sinus; Nipple pore; Suspensory ligaments of Cooper

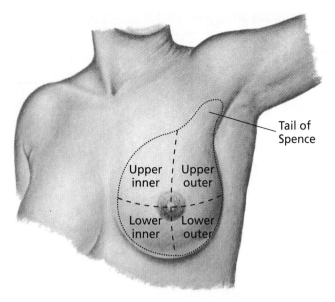

Fig. 16-2   Quadrants of the left breast and axillary tail of Spence. *(From Seidel et al, 1995.)*

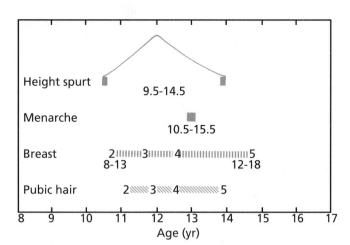

Fig. 16-3   Summary of maturational development of girls. See Fig. 16-4 for explanation of numbers 2 through 5. Number ranges in graph (e.g., 9.5—14.5) indicate average or common range of age for development of characteristic. *(From Marshall WA, Tanner JM: Arch Dis Child 44:291, 1969.)*

DEVELOPMENTAL CONSIDERATIONS

INFANTS AND CHILDREN

The function and structure of the breast changes throughout life. Breast development is latent during childhood and adolescence, with only minimal branching of primary ducts occurring. Before age 10 little difference exists in the appearance of male and female breasts. The nipples are small and slightly elevated. No palpable glandular tissue or areolar pigmentation exists.

ADOLESCENTS

Thelarche (breast development) represents an early sign of puberty in adolescent girls. At this time the estrogen hormones stimulate breast changes. Between the ages of 10 and 14, the mammary tissue beneath the areola begins to grow. The diameter of the areola increases, and a "mammary bud" is formed. The nipple and breast protrude as a single mound. Eventually the nipple begins to separate from the areola as the breasts become further elevated.

Tanner (1962) has described the five stages of maturational development in the female (Fig. 16-3). The full development of the breast from stages 2 to 5 takes an average of 3 years (range 1½ to 6 years). Stage 1 is the preadolescent stage.

The beginning of breast development in the female precedes the onset of menarche by approximately 2 years. Menarche begins when the breasts reach stages 3 or 4, usually just after the peak of the adolescent growth spurt, which is about age 12 (Fig. 16-4). Tanner developed the stages from studies conducted on British white females. Because of this, the nurse is cautioned about generalizing the stages to other cultural groups. For example, Harlan (1977) found that African-American girls developed secondary sex characteristics earlier than white girls of the same age.

By age 14, most girls have developed breasts that resemble those of the adult female. The continuing breast development, including size and form, is affected by heredity, nutrition, and individual sensitivity to hormones.

Throughout the reproductive years, the breasts undergo a cyclical pattern of size change, nodularity, and tenderness in response to hormonal changes during the menstrual cycle. The breasts are smallest during days four through seven of the menstrual cycle. Three to four days before the onset of menses, many women experience mammary tenseness, fullness, tenderness, and pain because of hormonal changes and fluid retention.

PREGNANT WOMEN

During pregnancy, dramatic changes occur in the breasts. The lactiferous ducts multiply rapidly, and the alveoli increase greatly in size and number in response to luteal and placental hormones. As a result, the breasts may enlarge two to three times their prepregnancy size. Connective tissue is displaced by the increased glandular tissue, causing the tissue to become looser and softer. Near the end of pregnancy, as epithelial secretion increases, colostrum is produced, accumulating in the acini cells (alveoli).

During this time, the nipples and areolae become more prominent and deeply pigmented. Montgomery's glands or tubercles often become more apparent as sebaceous glands hypertrophy. Increased mammary vascularization causes veins to become engorged and visible as a blue network beneath the skin's surface.

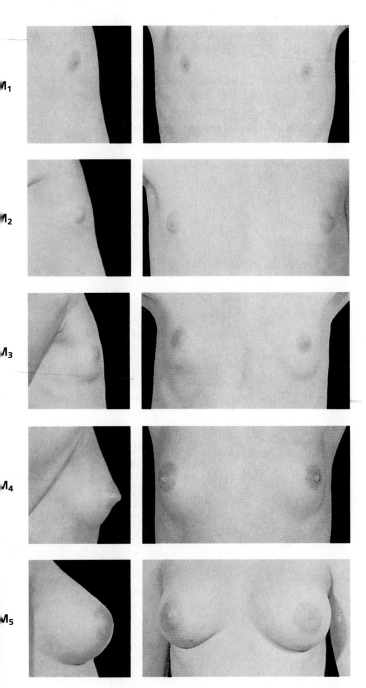

LACTATING WOMEN

Small amounts of colostrum are secreted from the breasts during the first few days after delivery. Colostrum contains more minerals and proteins than mature milk, as well as antibodies and other host resistance factors. Between 2 and 4 days after delivery, milk production to replace colostrum begins in response to surging prolactin levels, falling estrogen levels, and the stimulation of sucking. The breasts may become full and tense as the alveoli and lactiferous ducts fill. This, along with tissue edema and delayed ejection reflexes, results in breast engorgement.

Involution occurs over a period of about 3 months after the termination of lactation. Breast size decreases without loss of alveolar and lobular components. Rarely do the breasts return to their prelactation size.

OLDER ADULTS

Before menopause, a moderate decrease in glandular tissue and decomposition of alveolar and lobular tissue occurs. The glandular tissue continues to atrophy gradually after menopause and is replaced by fat deposits in the breast. A thickening of the inframammary ridge at the lower edge of the breast occurs. These tissues changes, and the relaxation of the suspensory ligaments, result in a tendency for the breast to hang more loosely from the chest wall. The nipples lose some erectile ability and become smaller and flatter.

THE MALE BREAST

The male breast consists of a thin layer of undeveloped tissue beneath the nipple. The areola of the nipple is small when compared with the female counterpart. The male breast undergoes some maturational changes during puberty. At this time the male's breast tissue may become enlarged, producing a temporary condition called *gynecomastia*. Although gynecomastia is usually unilateral, it may occur bilaterally. The older male may also have gynecomastia secondary to a decrease in testosterone.

Fig. 16-4 Five stages of breast development in females. M_1—Only the nipple is raised above the level of the breast, as in the child. M_2—Budding stage: bud-shaped elevation of the areola. On palpation, a fairly hard "button" can be felt, disk- or cherry-shaped. Areola increased in diameter and surrounding area slightly elevated. M_3—Further elevation of the mamma. Diameter of areola increases further. Shape of mammary tissue now visibly feminine. M_4—Increasing fat deposits. The areola forms a secondary elevation above that of the breast. This secondary mound apparently occurs in roughly half of all girls and in some cases presists in adulthood. M_5—Adult stage. The areola (usually) subsides to the level of the breast and is strongly pigmented. *(From Van Wieringen, et al, 1971. Reprinted by permission of Kluwer Academic Publishers.)*

HEALTH HISTORY | Breasts and Axillae

The history related to the breasts and axillae is directed toward current breast conditions, as well as toward evaluating the risk factors for breast cancer and assessing self-care routines. Every female client should have a risk profile developed and should be taught to perform breast self-examination. Both females and males should be questioned about breast changes.

QUESTIONS

RATIONALE

FEMALE

BREAST PAIN OR TENDERNESS

- Do you ever have pain or tenderness in your breasts? *If so:* When did you first become aware of it?
- Is the breast pain associated with a breast lump? Nipple discharge? Nipple retraction?
- Describe the pain. Is it like an ache? Sharp pain? Gnawing pain? Rate the severity of the pain on a scale from 1 (not very painful) to 10 (very painful).
- Where does it hurt? Is it in one breast or both? Is there a specific location or is the pain general? Can you point to the area that hurts? Is the area tender to the touch? Do you feel a burning or pulling in that area?
- Does the pain come and go in relation to your menstrual cycle?

- Have you noticed any specific activities that bring on the pain? For example, do you experience pain during sexual activity? When you wear underwire bras? When you exercise?
- How much chocolate and caffeine do you consume each day or each week?
- Have you noted any recent changes in your breasts? These changes may involve size, shape, overlying skin characteristics, or tenderness.

BREAST LUMP OR THICKENING

- Have you ever noticed a lump or a thickening of an area of the breast? *If so:* Where? When did you first notice it? Has it changed? *If so:* How?
- Is the lump tender to the touch?
- Does the lump appear related to your menstrual cycle?
- Have you noticed any change in the overlying skin, such as redness, warmth, dimpling, or swelling? Have you suffered any trauma to the breasts? Did swelling, a lump, or a skin break result?
- Do your breasts seem swollen at times? Is this just in one area or all over? Is the swelling related to your menstrual cycle, pregnancy, or breast-feeding? Have you had to change your size of bra because of the swelling?

◄ *Rapidly growing cysts may be painful. Cystic disease of the breast, as well as breast cancer, may not have any associated pain. On the other hand, some women with breast cancer report a burning or pulling sensation in addition to a vague pain.*

◄ *Cyclic pain commonly occurs with normal breasts with the use of oral contraceptives and with fibrocystic disease. Strenuous activity can bring on pain, as can the other specific causes noted.*

◄ *Although controversial, some experts believe that benign breast disease such as cystic disease of the breast may be associated with a high caffeine intake.*

◄ *Any lump should be thoroughly explored. One that has been present over a period of several years without change may be insignificant but still should be carefully examined. Any new lumps or changes in a lump should be of particular concern. Lumps resulting from an injury generally resolve shortly.*

NIPPLE CHANGES

■ Have you noticed any discharge from either nipple? *If so:* When? What color is the discharge? Is it thick or thin? Is there an odor associated with the discharge? Does the discharge occur at specific times, such as always before your menstrual period?

◄ *The most common types of discharge are* serous *and* bloody. *A serous discharge is thin and watery and may cause a yellowish stain on the client's bra. This type of discharge may occur secondary to intraductal papilloma in one of the larger subareolar ducts or to breast cancer. A bloody discharge associated with an intraductal papilloma may occur in pregnant and menstruating women.* Unilateral *bloody discharge, however, may also be associated with malignant intraductal papillary carcinoma.*

■ Is the discharge from one or both breasts?

◄ Bilateral *serous discharge may occur in women taking oral contraceptives.*

■ Are you taking any medications, such as oral contraceptives, phenothiazine, digitalis, diuretics, or steroids?

◄ *A bloody or blood-tinged discharge is always significant. If the discharge is associated with the presence of a lump, this also is significant. Note that several medications can cause clear nipple discharge, such as those previously listed.*

BREAST SKIN CHARACTERISTICS

■ Have you noted any rash on your breasts? *If so:* When? Did it start on the breast tissue, on the areola, or on surrounding skin?

◄ *Paget's disease begins with a small crust on the apex of the nipple and spreads to the areola. Eczema and other forms of dermatitis rarely begin on the nipple unless caused by breast-feeding. These skin disorders begin on surrounding skin and spread to the nipple area.*

AXILLA CHARACTERISTICS

■ Have you noted any tenderness or lumps in the area under your arms? *If so:* Where? Does this come and go or is it always present?
■ Do you have a rash in this area? *If so:* Please describe it. Is the rash related to a change in deodorant?

◄ *Note that breast tissue extends up under the arm. In addition, lymph nodes are located in this area.*

PAST MEDICAL HISTORY

■ Have you ever had breast problems such as fibrocystic disease or cancer? *If so:* What type? When? How was it diagnosed? How was it treated?
■ Is there a history of breast cancer or breast disease in your family? *If so:* In whom? At what age did this relative have breast cancer or disease? How was the cancer treated? What were the results?
■ Have you ever had surgery on a breast? *If so:* When was it and what was it for? Was it a biopsy? Mastectomy? Lumpectomy? Mammoplasty, either to reduce or augment your breast(s)?
■ How old were you at menarche and/or menopause?

◄ *A history of breast cancer increases the risk of recurrences. Fibrocystic disease complicates the evaluation of the breasts because the general lumpiness of the breast makes it difficult to detect new lumps. A family history of breast cancer occurring before menopause increases the risk for a woman having cancer.*

QUESTIONS

RATILONALE

Breast Cancer Risk Factors

- Age 40 years or older (80% of all breast cancer)
- Female
- Female family member with breast cancer history
- Menarche before 12 years of age
- Menopause after 55 years of age
- Has never given birth to a child
- Had first child after 30 years of age
- Previous personal history of any type of cancer

SELF-CARE PATTERN

- Do you understand and perform breast self-examination? *If so:* How often? When do you perform this each month?
- Have you ever had a mammogram? *If so:* When was your last mammogram? How frequently do you have a mammogram?

◀ *Evaluating self-care behaviors will help guide further education and encouragement of health-enhancing behaviors.*

MALE

- Have you noticed any enlargement or swelling to either of your breasts? *If so:* What is the change and when did it occur? Has the swelling been on one or both sides?
- Do you have any masses in either breast? *If so:* What are their locations? Are they tender or nontender?
- Have you noticed any discharge from either one or both of your nipples?

◀ *Gynecomastia is the enlargement of one or both breasts in the male. Although it may occur at any time, it is most prevalent during puberty and in the older adult man.*

◀ *Carcinoma of the breast affects approximately 1000 men in the United States each year. The average age of diagnosis is 59 years (Swartz, 1994).*

INFANTS

Newborns may have hypertrophic breast tissue with full raised areola buds. This is a normal phenomenon that lasts 1 to 2 months. If the hypertrophy lasts beyond 3 months, the parents should be asked if the infant has any other signs such as breast redness, firmness around the nipple, or an increased pigmentation around the areola.

CHILDREN

Generally, there are no specific questions for young children. Should the parents report that the young child has any breast symptoms such as breast redness or swelling or increased pigmentation around the areola, then further questioning about hormonal or systemic problems is necessary.

Preadolescent children, both boys and girls, should be questioned about breast changes. Specific questions to ask are as follows:

GIRLS

■ Have you noticed your breasts changing? *If so:* When did this start? Have you noted other changes in your body that come with growing up? What changes have you noticed?

Breast development is the most obvious sign of puberty, and girls focus a great deal of attention on this development. It occurs about the same time as the growth spurt and before the onset of pubic hair development and menarche.

■ How do you feel about these changes?

Evaluate the adolescent's perception of the changes she is undergoing and provide teaching and guidance as needed.

BOYS

■ Have you noticed any tenderness, redness, lumps, or inflammation in the breast area? *If so:* Is it only on one side or both sides?

Hypertrophy may be normal for stocky or heavy boys, but the symptoms noted should be evaluated for possible gynecomastia secondary to hormonal changes or systemic disease.

ADOLESCENTS

The history for the adolescent is an extension of the questioning discussed in the Children—Preadolescent section. History questions are primarily related to assessing the adolescent's developmental progress. In addition, once the teen has reached developmental maturity, the history questions related to the breast should be the same as for the adult. Adolescent developmental questions should include the following:

FEMALES

■ Describe the development of your breasts. Are they both developing at the same rate? Are your breasts the same size or is one larger than the other?

It is common for the adolescent's breasts to develop at different rates. Usually the breast size equalizes by the end of adolescence. Occasionally the asymmetry remains after puberty and must be surgically corrected.

■ Have you started your period yet? *If yes:* At what age did you begin?

Information about the onset of menarche will provide general information about the adolescent's maturational development.

■ Do you have any tenderness or pain in your breasts? Have you ever noticed any lumps or unusual areas of discoloration?
■ Do you have any discharge or drainage from either or both of your nipples? *If so:* How often does it occur and what does it look like?

Any report of a lump or localized area of tenderness requires further evaluation. If a mass is identified, it is most generally a benign tumor such as a fibroadenoma.

■ Are you sexually active? *If so:* Do you use oral contraceptives?

As with the adult, oral contraceptives may be a contributory factor to nipple discharge.

MALES

■ Have you notice any tenderness, redness, or lumps in the breast or nipple area? *If so:* Is the area tender or painful? Is it only on one side or both sides?

◄ *Hypertrophy may be normal for stocky or heavy boys, but the symptoms noted should be evaluated for possible gynecomastia secondary to hormonal changes or systemic disease.*

OLDER ADULTS

The incidence of breast cancer for both men and women rises steadily after the age of 40 and continues throughout the aging process. In addition to all of the questions in the adult section, inquire about the following:

FEMALES

■ At what age did you reach menopause? Since that time, have you taken hormone therapy? *If so:* What is the name and dosage of the medication? Do you take it every day or just at certain times of the month?

◄ *It is currently thought that an association exists between hormone therapy and breast cancer. Although hormone therapy is not thought to cause breast cancer, it may increase the speed of cancer growth should it occur.*

■ Do you have any irritation or rash under your breasts? *If so:* What do you do to treat it?

◄ *It is common, especially during warm weather, for pendulous breasts to cause skin-to-skin contact irritation.*

PREGNANT WOMEN

■ Do your breasts feel like they are enlarged or fuller? Have you noted any tenderness or tingling sensation? Do the veins appear more prominent on the surface of your breasts? Do the nipples seem more erect? Have you ever had inverted nipples? Does the nipple and areolar area seem darker? Can you express a thick yellow fluid from your breasts?

◄ *Breast changes are normal during pregnancy. Reassure the woman of this fact. Note that inverted nipples can present a problem with breast-feeding. The expression of colostrum is a late sign of pregnancy.*

■ Do you wear a supportive bra? *If yes:* Does it seem to provide adequate support for your breasts?

◄ *Because of the breast enlargement during pregnancy, it is important that the brassiere be large enough and be constructed to provide adequate support for the breasts.*

■ Do you plan to breast-feed? *If yes:* Have you received specialized breast-feeding education?

◄ *It is important to have plans and education in preparation for breast-feeding. If the woman has not made up her mind about breast-feeding, the nurse should encourage breast-feeding because of the positive health benefits for the newborn.*

QUESTIONS

RATIONALE

LACTATING WOMEN

Once the baby is born, a new series of problems and concerns arise related to the breasts. This is especially true if the woman is breast-feeding. The woman should be questioned about the care and condition of her breasts.

- Are you currently breast-feeding? *If so:* What is the average length and frequency of the feedings? How do you rotate the breasts? What positions do you use?
- Do you wear a nursing bra?
- Are your nipples tender, painful, cracking, bleeding, or retracted? *If so:* How does this interfere with your breast-feeding?

- Have you had or do you now have any problems with your breasts such as engorgement, nipple leaking, plugged ducts causing localized tenderness or a lump, fever, or infection? *If so:* What has been done to treat the problem?
- Has your baby had any mouth infections since being born, such as thrush (oral candida infection)?
- Do you pump your breasts? *If so:* How often and how much are you able to pump?

- How do you clean your breasts? What cleaning agent do you use?

- Are you currently taking any medications? *If so:* What are you taking and for how long?

◄ *Until the new mother develops a routine for breast-feeding and "toughens" her nipples, breast-feeding can cause the breasts to become sore and the nipples to become very irritated, crack, or bleed.*

◄ *Breast engorgement, pain, or infection can make the breast-feeding experience turn to disaster and may be a contributory factor in the woman giving up breast-feeding completely. It is important to determine the cause of the problem and institute corrective measures.*

◄ *Some soap products may remove the natural lubricants of the breast and nipple and may actually cause problems.*

◄ *Some medications—either prescription or nonprescription such as cimetidine and thiouracil—may cross the milk-blood barrier and be transmitted to the baby, causing potential side effects in the newborn. Lactating women should be educated about the possible risks of taking medications while breast-feeding.*

EXAMINATION Procedures and Findings

Guidelines To adequately examine the breasts of all clients regardless of age or gender, the client should ultimately be disrobed to the waist and sitting on the examining table facing the examiner. The examiner may provide the female client with a short gown that opens in the back. The gown, however, should be completely removed during the inspection of the breasts and the examination procedure. If the client is embarrassed or uncomfortable about disrobing, the examiner should be sensitive but also use a matter-of-fact approach to stress to the client that it is necessary to visualize both breasts at the same time so that an adequate evaluation and comparison of breasts may be done. It is an injustice to the client to permit the client to keep the gown on and only uncover one breast at a time for examination. In doing this, a thorough examination of the breasts is not possible.

Following the examination of the breasts, the examiner should be prepared to teach the female client breast self-examination. Men should also be taught to inspect their breasts regularly for evidence of masses or breast enlargement.

EQUIPMENT   Small pillow or towel (to place under the client's shoulder)
Ruler marked in centimeters (to measure lesions or masses)
Flashlight with transilluminator
Gloves (if there is suspicion of nipple discharge or tissue lesions)
Glass slide and cytologic fixative (if nipple discharge is present)
Teaching aids for breast self-examination (pamphlet may also
   be helpful)

TECHNIQUES and NORMAL FINDINGS

ABNORMAL FINDINGS

FEMALE

Initially, position the client so she is sitting on the examination table facing the nurse. She should be sitting erect with her gown dropped to the waist (Fig. 16-5). Following the breast inspection, assist the client into a supine position so the breasts and nipples may be palpated.

INSPECT both breasts, noting Size, Shape, and any Asymmetry. It is common for the breasts to be slightly unequal in size, with the right breast often slightly smaller than the left. Breast size may vary significantly, but symmetry or

■ A sudden increase in the size of one breast may signify inflammation or new growth.

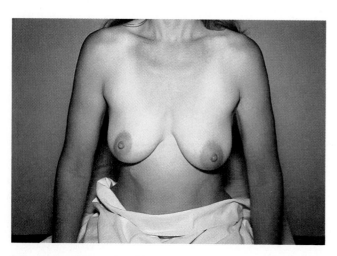

Fig. 16-5 Client should be seated, arms at sides, with gown dropped to the waist.

TECHNIQUES and NORMAL FINDINGS

only slight asymmetry should be considered normal. The breast contour should be smooth, convex, and even.

Gently lift each breast with your fingers and inspect the lower and outer aspects of each breast for dimpling or different characteristics.

INSPECT the skin of the breasts for Appearance, Color, Pigmentation, Vascularity, and Surface Characteristics. The skin of the breast should appear smooth and evenly pigmented.

ABNORMAL FINDINGS

■ Note evidence of marked asymmetry, dimpling, retraction or interruption of the curvature of the breast.

■ Note any localized or generalized areas of discoloration or change in surface characteristics such as dimpling or bulging. Note areas of redness or any moles that the client reports have changed in size or color.

■ Hyperpigmentation and erythema are abnormal (Fig. 16-6).

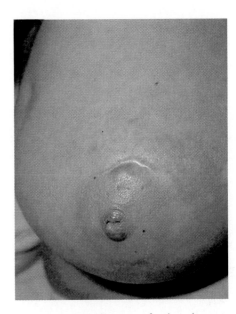

Fig. 16-6 Erythema of the breast. *(From Swartz, 1994.)*

TECHNIQUES and NORMAL FINDINGS

ABNORMAL FINDINGS

■ Note any roughened, tough skin, lesions, or thickening. Edema may give the skin a "peau d'orange" texture, like an orange (Fig. 16-7).

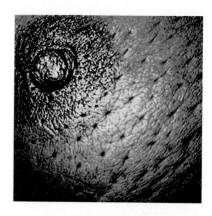

Fig. 16-7 Peau d'orange appearance caused by edema. *(From Gallager et al, 1978.)*

Also inspect the surface of the breast for lesions or vascular patterns in the skin. The venous patterns should be bilaterally similar. The venous pattern may be pronounced in obese or pregnant females.

■ Especially note any newly developed moles or those that have changed or are tender.
■ Inflammation in the tissue of the breast may cause surface redness or heat.
■ Unilateral venous patterns on the breast may occur secondary to dilated superficial veins from a increased blood flow to a malignancy.

INSPECT the areolae for Color and Surface Characteristics. The color of the areolae may vary depending on the client's skin color. Figure 16-8 shows the variations of areola color, ranging from pink to black.

■ Nipples that point in different directions are abnormal. Deviations include asymmetry, edema, redness, pigment changes, ulceration or crusting, erosion or scaling, and wrinkling or cracking. Note that any recently retracted nipple may signify acquired disease. Discharge of any type should be investigated further.

A   B   C

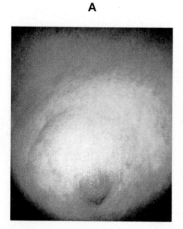 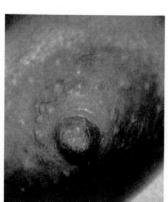 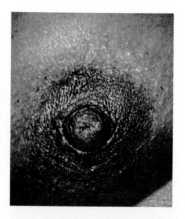

Fig. 16-8   Variations in color of areola. **A,** Pink. **B,** Brown. **C,** Black.   *(From Seidel et al, 1995.)*

TECHNIQUES and NORMAL FINDINGS

ABNORMAL FINDINGS

The areolae should be round or oval and should appear bilaterally similar. Montgomery's tubercles (Fig. 16-9) may appear as slightly raised bumps on the areola tissue. These are a normal variation.

■ Areolae that are unequal bilaterally, other than round or oval, with obvious masses or lesions and with pigment changes, either bilaterally or unilaterally, are abnormal.

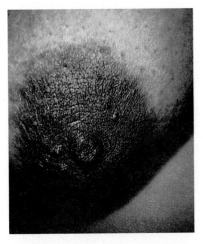

Fig. 16-9 Montgomery's tubercles. *(Modified from Seidel et al, 1995.)*

Next, **INSPECT the nipples for Position and Symmetry.** Most women's nipples protrude, although some may appear to be flat or actually inverted. All should be considered normal if they have remained unchanged throughout adult life.

Normal nipple inversion may be unilateral or bilateral and can usually be everted with manipulation (Fig. 16-10).

■ Nipples that point in different directions should be considered abnormal.

■ Recent changes in the nipple such as inversion or retraction (Fig. 16-11) is suggestive of malignancy, and the client should be referred for further evaluation.

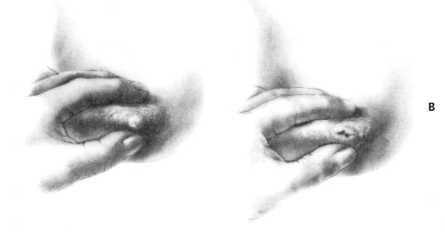

Fig. 16-10 A, Normal nipple everts with gentle pressure. **B,** Inverted or tied nipple inverts with gentle pressure. *(From Lawrence, 1994.)*

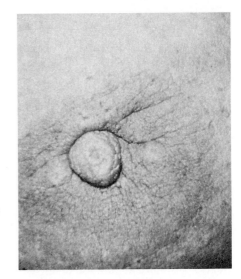

Fig. 16-11 Nipple retraction. *(From Gallager et al, 1978.)*

TECHNIQUES and NORMAL FINDINGS

ABNORMAL FINDINGS

INSPECT the nipples for Intactness, Evidence of Scaling, Lesions, Bleeding, or Discharge. *If the nipple appears to have drainage or a lesion, put on gloves before actually touching the nipple.*

Finally, inspect the nipples for evidence of any *supernumerary nipples,* or extra nipples (Fig. 16-12). The nipples appear as pink or brown areas. They are small and are commonly mistaken for moles. Infrequently a small amount of glandular tissue may accompany the nipple.

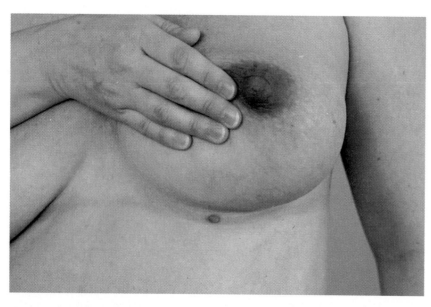

Fig. 16-12 Supernumerary nipple without glandular tissue. *(From Seidel et al, 1995.)*

■ Recent development of nipple discharge, either serous or bloody, should be considered abnormal until further evaluation. Any discharge should be saved for cytologic examination.

■ A red, scaly nipple with discharge and crusting that lasts more than a few weeks could indicate a rare type of breast cancer called Paget's disease (Fig. 16-13).

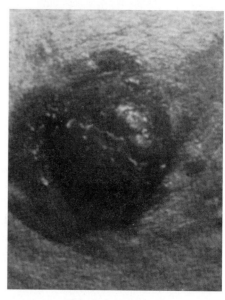

Fig. 16-13 Flaky nipple resulting from Paget's disease, which also causes a deeper reddening of the nipple than is normal. *(From Isaacs, 1992.)*

Preparation of Nipple Discharge for Cytologic Evaluation

Equipment: Gloves
Cotton-tipped
applicator
Clear microscopic
slide
Cytologic fixative

Steps: 1. Wearing gloves, gently squeeze the nipple to express a small amount of discharge.
2. Use a cotton-tipped applicator to collect a small sample of the discharge.
3. Using a rolling technique, smear the specimen on the slide and spray with the cytologic fixative.
4. Label the specimen with the client's name, date, and source—right or left breast. On the requisition, describe the characteristics of the discharge and other relevant clinical information, such as duration of discharge.

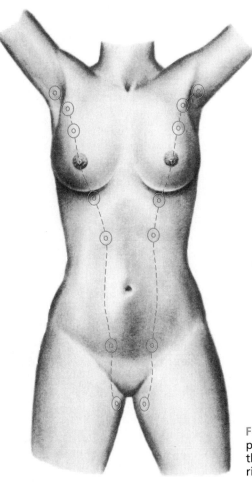

Fig. 16-14 Supernumerary nipples and tissue may arise along the "milk line," an embryonic ridge. *(From Thompson et al, 1993.)*

These nipples and related tissue generally appear along the "milk line," which is an embryonic ridge (Fig. 16-14).

 Racial Variation

Supernumerary nipples are more prevalent in African-American women than in white women.

INSPECT the breasts in various postures for Bilateral Pull, Symmetry, and Contour. Ask the client to remain seated and raise her arms over her head (Fig. 16-15, *A*). This position adds tension to the suspensory ligaments and will accentuate dimpling or retractions.

Observe and compare all of the areas already mentioned. Then evaluate for any bilateral pull on the suspensory ligaments. It should be equal on both sides, so that the breasts are bilaterally symmetric.

With her arms still raised, have the client lean forward (Fig. 16-15, *B*). It may be helpful for the examiner to hold onto the client's hands to provide balance.

Inspect the breasts for symmetry and bilateral pull, as previously described. The breasts should hang equally with a smooth contour, and pull should be symmetric. This is an especially useful technique if the client has large and pendulous breasts, because the breasts will fall away from the chest wall and will hang freely.

■ Note any asymmetry, shortening, or appearance of attachment (fixation) of either breast.

■ Note asymmetry or any bulging retraction. Note fixation as described previously.

A
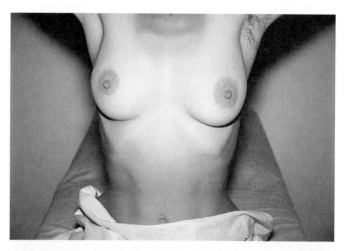

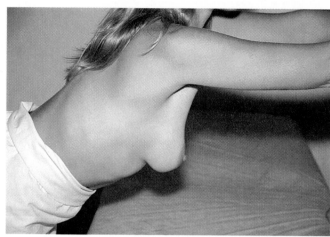
B

C
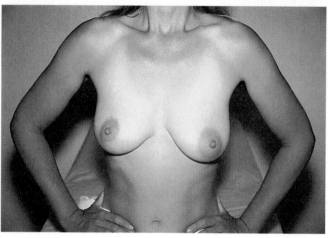

Fig. 16-15 **A,** Client with arms extended overhead. **B,** Client with arms raised and leaning forward. **C,** Client sitting and pressing her hands on hips.

Next, inspect the breasts while the seated client pushes her hands onto her hips or pushes her palms together, thus contracting the pectoral muscles (Fig. 16-15, *C*). Observe for deviations in contour and symmetry.

INSPECT the axillae for evidence of Rash, Lesions, or Masses. While the client is still in the sitting position, instruct the client to lift each arm. Next, instruct the client to relax both arms at her sides. Using your hand (generally your left if you are right-handed), lift one of the client's arms and support it so that her muscles are loose and relaxed (Fig. 16-16). While in this position, use your other hand (right if you are right-handed) to palpate each axilla. Repeat with the client's other arm.

Reach your fingers deep into the axilla and slowly and firmly slide your fingerpads along the client's chest wall, first down the middle of the axilla, then again along the anterior border of the axilla, and finally along the posterior border. Then turn your hand over and examine the inner aspect of the client's upper arm. During all maneuvers, position the client's arm with your other hand to maximize the examining area. In all positions, palpate for areas of enlargement, masses, lymph nodes, or isolated areas of tenderness. *If the client has a rash or lesion in the axilla, be sure to wear examining gloves during the palpation.*

CAUTION: *You must have short fingernails to adequately perform this maneuver.*

■ Infections in the breast, arms, and even the hand may have lymphatic drainage into the axillary area. Swellings in the axilla may indicate such an infection. Hard, fixed nodules or masses may suggest metastatic carcinoma or lymphoma.

TECHNIQUES and NORMAL FINDINGS

ABNORMAL FINDINGS

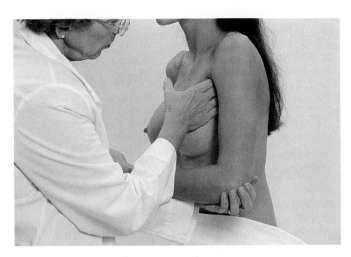

Fig. 16-16 Raise and support client's arm while palpating axilla.

Positioning Options for Breast Palpation

The breasts may be palpated with the client in either a seated or lying position or both. It is generally recommended that the palpation occur initially while the client is lying down. This position permits the breast tissue to be evenly spread over the chest wall; it also provides a firm chest wall surface against which to palpate. The sitting position may be used if the client is young and has very small breasts or if the client has difficulty lying down. The seated position may also be used in addition to the supine position when the client has very large, pendulous breasts. In the seated position, the breast tissue may be actually palpated between the examiner's two hands.

Palpating the Breast. *General technique.* Assist the client into a supine position and place a small pillow or towel under the shoulder of the breast to be examined. Instruct the client to place her arm over her head. The combination of the slight shoulder elevation and the arm positioning flattens the breast tissue evenly over the chest wall.

■ Abnormal findings during the breast palpation include masses or isolated areas of tenderness or pain. If a mass is identified, note its specific location, shape, size, consistency, tenderness, mobility, delineation of borders, and retraction. Transillumination may be used to confirm the presence of fluid in superficial masses.

 Racial Variation

In some cases, especially in white women, supernumerary nipples may be associated with congenital renal or cardiac anomalies.

TECHNIQUES and NORMAL FINDINGS

Using the finger pads of the first two three fingers of your examining hand, gently, firmly, and systematically palpate all four quadrants of the breast and the tail of Spence (see Fig. 16-2).

Several motions may be used for palpation. The most common is a circular technique moving from the center area of the breast near the nipple to the outer sections and ending with the tail of Spence (Fig. 16-17, *A*).

The second common technique is a wedge palpation, where the examiner systematically divides the breast into spokes and palpates the breast in a radial fashion from the center to the periphery (Fig. 16-17, *B*). The third technique is the vertical strip method (Fig. 16-17, *C*) (see box on p. 419).

Whatever technique is used, it is imperative that the examiner develop a systematic approach that always begins and ends as a designated point. This will ensure that all areas of the breast are systematically examined.

The breast should feel firm, smooth, and elastic. After pregnancy or menopause, the breast tissue may feel softer and looser. During the premenstrual period, the client's breasts may be engorged, slightly tender, and have generalized nodularity.

ABNORMAL FINDINGS

Breast Mass Characteristics

Note and record the following:

- *Location:* Which breast; which quadrant (may describe as position on the clock or draw on chart to show location)
- *Size:* Measure the width, length, and thickness in centimeters?
- *Shape:* Is the mass oval, round, lobed, irregularly shaped, or indistinct?
- *Consistency:* Is the mass hard, soft, or firm?
- *Tenderness:* Is the mass tender during palpation?
- *Mobility:* Does the lump move during palpation or is it fixed to the overlying skin or the underlying chest wall?
- *Borders:* Are the edges of the mass discrete or poorly defined?
- *Retractions:* Is there any dimpling of the tissue around the mass?

From Seidel et al: Mosby's guide to physical examination, *ed 3, St. Louis, 1995, Mosby.*

A
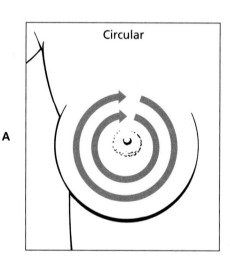
Circular

B
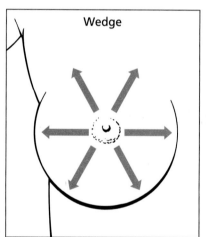
Wedge

C
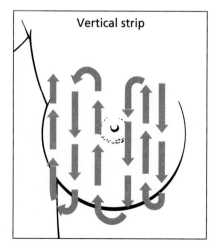
Vertical strip

Fig. 16-17 Methods for palpation of the breast. **A,** Concentric circles. **B,** Wedge section. **C,** Vertical strip. *(From Belcher, 1992.)*

TECHNIQUES and NORMAL FINDINGS

ABNORMAL FINDINGS

Methods for Breast Palpation

Circular Method
Place the finger pads of your middle three fingers against the outer edge of the breast. Press gently in small, circular motions around the breast. Move your fingers in smaller circles around the breast until you reach the nipple. Try not to lift your fingers off the breast as you move from one point to another.

Wedge Method
Place the finger pads of your middle three fingers against the outer edge of the breast. Press gently from the outer edge in a straight line toward the nipple. Move your fingers in parallel lines around the breast until each area is covered.

Vertical Strip Method
Place the finger pads of your middle three fingers against the top outer edge of the breast. Press gently from the top outer edge down to the bottom edge. Continue up and down until you reach the inner aspect of the breast.

During the palpation, feel specifically for masses, nodules, or areas of localized tenderness not related to the menstrual cycle (Fig. 16-18). Press firmly enough to get a good sense of the underlying tissue, but not so firmly that the tissue is compressed against the rib cage, giving a false sense of a mass. Try not to lift your fingers from the chest wall during the palpation. This will break the continuity of the palpation. Instead, gently slide your fingers over the breast tissue, moving along the designated pattern of palpation.

When the palpation of the first breast is completed, place the towel or pillow under the other shoulder, instruct the client to lift her arm above her head, and repeat the entire procedure.

Most women have a firm transverse ridge along the lower edge of the breast called the *inframammary ridge.* This firm ridge is normal and should not be mistaken for a breast mass.

A
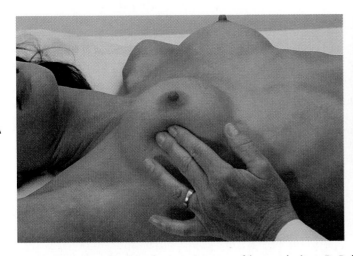

B
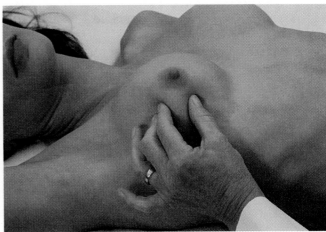

Fig. 16-18 A, Palpating for consistency of breast lesion. **B,** Palpating for delineation of borders and mobility of breast mass.

If the client has very large breasts and if it is difficult to palpate the breasts while she is in a supine position, assist her to a sitting position and instruct her to lean slightly forward. Take the breast between your hands and, while supporting the inferior side of the breast with one hand, use the other hand to palpate the breast (Fig. 16-19). Start at the top of the breast and slowly and purposefully feel the underlying breast tissue while sliding the top examining hand's fingerpads down the breast. Repeat the technique until all breast tissue is examined. As with the previously described techniques, do not lift your fingers during the palpation. Be sure to include the tail of Spence in the palpation.

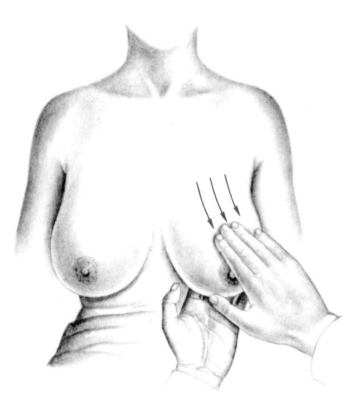

Fig. 16-19   Manual palpation of large breasts.   *(From Seidel et al, 1995.)*

PALPAGE the nipples for Surface Characteristics and Discharge. With the client in the supine position, palpate the nipples. To do this, gently compress the nipple between your index finger and thumb (Fig. 16-20). Inspect the nipple for discharge. If a discharge is present, note the color, consistency, and odor. Gently palpate the area around the nipple to determine if the origin of the discharge can be ascertained.

NOTE: *It is advisable to wear gloves during the nipple palpation to protect the examiner from possible discharge contamination.*

■ Nipple discharge may occur secondary to fluid retention of the ducts, infection, hormonal flux, or carcinoma. If a nipple discharge is present, a specimen should be sent for cytologic evaluation. (The directions for preparing a smear are previously discussed.)

TECHNIQUES and NORMAL FINDINGS

ABNORMAL FINDINGS

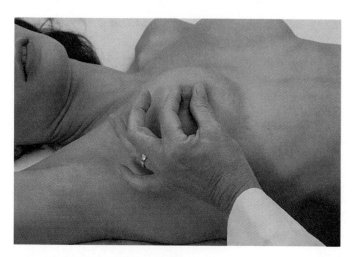

Fig. 16-20   Palpating the nipple.

TEACH Breast Self-Examination. Finally, the woman should be taught breast self-examination. If she states that she already does this, have her briefly show you what she does and how often she does it and what she looks or feels for during the self-assessment. (See a full discussion of the breast self-examination procedures below).

Teaching Breast Self-Examination

Teach the client to do breast self-examination by instructing the following:

1. Undress and stand in front of a mirror with your arms at your sides. Look for any changes in the shape or size of your breasts or anything unusual, such as discharge from the nipples or puckering or dimpling of the skin.

2. Raise your arms above and behind your head, and press your hands together. Look for the same things as in Step 1.

3. Place the palms of your hands firmly on your hips; look again for any changes.

4. Raise your left arm over your head. Examine your left breast by firmly pressing the fingers of your right hand down and around in a circular motion until you have examined every part of your breast. You may use the wedge section, circular, or vertical strip examination method *(instruct the client in one of these three techniques; see pp. 418-419 for directions).* Be sure to include the area between your breast and armpit and the nipple itself. You are feeling for any lump or mass under the skin. If you find a lump, notify your health provider.

5. Gently squeeze the nipple and look for any discharge. If there is any, notify your health care provider.

6. Repeat Steps 4 and 5 on your right breast. (You may also perform Steps 4 and 5 in the shower.)

7. Now, lie down on your back with a pillow under your right shoulder. Put your right arm over your head. This position flattens the breast and makes it easier to examine. Examine your right breast just as you did in Steps 4 and 5. Repeat the examination on your left breast.

From Mosby's patient teaching guides, *St. Louis, 1995, Mosby, p. 162.*

TECHNIQUES and NORMAL FINDINGS

ABNORMAL FINDINGS

MALE

As part of a comprehensive examination, it is essential to examine the male client's breasts.

INSPECT the Breasts. With the client in a seated position, inspect both breasts, looking for breast symmetry, color, skin lesions, and enlargement. The breasts should be flat and without rashes or lesions. Men who are overweight often have a thicker fatty layer of tissue on the chest, giving the appearance of breast enlargement. If this is noted, it is important to assess the client's situation with a careful history of weight gain. If the client reports that his breasts became full as he gained weight, the condition is most likely within normal limits. If, on the other hand, the client reports a sudden bilateral or unilateral breast enlargement with associated tenderness, the examiner should consider the situation possibly abnormal and should send the client for further evaluation.

Inspect the male breast while the client is seated with his arms at his sides. The nipple and areolar areas should be intact, smooth, and of equal color, size, and shape bilaterally.

- Note any asymmetry or distinct differences between the two sides. Note any ulcerations, masses, or swelling.
- Unilateral or bilateral breast enlargement in men may be *gynecomastia*, which may occur secondary to a hormonal imbalance, liver failure, or certain medications. (See Common Problems/Conditions later in this chapter for a more detailed discussion.)

PALPATE the Breasts. With the client in the same position, palpate. the breasts and areolar areas. The tissue should feel smooth, intact, and nontender. Note evidence of tenderness, unilateral enlargement, or masses.

PALPATE the Axilla. If not already done as part of the lymphatic assessment, palpate the client's axillary area for tenderness or lymphatic enlargement.

PALPATE the Nipples. Gently compress the nipples of both breasts to assess for nipple discharge.

- Although not common, breast cancer in men may be assessed as a hard, painless, irregular nodule often fixed to the area under the nipple or in the upper outer quadrant of the breast.

AGE-RELATED VARIATIONS

INFANTS/NEWBORNS

■ APPROACH

The examination of the newborn's breasts may be done quickly and easily. The infant should be lying supine and be undressed to the waist.

■ FINDINGS

Newborns of both genders may have full, slightly enlarged breasts secondary to the mother's estrogen level before the infant was born (Fig. 16-21). The newborn may have a small amount of watery or milky nipple discharge, also secondary to maternal hormones. This discharge has been commonly referred to as "witch's milk." Both the discharge and breast swelling are transient and should last only a few days to a few weeks.

The nurse should also carefully examine the infant's breasts for abnormalities such as mastitis. If this is present, the breasts will appear reddened and warm to the touch.

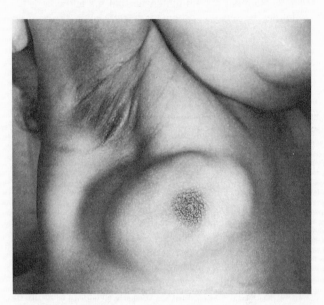

Fig. 16-21 Marked enlargement of breast bud in neonate. This is an exaggerated response to maternal hormones. *(From Gallager et al, 1978.)*

CHILDREN

■ APPROACH

Children should also be disrobed for the breast and chest examination. With a little encouragement, young children will generally readily remove their tops, exposing the chest and breast area. School-age girls may show increasing shyness as they get older. The examiner should be sensitive to this but should also provide a gown for the girl and then use a matter-of-fact approach to expose the girl's entire chest area for a complete breast examination.

School-age boys will usually have no qualms about exposing their chest. If the boy is obese and has slightly enlarged breast tissue, he may be self-conscious. In this case, the nurse should acknowledge the child's sensitivity and reassure him that, as he matures, this condition will most likely subside.

■ FINDINGS

Although the breast should be examined at each well-child evaluation, no significant findings are generally noted until puberty. As noted above, obese children may have slightly full bilateral breast tissue. Any unilateral breast enlargement or changes should be further evaluated.

As the girl reaches prepubertal age, sometimes as young as age 8, her breasts will show prepubertal budding

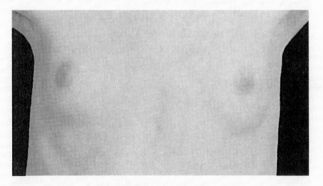

Fig. 16-22 Preteen female with budding breasts. *(From Van Wieringen et al, 1971. Reprinted by permission of Kluwer Publishers.)*

(Fig. 16-22). At this time the breasts change from flat to slightly convex. Although both breasts may not appear exactly alike, they should both show maturational development. If only one breast shows development, other causes for the enlargement such as a cyst or hormonal imbalance must be evaluated.

ADOLESCENTS

■ APPROACH

The examiner should anticipate that the adolescent female may be sensitive to having her breasts exposed. The nurse should take time to reassure the client that while her privacy is important, it is also important to adequately expose the chest for a complete breast examination. The examiner should use the same breast examination techniques as discussed in the adult section. Adolescence is also the time to teach breast self-examination techniques and to stress the importance of regular self-examination.

Male adolescents should be taught that breast examination is also important for them and that, although infrequent, they may also develop diseases of the breast such as gynecomastia and breast cancer.

■ FINDINGS

During inspection of the girl's breasts, note the developmental stage of the client. The right and left breasts may develop at different rates. It is important to reassure the client that this is very common and, in time, the development will equalize. The breast examination should include all of the breast examination components as presented in the discussion of the adult female examination. The breast tissue in the adolescent female should feel uniform throughout and be firm and elastic. Refer to the anatomy section of this chapter for a review of the developmental stages of the female breast to ensure that the client is adequately developing. This is also an excellent time to teach breast self-examination.

Male adolescents, especially obese males, may have transient unilateral or bilateral subareolar masses (Fig. 16-23). These firm and sometimes tender masses may be of great concern. Reassure the teen that these are generally transient and should disappear within a year or so. Gynecomastia, on the other hand, is an unexpected enlargement of one or both breasts in the male that may occur secondary to a hormonal imbalance, testicular or pituitary tumors, or illicit or prescription medications.

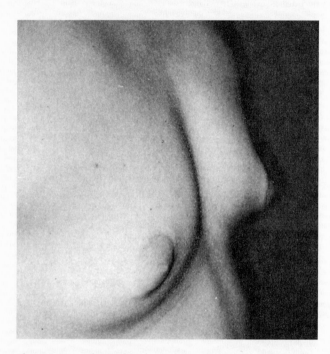

Fig. 16-23   Bilateral pubertal gynecomastia in 13-year-old boy.   *(From Gallager et al, 1978.)*

OLDER ADULTS

■ APPROACH

Postmenopausal women should continue to have regular breast examinations. Because the women are no longer subject to hormonal changes and menstruation, it may be difficult for the woman to remember to perform breast self-examination. The woman should be taught to pick one day each month (such as the date of her birth date) to perform the examination. Likewise, she should be encouraged to receive regular, professional breast examinations and mammograms.

Older males should also have a systematic breast examination. Most breast cancer in men occurs in men over the age of 60.

■ FINDINGS

The breasts in postmenopausal women may appear flattened and elongated or pendulous secondary to a relaxation of the suspensory ligaments. They tend to have increased adipose tissue and decreased subcutaneous fat. Although women after menopause tend to have decreased chronic cystic disease, they also have an increased incidence of breast cancer.

The techniques for examining the breasts in older women are the same as for younger women. Palpation findings that may be normal variations in the older adult include a granular feeling of the glandular tissue of the breast. If the woman had cystic disease earlier in life, her breasts are now more likely to feel smoother and less cystic. The inframammary ridge thickness may now be more prominent, and the nipples may be smaller and flatter.

The techniques for examining the older adult man's breasts are the same as for the younger man. Any absence of these changes or presence of other findings should be investigated.

CLIENTS WITH SITUATIONAL VARIATIONS

PREGNANT WOMEN

■ APPROACH

Many of the changes that occur during pregnancy are transitional and will disappear following the child's birth; other changes, such as striae, will permanently alter the breast characteristics. It is most important to encourage the woman to increase her brassiere size during the pregnancy so as to provide adequate support to her changing breasts. This may need to be done several times during the pregnancy.

■ FINDINGS

During the first trimester the breasts will become fuller, tender, increase in size, and may have a tingling sensation. The nipples may become somewhat flattened or inverted. The areolar area borders become darker and Montgomery's tubercles may appear. A small amount of crusting caused by dried colostrum may be noted on the nipple. A subcutaneous venous pattern secondary to dilated veins may be seen as a network of blue tracings across the breasts. Later in pregnancy, the stretching of the breast tissue may cause striae to appear. Palpation of the breasts reveal fullness and coarse nodularity. Following the first trimester, colostrum may be expressed from the breast as a thick yellow discharge. (*Note:* The examiner should be wearing gloves during this procedure).

Late during pregnancy, an increase in circulating estrogen may cause vascular spiders to appear on the client's upper chest, arms, neck, and face. These spiders have a "bluish" tinge and will not blanch with direct pressure.

Breast self-examination should be performed by the woman at regular times during pregnancy, just as it is at times when she is not pregnant.

Following the delivery of the child, the breasts will undergo a period of engorgement that may occur about the third postpartum day secondary to milk production. This is most pronounced in women who are not breast-feeding. Eventually the breasts will return to a somewhat prepregnancy state. They will most likely remain larger than they were before the pregnancy and will be less firm than in their prepregnancy state. The areolae and nipples tend to retain their darker color and will usually not return to their prepregnancy color.

LACTATING WOMEN

■ APPROACH

Breast engorgement following the delivery is most helped by frequent nursing. This helps to drain the ducts and sinuses of the breast and stimulate milk production. Care must be taken to carefully assess the woman's current condition, breast-feeding concerns and techniques, and the actual condition of the breasts. It is important to continue to assess whether the breasts are adequately supported by a properly fitting bra.

■ FINDINGS

Breast engorgement will be at its peak about the third day following delivery. The breasts may become engorged, appear enlarged, reddened, and shiny, and feel warm and hard (Fig. 16-24). Engorged breasts may be very uncomfortable and actually painful. Engorgement or breast pain that lasts beyond 4 days, or breasts that become engorged or painful after that time, must be assessed for possible infection or mastitis. Other clinical signs of mastitis include fever, headache, malaise, chills, and other flulike symptoms. Treatment generally includes rest, antibiotics, local heat, and frequent nursing.

An isolated tender spot or lump on the breast may be a clogged milk duct. If this is the case, frequent nursing or expression of milk, along with the application of moist heat, may help to unclog the duct. A clogged duct may occur secondary to inadequate emptying of the breast or a bra that is too tight. If the clogged duct is left unattended, it may result in mastitis.

The nipples of lactating women require careful assessment, especially during the early period following delivery of the infant and the beginning of breast-feeding. Repeated infant sucking may cause the client's nipples to become irritated, red, and tender. If left unattended, they may become blistered and actually crack and bleed (Fig. 16-25). If this is evident, it must be attended to and healed so that successful breast-feeding may continue. Healing of cracked nipples will usually occur rapidly if they are kept dry and exposed to the air. Frequent and short nursing periods may also help nipple soreness. If left unattended, nipples may become infected and breast-feeding will most likely fail.

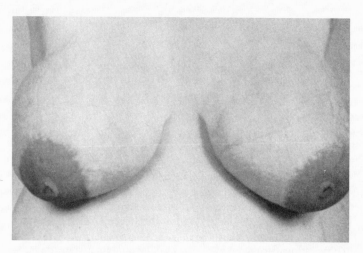

Fig. 16-24 Breast engorgement. *(From Isaacs, 1992.)*

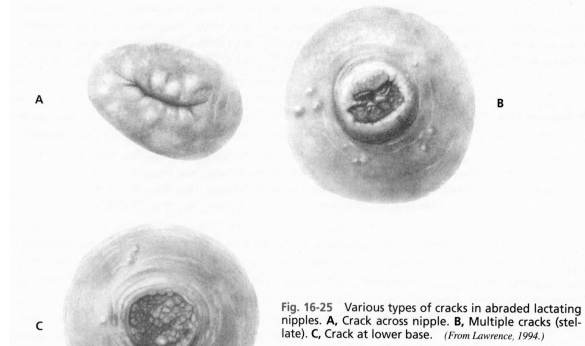

Fig. 16-25 Various types of cracks in abraded lactating nipples. **A,** Crack across nipple. **B,** Multiple cracks (stellate). **C,** Crack at lower base. *(From Lawrence, 1994.)*

CLIENTS WITH A MASTECTOMY

■ APPROACH

Women who have had a mastectomy require the same careful breast assessment as all other women. Likewise, they should be encouraged to routinely perform breast self-examination and have mammograms on a regular basis.

The woman may feel self-conscious about removing her brassiere and prosthesis, if she wears one. The examiner should be sensitive to this but should also reassure the client that it is necessary to perform a comprehensive examination.

■ FINDINGS

In addition to examining the remaining breast in the usual manner, careful assessment should be made of the mastectomy site, including the area of the scar. If a malignancy recurs, it may be at the scar site. The mastectomy site and axilla should be inspected for color changes, redness, rash, irritation, and visible signs of swelling, thickening, or lumps. Note areas that may have had muscle resection. Also note any signs of proximal or distal lymphedema.

Using the fingerpads of your examining hand, carefully palpate the side with the mastectomy, especially around the area of the scar. Use a small circular motion assessing for thickening, lumps, swelling, or tenderness, then use a sweeping motion to palpate the entire chest area on the affected side to ensure that nothing has been missed. Finally, palpate the axillary and supraclavicular areas for lymph nodes.

If the client has had breast reconstruction or augmentation, perform the breast examination in the usual manner. Pay particular attention to any scars and new tissue.

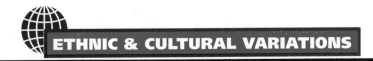

ETHNIC & CULTURAL VARIATIONS

■ FINDINGS

Breast size, shape, and symmetry vary widely with individual women. Asian women tend to have smaller breasts and African-American women have a higher prevalence of supernumerary nipples, but other racial differences in breasts are not well documented. African-American adolescents develop secondary sex characteristics, most notably breasts and axillary hair, at an earlier age. But the onset of puberty in adolescent females continues to occur at a younger age across all racial groups in the United States.

Breast cancer is a major health problem for women and is the number one killer of women in the 35 to 54 year age range. Incidence of breast cancer varies widely across cultural lines for reasons that are not well understood. Environmental influences such as diet are thought to play a role, but no hard evidence yet exists to support these suppositions. Hawaiian native women have the highest incidence, closely followed by white and African-American women. Hispanic and Asian women are in the midrange and with American Indian and Alaskan Native women have the lowest incidence.

EXAMINATION SUMMARY

Breasts and Axillae

Female *(pp. 410-421)*
Examination of the Breast and Axilla

- Inspect the breasts for:
  Size
  Shape
  Symmetry
- Inspect the skin of the breasts for:
  Appearance
  Color
  Pigmentation
  Vascularity
  Surface characteristics
- Inspect the areolae for:
  Color
  Surface characteristics
- Inspect the nipples for:
  Position and symmetry
  Intactness

  Evidence of scaling, lesions, bleeding, or discharge
- Inspect the breasts in various positions for:
  Bilateral pull
  Symmetry
  Contour
- Inspect the axillae for:
  Evidence of rash, lesions, or masses
- Palpate the breasts and axillae for:
  Surface characteristics
  Masses, nodules, tenderness
- Palpate the nipples for:
  Surface characteristics
  Discharge
- Teach breast self-examination

Male *(p. 422)*

COMMON PROBLEMS/CONDITIONS
associated with the Breast and Nipple

FEMALES

■ *Fibrocystic disease of the breast:* A benign, generally bilateral cystic condition caused by ductal enlargement (Fig. 16-26). The cysts are filled with fluid, which may be aspirated for diagnostic purposes. Premenstrually, the breasts may be tender and have heavy dull pain. The disease is most prevalent in women ages 30 to 55 and will decrease after menopause (see Table 16-2).

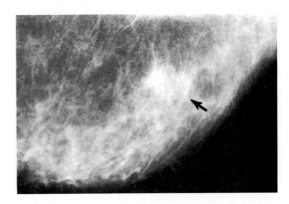

Fig. 16-26 Typical fibrocystic condition in right breast. *(From Stark, Bradley, 1992.)*

■ *Fibroadenoma:* A common benign breast tumor that occurs most frequently in young women (Fig. 16-27). The lump, which consists of dense epithelial and fibroblastic tissue, is nontender and does not change premenstrually. It is generally freely moveable and slippery to the touch. Surgical excision or biopsy is generally performed to rule out cancer. The lesion is most prevalent in young women less than 25 years of age but may be seen until menopause (see Table 16-1).

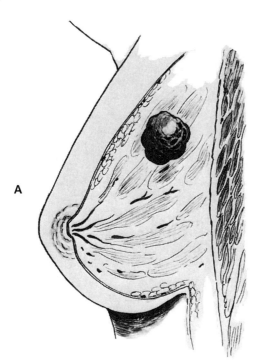

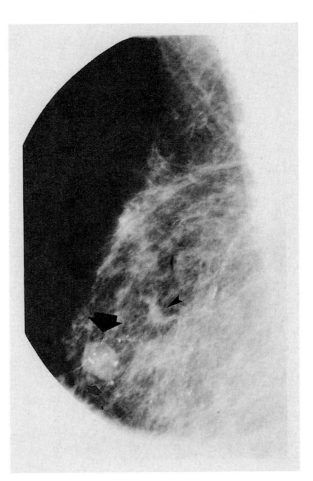

Fig. 16-27 Fibroadenoma. **A,** Clinical findings in solid tumor such as cancer, fibroadenoma, or lipoma. **B,** Fibroadenoma with typical coarse calcifications *(arrows).* Small, nonpalpable, edematous carcinoma is also present *(arrowhead).* *(From Gallager et al, 1978.)*

■ *Malignant tumors:* Usually a solitary, unilateral, nontender lump, thickening, or mass (Fig. 16-28). As the mass grows, there may be breast asymmetry, discoloration (erythema or ecchymosis), unilateral vein prominence, peau d'orange, ulceration, dimpling, puckering, or retraction of the skin. The nipple may be inverted or diverted to one side. The lesion is sometimes fixed to underlying tissue. Its borders are irregular and poorly delineated. There may be crusting around the nipple or erosion of the nipple or areola. Breast cancer is most prevalent in women ages 40 to 60 years (see Table 16-1).

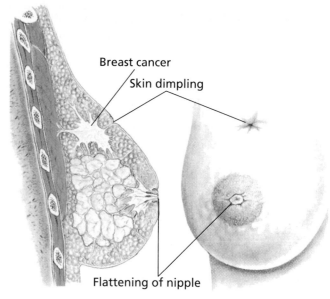

Breast cancer

Skin dimpling

Flattening of nipple

Fig. 16-28   Clinical signs of breast cancer: nipple retraction and dimpling of skin.   *(From Seidel et al, 1995.)*

■ *Intraductal papilloma:* A 2- to 3-cm tumor of the subareolar duct. It may consist of a single or multiple tumors. Clinically, no mass is usually palpable, but there is serous or bloody discharge from the nipple. The tumors should be removed surgically and cytologically examined for malignancy.

■ *Paget's disease of the breast:* A surface manifestation on the nipple and areolar area of an underlying intraductal carcinoma of the breast (Fig. 16-29). In the early stages, the nipple and areola becomes friable, dry, and scaling. As the condition worsens, the nipple becomes reddened, excoriated, and finally ulcerated. The condition may be differentiated from more common dermatologic conditions such as eczema because it appears unilaterally.

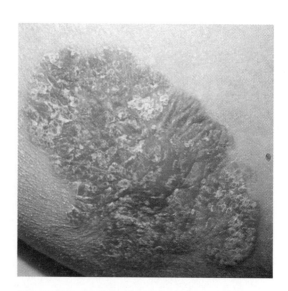

Fig. 16-29   Paget's disease.   *(From Habif, 1990.)*

TABLE 16-1	Differentiation of Breast Masses		
	FIBROCYSTIC DISEASE	**FIBROADENOMA**	**CANCER**
Age	20–49	15–55	30–80
Occurrence	Usually bilateral	Usually bilateral	Usually unilateral
Location	Upper outer quadrant	No specific location	48% occur in the upper outer quadrant, but may occur in any part of the breast or axillary tail
Nipple discharge	No	No	If present, may be bloody or clear
Pain	Yes	No	Usually none
Number	Multiple or single	Single; may be multiple	Single
Shape	Rounded	Rounded or discoid	Irregular or stellate
Consistency	Soft to firm; tense	Firm, rubbery	Hard, stonelike
Mobility	Mobile	Mobile	Fixed
Retraction signs	Absent	Absent	Often present
Tenderness	Usually tender	Usually nontender	Usually nontender
Borders	Well delineated	Well delineated	Poorly delineated; irregular
Variations with menses	Yes	No	No

From Seidel et al: Mosby's guide to physical examination, *ed 3, St. Louis, 1995, Mosby; and Fogel and Woods, editors:* Health care of women: a nursing perspective, *1981.*

■ ***Mastitis:*** An inflammatory condition of the breast usually caused by a bacterial infection. The infection generally occurs in one area of the breast, which appears as red, swollen, tender, warm to the touch, and hard. The condition occurs most frequently in lactating women secondary to milk stasis or a plugged duct.

■ ***Galactorrhea:*** Lactation not associated with childbearing. It occurs most frequently in women taking medications such as phenothiazine, tricyclic antidepressants, estrogens, and select antihypertensive agents. It may also occur secondary to diseases such as hypothyroidism, Cushing's syndrome, hypoglycemia, and in prolactin-secreting tumors.

MALES

■ *Gynecomastia:* A noninflammatory enlargement of one or both male breasts (Fig. 16-30). At puberty the condition is idiopathic and transient. In men at older ages, however, it may occur secondary to hormonal imbalances (such as hormone-secreting tumors—testicular, prostate, or pituitary), liver disease (such as cirrhosis of the liver), leukemia, or occasionally medications containing estrogens or steroids.

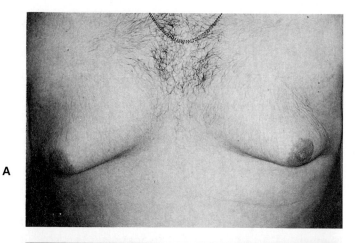

A

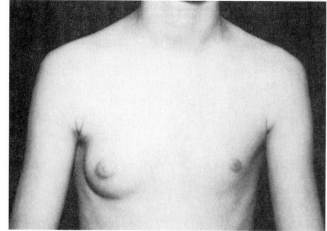

B

Fig. 16-30 Gynecomastia. **A,** Bilateral idiopathic gynecomastia in 34-year-old man. **B,** Idiopathic unilateral gynecomastia in a 15-year-old boy. *(A from Gallager et al, 1978; B from Isaacs, 1992.)*

■ *Cancer of the breast:* Uncommon in men but accounts for 1% to 2% of all breast cancers (Fig. 16-31). The lesions occurs most frequently around the nipple as a hard, irregular, and nontender mass.

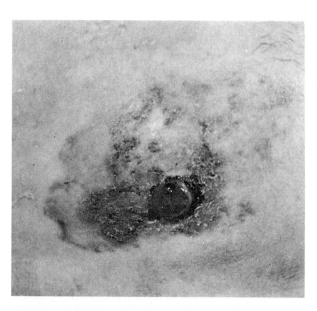

Fig. 16-31 Carcinoma of breast has infiltrated overlying skin, producing ulceration of nipple and areola. *(From Crichlow et al, 1972.)*

Sample Documentation & Nursing Diagnosis

CASE 1 52-year-old Hispanic woman with reported breast lump

Subjective

A tearful 52-year-old Hispanic woman reports finding a lump on her left breast while bathing. The mass was found 4 weeks ago. The client reports having a previous lump in the right breast approximately 5 years ago that was surgically removed and reported as benign. Client reports that she had a mammogram 4 years ago but has had none since that time. She also reports performing breast self-examination occasionally. Client is approximately 2 years postmenopausal and currently takes premarin 0.625 mg and provera 10 mg. There is no reported family history of breast cancer. Client reports that she believes that she is not responsible for her health; believes that external forces influence her life.

The client reports that the lump is in the upper outer quadrant of the left breast. It feels hard and is not tender. She denies nipple retraction or nipple discharge.

Objective

Inspection The breasts appear symmetric and full. There is no evidence of retractions, dimpling, bulging, breast discoloration, asymmetric vascularity, or nipple discharge.

Palpation The right breast is smooth and soft and without evidence of nodularity, masses, or tenderness throughout. The left breast is smooth, soft, and without tenderness. A single 2-cm, hard, nontender nodule is palpable at the 2 o'clock position in the upper outer quadrant approximately 5 cm from the nipple. The mass has a discrete border and is slightly moveable with palpation.

Nipple Palpation There is no evidence of nipple discharge, lesions, or crusting.

. . . .

Nursing Diagnosis #1

Fear related to whether breast mass is benign or malignant.

Defining Characteristics: Lump in left breast; history of previous lump.

Nursing Diagnosis #2

Altered health maintenance related to inability to seek help to maintain health secondary to health beliefs.

Defining Characteristics: External locus of control; performs breast self-examination inconsistently.

Sample Documentation

*&*Nursing Diagnosis

CASE 2   12-year-old African-American male with complaint of a big breast

Subjective

Client reports that approximately 1 month ago he noticed that his left breast was "getting big." He denies any previous episodes of breast enlargement or health problems. The client denies any use of medications or illicit drugs. He denies any nipple discharge or breast tenderness. Boys in the client's physical education class laugh at him. Client also reports poor diet that lacks intake of fruits and vegetables.

Objective

Height 4′11″ (1.5 m) ***Weight*** 160 pounds (72.7 kg)

Obese black male who appears to be stated age. Chest/breast appearance provides evidence of an enlarged left breast area. The right breast shows only slight fullness congruent with body weight. Palpation of the left breast feels smooth and slightly firm. There is no evidence of a mass or nodularity. There is no tenderness with palpation and no nipple discharge.

Nursing Diagnosis #1

Body image disturbance related to disfigurement of body.

Defining Characteristics: Left breast is "getting big" and others at school are teasing client.

Nursing Diagnosis #2

Altered nutrition: more than body requirements related to excessive intake in relation to metabolic need.

Defining Characteristics: Lack of exercise; diet deficit of fruits and vegetables; height 4′11″; weight 160 lbs.

HEALTH PROMOTION

■ **Breast Cancer Prevention and Screening** Instruct the client to reduce the amount of fat in the diet to no more than 30% of the total daily caloric intake. Instruct the client to participate in comprehensive breast screening on a regular basis. The comprehensive screening of the breast includes a triad of activities: professional clinical examination, breast self-examination, and mammography. Most authorities agree that all three methods of screening are important and necessary health promotion. See Table 16-2.

■ **Professional Clinical Examination** The American Cancer Society (1992) recommends that women ages 20 to 40 years have a manual clinical examination of the breasts at least every 3 years. After age 40, a professional examination is recommended annually.

■ **Breast Self-Examination** It is widely recommended that all women be taught and encouraged to perform breast self-examination. See box on p. 421 for the techniques of teaching breast self-examination.

■ **Mammography** The American Cancer Society (1988) and the National Cancer Institute (1987) recommend that baseline mammography should be done between ages 35 and 40, followed by annual or biennial mammograms from ages 40 to 49 and annual mammograms beginning at age 50. Other groups recommend annual clinical breast examinations until the woman reaches age 50 and then recommend mammograms every 1 to 2 years thereafter, concluding at approximately age 75 unless pathology has been detected (U.S. Preventive Services Task Force, 1989; Canadian Task Force, 1986; American College of Physicians, 1985). It may be prudent to begin mammography at an earlier age for women at increased risk for breast cancer. It has been estimated that mammography can detect a malignant mass as much as 2 years before it is detectable by palpation.

■ **Breast-Feeding** Women who are breast-feeding should be carefully assessed for problems with lactation. In addition, these women should be encouraged not to use over-the-counter medications, recreational drugs, alcohol, or tobacco.

TABLE 16-2	Breast Screening Recommendation		
	20–39 YEARS	**40–49 YEARS**	**50 YEARS AND OLDER**
Professional examination	every 3 years*	every year	every year
Breast self-examination	every month	every month	every month
Mammography	baseline age 35–39	every 1–2 years*	every year*†

* More frequently if clinically indicated
† Some sources do not recommend mammography beyond age 75

??????? STUDY QUESTIONS ???????

1. Describe the composition of the female breast.

2. Trace the routes of the three types of lymphatic drainage from the breast.

3. Identify four changes that occur during adolescent female breast development. How long does breast development take?

4. Describe the changes that take place in breast tissue during pregnancy.

5. Describe the changes that occur in the breasts of lactating women.

6. Describe the appearance of the breast after menopause.

7. How does the male breast differ from the female breast? What condition of the male breast is sometimes seen in adolescence or with a decrease in testosterone levels?

8. An individual presents with the complaint of breast tenderness. What specific questions would you ask when taking a history?

9. What information do you want to gather from an individual who has a lump in the breast? Discharge from the left nipple?

10. Identify the known risk factors for breast cancer. What racial group is at greatest risk for breast cancer? How prevalent is breast cancer in women?

11. How would you evaluate a woman's self-care behaviors when screening for breast cancer?

12. A client is breast-feeding for the first time. She complains of tenderness and pain in both breasts. What specific information would you need to obtain when taking her history?

13. What general guidelines should be considered before examination of an individual's breast? What equipment do you need?

14. Describe the steps and expected findings in a general inspection of the female breast, nipple, and areola.

15. A patient has a discharge from the nipple. What procedure is used to obtain a cytologic specimen?

16. List and describe the various arm positions used for breast examination.

17. Describe how to palpate the axilla. For what are you looking?

18. Describe the different methods that may be used for palpation of the breast.

19. Describe the common characteristics of breast masses.

20. A client has pendulous breasts. What specific techniques should be used for this examination?

21. Describe the procedure that should be used for examination of the male breast.

22. When examining an infant's breast, what normal findings might be expected? For what abnormalities are you looking?

23. Describe expected findings when examining the breasts of a lactating woman.

24. Describe the specific variations in the examination of the breast area of a woman who has had a mastectomy.

25. List common characteristics of malignant breast tumors. How are they distinguished from benign tumors such as fibroadenomas or fibrocystic disease?

26. Match the disease with the appropriate sign or symptom.

Intraductal papilloma	*Milk discharge from nipple*
Paget's disease	*Hard, red, swollen breast*
Galactorrhea	*Dry, scaly nipple*
Mastitis	*Serous nipple discharge*

27. Identify four health promotion behaviors and the associated recommended guidelines for improving breast health.

28. Outline the approach you would use to teach breast self-examination. Do males need to engage in breast self-examination?

CHAPTER 17

Abdomen and Gastrointestinal System

ANATOMY AND PHYSIOLOGY

The abdominal cavity, the largest cavity in the human body, contains vital organs, including the stomach, small and large intestines, liver, gallbladder, pancreas, spleen, kidneys, adrenal glands, and the uterus and ovaries in women, as well as major vessels. Lying outside the abdominal cavity, but a vital part of the gastrointestinal (GI) system, is the esophagus (Fig. 17-1). Support for the abdominal cavity is provided by the spine and rib cage, and protection by the peritoneum membrane and a muscular structure.

PERITONEUM, MUSCULATURE, AND CONNECTIVE TISSUE

The abdominal lining, the peritoneum, is a serous membrane forming a protective cover. It is divided in two layers, the parietal and the visceral peritoneum. The parietal peritoneum lines the abdominal wall, while the visceral peritoneum covers organs. The space between the parietal and visceral peritoneum is the peritoneal cavity. It usually contains a small amount of serous fluid to reduce friction between abdominal organs and their membranes.

The recti abdomini muscles form the anterior border of the abdomen, while the vertebral column and lumbar muscles form the posterior border. Lateral support is provided by the internal and external oblique muscles. A tendinous band, the linea alba, protects the midline of the abdomen between the recti abdomini. This band extends from the xiphoid process to the symphysis pubis. The abdomen is bordered superiorly by the diaphragm and inferiorly by the superior aperture of the lesser pelvis. The inguinal ligament, also called the Poupart

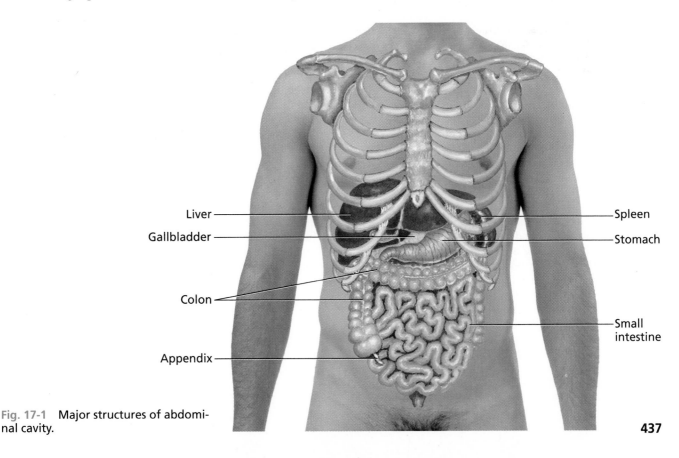

Liver

Gallbladder

Colon

Appendix

Spleen

Stomach

Small intestine

Fig. 17-1 Major structures of abdominal cavity.

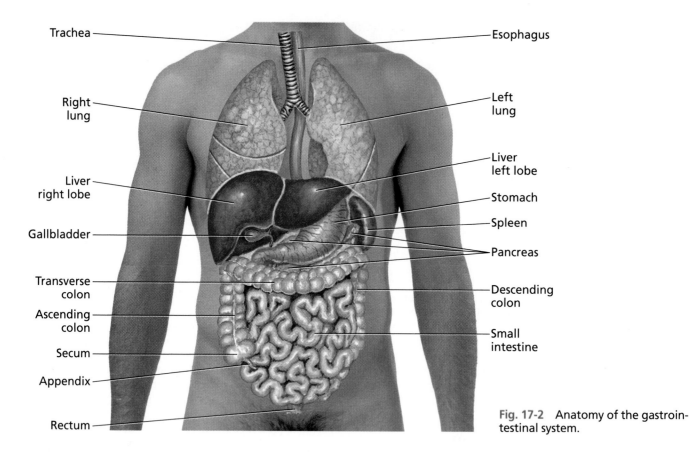

Trachea

Right lung

Liver right lobe

Gallbladder

Transverse colon

Ascending colon

Secum

Appendix

Rectum

Esophagus

Left lung

Liver left lobe

Stomach

Spleen

Pancreas

Descending colon

Small intestine

Fig. 17-2 Anatomy of the gastrointestinal system.

ligament, extends from the anterior superior iliac spine to the pubis on each side.

ALIMENTARY TRACT

The digestive system can be thought of as one long tube, the alimentary tract. From the mouth to the anus, the adult alimentary tract extends 27 feet (8 m) and includes the esophagus, stomach, small intestine, and large intestine (Fig. 17-2). One of its main functions is to ingest and digest food, absorbing nutrients, electrolytes, and water. Its other main function is to excrete resultant waste products. Products of digestion are moved along the digestive tract by peristalsis, under the control of the autonomic nervous system. The esophagus is a collapsible tube about 10 inches long connecting the pharynx to the stomach, passing just posterior to the trachea, through the mediastinal cavity and diaphragm.

Stomach. The stomach is located directly below the diaphragm in the left upper quadrant. It is a hollow, flask-shaped, muscular organ that stores food during eating, secretes digestive juices, and mixes food with the digestive enzymes and hydrochloric acid to break down fats and proteins (Fig. 17-3). Pepsin breaks down proteins, converting them to peptones and amino acids, while gastric lipase acts on emulsified fats to convert triglycerides to fatty acids and glycerol. The stomach also liquifies food into chyme and propels it into the duodenum of the small intestine.

Two sphincters control the flow of contents into and out of the stomach. The cardiac sphincter controls the flow of food from the esophagus into the stomach, and the pyloric sphincter regulates the outflow of chyme into the duodenum. The gastric mucosa contains parietal cells which absorb vitamin

B_{12}, necessary for erythrocyte production. The acidity of the stomach facilitates absorption of iron from the diet.

Small intestine. The longest section of the alimentary tract, the small intestine, is about 21 feet (6.3 m) long, beginning at the pyloric orifice and joining the large intestine at the ileocecal valve. In the small intestine, ingested food is mixed, digested, and absorbed. The small intestine is divided into three segments: the duodenum, jejunum, and ileum. The duodenum occupies the first foot (30 cm) of the small intestine and forms a C-shaped curve around the head of the pancreas. At the duodenum, bile and pancreatic secretions are received from the common bile duct for digestion; absorption then takes place through the walls of the small intestine.

The jejunum is 8 feet (2.5 m) long and the ileum is 12 feet (3.5 m) long. The ileocecal valve between the ileum and the large intestine prevents backward flow of fecal material.

Large intestine (colon) and rectum. The large intestine begins at the cecum, a small blind pouch that receives chyme from the ileum, and ends at the anus. It is about 4.5 to 5 feet (1.5 m) long, consisting of cecum, appendix, colon, rectum, and anal canal. The ileal contents empty into the cecum through the ileocecal valve; the appendix extends from the base of the cecum. The colon is divided into three parts: the ascending, transverse, and descending colon. The end of the descending colon turns medially and inferiorly to form the S-shaped sigmoid colon. The rectum extends from the sigmoid colon to the pelvic floor, where it continues as the anal canal, terminating at the anus.

Liver. The liver, gallbladder, and pancreas all secrete substances necessary for the digestion of chyme (Fig. 17-4). The largest organ in the body, weighing 3 to 4 lbs (1.5 kg), the liver

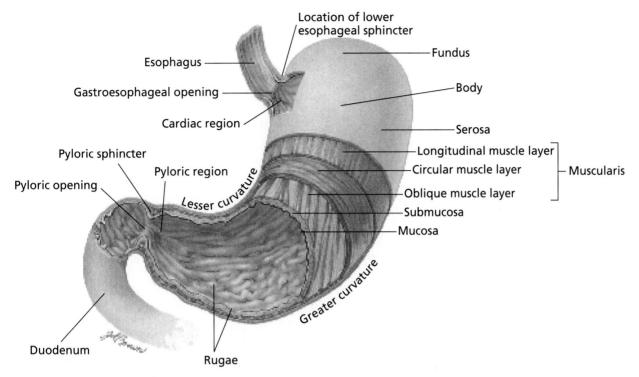

Fig. 17-3 Gross anatomy of the stomach. Cutaway section reveals muscular layers and internal anatomy. *(From Seeley, Stephens, and Tate, 1995.)*

lies under the right diaphragm, spanning the supper quadrant of the abdomen from the fifth intercostal space to slightly below the costal margin. The rib cage covers a substantial portion of the liver; only the lower margin is exposed beneath it. The liver is divided into right and left lobes. This complex organ has a variety of functions, including the following:

- Bile production and secretion, to emulsify fat
- Transfer of bilirubin from the blood (conjugated or direct) to the duodenum (unconjugated or indirect)
- Protein, carbohydrate, and fat metabolism
- Glucose storage in the form of glycogen
- Production of clotting factors and fibrinogen for coagulation
- Synthesis of most plasma proteins (albumin and globulin)
- Detoxification of a variety of substances, including drugs and alcohol
- Storage of certain minerals (iron and copper) and vitamins (A, B_{12}, and other B-complex vitamins).

Gallbladder. The gallbladder is a pear-shaped sac, 3 inches (7.6 cm) long, attached to the inferior surface of the liver (Fig. 17-4). It concentrates bile produced in the liver by absorbing excess water through its walls, then storing the bile, particularly between meals. The cystic duct combines with the hepatic duct to form the common bile duct, which drains bile into the duodenum. The presence of bile in the feces is evident by the brown color.

Pancreas. The pancreas lies in the upper left abdominal cavity, immediately under the left lobe of the liver, behind the stomach (Fig. 17-4). It is one of those rare glands with both endocrine and exocrine function. First, it produces endocrine enzymes such as insulin, glucagon, and gastrin for carbohydrate metabolism. Its exocrine secretions contain bicarbonate and pancreatic enzymes used to break down proteins, fats, and carbohydrates for absorption in the small intestine. The pancreatic duct empties into the duodenum.

Spleen. The concave, encapsulated spleen is a small organ about the size of a fist. It is located in the upper left abdominal cavity, posterior to the greater curvature of the stomach, in front of the first and second lumbar vertebrae (Fig. 17-4). Its main functions include the following:

- Storage of 1% to 2% of erythrocytes and platelets
- Removal of old or agglutinated erythrocytes and platelets by macrophages
- Activation of B and T lymphocytes
- Production of erythrocytes during bone marrow depression

Urinary Tract. The urinary tract includes the kidneys, ureters, urinary bladder, and urethra. Together, they remove water-soluble waste materials. In addition, the kidneys interact with other body systems to regulate fluid and electrolyte balance through elaborate microscopic filter and pressure systems that eventually produce urine. Kidneys also influence red cell production by secreting erythropoietin, influence blood pressure by secreting renin, and produce the biologically active form of vitamin D.

Kidneys. The kidneys are located in the posterior abdominal cavity on either side at the spinal levels of T12 through L3, where they are covered by the peritoneum and attached to the posterior abdominal wall. Each kidney is approximately 11 by 6 by 3 cm (4 inches × 2 inches × 1 inch) and partially protected

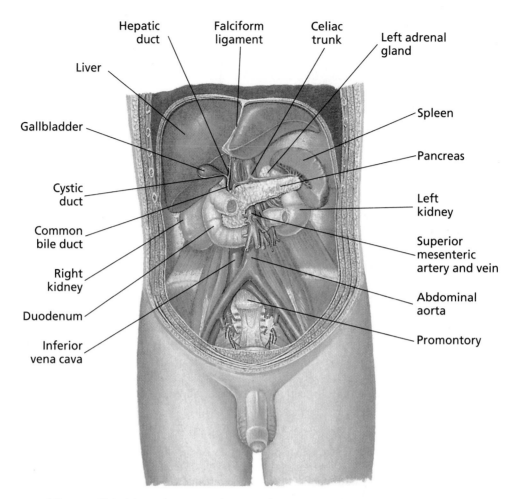

Fig. 17-4   Anatomy of liver, gallbladder, pancreas, spleen, and major vessels of abdominal cavity.   *(From Seidel et al, 1995.)*

by the ribs and a cushion of fat and fascia. The right kidney is slightly lower than the left, due to displacement by the liver.

Ureters. The urine formed in the nephron flows from the distal tubes and collecting ducts into the ureters and on into the bladder through peristaltic waves. Each ureter is composed of long, intertwining muscle bundles. The ureters extend for approximately 12 inch (30 cm) to insertion points at the base of the bladder.

Bladder. The bladder, a sac of smooth muscle fibers, is located behind the symphysis pubis in the anterior half of the pelvis. The bladder contains an internal sphincter, which relaxes in response to a full bladder. As a rule, when the bladder's urine volume reaches about 300 ml, moderate distention is felt; a level of 450 ml causes discomfort. On voiding, the urine exits the body through the urethra, which extends out of the base of the bladder to the external meatus.

Vasculature of the abdomen.   In the abdomen, the descending aorta travels from the diaphragm just to the left of midline until it branches into the two common iliac arteries at about the level of the umbilicus. The splenic and renal arteries also branch off within the abdomen.

PREGNANT WOMEN

A variety of abdominal changes occur during pregnancy. Changes in hormone levels contribute to gastrointestinal symptoms. A rise in chorionic gonadotrophin causes nausea and vomiting early in pregnancy, often referred to as "morning sickness." Later in the pregnancy, increased progesterone levels cause esophageal regurgitation, and a decreased emptying of the stomach may occur due to a decrease in smooth muscle tone and motility.

As the uterus enlarges, the abdominal muscles must stretch and lose some of their tone. During the third trimester, the recti abdomini muscles may separate, allowing the abdominal contents to protrude at the midline, creating a condition known as *diastasis recti*. Although the muscles gradually regain their tone after pregnancy, diastasis recti may persist. As the abdomen expands, the umbilicus flattens or protrudes. Striae and a midline stripe of pigmentation (linea nigra) may develop.

During pregnancy, both the appendix and colon are displaced upward and laterally. As the colon moves toward the back, peristaltic activity is decreased. Thus, in the third trimester, the woman may experience constipation, gastric burning, and flatus from loss of gastrointestinal tract tone and increased uterine pressure. Hemorrhoids are common, caused by increased pelvis vascularity and pressure. Also in the third trimester, there is an upward displacement of the stomach, with 15% to 20% of clients experiencing stomach herniation through the diaphragm.

Increased incidence of gallstones during pregnancy may be due to a combination of gallbladder distention, decreased emptying time, bile thickening, and hypercholesterolemia.

OLDER ADULTS

Changes in the structure and function of the gastrointestinal system occur with aging. Motility of the esophagus is reduced, due to a decreased number of cells causing dilation of the lower end of the esophagus. As aging occurs, less gastric acid is secreted; however, sufficient enzymes are available for di-gestion. Decreased motor activity delays the emptying of the stomach into the duodenum. With degeneration of the gastric mucosa, there is a reduction in parietal cells, which normally secrete intrinsic factor needed for vitamin B_{12} absorption.

The small intestine contains fewer absorbing cells, but this usually does not affect function. A decrease in lipase produc-tion may contribute to an intolerance of fatty foods. In the large intestine, weakened muscle and decreased peristalsis contribute to constipation. Bacterial flora in the intestines be-come less biologically active, contributing to food intolerance and impaired digestion. For example, older adults may have faulty absorption of vitamins B_1, B_{12}, calcium, and iron.

The liver decreases in size after age 50, reducing its stor-age capacity and ability to synthesize proteins. A decrease in cardiac output reduces the blood flow to the liver. As a result, the livers metabolism of drugs, hormones, and alcohol is less efficient (Lueckenotte, 1994).

Questions regarding nutrition and eating habits are asked in the general evaluation of the client (see Chapter 7). Specific areas to be covered in the assessment of the abdomen and GI system include abdominal pain, nausea and vomiting, jaundice, abdominal distention, urination, weight changes, and personal habits.

QUESTIONS

RATIONALE

ABDOMINAL PAIN

■ Do you have abdominal pain? How long have you had this pain? Where is it located? When did you first feel the pain? What were you doing at that time?

◄ *Time and activity at time of pain are important. Sudden, severe pain that awakens the client may be associated with acute perforation, inflammation, or torsion of an abdominal organ.*

■ Describe the pain. It is sharp? Burning? Cramping? Is it constant or does it come and go? Have you had episodes of this pain before? Did the pain start suddenly? Have you ever had gallstones or kidney stones?

◄ *Pain description is important. Intense pain may be caused from a stone in the biliary tract or ureter, rupture of a fallopian tube from an ectopic pregnancy, perforation of a gastric ulcer, peritonitis, or acute appendicitis.*

■ Has the pain changed its location since it started? Do you feel the pain in any other parts of your body?
■ Is it worse when your stomach is empty? Is it affected by eating?
■ Is the pain worse at night or during the day?

◄ *Diffuse, deep, and dull pain is visceral in origin, due to localized distention, inflammation, or ischemia. Sharp localized pain is parietal or peritoneal, due to generalized inflammation. Pain radiation patterns are shown in Table 17-3. Pain from acute appendicitis starts around the umbilicus and travels to the right lower quadrant. Pain from an abdominal aneurysm may start in the chest and travel to the abdomen. Back pain is associated with abdominal aneurysms also.*

■ Is there any particular position that relieves the pain?

◄ *Pancreatitis pain is relieved in the knee-chest position. Colicky (sharp visceral) pain (gallbladder or kidney stone) is relieved with restless movement. Pain of appendicitis is relieved by lying very still.*

■ Is pain associated with other factors, such as stress, fatigue, nausea and vomiting, gas, eating certain foods, fever, chills, constipation, diarrhea, rectal bleeding, frequent urination, or vaginal or penile discharge? What relieves the pain? What makes it worse? What have you done to relieve the pain?
■ Is the pain associated with your menstrual period? When was your last menstrual period?

◄ *Identifying symptoms associated with pain may assist in determining the cause.*

NAUSEA AND VOMITING

■ Have you been experiencing nausea or vomiting? How often? For how long? How much do you vomit?

◀ *Vomiting is usually caused by severe irritation of the peritoneum, caused by (1) obstruction of the intestine, bile duct, or ureter, (2) toxins, or (3) perforation of an abdominal organ (Swartz, 1994).*

■ What does it look like? Does it have an odor?

◀ *The characteristics of the vomitus may help to determine its cause. Acute gastritis leads to vomiting of stomach contents, whereas obstruction of the bile duct results in greenish-yellow vomitus, and an intestinal obstruction may have a fecal odor to the vomitus. Vomiting stomach contents is associated with acute gastritis.*

■ Are you taking any new medications? Could you be pregnant?

◀ *Many medications produce nausea or vomiting as a side effect. These symptoms are also associated with pregnancy and GI disease.*

■ Does vomitus contain blood?

◀ *Consider stomach or duodenal ulcers or esophageal varices when vomitus contains blood.*

■ Do you have nausea without vomiting?

◀ *Nausea without vomiting is a common symptom of pregnant clients or those with metastatic disease.*

■ Have you noticed a change in your hearing ability? Do you have ringing in your ears?

◀ *Clients with Meniere's disease may have nausea accompanied by hearing loss and tinnitus (see Chapter 12).*

■ Do you have other symptoms with the nausea or vomiting? Pain? Constipation? Diarrhea? Change in color of stools? Change in color of urine? Fever or chills?

◀ *Liver disease may change stool color. Infection may cause fever and chills.*

■ Did the symptoms begin over the last 24 hours? What foods did you eat over this period? Where did you eat? At home? At a restaurant? How long after you ate did you vomit? Has anyone else in your family exhibited these symptoms over the same time period?

◀ *Food poisoning, stomach influenza, or pregnancy may cause these symptoms.*

JAUNDICE (Icterus)

■ How long have you had a yellow discoloration of the skin, mucous membrane, or sclera? Did it occur rapidly? Is it associated with abdominal pain? Loss of appetite? Nausea? Vomiting? Do you drink alcohol? If so, how much? How often?

◀ *Jaundice indicates liver disease or obstruction of bile flow.*

■ In the last year, have you had a blood transfusion or tattoos? Are you using any intravenous drugs? Do you eat raw shellfish, for example, oysters? Have you traveled abroad in the last year? Where? Did you drink unclean water?

◀ *Hepatitis infection can result from blood transfusions, use of unsterile needles, or ingestion of contaminated shellfish or unclean water.*

■ Has your urine or stools changed color?

◀ *Urine changing from amber to brown and stools changing from brown to clay-colored suggest high serum bilirubin from liver disease.*

QUESTIONS   ## RATIONALE

ABDOMINAL DISTENTION

■ How long has your abdomen been distended? Does it come and go? Is it related to eating? Is the distention relieved by passing gas? By burping? Is the distention associated with vomiting or loss of appetite? Weight loss? Change in bowel habits? Shortness of breath?

◄ *Distention associated with eating is intermittent and relieved by passing gas. Distention caused by ascites is a progressive process and increases abdominal girth. Loss of appetite is associated with cirrhosis and malignancy. Shortness of breath and ascites are associated with heart failure or some other cause of ascites.*

URINATION

■ Have you felt any pain or burning when urinating? Have you had the urge to urinate, but been unable to?
■ Is there any blood in the urine?

◄ *Pain, burning, or frequency may indicate a bladder infection.*
◄ *Blood in the urine is associated with menstrual periods in women or with kidney disease.*

■ Describe the color of the urine.

◄ *Dark amber urine is associated with kidney disease.*

■ Have you had fever or chills?

◄ *Fever and chills may indicate bladder or kidney infection.*

■ Have you had any pain in your back on the right or left side?

◄ *Back pain may be an indication of costovertebral angle (CVA) tenderness, which accompanies kidney infections.*

WEIGHT CHANGES

■ Have you noted any change in your appetite, either an increased hunger or a lack of appetite? What have you eaten in the last 24 hours? Have you noted any weight gain or loss? How much weight have you gained (lost)? *If client does not weigh self, ask:* Do your clothes seem tight or loose? Over what period of time? Have you been dieting?
■ Does eating relieve your depression or stress? Does eating relieve physical symptoms?

◄ *Decreased appetite may occur as a side effect of medications, during pregnancy, or with psychological problems or cancer.*

◄ *Eating can be a response to psychologic variables (depression, anxiety, multiple lifestyle changes, stress) or physical variables (ill health, alterations in physical activity, allergies or food idiosyncracies, mouth or dental problems).*

■ Have you had any difficulty swallowing? How long has this been happening? What have you done to help it?

◄ *Dysphagia can occur with throat or esophageal disorders or when objects are stuck in the throat or esophagus such as a piece of meat.*

■ Are there foods that you do not or cannot eat? What happens when you eat them?

◄ *Food intolerance can be the result of personal habits (likes and dislikes), cultural and religious values, allergies, or physical conditions (e.g., lactose intolerance can make a person unable to digest milk).*

■ Does your stomach feel bloated or uncomfortably full after eating? Do you have indigestion? Do you take any antacid products on a regular basis? When was your last bowel movement? Describe its consistency and color.

◄ *Fullness could be caused by gas or overeating.*
◄ *Constipation can contribute to distention.*

QUESTIONS   RATIONALE

PERSONAL HABITS

■ What medications are you currently taking? Do you drink alcohol? How much? How often? When did you last have an alcoholic beverage?

◄ *Both medications and alcohol have definite effects on the GI system.*

■ Do you smoke? How much? When did you start smoking?

◄ *Cigarette smoking is a risk factor for gastric ulcers.*

■ What have you eaten over the last 24 hours, or since breakfast yesterday?

◄ *A 24-hour recall is needed to evaluate nutritional status.*

INFANTS

■ Is the baby being breast-fed or bottle-fed? If bottle-fed, how is the baby tolerating the formula? Does the baby spit up frequently?

◄ *Frequent regurgitation is associated with gastroesophageal reflux.*

■ Have you changed the baby's formula? What new foods do you feed the baby? How does the baby tolerate these foods? How many bowel movements does the baby have daily? Describe.

◄ *Formula with iron may be a cause of irritation. New foods can be allergens (especially wheat and corn), and should be added to the infant's diet one at a time until acceptance has been evaluated.*

CHILDREN

■ Does your toddler eat regular meals? How often? How do you feel about your child's eating habits?

◄ *Parents can be anxious about their toddler's eating habits, although irregular and unpredictable patterns are common at this time. As long as the child's growth and development are normal, parents should be reassured.*

■ What foods does your child snack on?

◄ *Offering nutritious snacks will help the child make good choices.*

■ What has your child eaten over the past 24 hours?

◄ *Evaluation of the child's diet requires a 24-hour recall.*

■ Does your child ever eat things that are not food, such as paint chips, dirt, paper, or grass?

◄ *By the age of 2, children should know what is edible. Pica is the eating of nonedible materials. At this age children are at risk for lead poisoning.*

■ Does your child have abdominal pain? What is the pain like? When did it start? Where is it located?

◄ *Although this symptom is difficult to assess in young children, it often accompanies inflammation of the bowel, constipation, urinary tract infection, and anxiety. Note that children do not always differentiate the stomach from the abdomen in reporting pain.*

ADOLESCENTS

■ What do you generally eat at regular meal times? Do you eat breakfast? What foods do you snack on?

◀ *Adolescent eating behaviors are under the adolescent's control and may reflect rejection of familial values or practices. Problems such as being overweight, underweight, anemic, fatigued, or having systemic disease, will require further evaluation.*

Determining Risk for Anorexia Nervosa

Cluster four of the following:
■ Distorted body image
■ Periods of amenorrhea
■ Periods of hyperactivity
■ History of being overweight
■ Denial of hunger
■ Denial of fatigue
■ History of self-induced vomiting to stay thin
■ Morbid fear of obesity
■ Preoccupation with food

■ How many calories do you believe you consume? Do you eat food high in fat or salt? How much exercise do you get?

◀ *It is important to assess the adolescent's knowledge of good nutrition and exercise and supply educational facts where needed.*

■ Have you lost weight recently? How much? Did you do this through diet, exercise, or another method? Do you eat when you are not hungry? When you feel depressed or stressed? Do you ever use laxatives or vomiting to control weight?

◀ *Thin teenaged girls should be evaluated for anorexia nervosa, a serious psychosocial disorder that involves loss of appetite, voluntary starvation, and severe weight loss. Self-induced vomiting and laxatives may be used to control weight by individuals with anorexia nervosa and bulimia.*

■ Do you ever eat large amounts of food at one time? How often?

◀ *These are characteristics of bulimia. Half of the individuals with anorexia nervosa are bulimic as well.*

■ In general, how do you feel about yourself? Do you feel attractive?

◀ *Body image is distorted in anorexia nervosa and other eating disorders.*

■ Are you active? Do you feel tired? Are your menstrual periods normal? How do your parents feel about your eating habits? Your friends?

◀ *Other signs of anorexia nervosa include hyperactivity, irregular menstrual periods or amenorrhea, and denial of hunger or fatigue. Anorexia nervosa is a control disorder and the client should be referred to a physician.*

OLDER ADULTS

■ Do you need any assistance getting groceries or preparing meals?

◀ *Nutritional deficiencies among the elderly can result from lack of access to grocery stores, limited income, or physical disabilities.*

■ Do you eat alone or share mealtime with others?

◀ *Social isolation, including living alone, can lead to the older adult not bothering to prepare meals at all and then suffering malnutrition.*

QUESTIONS

■ What did you eat for breakfast yesterday? For lunch? For dinner? How did you fix the food (e.g., did you fry food in butter)?

■ Do you have any difficulty eating? Does this involve swallowing? Loose or missing teeth? Do you wear dentures?

■ Do you walk after a meal or lie down to rest? Do you have difficulty with constipation? How do you define constipation? How much liquid do you drink a day? How much bulk or fiber do you eat? Do you take any laxatives for constipation? Which ones? How often?

■ What medications do you take?

RATIONALE

◀ *A 24-hour recall is the best method for evaluating nutritional status. However, with older adults the pattern may vary with the time of the month (with money running out before the end of the month), so the examiner may want to ask about weekly variations.*

◀ *Any of these problems may contribute to poor nutrition.*

◀ *It is important to evaluate the GI side effects of all medications for older adults.*

EXAMINATION Procedures and Findings

Guidelines **Strong overhead light should be provided for this examination, in addition to a second light source. The abdomen should be fully exposed, with genitalia and breasts (if client is female) draped. Make sure that the client's bladder has been recently emptied, his or her arms are alongside the torso, a small pillow is under the head, and the client's knees are slightly flexed. (A pillow may be placed under the knees.) The room, the stethoscope, and the examiner's hands should be warmed and fingernails should be short and smooth.**

Assessment of the abdomen uses the four assessment techniques; however, auscultation is performed before percussion and palpation, since these latter techniques may alter the presence or absence of bowel sounds or pain. To accurately describe the location of findings, the abdomen can be divided into four quadrants (Fig. 17-5; see box below for anatomic correlates) or nine regions (Fig. 17-6; see box on facing page for anatomic correlates). Specific anatomic landmarks are used to facilitate description of signs and symptoms (Fig. 17-7). These landmarks include the xiphoid process of the sternum, the costal margin, the midline from the tip of the sternum through the umbilicus to the pubic bone, the left and right midclavicular lines (RMCL, LMCL), the left and right midaxillary line (LMAL, RMAL), the umbilicus, the anterosuperior iliac spine, Poupart's (inguinal) ligament, and the superior margin of the pubic bone.

EQUIPMENT **Stethoscope**
Small ruler
Marking pencil or pen
Tape measure
Penlight or other light source

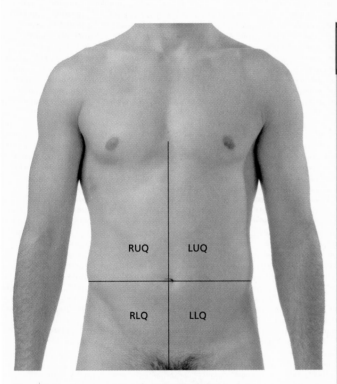

Fig. 17-5   Four quadrants of the abdomen.

Anatomic Correlates of the Four Quadrants of the Abdomen

Right Upper Quadrant	**Left Upper Quadrant**
Liver and gallbladder	Left lobe of liver
Pylorus	Spleen
Duodenum	Stomach
Head of pancreas	Body of pancreas
Right adrenal gland	Left adrenal gland
Portion of right kidney	Portion of left kidney
Hepatic flexure of colon	Splenic flexure of colon
Portions of ascending and transverse colon	Portions of transverse and descending colon
Right Lower Quadrant	**Left Lower Quadrant**
Lower pole of right kidney	Lower pole of left kidney
Cecum and appendix	Sigmoid colon
Portion of ascending colon	Portion of descending colon
Bladder (if distended)	Bladder (if distended)
Ovary and salpinx	Ovary and salpinx
Uterus (if enlarged)	Uterus (if distended)
Right spermatic cord	Left spermatic cord
Right ureter	Left ureter

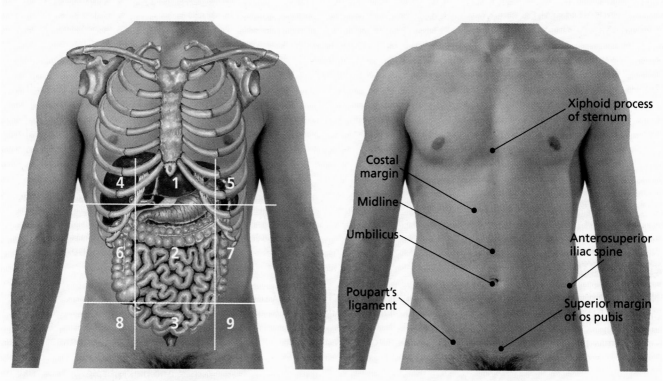

Fig. 17-6   Nine regions of the abdomen.

Fig. 17-7   Landmarks of the abdomen.

Anatomic Correlates of the Nine Regions of the Abdomen

Right Hypochondriac	Epigastric	Left Hypochondriac
Right lobe of liver	Pyloric end of	Stomach
Gallbladder	stomach	Spleen
Portion of duodenum	Duodenum	Tail of pancreas
Hepatic flexure of colon	Pancreas	Splenic flexure of colon
Portion of right kidney	Portion of liver	Upper pole of left kidney
Suprarenal gland		Suprarenal gland
Right Lumbar	**Umbilical**	**Left Lumbar**
Ascending colon	Lower duodenum	Descending colon
Lower half of right kidney	Jejunum and ileum	Lower half of right kidney
Portion of duodenum		Portions of jejunum
and jejunum		and ileum
Right Inguinal	**Hypogastric**	**Left Inguinal**
Cecum	Ileum	Sigmoid colon
Appendix	Bladder	Left ureter
Ileum (lower end)	Uterus (in pregnancy)	Left spermatic cord
Right ureter		Left ovary
Right spermatic cord		
Right ovary		

TECHNIQUES and NORMAL FINDINGS

Observe the client's general behavior and appearance. He or she should appear relaxed, lying quietly, with slow, even respirations.

ABDOMEN

INSPECT the abdomen for Skin Color, Surface Characteristics, Contour, and Surface Movements. Direct a light source at a right angle to the client's long axis.

Color may be paler than other parts of the skin, due to lack of exposure.

Surface characteristics should be smooth, with silver-white striae possibly present; scars; and a very faint, fine vascular network. Note the umbilicus should be centrally placed, contour is usually sunken, although it may protrude slightly, and should be smooth and noninflamed.

Contour of the abdomen may be enhanced by adjusting the light source to form shadows that highlight small changes in the contour. Contour should be flat to slightly rounded. Evaluate symmetry of features by viewing the abdomen at eye level from the side, as well as from behind the client's head.

Observe for *surface movements*. Peristalsis is usually not visible, but there may be an upper midline pulsation visible in thin individuals. Generally, the abdomen should move smoothly and evenly with respirations. Generally females exhibit costal movements and males abdominal movements.

Ask the client to take a deep breath and hold it. The contour of the abdomen should remain smooth and symmetric.

Ask the client to raise his or her head without using the arms for support. The rectus abdominis muscles become prominent and a midline bulge may appear.

ABNORMAL FINDINGS

■ Emaciation, obesity, marked restlessness, marked immobility or a rigid posture, the knees drawn up, facial grimacing, and rapid, uneven, or grunting respirations should be noted as abnormal. Clients with pancreatitis prefer knee-chest position; those with peritonitis or appendicitis will lie very still; those with colicky gallstones or ureteral stones may rock.

■ Jaundice, redness (inflammation), lesions, bruises, discoloration, cyanosis, rashes, and pink, purple, or red striae indicate abnormalities.

■ Note prominent venous patterns or engorgements of the veins around the umbilicus. Glistening or taut appearance is associated with ascites. The umbilicus should not be displaced upward, downward, or laterally, nor should a hernia be visible around or slightly above the umbilicus. Note if the umbilicus is inflamed or has drainage.

■ Check for distention or marked concavity, which is associated with general wasting signs or anteroposterior rib expansion. No masses or bulges should be visible in any area of the abdominal surface. Abdominal distention may result from the 7 "Fs"—fat (obesity), fetus (pregnancy), fluid (ascites), flatulence (gas), feces (constipation), fibroid tumor, or fatal tumor.

■ Note visible peristalsis or marked pulsations. Grunting or labored movements or restricted abdominal movements with respirations should be recorded.

■ Note any bulges or masses, particularly of the liver or spleen.

■ Areas where bulges are apparent through the muscle layer may result from pregnancy or marked obesity and are not pathologic. However, bulges may be caused by abdominal or incisional hernias.

TECHNIQUES and NORMAL FINDINGS

AUSCULTATE the abdomen for Bowel Sounds. Be sure to auscultate *before* palpating and percussing the abdomen. A quiet environment may be necessary. Auscultate the four abdominal quadrants and the epigastrium for bowel sounds. Use the diaphragm of the stethoscope and press lightly. Listen in a systematic progression, such as from right upper quadrant (RUQ) to left upper quadrant (LUQ) to left lower quadrant (LLQ) and finally to right lower quadrant (RLQ). Bowel sounds should be noted every 5 to 15 seconds. The duration of a single bowel sound may range from 1 second to several seconds. The sounds are high-pitched gurgles or clicks, although this varies greatly.

AUSCULTATE the abdomen for Arterial and Venous Vascular Sounds. Listen for arterial vascular sounds with the bell of the stethoscope. Normally vascular sounds are not heard. Listen over the aortic, renal, iliac, and femoral arteries for bruits that make "swishing" sounds, are systolic in timing, and continuous as the client is moved into various positions (Fig. 17-8).

ABNORMAL FINDINGS

■ Palpation of the abdomen before auscultation may alter the presence or absence of bowel sounds or pain.

■ Report any absence of sound after listening for several minutes in each quadrant. *Decreased* or absent bowel sounds occur with inflammation, paralytic ileus, and following general anesthesia. Decreased bowel sounds are associated with peritonitis and bowel obstruction. *Increased* bowel sounds, also called borborygmi, are high-pitched "tinkles" associated with increased peristalsis from diarrhea, use of laxative, gastroenteritis, or an area anterior to an early intestinal obstruction.

■ Bruits indicate a turbulent blood flow caused by narrowing of the vessel. Bruits over the aorta suggest an aneurysm. Two sound patterns may indicate renal arterial stenosis: soft, medium-to-low-pitched murmurs heard over the upper midline or toward the flank, or epigastric bruits that radiate laterally.

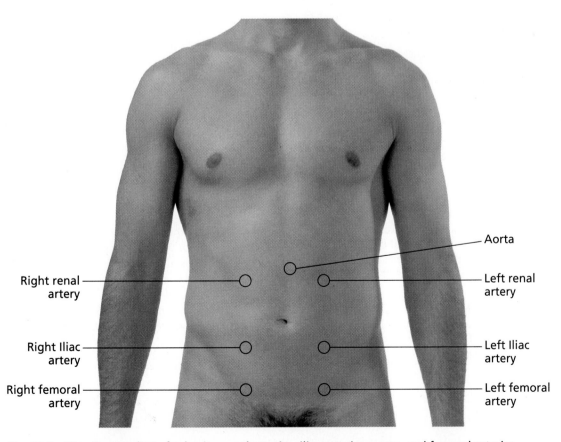

Aorta

Right renal artery — Left renal artery

Right Iliac artery — Left Iliac artery

Right femoral artery — Left femoral artery

Fig. 17-8 Sites to auscultate for bruits: renal arteries, iliac arteries, aorta, and femoral arteries.

Also listen with the bell over the epigastric region and around the umbilicus for a venous hum, a soft, low-pitched, and continuous sound.

PERCUSS the abdomen for Tones. Percuss all four quadrants for tones, using indirect percussion to assess density of abdominal contents. (Develop a system or routine for the percussion process to ensure that all areas are covered)(Fig. 17-9). Percuss in each quadrant for tympany and dullness. Tympany is the most common percussion tone found due to the presence of gas. The suprapubic area may be dull when the urinary bladder is distended. See Chapter 6 for the procedures for percussion.

◼ Venous hums are rare, but associated with portal hypertension and cirrhosis.

◼ Note any marked dullness in a localized area.

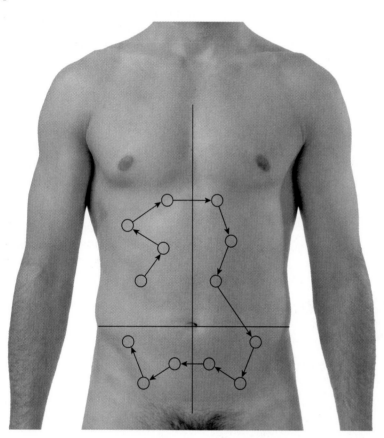

Fig. 17-9   Systematic route for abdominal percussion.

PERCUSS the liver to determine Span.
Midclavicular liver span. 1. Beginning below the level of the umbilicus at the (RMCL); percuss upward over the tympanic area until dull percussion tone indicates the liver border. Mark the border with the marking pencil or pen. The lower border is usually at the costal margin or slightly below it (Fig. 17-10, *A*).

2. Beginning over the lung in the RMCL, percuss downward until percussion tone changes from resonant to dull, indicating the upper liver border. Mark the location with the marking pencil or pen. The upper border usually begins in the fifth to seventh intercostal space (Fig. 17-10, *B*).

◼ Note when the lower border of the liver exceeds 0.75 to 1 inch (2 to 3 cm) below the costal margin. This indicates an enlarged liver, which is associated with cirrhosis and hepatitis.

◼ Note when dullness extends above the fifth intercostal space indicating an enlarged liver.

TECHNIQUES and NORMAL FINDINGS

3. Estimate the midclavicular liver span. Normal is 2.5 to 4.5 inches (6 to 12 cm), with men having a greater liver span than women (Fig. 17-10, *C*). Taller individuals have a greater span also.

4. Ask the client to take a deep breath and hold; then percuss upward in the right MCL again to estimate the liver descent. The lower border of the liver should descend inferiorly 2 to 3 cm.

■ Note any span exceeding 4.5 inches (12 cm). Enlarged liver is called *hepato-megaly* and is associated with cirrhosis. Also, clients with chronic obstructive pulmonary disease may have a flat diaphragm, which makes percussion of the upper border of the liver difficult. Obesity can make percussion difficult.

■ Note if the liver fails to move with inspiration or if movement is less than 2 cm.

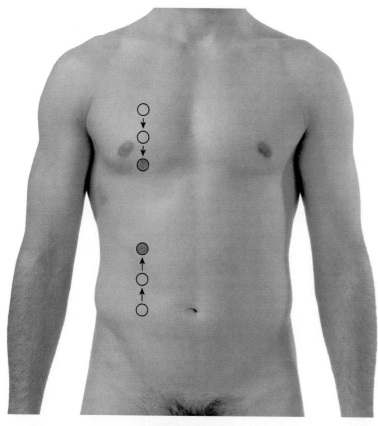

A

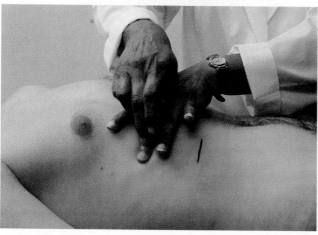

B

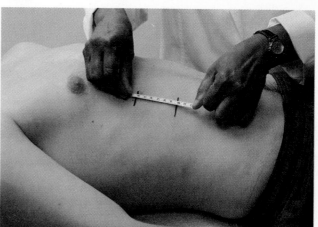

C

Fig. 17-10 **A,** Liver percussion route. **B,** Percussion method of estimating size of liver in the midclavicular line. **C,** Distance between the two marks measured in estimating the liver span in midclavicular line is usually 6 to 12 cm.

TECHNIQUES and NORMAL FINDINGS

ABNORMAL FINDINGS

PERCUSS the spleen for Size. Percuss from the seventh to the eleventh rib at about the left midaxillary line (Fig. 17-11). Begin in the left midaxillary line (MAL) at about the tenth rib. Try to outline the spleen by percussing in several directions from dullness to resonance or tympany. A small area of splenic dullness may be heard at the sixth to the tenth rib.

Percuss the lowest intercostal space in the left anterior axillary line before and after the client takes a deep breath. The area is usually tympanic.

■ Splenic enlargement may indicate infection or trauma.

■ Note whether the tympany changes to dullness on inspiration. An enlarged spleen is brought forward on inspiration to produce a dull percussion note. *Caution:* A full stomach or feces-filled intestine may create dullness in this area also.

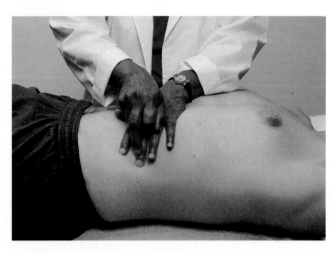

Fig. 17-11   Percussion of the spleen

PERCUSS the stomach for Tympany. Percuss over the left lower rib cage. A gastric "bubble" may be noted that is tympanic and varies in size.

PALPATE the abdomen lightly for Tenderness, Muscle Tone, and Surface Characteristics. Palpate all four quadrants of the abdomen. Use the pads of the fingertips to depress abdomen 1 to 2 cm (Fig. 17-12). No tenderness should be present, and the abdominal muscles should be relaxed, although anxious clients may have some muscle resistance on palpation. Note consistent tension as you move across the smooth surface. Detect hypersensitivity in two ways. Gently lift a fold of skin away from underlying tissue or use a pin to stimulate the skin (Fig. 17-13, *A* and *B*).

Ask client to describe the sensation (Fig. 17-14).

■ Dullness over the stomach may indicate ascites.

■ Note any cutaneous tenderness or area of hypersensitivity, as well as any involuntary resistance that cannot be relaxed on command. Note superficial masses or localized areas of rigidity or increased tension. Rigidity is associated with peritoneal irritation, and may be diffuse or localized.
■ Client may describe pain as an exaggerated sensation, which may indicate peritoneal irritation.

TECHNIQUES and NORMAL FINDINGS   **ABNORMAL FINDINGS**

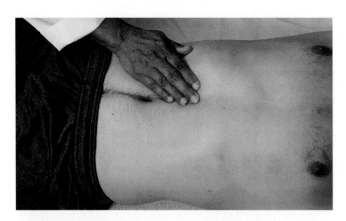

Fig. 17-12   Light palpation of the abdomen.

A 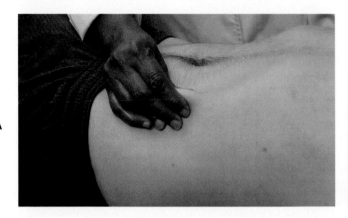 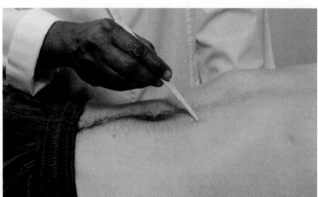 B

Fig. 17-13   Testing for cutaneous hypersensitivity. **A,** Lift a fold of skin away from underlying muscle, or **B,** stimulate the skin with the sharp point of a broken tongue blade.

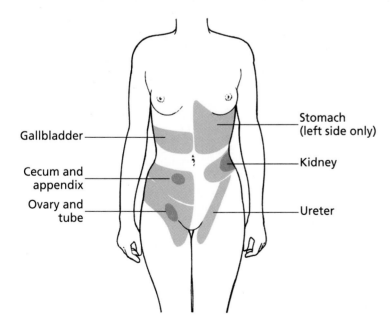

Fig. 17-14   Areas of cutaneous hypersensitivity.   *(From Seidel et al, 1995.)*

TECHNIQUES and NORMAL FINDINGS

PALPATE the abdomen deeply for Tenderness, Masses, and Aorta Pulsation. Palpate all four quadrants. Use either the distal flat portions of the finger pads (Fig. 17-15) pressing gradually and deeply (4 to 6 cm) into the palpation areas, or use a bimanual technique, with the lower hand resting lightly on the surface and the upper hand exerting pressure for deep palpation (Fig. 17-16). Observe for facial grimaces during palpation that may indicate areas of tenderness.

ABNORMAL FINDINGS

■ Note any pain that is present in local or generalized areas. The client may respond to pain by using muscle guarding, facial grimaces, or pulling away from the examiner (Table 17-1). Note any masses.

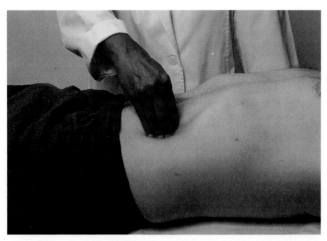

Fig. 17-15 Deep palpation of the abdomen.

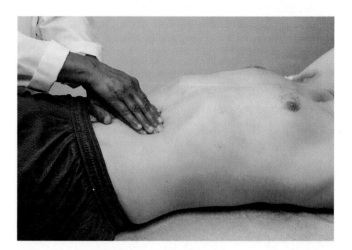

Fig. 17-16 Deep bimanual palpation.

TABLE 17-1	Differentiation of Abdominal Pain		
CAUSE	**CLIENT CHARACTERISTICS**	**PAIN TYPE**	**PAIN LOCATION**
Gastroesophageal reflux	Any age	Gnawing, burning	Midepigastric; may radiate to jaw
Gastroenteritis	Any age	Crampy	Diffuse
Gastritis	Alcoholism	Constant, burning	Epigastric
Peptic ulcer	30-50 years; more males than females	Gnawing, burning	Epigastric radiating to sides, back, right shoulder
Pancreatitis	Alcoholism, cholelithiasis	Steady, severe to mild, knife-like, sudden onset	LUQ and epigastric; radiates to back
Appendicitis	Any age; peak 10-20 yrs.	Colicky, progressing to constant	Umbilicus moving to RLQ
Cholecystitis	Adults; more females than males	Colicky, progressing to constant	RUQ radiates to right scapula
Ectopic pregnancy	History of menstrual irregularity	Sudden onset, persistent pain	Lower quadrant
Diverticular disease	Elderly	Intermittent cramping	LLQ
Irritable bowel disease	Young women	Crampy, recurrent, sharp, burning	LLQ
Intestinal obstruction	Elderly; those with prior abdominal surgery	Colicky, sudden onset	May be localized or generalized

TECHNIQUES and NORMAL FINDINGS

Tenderness is often present in the midline near the xiphoid process, over the cecum, and possibly over the sigmoid colon. Ask the client to breathe through the mouth to facilitate muscle relaxation.

The aorta is often palpable at the epigastrium, as well as above and slightly to the left of the umbilicus (Fig. 17-17). It pulsates in a forward direction. The borders of the rectus abdominis muscles can be felt, as can the sacral promontory and feces in the ascending or descending colon.

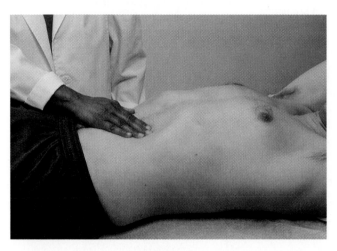

Fig. 17-17 Palpating the aorta.

ABNORMAL FINDINGS

■ Abnormal findings include masses that descend during inspiration, lateral pulsatile masses (abdominal aortic aneurysm), laterally mobil masses, and fixed masses.

ASSOCIATED SYMPTOMS	AGGRAVATED BY	AMELIORATED BY	FINDINGS
Weight loss	Recumbency, bending, stooping	Antacids, sitting up	
Nausea and vomiting, fever, diarrhea	Food	Some relief with vomiting, diarrhea	Hyperactive bowel sounds
Hemorrhage, nausea and vomiting, diarrhea, fever	Alcohol, food, salicylates	Antacids	
	Empty stomach, stress, alcohol, recumbency	Food, antacids	Epigastric tenderness to palpation or percussion
Nausea and vomiting, diaphoresis	Lying supine	Leaning forward	Abdominal distention, ↓ bowel sounds, diffuse rebound
Vomiting, constipation, fever	Worse with moving, coughing	Lying still	Rebound tenderness RLQ, positive obturator, positive iliopsoas
Nausea and vomiting, dark urine, light stools, jaundice	Fatty foods, drugs		Tender to palpation or percussion of RUQ
Tender adnexal mass, vaginal bleeding			Palpable mass on affected side
Constipation, diarrhea	Eating	Bowel movement, passing flatus	Palpable mass LLQ
Mucus in stools		May be relieved by defecation	Colon tender to palpation
Vomiting, constipation			Hyperactive bowel sounds in small obstruction

PALPATE around the umbilicus for Bulges, Nodules, and the Umbilical Ring. The ring should be round with no irregularities or bulges. The umbilicus itself may be inverted or slightly everted.

PALPATE the liver for Lower Border and Tenderness. Deeply palpate at the right costal margin before and during deep inspiration and after complete expiration. Place the left hand under the eleventh and twelfth ribs and lift upward, while the right hand is parallel to the right costal margin (Fig. 17-18). Ask the client to inhale deeply and then exhale. The border and contour of the liver is often not palpable. It may "bump" against the fingers during inspiration, especially in thin clients. The border of the liver should feel smooth, and no tenderness should be present.

■ Note if the umbilical ring is incomplete or soft in the center.

■ A very enlarged liver may lie under the examiner's hand as it extends downward into the abdominal cavity.

■ Note any irregular surfaces or edges as well as any tenderness. With pain, the client may abruptly stop inspiration.

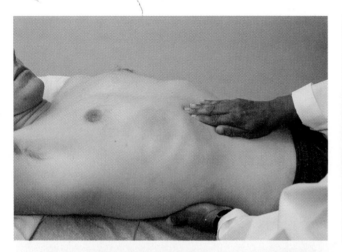

A

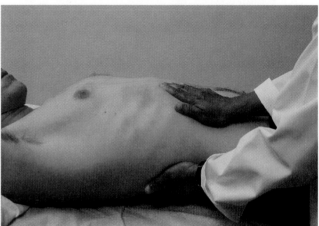

B

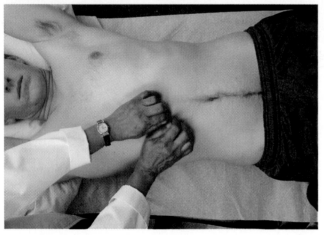

C

Fig. 17-18   Methods of palpating the liver. **A,** Fingers are extended, with tips on right midclavicular line below the level of liver tenderness and pointing toward the head. **B,** Fingers parallel to the costal margin. **C,** Fingers hooked over the costal margin.

PALPATE the gallbladder for Tenderness. Palpate below the liver margin at the lateral border of the rectus abdominus muscle for the gallbladder. A healthy gallbladder is not palpable.

■ A palpable, tender gallbladder may indicate cholecystitis. Test for cholecystitis by asking the client to take in a deep breath during deep palpation. Cholecystitis is suspected if the client experiences pain and abruptly stops inhaling during palpation. This is called Murphy's sign. A nontender, enlarged gallbladder suggests common bile duct obstruction.

PALPATE the spleen for Border and Tenderness. Standing at the client's right side, place the left hand under the client's left costovertebral angle and exert pressure upward to move the spleen anteriorly. Press the right hand gently under the left anterior costal margin (Fig. 17-19).

Ask the client to take a deep breath and then exhale. With the exhalation, follow the tissue contour under the border of the ribs to try to palpate the spleen; normally it is not palpable.

An alternate strategy for spleen palpation is to perform the procedure with the client lying on the right side with the legs and knees somewhat flexed. Stand on the client's right and place your left hand over the client's left costovertebral angle while pressing your right hand under the left anterior costal margin.

■ A palpable will feel like a firm mass that bumps against examiner's fingers. Spleen tenderness may indicate infection or trauma.

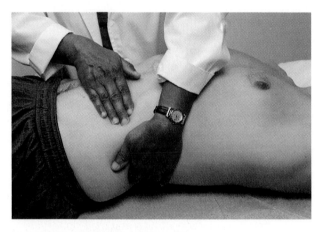

Fig. 17-19 Palpation of the spleen.

PALPATE the kidneys for Presence, Contour, and Tenderness.

1. *Left kidney.* Stand to the client's right with client in a supine position. Place the left hand at the left posterior costal angle (left flank) and the right hand at the client's left anterior costal margin. Ask the client to take a deep breath and exhale completely. With exhalation, elevate the client's left flank with your left hand and palpate deeply with your right hand (Fig. 17-20). Occasionally the lower pole of the kidney can be felt in thin clients, but rarely in the average client. The contour should be smooth with no tenderness.

2. *Right kidney.* Repeat the same maneuver on the right side, which is easier to palpate since it lies lower than the left kidney (Fig. 17-21). The lower pole of the right kidney may be palpated during inspiration as smooth, firm and nontender.

■ Tenderness is associated with kidney trauma or infection, for example, pyelonephritis.

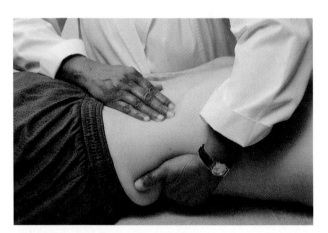

Fig. 17-20 Palpation of left kidney.

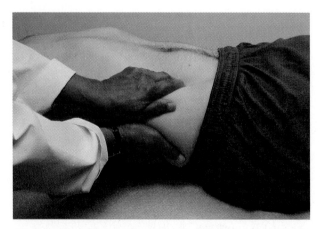

Fig. 17-21 Palpation of right kidney.

PALPATE the inguinal nodes for Size, Tenderness, Mobility, and Contour. With the finger pads, lightly palpate the inguinal areas just below the inguinal ligament and the inner aspect of the upper thigh at the groin for horizontal and vertical inguinal nodes (Fig. 17-22). If palpable nodes should be small and mobile; nontender nodes are often present. The contour is smooth or nonpalpable, and the nodes seem soft or cannot be palpated. The femoral pulse, located lateral to the inguinal nodes, may be palpated at this time.

■ Note any enlarged, tender, or hard nodes which may indicate inflammation.

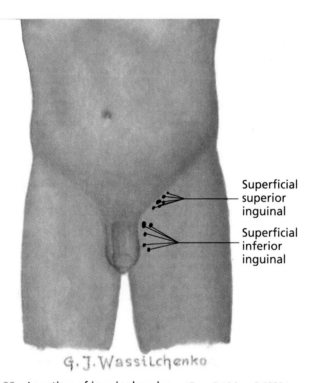

G. J. Wassilchenko

Fig. 17-22   **Location of inguinal nodes.**   *(From Seidel et al, 1995.)*

Superficial superior inguinal

Superficial inferior inguinal

TECHNIQUES and NORMAL FINDINGS	**ABNORMAL FINDINGS**

ELICIT abdominal reflexes for Presence. Elicit the abdominal reflexes by stroking each quadrant with the end of a reflex hammer or tongue blade (Fig. 17-23). For upper abdominal reflexes, stroke upward and away from the umbilicus; for lower abdominal reflexes, stroke downward and away from the umbilicus. The expected response to each stroke is contraction of the rectus abdominis muscle and movement of the umbilicus toward the side stroked.

■ Diminished reflexes may be found in clients who are obese or have been pregnant. An absence of reflexes is associated with disease of the motor tracts of the spinal cord.

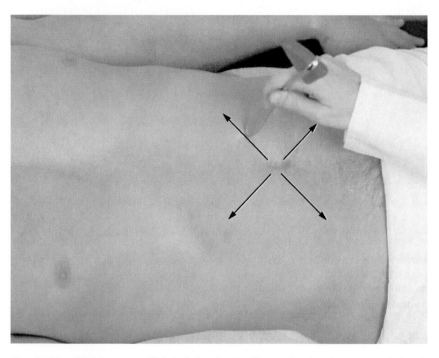

Fig. 17-23   Eliciting superficial abdominal reflexes. Stroke the upper abdominal area upward, away from the umbilicus, and the lower umbilicus area downward, away from the umbilicus.   *(From Seidel et al, 1995.)*

ADDITIONAL ASSESSMENT TECHNIQUES FOR SPECIAL CASES

PERCUSS the kidneys for Costovertebral Angle (CVA) Tenderness. Approach the client from behind as he or she is seated. Use direct percussion to tap each CVA with the ulnar surface of the dominant fist (Fig. 17-24, *A*). An alternative method is to use indirect percussion. Place the palmar surface of the nondominant hand over the CVA and tap the dorsum of that hand with the dominant fist (Fig. 17-24, *B*). The client should perceive a thud.

■ CVA tenderness or severe pain may indicate pyelonephritis.

TECHNIQUES and NORMAL FINDINGS

ABNORMAL FINDINGS

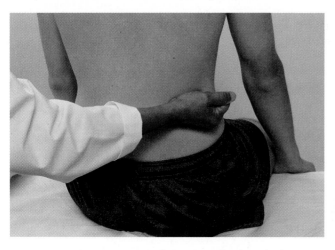
A

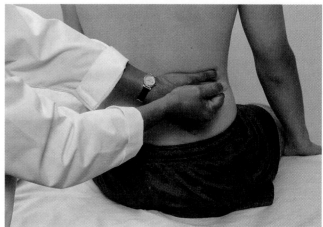
B

Fig. 17-24   Fist percussion of costovertebral angle for kidney tenderness. **A,** Direct percussion. **B,** Indirect percussion.

ASSESS the abdomen for Fluid. If fluid is suspected within the abdomen, perform the following tests:

1. *Shifting dullness.* Ask the client to lie supine so that any fluid will pool in the lateral (flank) area. Percuss the abdomen. Draw lines on the abdomen to indicate the midline tympany percussion area in contrast to lateral dullness. Then have the client turn to the right side and listen as the tympanic sound shifts to the upper (left) side and the area of dullness rises toward the midline (Fig. 17-25). Finally, have the client turn to the left lateral position and listen as the dullness rises toward the midline.

■ Movement of dullness as the client shifts position reflects the shift of fluid in the abdomen (ascites).

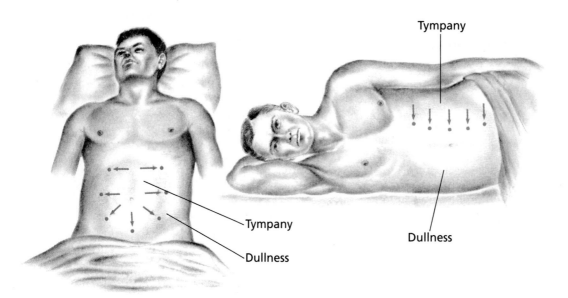

Fig. 17-25   Testing for shifting dullness. Dullness shifts to the dependent side.   *(From Seidel et al, 1995.)*

2. *Fluid wave.* Another examiner's or client's hand is placed sideways in the middle of the client's abdomen to stop the transmission of a tap across the skin (Fig. 17-26). The examiner then taps one flank while palpating the other side. If ascites is present, the tap will cause a fluid wave through the abdomen, and the examiner will feel the fluid with the other hand on the opposite side of the abdomen.

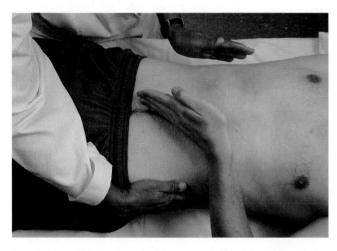

Fig. 17-26 Testing for fluid wave. Strike one side of the abdomen sharply with the fingertips. Feel for the impulse of a fluid wave with the other hand.

ASSESS the abdomen for Pain. If the client has abdominal pain, test for rebound tenderness as follows: Press down firmly and slowly over the area of discomfort (Fig. 17-27), then release the hand suddenly. Ask the client which pain is worse while pressing down or releasing. Rebound tenderness is present if the client experiences more pain when pressure is released than with pressure.

■ Rebound tenderness indicates peritoneal irritation or appendicitis.

A

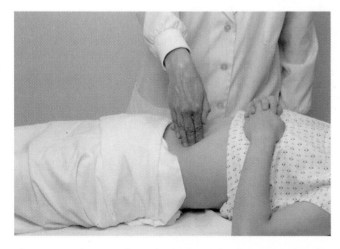

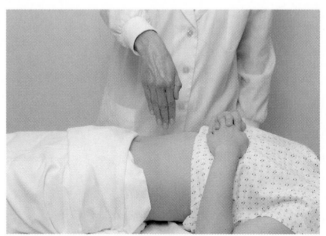

B

Fig. 17-27 Testing for rebound tenderness. **A,** Press deeply and gently into the abdomen; then **B,** rapidly withdraw the hands and fingers.

TECHNIQUES and NORMAL FINDINGS

ABNORMAL FINDINGS

Perform the *iliopsoas muscle test* when acute appendicitis is suspected. With the client supine, the examiner places his or her hand over the lower right thigh. Ask the client to raise the right leg, flexing at the hip. The examiner pushes down to resist the raising of the leg (Fig. 17-28). When the client reports no pain from the pressure on the iliopsoas muscle, the test is negative.

■ An inflamed appendix may irritate the lateral iliopsoas muscle. When the client reports LLQ pain to pressure against the raised leg, the iliopsoas muscle test is positive.

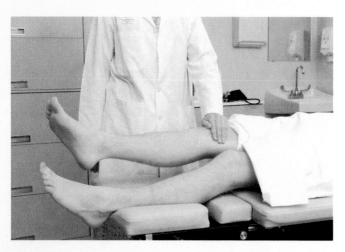

Fig. 17-28   Iliopsoas muscle test.   *(From Doughty, 1993.)*

Perform the *obturator muscle test* when a ruptured appendix or pelvic abscess is suspected. The client lies supine and flexes the right hip and knee to 90°. The examiner, holding the leg just above the knee and at the ankle, rotates the leg medially and laterally (Fig. 17-29). If the client has no pain, the test is negative.

■ Pain in the hypogastric region is a positive sign indicating irritation of the obturator muscle, which may be caused by a ruptured appendix or pelvic abscess.

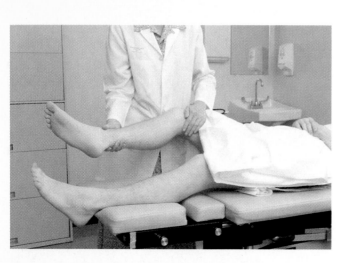

Fig. 17-29   Obturator muscle test.   *(From Doughty, 1993.)*

ASSESS abdomen for Floating Mass. *Ballottement* is a palpation technique used to determine a floating mass, such as the fetal head. Ballottement can be performed with one or two hands.

The examiner places one hand perpendicular to the abdomen and pushes in toward the mass with fingertips (Fig. 17-30, *A*). A freely moveable mass will float upward and touch the fingertips as fluids and other structures are displaced.

When using the bimanual method, the examiner places one hand on the anterior abdomen to push down. The other hand is placed against the flank to push up and palpate the mass to determine presence and size (Fig. 17-30, *B*).

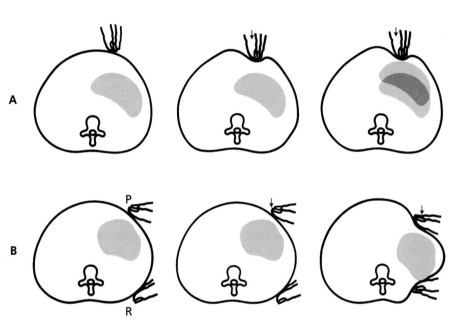

Fig. 17-30 Ballottement technique. **A,** Single-handed ballottement. Push inward at a 90° angle; if the object is freely movable, it will float upward to touch the fingertip. **B,** Bimanual ballottement: *P,* pushing hand; *R,* receiving hand. *(From Seidel et al, 1995.)*

AGE-RELATED VARIATIONS

INFANTS

■ APPROACH

The abdominal examination is easy and straightforward, with the infant lying supine on an examining table. Hearing bowel sounds may be a challenge with the very active infant.

■ FINDINGS

Follow the same procedures for examining the abdomen as for adults. The normal infant abdomen is symmetric, soft, and round with a slight protrusion, and no masses are present. Diastasis swelling and a gap between the rectus muscles may be noted during crying. Note any distention, masses, and concave, sunken, or flat appearance. A scaphoid, turnip-shaped abdomen suggests diaphragmatic hernia. Report distention and vomiting, which may suggest intestinal obstruction.

Evaluate the liver, spleen, and kidneys as described for adults. The edge of the liver should be 1 to 2 cm (0.5 to 0.75 inch) below the right rib cage (costal margin). The spleen is generally not palpable, although the tip may be felt in the left upper quadrant (far left costal margin). The left kidney is noted with deep palpation; both should be 1 to 2 cm (0.5 to 0.75 inch) above the umbilicus. Bladder ballottement is noted above the symphysis pubis. *Abnormal findings* include an enlarged liver 3 cm or more below the margin, palpable spleen, masses near the kidneys, and enlarged kidneys.

Evaluate the umbilicus in the newborn. Immediately after the umbilical cord is cut, two veins and one artery should be noted. After the cord is clamped, it will change from white to black as it dries; it should be dry in 5 days and fall off spontaneously in 7 to 14 days. *Abnormal findings* include discharge, odor, or redness around the umbilicus; a protrusion or nodular appearance of the umbilicus; thick Wharton's jelly; and a thin or green cord.

CHILDREN

■ APPROACH

Children may resist palpation because they are ticklish. Have them put a hand on their own abdomen for self palpation. Place your hand over their fingers and slowly move your fingers to their abdomen for your palpation.

■ FINDINGS

Evaluation in children is generally the same as for adults, with the following areas to be noted.

Evaluate any umbilical hernia. This is common in African-American children until 7 years of age and considered normal in white children under 2 years of age. Note any hernia still present beyond the ages noted.

Inspect the contour of the abdomen. It is normally rounded (a "pot belly") in toddlers both while standing and while lying down. School-age children may show this roundedness until about 13 years of age when standing; when lying, the abdomen should be scaphoid. Note any scaphoid abdomen in toddlers and any generalized distention.

Note movement of the abdomen on respiration. Until about age 7, children are abdominal breathers; after age 7, boys exhibit chiefly abdominal movement whereas girls exhibit chiefly costal movement. Note any grunting or labored breathing accompanied by restricted abdominal movement.

Check the tenseness of the abdominal muscles. The condition of diastasis recti abdominis (two rectus muscles fail to approximate one another) is common in African-American children but should disappear during the preschool years. Note if the condition is present beyond preschool or is accompanied by hernia.

Percuss the liver for tone and span. Averages vary by age, as follows: 5 years of age = 2.75 inches (7 cm); 12 years of age = 3.5 inches (9 cm). Percuss for spleen tone and span. In young children the area of dullness may extend to 0.5 to 0.75 inches (1 to 2 cm) below the costal margin.

Palpate the liver to locate the border. Location varies by age, as follows: birth to 6 months of age = 0 to 3 cm (0 to 0.25 in.) below costal margin; 6 months to 4 years of age = 1 to 2 cm (0.5 to 0.75 inches) below costal margin; over 4 years = 1 to 2 cm (0.5 to 0.75 inches) or not palpable below the right costal margin.

Palpate the spleen. It may be felt at the costal margin or slightly under the ribs in small children; note that only the tip (which should feel like a small tongue) should be palpable. Finding a palpable spleen in an older child who also appears ill or who has multiple other symptoms is abnormal.

Palpate the bladder. The bladder is frequently felt as a smooth mass that extends along the midline, somewhere between the pubis and the umbilical area. It may not be palpable after urination. Note if there is still bladder distention after voiding.

■ APPROACH

The evaluation of older adults is generally the same as for other adults.

■ FINDINGS

Elderly individuals may have increased fat deposits over the abdominal area even with decreased subcutaneous fat over the extremities. Note any marked distention or concavity associated with general wasting signs or antero-posterior rib expansion.

Elderly clients often have a more lax abdominal tone. They may not manifest a rigidity response to the extent that a younger client does; rigidity may be replaced by distention.

CLIENTS WITH SITUATIONAL VARIATIONS

PREGNANT WOMEN

■ APPROACH

Physical examination of the pregnant woman depends on the stage of gestation. Unique assessment skills for evaluating the pregnant woman include measuring the fundal height and using Leopold's maneuvers to help determine fetal presentation and position. When auscultating the abdomen, count fetal heart beats for an entire minute.

■ FINDINGS

Several expected findings during an abdominal examination are unique to pregnancy. The bowel sounds are decreased as a result of reduced peristaltic activity. Nausea and vomiting may occur during the first trimester due to the rise in chorionic gonadotrophin hormone. Striae and a linea nigra (a line of dark pigmentation through the midline) may be observed as the uterus grows, stretching the abdominal wall. Later in the pregnancy, as fetal growth expands the uterus, pressure on the intestine contributes to constipation, which is commonly reported, and to hemorrhoids.

The enlarged uterus may separate the muscles (diastasis recti). Venous patterns may be seen throughout the abdomen.

Palpate the fundus (top of the uterus), it should be in the midline or slightly to the right (Fig. 17-31). Fetal movements (quickening) may be reported at 16 to 20 weeks; movement can be evaluated by placing the hand over the abdomen. When tapped, the fetus may rebound in amniotic fluid.

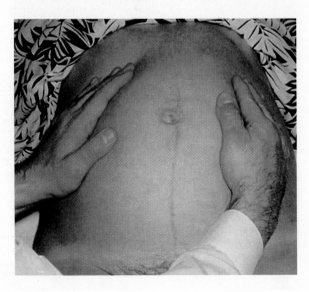

Fig. 17-31 Palpating uterine fundus. *(From Al-Azzawi, 1990.)*

Measure fundal height from the symphysis pubis to the top of the fundus (Fig. 17-32). By week 12 of pregnancy the fundus is palpable just above the symphysis pubis; at 16 weeks the fundus is approximately halfway between the symphysis and umbilicus; at 20 weeks the fundus is at the umbilicus; at 28 weeks the fundus is halfway between the umbilicus and the xiphoid; and at 34 weeks the fundus is at the xiphoid (Fig. 17-33). Measurement of fundal height is an estimate and may vary among examiners by 1 to 2 cm. After week 20 the fundus should increase in size about 1 cm (0.5 inch) per week. Uterine size should correlate with gestational age. Any discrepancy between fundal height and the estimate of gestational age based on last menstrual period (LMP) should be evaluated further. A uterus that is larger than expected may be due to inaccurate date of LMP, more than one fetus, gestational diabetes, or polyhydramnios. A uterus that is smaller than expected for gestational age may be due to inaccurate date of LMP or a poorly growing fetus.

Palpate fetal position for fetal attitude, lie, presentation, position, and size. The outline of the fetus can be determined after 26 to 28 weeks. The *attitude* is the relationship of the fetal head and limbs to the body. The expected attitude is moderate flexion of the head, flexion of the arms onto the chest, and flexion of the legs. The *lie* is the relationship of the long axis of the fetus to the long axis of the uterus. The lie can be longitudi-

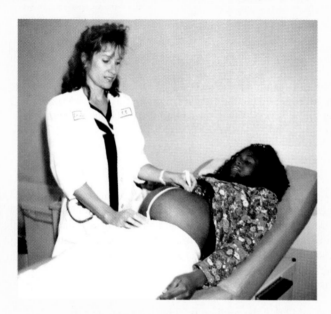

Fig. 17-32 Measuring fundal height. *(From Dickason, Silverman, Schult, 1994.)*

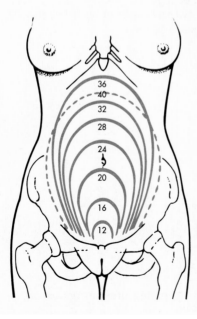

Fig. 17-33 Changes in fundal height with pregnancy. Weeks 10-12, uterus within pelvis; fetal heartbeat can be detected with Doppler. Week 12, uterus palpable just above symphysis pubis. Week 16, uterus palpable halfway between symphysis and umbilicus; ballottement of fetus is possible by abdominal and vaginal examination. Week 20, uterine fundus at lower border of umbilicus; fetal heartbeat can be auscultated with fetoscope. Weeks 24-26, uterus changes from globular to ovoid shape; fetus palpable. Week 28, uterus approximately halfway between umbilicus and xiphoid; fetus easily palpable. Week 34, uterine fundus just below xiphoid. Week 40, fundal height drops as fetus begins to engage in pelvis. *(From Seidel et al, 1995.)*

nal, oblique, or transverse (Fig. 17-34). The *presentation* is determined by the fetal lie and by the body part of the fetus that enters the pelvic passage first. The presentation may be vertex, brow, face, shoulder, or breech (Fig. 17-35). *Position* refers to the relationship of the landmark on the presenting fetal part to the front, sides, or back of the maternal pelvis. The landmark on the fetal presenting part is related to four imaginary quadrants of the pelvis: left anterior, right anterior, left posterior, and right posterior. These quadrants indicate whether the presenting part is directed toward the front, back, left, or right of the pelvic passage.

A   B   C

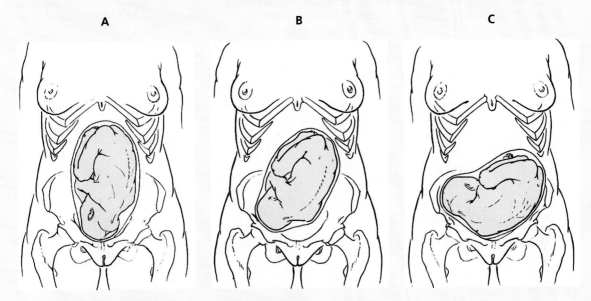

Fig. 17-34 **Examples of fetal lie. A,** Longitudinal lie. **B,** Oblique lie. **C,** Transverse lie. *(From Barkauskas et al, 1994)*

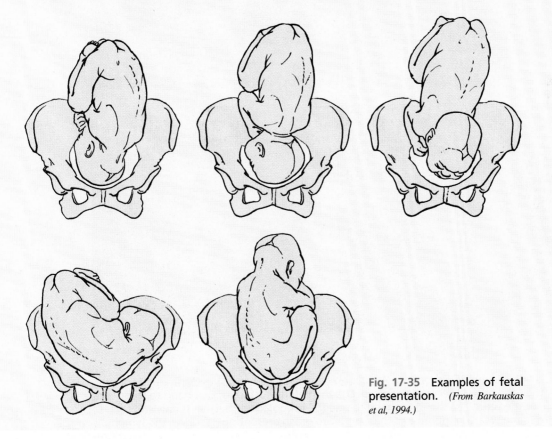

Fig. 17-35 **Examples of fetal presentation.** *(From Barkauskas et al, 1994.)*

Palpate the fundus using Leopold's maneuvers. The client should be lying supine, with head slightly elevated and knees flexed slightly. Using the palmer surface of both hands on the uterine fundus, apply firm, smooth pressure to identify the fetal parts. The first maneuver is to detect the head; it is round, firm and movable. The buttocks feel softer and less mobile. The second maneuver is to palpate the spine of the fetus. It is smooth and convex, as compared to irregular feel on the other side of the fetus—the hands, elbows, knees, and feet. The third maneuver is to gently grasp the presenting anatomic part over the symphysis pubis using your dominant hand. The head feels firm and movable from side to side if not engaged. The buttocks feel soft and irregular. The fourth and final maneuver is to use both hands to identify the outline of the fetal head. If it is the presenting part, only a small portion may be felt (Fig. 17-36, *A-D*).

 ## Racial Variation

African-American women have an average gestational period of 273 days, which is 9 days shorter than the average gestational period in white women.

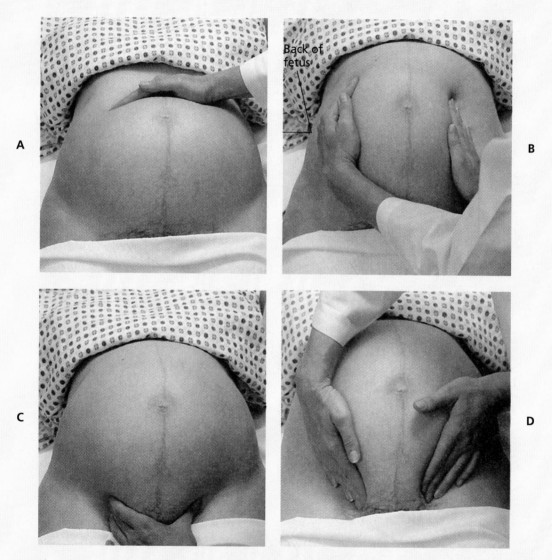

Fig. 17-36 Leopold maneuvers. **A,** First maneuver. Place hand(s) over fundus and identify the fetal part. **B,** Second maneuver. Use the palmar surface of one hand to locate the back of the fetus. Use the other hand to feel the irregularities, such as hands and feet. **C,** Third maneuver. Use thumb and third finger to grasp presenting part over the symphysis pubis. **D,** Fourth maneuver. Use both hands to outline the fetal head. With a head presenting deep in the pelvis, only a small portion may be felt. *(From Seidel et al, 1994.)*

Fetal heart tones are heard by Doppler at about 10 to 12 weeks and by fetoscope at 17 to 19 weeks. An expected range is 140 to 160 beats per minute. Note if these sounds are not appropriate. The fetal head will move into the maternal pelvis before delivery (lightening), causing maternal bowel sounds to decrease.

After delivery, evaluate muscle tone and resolution of problems associated with pregnancy. Abdominal muscle tone returns in a few weeks. Rectus muscles may remain separated. Hemorrhoids usually resolve in 1 to 2 weeks; constipation remains common for the first 3 or 4 days. Thirst may be prominent during the early puerperium as a result of dehydration during labor or postpartum diuresis.

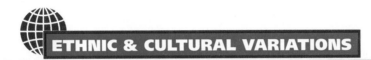

ETHNIC & CULTURAL VARIATIONS

■ **FINDINGS**

Documented racial variations of the abdomen and gastrointestinal system are few. Gestational periods are generally shorter for pregnant African-American women. American Indians and Alaskan Natives have a higher incidence of liver and gallbladder disease.

EXAMINATION SUMMARY
Abdomen and Gastrointestinal System

Abdomen *(pp. 450-461)*
- Inspect the abdomen for:
  Skin color
  Surface characteristics
  Contour
  Surface movements
- Auscultate abdomen with diaphragm of stethoscope for:
  Bowel sounds
- Auscultate abdomen with bell of stethoscope for:
  Arterial (aortic, renal, iliac, femoral) bruits
  Venous hum
- Percuss abdomen for:
  Tones in all quadrants
- Percuss liver for:
  Span
- Percuss spleen for:
  Size
- Percuss stomach for:
  Tympany
- Palpate abdomen lightly in all quadrants for:
  Tenderness
  Muscle tone
  Surface characteristics
- Palpate abdomen deeply for:
  Tenderness
  Masses
  Aorta pulsation
- Palpate around the umbilicus for:
  Bulges
  Nodules
  Umbilical ring

- Palpate the liver for:
  Lower border and tenderness
- Palpate gallbladder for:
  Tenderness
- Palpate spleen for:
  Border
  Tenderness
- Palpate kidneys for:
  Presence
  Contour
  Tenderness
- Palpate inguinal nodes for:
  Size
  Tenderness
  Mobility
  Contour
- Elicit abdominal reflexes for:
  Presence

Additional Assessment Techniques for Special Cases *(pp. 461-465)*
- Percuss kidneys for costovertebral angle tenderness
- Assess abdomen for fluid:
  Shifting dullness
  Fluid wave
- Assess abdomen for pain:
  Rebound tenderness
  Iliopsoas test
  Obturator test
- Assess abdomen for floating mass:
  Ballottement

COMMON PROBLEMS/CONDITIONS
associated with the Abdomen and Gastrointestinal System

ALIMENTARY TRACT

■ *Gastroesophageal reflux:* Flow of gastric secretions up into the esophagus. Causes epigastric pain and heartburn, aggravated by lying down and relieved by sitting up, antacids, and eating.

■ *Hiatal hernia:* A protrusion of the stomach through the esophageal hiatus of the diaphragm into the mediastinal cavity. Muscle weakness is a primary factor in developing this type of hernia. It is associated with pregnancy, obesity, and ascites, and occurs more frequently in women and older adults.

■ *Peptic ulcer:* An ulcer occurring in the lower end of the esophagus; in the stomach, usually along the lesser curvature; or the duodenum. *Duodenal ulcer* is the most common form, caused by a break in the duodenal mucosa that scars with healing (Fig. 17-37). Ulcers may result from infection with *Helicobacter pylori* and cause increased gastric secretion. Clients complain of localized epigastric pain when the stomach is empty, which is relieved by food or antacids. Gastric bleeding may occur as a result of the ulcer, causing signs of hematemesis, melena, dizziness, hypotension, or tachycardia. Perforation of a duodenal ulcer may be life-threatening. Ulcers on the anterior walls are more likely to perforate, while ulcers on the posterior wall are more likely to bleed.

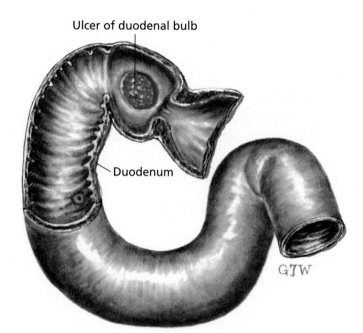

Fig. 17-37   Duodenal peptic ulcer.   *(From Doughty, 1993.)*

■ *Crohn's disease:* A chronic inflammatory bowel disease of unknown origin (Fig. 17-38). Inflammation may occur anywhere along the GI tract from mouth to anus, but it most commonly affects the terminal ileum and colon and produces ulcers, fibrosis, and malabsorption. Diseased sections become thicker, which narrows the lumen. The mucosa is ulcerated, with formations of fistulas, fissures, and abscesses. Diseased sections may be separated by normal bowel segments. Clients complain of severe abdominal pain, cramping, diarrhea, nausea, fever, chills, weakness, anorexia, and weight loss. It is also called regional enteritis or regional ileitis.

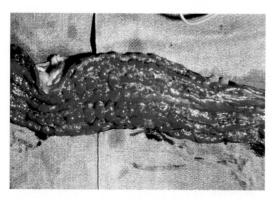

Fig. 17-38   Crohn's disease showing deep ulcers and fissures, creating "cobblestone" effect.   *(From Doughty, 1993.)*

■ *Ulcerative colitis:* A chronic, episodic inflammatory disease that starts in the rectum and progresses through the large intestine (Fig. 17-39). The submucosa becomes engorged, and mucosa becomes ulcerated and denuded with granulation tissue. Ulcerative colitis is characterized by profuse watery diarrhea of blood, mucus, and pus, and may progress to colon cancer. Clients complain of severe abdominal pain, fever, chills, anemia, and weight loss.

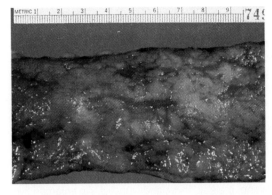

Fig. 17-39 Ulcerative colitis showing severe mucosal edema and inflammation with ulcerations and bleeding. *(From Doughty, 1993.)*

■ *Diverticulitis:* Inflammation of diverticula (pouch-type herniations through the muscular wall) in the colon (Fig. 17-40). Presence of fecal material through the thin-walled diverticula causes inflammation and abscess in the tissues around the rectum. It is probably secondary to a diet low in fiber. Clients complain of cramping pain in the LLQ, nausea, vomiting, and altered bowel habits, usually constipation. The abdomen may be distended and tympanic, with decreased bowel sounds and localized tenderness.

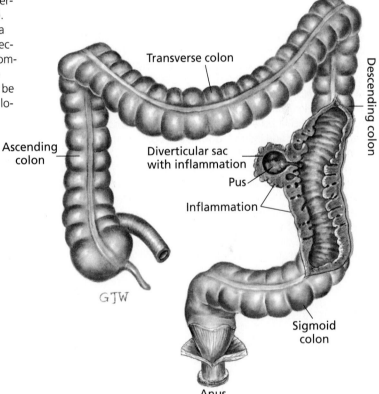

Fig. 17-40 Diverticulosis (diverticulitis). *(From Doughty, 1993.)*

HEPATOBILIARY SYSTEM

■ ***Viral hepatitis:*** Inflammation of the liver resulting from different hepatitis viruses. Table 17-2 shows modes of transmission and incubation period for common types of hepatitis. Pathologic changes in the liver are similar regardless of the causative virus. Edema and cell infiltration in parenchyma and portal ducts, hepatic cell necrosis, Kupffer cell proliferation, and accumulation of necrotic debris produce changes in the lobules and ducts that ultimately disturb bilirubin excretion. Symptoms range from mild to severe, with hepatitis B being the most serious. Common symptoms are anorexia, vague abdominal pain, nausea, vomiting, malaise, fever, and jaundice. An enlarged liver and spleen are classic findings. The liver inflammation alters the bilirubin conjugation so that the stools appear clay-colored and urine is dark amber.

TABLE 17-2	Comparison of Hepatitis A, B, and C		
	HEPATITIS A	**HEPATITIS B**	**HEPATITIS C**
Mode of transmission	fecal-oral route	Contact with infected blood or body fluids	Parenteral and non-parenteral routes
Incubation period	14-42 days	50-180 days	14-150 days
Chronicity	Does not result in chronic liver disease	May result in chronic liver disease (6%-10%)	May result in chronic liver disease (50%)
Vaccine	No vaccine	Vaccine	No vaccine

From Doughty DB, Jackson DB: Gastrointestinal disorders, *St. Louis, 1993,* Mosby.

■ ***Cirrhosis:*** A chronic degenerative disease of the liver in which diffuse destruction and regeneration of hepatic parenchymal cells have occurred (Fig. 17-41). Lobes of the liver become fibrotic and infiltrated with fat. A diffuse increase in connective tissue results in disorganization of the lobular and vascular structure. Causes of cirrhosis include viral hepatitis, biliary obstruction, and alcohol abuse. The liver becomes palpable, hard, and nontender. The proliferation of connective tissue spreads throughout the liver, changing the normal lobular structure. Associated signs include ascites, jaundice, cutaneous spider angiomas, dark urine, clay-colored stools, and spleen enlargement. End-stage cirrhosis is characterized by hepatic encephalopathy and coma.

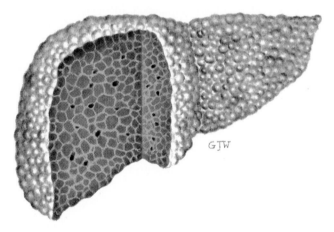

Fig. 17-41 Cirrhosis of the liver. *(From Doughty, 1993.)*

⊕ Cultural Note

Cirrhosis of the liver and other liver diseases are the fifth leading causes of mortality among American Indians and Alaskan Natives. Gallbladder disease is also disproportionately high among American Indians and Alaskan Natives.

■ **Cholecystitis with cholelithiasis:** Acute or chronic inflammation of the gallbladder with stone formation (Fig. 17-42). The bile duct becomes obstructed either by edema from inflammation of the gallbladder wall or by a stone. The primary symptom is RUQ colicky pain that may radiate to midtorso or right scapula. Other indications include indigestion and mild transient jaundice.

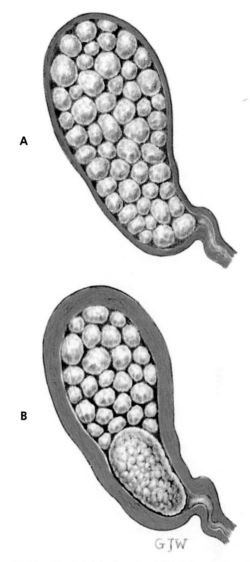

Fig. 17-42 Cholelithiasis. **A,** Multiple faceted stones. **B,** Large and numerous small stones in chronic cholecystitis. *(From Doughty, 1993.)*

PANCREAS

■ **Pancreatitis:** Acute or chronic inflammation of the pancreas resulting from autodigestion of the organ. The flow of pancreatic digestive enzymes into the duodenum is obstructed, so that three enzymes act on the pancreas itself. Clients complain of pain, described as steady, boring, dull, or sharp, that radiates from the epigastrium to the back. Clients prefer the fetal position with knees to the chest. Other manifestations include nausea and vomiting, weight loss, steatorrhea, and glucose intolerance.

URINARY SYSTEM

■ *Glomerulonephritis:* Inflammation of the renal glomeruli caused by an autoimmune process. Clients complain of nausea, malaise, and arthralgia. Hematuria may occur.

■ *Pyelonephritis:* Infection of the kidney and renal pelvis caused by bacteria that spread by hematogenous or lymphatic means or by ascending from the lower urinary tract. It is one of a group of conditions called a urinary tract infection; the others are asymptomatic bacteriuria and cystitis. Clients complain of flank pain, bacteriuria, pyuria, dysuria, nocturia, and frequency. Costovertebral angle tenderness may be evident.

■ *Renal calculi:* Stones formed in the kidney pelvis. Formation of calculi is associated with obstruction and urinary tract infections. Renal calculi are made of calcium salts, uric acid, cystine, and struvite. Alkaline urine facilitates stone formation. Men develop renal calculi more often than women. Signs and symp-

toms include fever, hematuria, and flank pain that may radiate to the groin and genitals.

■ *Acute renal failure:* Sudden, severe impairment of renal function, causing an acute uremia episode. Impairment may be prerenal (e.g., reduced cardiac output), renal (e.g., acute pyelonephritis), or postrenal (e.g., acute urinary tract obstruction). Other major causes include acute tubular necrosis, acute glomerulonephritis, and nephrotoxic agents, including drugs. Urine output may be normal, decreased, or absent.

■ *Chronic renal failure:* Slow, insidious, and irreversible impairment of renal function. Uremia usually develops gradually. Major causes include diabetic nephropathy, glomerulonephritis, and polycystic kidney disease. The client complains of oliguria or anuria and has signs of fluid volume overload.

INFANTS

■ *Intussusception:* Prolapse of one segment of the intestine into another, causing intestinal obstruction. Occurs in infants aged 3 to 12 months. The cause is unknown. Manifestations include abdominal distention, intermittent abdominal pain, vomiting, and stools that are mixed with blood and mucus with a currant-jelly appearance. A mass is found on palpation of the upper quadrants,while the lower quadrants feel empty.

■ *Pyloric stenosis:* Obstruction of the pyloric sphincter by hypertrophy of circular muscle of the pylorus. It occurs during the first month after birth. Signs and symptoms include regurgitation, progressing to projectile vomiting and failure to gain weight with signs of dehydration.

■ *Meconium ileus:* Obstruction of the lower intestine, caused by thickening and hardening of meconium. It is characterized by

failure of the newborn to pass a meconium stool in the first 24 hours after birth and abdominal distention.

■ *Biliary atresia:* Congenital obstruction or absence of some or all of the bile duct system. Signs include jaundice, hepatomegaly, abdominal distention, and failure to gain weight. Urine is a dark color, while stools are clay-colored.

■ *Meckel diverticulum:* Outpouching of the ileum proximal to the ileocecal valve. It is the most common congenital anomaly of the GI tract. Signs and symptoms, if present, resemble intestinal obstruction, diverticulitis, or appendicitis. There may be bright or dark bleeding with little abdominal pain.

PREGNANT WOMEN

■ *Hydramnios (polyhydramnios):* An excessive quantity of amniotic fluid, which can range from 2 to 15 liters (≅ 2–15 quarts). Hydramnios is common in twin pregnancies, but in single pregnancies it is associated with fetal malformation of the central nervous system and GI tract. Symptoms are due to pressure on the surrounding organs and include dyspnea, edema, and pain. Hydramnios may result in perinatal mortality from premature labor and fetal abnormalities.

Nursing Diagnosis

CASE 1 11-year-old Hispanic male seeks health care for a physical examination for summer camp.

Subjective

Alert, timid, obese child is accompanied by mother. He just completed the fifth grade and will attend middle school next year. He liked physical education class in elementary school and decided to attend a basketball camp at a local university this summer. He reported that he liked school and made good grades. His mother reported he would rather read books than play outside. He reports other children making fun of him because he is overweight. Child rarely makes eye contact with examiner. He reports no medical problems. The family history is noncontributory. His mother is obese also.

Twenty-four hour diet recall: Breakfast: pop-tart, milk, juice
Lunch: pizza, soft drink, candy bar
After school snack: chips or cookies, soft drink
Dinner: meat, rice, beans, milk, dessert
Bedtime snack: cake, ice cream, cookies

Objective

Height 4'9" (150 cm).

Weight 175 lbs. (79.5 kg) (80th percentile of boys his age).

(Recording of assessment of other body systems in other chapters.)

Abdomen Obese, symmetric, without distension; no lesions, scars, masses, or peristalsis observed. Skin smooth. Umbilicus midline and protruding without herniation. Bowel sounds present in all quadrants, aorta midline without bruit. No bruits in iliac, renal, or femoral arteries. tympanic tones over abdomen. Liver span 7 cm (2.5 inches) RMCL. Abdomen soft, nontender, no masses. Spleen and kidneys nonpalpable. Superficial reflexes intact. No CVA tenderness.

• •

Nursing Diagnosis #1

Nutrition greater than body requirements related to food choices and lack of exercise.

Defining Characteristics Little physical activity, 24-hour recall of nutrition; height: 4'9" (150 cm), weight 175 lb (79.5 kg).

Nursing Diagnosis #2

Self-esteem disturbance related to body weight.

Defining Characteristics Obese, timid, little eye contact; children make fun of his weight.

&Nursing Diagnosis

CASE 2   55-year-old Native American Indian man presenting with epigastric pain.

Subjective

Alert, cooperative man with hand on stomach. Reports 2-week episode of gnawing epigastric pain that does not radiate. Pain is worse before meals and relieved somewhat after meals. He denies nausea and vomiting. He has taken antacids with some relief. He takes nonsteroidal anti-inflammatory drugs (NSAID) daily for arthritis; has smoked 1 pack of cigarettes per day for 40 years; drinks a fifth of whiskey per week. He is employed full-time at an insurance company; he is married with two children. Reports occasional stress at work, minimal stress at home.

Objective

BP   140/80.

Pulse   88.

Respirations   18.

Temperature   98.8° F (37° C).

Height   6'3" (190 cm).

Weight   180 lb (82 kg).

Abdomen   Scaphoid, soft, no scars; aorta midline with bruit; no bruit in iliac, renal, or femoral arteries; bowel sounds heard in all quadrants, epigastric tender to deep palpation; liver span 9 cm (3.5") RMCL; liver palpable 2 cm (¾ inches), nontender, spleen and kidneys nonpalpable; superficial reflexes intact; no CVA tenderness.

• •

Nursing Diagnosis #1

Acute pain related to gastric hypersecretion.

Defining Characteristics   Report 2-week episode of gnawing epigastric pain that does not radiate; pain is worse before meals and relieved somewhat after meals; client smokes 1 pack per day; drinks a fifth of alcohol per week; takes NSAID daily; epigastric tender to light and deep palpation.

Nursing Diagnosis #2

Altered health maintenance related to inadequate information about effect of smoking and alcohol on abdominal pain.

Defining Characteristics   Client has gastric hypersecretion, smokes, drinks alcohol.

HEALTH PROMOTION

■ **Nutrition** Healthy food choices, as discussed in Chapter 7, help to promote health. Dietary factors are related to 5 of the 10 leading causes of death in the United States, including heart disease, some cancers, stroke, non–insulin-dependent diabetes mellitus, and atherosclerosis. Discuss with client and family not only what foods to select, but also atmosphere during meal time and any behavioral or emotional cues that prompt eating. Clients need to maintain or develop habit of selecting foods from the food pyramid, remembering that a serving is ½ cup or 3 oz. of food. Periodic measurement of height and weight are recommended. Developing nutritionally sound behaviors early in life help to ensure a healthier diet.

■ **Immunizations** Parents need education about the importance of immunizing their children. Hepatitis B vaccine is started at birth or by 2 months of age. The second injection is due 1 month after the first, and the third and final injection is due 6 months after the first.

■ **Food Poisoning** Prevent food poisoning by refrigerating foods containing eggs and milk products and cooking meat and fish thoroughly before eating.

■ **Lead Poisoning*** Since all children are at risk for lead poisoning, universal screening is recommended. Priority is given to screening children ages 6 to 72 months who are at highest risk: (1) those who live in houses built before1960, and some before 1980, that are deteriorating or are being remodeled; (2) those whose siblings or close peers have lead poisoning; and (3) those whose household members have lead-related occupations (e.g., automotive repair, construction) or hobbies (e.g., stained glass or jewelry making) or who live near lead-related industries. Lead enters the system by inhalation or ingestion. Infants and toddlers are at risk because they explore their environment by putting objects in their mouths. Effects of lead poisoning include behavioral problems, shortened attention span, and poor reading ability, as well as slowed growth, impaired hearing, and kidney damage. Children under the age of 6 absorb lead up to eight times faster than adults. Once the lead poisoning has occurred, the damage to the child cannot be reversed. Preventing lead poisoning includes making sure children not have access to peeling paint or chewable surfaces painted with lead-based paint, such as window sills. Washing and drying the child's hands and face frequently are important, especially before eating. Further information about lead poisoning is available from local and state health departments.

*Centers for Disease Control: *Preventing lead poisoning in young children*, Atlanta, Georgia, 1991, the Centers.

??????? STUDY QUESTIONS ???????

1. What eight organs are found within the abdominal cavity?

2. List each of the four major parts to the digestive system and describe the role they play in the process of providing nutrition to the body.

3. List at least two functions for each of the following organs: liver, gallbladder, spleen, pancreas.

4. What causes morning sickness?

5. What changes occur with pregnancy that affect the abdomen, other than morning sickness?

6. Identify the changes that occur in the structure and function of the gastrointestinal tract with aging.

7. What questions would you ask of an individual presenting with each of the following complaints? (1) Difficulty in swallowing; (2) vomiting; (3) bloated belly; (4) yellow conjunctivae.

8. The mother of a 3-month-old infant complains of the baby spitting up frequently. What additional information is needed?

9. How would you assess a toddler's eating habits?

10. If an extremely underweight teenager is seen, what is your major concern? How would you assess whether this concern is justified?

11. List four factors that may contribute to nutritional deficiencies in the elderly.

12. What is the correct sequence of the four techniques for assessment of the abdomen? What is the rationale for the sequence?

13. Identify the anatomic landmarks of the abdomen.

14. How would you describe a normal abdomen ?

15. Should there normally be movements noted on the surface of the abdomen? If so, what would they look like?

16. Describe how you would auscultate bowel sounds. How often should bowel sounds occur? What are some factors that may influence the frequency of bowel sounds?

17. What is the proper technique for percussion of the abdomen? What common sounds are expected when percussing?

18. Describe the techniques used for percussion of the liver and the spleen.

19. Describe the difference between light and deep palpation techniques of the abdomen. What is each used for?

20. Describe a technique used to evaluate costovertebral angle tenderness.

21. What assessment techniques would you employ for an individual with suspected abdominal fluid?

22. How does your palpation technique differ when an individual presents with pain in the abdomen?

23. How does an abdominal exam of an infant or a child differ from that of an adult?

24. What is the normal contour of the abdomen in a child?

25. List two age-related differences that you would expect when examining the abdomen of a 76-year-old woman.

26. How is the fundal height measured on a pregnant woman?

27. When palpating fetal position, what five factors are important? Define each.

28. At what point in pregnancy should fetal heart tones be auscultated by Doppler?

29. Match the alimentary tract condition with the appropriate sign/symptom:

Peptic ulcer	*Severe abdominal pain*
Ulcerative colitis	*Hematemesis*
Diverticulitis	*Bloody, watery diarrhea*
Crohn's disease	*Constipation*

30. Match the hepatobiliary or pancreatic condition with the appropriate sign or symptom:

Hepatitis	*Boring pain radiating to back*
Cirrhosis	*Clay-colored stool*
Cholecystitis	*Nontender, palpable liver*
Pancreatitis	*Colicky pain radiating to shoulder*

31. Describe the following abdominal conditions found in infancy: intussusception, pyloric stenosis, meconium ileus, biliary atresia, and Meckel diverticulum.

32. When is hydramnios a concern in pregnancy? What is it indicative of? What may hydramnios lead to?

CHAPTER 18

Female Genitalia and Reproductive System

ANATOMY AND PHYSIOLOGY

EXTERNAL GENITALIA

The external female genitalia, collectively called the *pudendum* or *vulva,* include the mons pubis, clitoris, labia majora, labia minora, vaginal vestibule, vestibular glands, vaginal orifice, and urethral opening (Fig. 18-1). The mons pubis (or mons veneris) is a fatty pad that covers the symphysis pubis. After puberty this surface is covered with coarse hair

that extends down over the outer labia to the perineum. The labia majora are adipose folds that extend downward from the mons pubis, surround the vestibule, and meet at the perineum. The inner surfaces are hairless, smooth, and moist.

Lying inside the labia majora are two darker, hairless folds called the labia minora. The labia minora meet at the anterior of the vulva where each labium divides into two lamellae, the lower pair fusing to form the frenulum of the

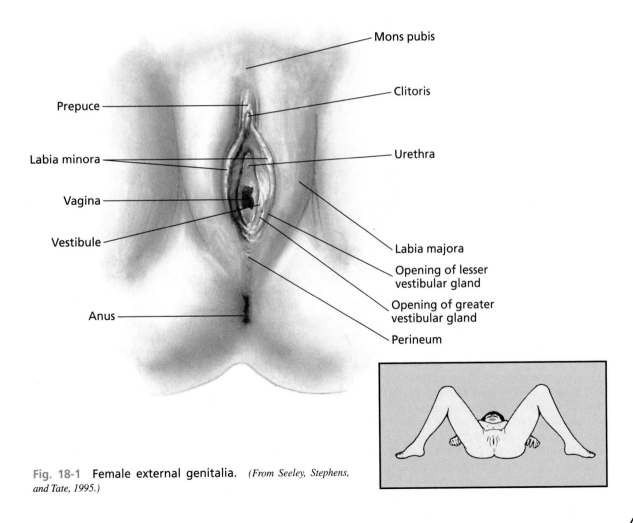

Fig. 18-1 Female external genitalia. *(From Seeley, Stephens, and Tate, 1995.)*

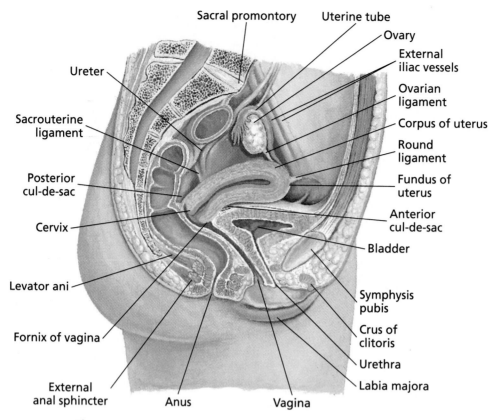

Fig. 18-2   Midsagittal view of female pelvic organs.   *(From Seidel et al, 1995.)*

clitoris and the upper pair forming the prepuce. The clitoris is a small, cylindrical bud of erectile tissue, homologous to the male penis and a primary center of sexual excitement. It is approximately 2 cm (0.8 inch) in length and 0.5 cm (0.2 inch) in diameter.

The labia minora enclose the vestibule, an area which contains the urethral (urinary) orifice, the vaginal orifice (introitus), and hymenal tissue. The urethral opening is located about 2 cm (0.8 inch) posterior and inferior to the clitoris and appears as an irregularly shaped slit. The vaginal orifice lies immediately inferior to the urethral orifice and varies in size and shape, depending on the condition of the hymen. The hymen is a fold of mucous membrane lying over the vaginal opening. When unperforated, it is usually a continuous membrane. The insertion of a tampon or the act of coitus enlarges the opening or tears the hymenal tissue, leaving small, irregular, fleshy projections around the introitus.

Also opening on the vulva are the ducts of two types of vestibular glands: Skene glands, with ducts that lie on each side of the urethral meatus, and Bartholin glands, with ducts located on either side of the introitus. Skene ducts drain a group of urethral glands; the ductal openings may be visible. Bartholin glands open onto the sides of the vestibule in the space between the hymen and the labia minora. The ductal openings are usually not visible. During sexual excitement, Bartholin glands secrete a mucoid material into the vaginal orifice for lubrication.

The perineal surface is the triangular-shaped area between the vaginal opening and the anus.

The pelvic floor consists of a group of muscles that form a suspended sling supporting the pelvic contents. These muscles attach to various points on the bony pelvis and form functional sphincters for the vagina, rectum, and urethra.

INTERNAL GENITALIA

The internal genitalia include the vagina, uterus, fallopian tubes, and ovaries. They are supported by four pairs of ligaments: the cardinal, uterosacral, round, and broad ligaments (Fig. 18-2).

Vagina.   The vagina is a musculomembranous tube extending posteriorly from the vestibule to the uterus. It inclines posteriorly at an angle of approximately 45° to the vertical plane of the body. Its posterior length is approximately 9 to 10 cm, and its anterior length is 6 to 8 cm. The tube is transversely rugated in the reproductive years, lined with a moist mucous membrane. The uterine cervix juts superiorly and anteriorly into the vaginal cavity to form a circular pocket, or fornix, around the cervix. This pocket is divided into anterior, posterior, and lateral fornices, through which the internal pelvic walls can be palpated. The vagina carries menstrual flow from the uterus and is the receptive organ for the penis during sexual intercourse. During birth, the vagina becomes the terminal portion of the birth canal.

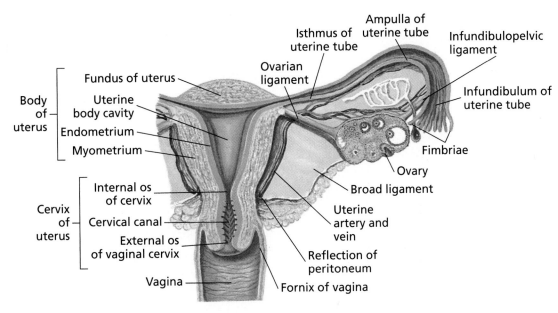

Fig. 18-3 Cross-sectional view of internal female genitalia and pelvic contents. *(From Seidel et al, 1995.)*

Uterus. The uterus is a thick, pear-shaped, muscular organ suspended and stabilized in the pelvic cavity by four sets of ligaments. It is fairly mobile, usually loosely suspended in an anteverted position between the bladder and rectum; the exact positions of the organ may normally vary in individuals. Like the vagina, the uterus is inclined at an angle of about 45°; however, while the vagina is angled posteriorly, the uterus is usually inclined forward. Still, the angle may vary and can normally be found in any of the following positions: anteverted, anteflexed, retroverted, or retroflexed.

The uterus is approximately 5.5 to 8 cm (2.2 to 3.2 inches) long, 3.5 to 4 cm (1.4 to 1.6 inches) wide, and 2 to 2.5 cm (0.8 to 1.0 inches) thick. The two main parts of the uterus are the cervix and the corpus. The corpus is further composed of three sections: the fundus, which is the bulbous top portion between the points of insertion of the fallopian tubes; the main body, or corpus, which extends to the lower section; and the isthmus, the narrow neck from which the cervix extends into the vagina (Fig. 18-3). The thick, smooth fundus, which is usually palpable at the level of the pubis, maintains its anterior position by the attached round ligaments, which are occasionally palpable on either side of the uterus.

The inner lining of the uterus (endometrium) proliferates and sloughs in response to sex hormones on a monthly cycle to produce menstruation. The endometrial layer extends to the cervical os, which is lined with columnar epithelial cells. This layer may be visible to the examiner and appears as a symmetric, circumscribed, reddened area surrounding the os. The columnar mucosa joins the squamous epithelium, which lines the vagina at the endocervical canal. This is called the *squamo-columnar junction,* and is a common site for cervical cancer.

Fallopian (uterine) tubes. The fallopian tubes extend laterally from the uterine body to a space under the ovaries for a total length of anywhere from 8 to 14 cm (3.1 to 5.5 inches). The fringed ends of the fallopian tubes open into the pelvic cavity to capture and draw ova into the tube

for fertilization. The ova are transported to the uterus by rhythmic contractions of the tubal musculature. The fallopian tubes are not palpable.

Ovaries. The ovaries, a pair of oval organs on the lateral pelvic wall, are connected to the uterine body by the ovarian ligaments. They secrete estrogen and progesterone, which have several functions, including control of the menstrual cycle and pregnancy support. They are usually located at the level of the anterosuperior iliac spine. The ovaries are approximately 3 cm (1.2 inches) in length, 2 cm wide (0.8 inch), and 1 cm (0.4 inches) thick during the reproductive years; they are often palpable in the lower, lateral abdominal quandrants.

MENSTRUAL CYCLE

The hypothalamus and pituitary in the brain and the ovaries in the pelvis are the main sites of regulation of the menstrual cycle. The cycle moves predictably through a 28-day cycle. Table 18-1 and Figure 18-4 detail the stages.

BONY PELVIS

The bony pelvis is structured to accommodate both fetal growth and the birth process. It is composed of four bones: two innominate (each consisting of ilium, ischium, and pubis); the sacrum; and the coccyx. The pelvis contains four joints of very limited movement: the symphysis pubis, the sacrococcygeal, and two sacroiliac joints. The pelvis is divided into two parts: the false pelvis (the shallow upper section) and the true pelvis (the lower curved bony canal, including the inlet, cavity, and outlet) (Fig. 18-5). The fetus will pass through this lower canal during birth. The lower border of the outlet is bounded by the pubic arch and the ischial tuberosities. The upper border of the outlet is at the level of the ischial spines. These project into the pelvic cavity and are important landmarks during labor.

Text continued on p. 486.

TABLE 18-1	The Menstrual Cycle

Menstrual phase: Days 1 to 4

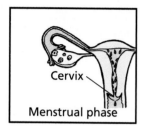

Cervix

Menstrual phase

Ovary	Estrogen levels begin to rise, preparing follicle and egg for next cycle.
Uterus	Progesterone stimulates endometrial prostaglandins that cause vasoconstriction; upper layers of endometrium shed.
Breast	Cellular activity in the alveoli decreases; breast ducts shrink.
Central nervous system (CNS) hormones	FSH and LH levels decrease.
Symptom	Menstrual bleeding may vary, depending on hormones and prostaglandins.

Postmenstrual, preovulatory phase: Days 5 to 12

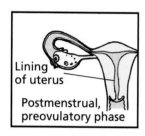

Lining of uterus

Postmenstrual, preovulatory phase

Ovary	Ovary and maturing follicle produce estrogen. *Follicular phase*—egg develops within follicle.
Uterus	*Proliferative phase*—uterine lining thickens.
Breast	Parenchymal and proliferation (increased cellular activity) of breast ducts occurs.
CNS hormone	FSH stimulates ovarian follicular growth.

Ovulation: Day 13 or 14

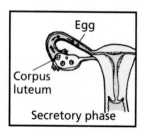

Egg

Ovulation

Ovary	Egg is expelled from follicle into abdominal cavity and is drawn into the uterine (fallopian) tube by fimbriae and cilia; follicle closes and begins to form corpus luteum. Fertilization of egg may occur in outer one third of tube if sperm are unimpeded.
Uterus	End of proliferative phase; progesterone causes further thickening of the uterine wall.
CNS hormones	LH and estrogen levels increase rapidly; LH surge stimulates release of egg.
Symptom	Mittelschmerz may occur with ovulation; cervical mucus is increased and is stringy and elastic (spinnbarkeit).

Secretory phase: Days 15 to 20

Egg

Corpus luteum

Secretory phase

Ovary	Egg (ovum) is moved by cilia into the uterus.
Uterus	After the egg is released, the follicle becomes a corpus luteum; secretion of progesterone increases and predominates.
CNS hormones	LH and FSH decrease.

Premenstrual, luteal phase: Days 21 to 28

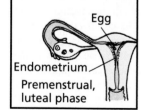

Egg

Endometrium

Premenstrual, luteal phase

Ovary	If implantation does not occur, the corpus luteum degenerates. Progesterone production decreases, and estrogen production drops and then begins to rise as a new follicle develops.
Uterus	Menstruation starts around day 28, which begins *day 1* of the menstrual cycle.
Breast	Alveolar breast cells differentiate into secretory cells.
CNS hormones	Increased levels of GnRH cause increased secretion of FSH.
Symptoms	Vascular engorgement and water retention may occur.

From Edge V, Miller M: Women's health care, *St. Louis, 1994, Mosby.*

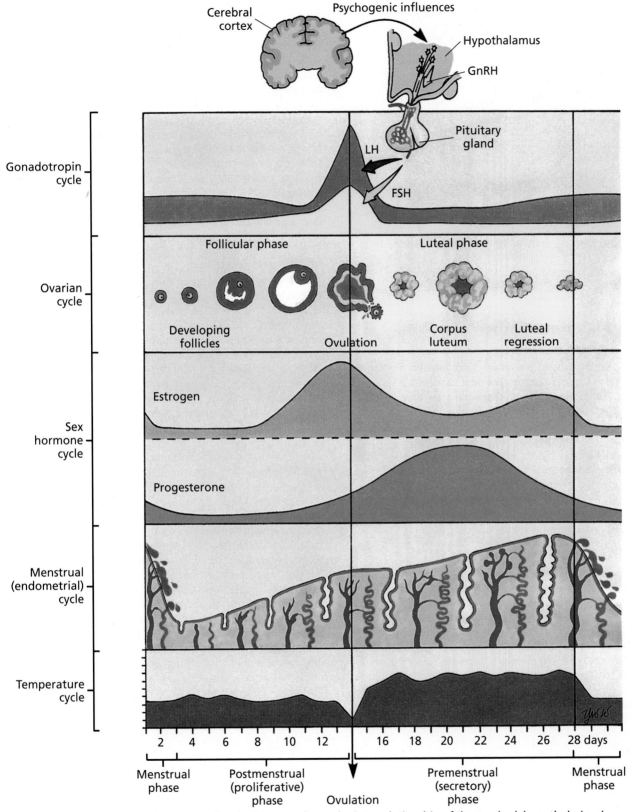

Fig. 18-4   Female menstrual cycle. Diagram shows the interrelationship of the cerebral, hypothalmic, pituitary, and uterine functions throughout a standard 28-day menstrual cycle. The variations in basal body temperature are also shown.   *(From Thibodeau and Patton, 1994.)*

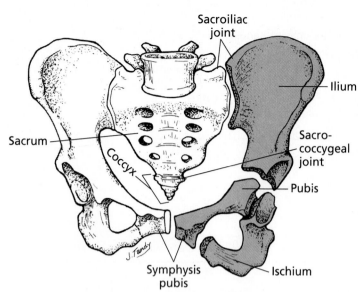

Fig. 18-5 Adult female pelvis. Note the pelvic joints. *(From Bobak and Jensen, 1993.)*

DEVELOPMENTAL CONSIDERATIONS

INFANTS AND CHILDREN

The female infant possesses functionally immature ovaries, and the cervix constitutes about two thirds of the entire uterus. The vagina is simply a small narrow tube with few epithelial folds. No pubic hair will develop until late preadolescence, and the nonprominent labia majora have a smooth, dry appearance. The thin, avascular labia minora are much more prominent and lighter in color than in the adolescent and adult. It is not unusual for the infant or child to exhibit an irregular urethral opening. The clitoris is very small. The hymen, a thin diaphragm just inside the introitus, may or may not be across the vaginal opening. It may demonstrate a crescent-shaped opening in the midline.

PREADOLESCENTS AND ADOLESCENTS

Pubescence is the prepubertal growth that usually occurs in spurts during the 2 years preceding puberty. *Puberty* is the age of sexual maturity. The age of menarche has decreased over the past three or four decades, for reasons not fully understood. Puberty in girls occurs between the ages of 8 and 14 years. During puberty *thelarche* (breast development) occurs, usually followed in 2 to 6 months by *adrenarche,* or the development of axillary and pubic hair (Table 18-2). Menstruation usually begins between ages 8 and 14, at the time when the breast and pubic hair development is in Tanner's developmental stages 3 or 4.

At the time of puberty, the external genitalia become larger, gaining adult proportions and adult functional maturation. In particular, the labia majora and mons pubis become prominent and develop pubic hair, while the labia minora darken and recede. These phenomena tend to occur simultaneously with breast development. During this time, the vagina also lengthens with a thickening of its epithelial layers; if the hymen is intact, the vaginal opening will be about 1 cm (0.4 inch) in diameter.

The internal reproductive organs also grow larger. The main reason for the darkening pigmentation evidenced in the labia minora is the increased vascular supply, especially to the uterus. In preparation for the onset of menstruation, the endometrial lining thickens. For 2 to 3 years before the onset of menstruation, a watery discharge will be present; within 1 year after onset, the discharge will become the same as that observed in the adult. In particular, vaginal secretions become acidic.

PREGNANT WOMEN

As a rule, pregnancy begins with amenorrhea, missed period, nausea, and breast tenderness.

During pregnancy the pelvic ligaments become stronger and more elastic, and the cartilage softens; these changes occur because of an increase in the levels of estrogen and relaxin. This allows separation and more mobility in these joints, in preparation for fetal growth and birth. Later in pregnancy, the wider separation of the symphysis pubis may cause discomfort in walking, and the forward tilt of the pelvis may place additional strain on the back and sacroiliac joints.

The most noticeable change during pregnancy, of course, is uterine growth. Over the course of the average pregnancy, uterine weight—excluding the fetus and placenta—will have increased more than tenfold, to a weight of about 1000 gm (35.3 oz). During the first trimester of pregnancy this uterine enlargement is due to the increased levels of estrogen and progesterone; the uterus also becomes more anteflexed, soft, and spongy, largely as a result of an increase in uterine blood flow and lymph; the cervix also takes on a bluish color. After the third month, uterine growth will be largely due to pressure from the growth of the fetus. Hormonal activity also contributes to a softening and strengthening of the pelvic ligaments, allowing the pelvic joints to separate slightly for increased mobility. As the uterus becomes larger and more ovoid, with its muscular walls becoming stronger and more elastic, it rises out of the pelvis into the abdomen. Breathing may become more difficult until the fetus shifts into the pelvis—a phenomenon referred to as "lightening." The signs of pregnancy, uterine growth, and distension during pregnancy can be mapped (Table 18-3).

TABLE 18-2	Tanner's Sex Maturity Development

STAGE		PUBIC HAIR DEVELOPMENT
Stage 1		No growth of pubic hair
Stage 2		Initial, scarcely long, straight, downy and slightly pigmented hair, especially along the labia
Stage 3		The hair is darker, coarser, and curly, and spread sparsely over the entire pubis in the typical female triangle
Stage 4		Pubic hair is denser, curled, and in an adult distribution, but less abundant and restricted to the pubic area
Stage 5		The pubic hair is adult in quantity, type, and pattern, with lateral spreading to the inner aspect of the thighs
Stage 6		Further extension laterally, upward, or over the upper thighs (this stage may not occur in all women)

Photographs from Van Wieringen, 1971. Reprinted by permission of Kluwer Academic Publishers.

TABLE 18-3	Signs and Stages of Pregnancy

FINDING	GESTATIONAL AGE IN WEEKS
Softening of the cervix	4 to 6 weeks
Softening of the uterine isthmus	6 to 8 weeks
Fundus flexes easily on the cervix	7 to 8 weeks
Fullness and softening of the fundus near the site of the implantation	7 to 8 weeks
Bluish color of the cervix, vagina, and vulva	8 to 12 weeks
Fundus of the uterus is one finger-breadth above the symphysis pubis	12 weeks
Fundus is between the symphysis and the umbilicus	16 weeks
Fundus is at the level of the umbilicus	20 to 22 weeks
Fundus is between the umbilicus and the xiphoid process	28 weeks
Fundus is at the xiphoid process	36 weeks

Vaginal changes are similar to cervical changes, giving the vaginal mucosa a violet color and a thickening of the vaginal walls. The vulva and perianal area also darken. Vaginal secretions increase and have a more acidic pH due to the increase in lactic acid production.

After delivery, pigmented changes may fade. Lochia (discharge) after delivery will be red for 1 to 3 days, then pink-brown with no clots for 5 to 7 days, then yellow-brown and odorless for 1 to 3 weeks. Breast-feeding women may progress through these stages a little faster; after cesarean section, there will be less lochia, because of suctioning or surgery.

Urinary changes are also noticed during pregnancy. Initial increased frequency will subside when the uterus moves out of the pelvis (again, with lightening). However, an increase in the amount of urine remains consistent throughout pregnancy. Stress incontinence may occur. Lactosuria occurs as a result of mammary gland production.

After delivery, the urge to void should decrease. This may occur because of a decrease in pressure or because of anesthesia. However, this will be short-lived; generally, excess fluid will cause an increase in urination for a few days after delivery. Lactosuria will increase during early lactation.

OLDER ADULTS

Ovarian function begins to diminish during a woman's 40s, with a cessation in menstrual periods between the ages of 40 and 55. However, fertility may continue during this time. Menopause is considered complete after the woman has experienced an entire year with no menses. Ovulation usually ceases 1 to 2 years before menopause.

During menopause, the labia and clitoris become smaller and paler in color, and the epithelial layers become thinner and flatter, losing their subcutaneous fat as a result of decreased estrogen levels. Pubic hair grays and thins. The vaginal introitus may diminish in size, with a shortening and narrowing of the vagina; a thinning and drying of the mucosa may result in dyspareunia. The cervix, too, becomes smaller and paler. The uterus and ovaries also decrease in size, with the ovarian follicles gradually disappearing.

Finally, in some women, the ligaments and connective tissue of the pelvis may lose their muscle tone and elasticity, resulting in less structural support for the pelvic contents, including the vaginal walls.

HEALTH HISTORY | Female Genitalia and Reproductive System

The history should include questions about menstruation, obstetric issues, menopause, urinary symptoms, vaginal discharge, sexual relations and contraceptive use, sexually transmitted diseases, including HIV exposure, and self-care behaviors.

QUESTIONS

RATIONALE

MENSTRUATION

- What was the date of your last menstrual period?
- How old were you when you started having periods?

- How often do you have periods? How long do they usually last?
- How would you describe your usual amount of flow—light, moderate, heavy? How many pads or tampons do you use over the course of a day? An hour? Have you noted any change in your periods recently?

- Have you noted any clotting during your periods? If so, is it becoming worse over time? Have you talked with a health care provider about this?
- Do you have cramps or other pains associated with your period? What relieves the discomfort? Do the cramps or pains interfere with your normal activities?
- Do you ever have spotting between periods?
- What part of the menstrual cycle are you in right now? Do you use a vaginal douche? How often? Do you use feminine hygiene spray? Do you wear tight, nonventilating underpants or pantyhose? Do you have a vaginal discharge? If so, have you treated the discharge with anything? What result was obtained?

The exact date should be noted. Normal onset of menarche is between ages 12 and 14 years, although the range spans ages 8 to 16. Onset between ages 16 and 17 suggests an endocrine problem.

Normal cycle is every 18 to 45 days, and normal duration is 3 to 7 days. Normal flow is difficult to determine, but any change from what is "normal" for the client should be noted.

This may indicate a heavy flow or vaginal pooling.

All of these factors can affect the discharge by increasing glycogen content, altering pH, or producing local irritation or contact dermatitis.

PREMENSTRUAL SYMPTOM PROBLEMS

- Do you have any other problems or symptoms associated with menses, such as headaches, bloated feeling, weight gain, breast tenderness, irritability, or moodiness? Does this seem to be associated with all of your periods or just periodically? Does it interfere with your activities of daily living? What do you do to treat the problem? Does the treatment work?

Hormonal fluxuation associated with the menstrual cycle may cause the client to have symptoms that are frequently referred to as "premenstrual syndrome" (PMS).

LOWER ABDOMINAL OR PELVIC PAIN

- Do you ever experience pain either associated with your periods or between your periods? If so, describe the discomfort, and try to remember if the pain is associated with any other activity or function such as menstruation, sexual activities, having a bowel movement, urinating, exercise, walking, etc.
- Describe the characteristics of the pain; is it sharp? Aching? Nagging? Dull? How long has the pain been going on? Is it getting better or worse?
- Do you have associated systems such as vaginal discharge or bleeding, gastrointestinal symptoms, abdominal distention or tenderness, or pelvic fullness? Are you able to put your finger on the place where the pain is or is the discomfort more generalized?
- What have you done to treat the pain?

Lower abdominal pain or discomfort may be caused by many problems. It may include problems with the gastrointestinal tract, the urinary tract, or the reproductive system. If the client is having discomfort, it is important to try to determine the etiology of the pain. Common problems may be associated with the uterus, the ovaries, or the vagina.

QUESTIONS

RATIONALE

VAGINAL DISCHARGES

- Do you have any unusual vaginal discharge? Do you feel that there is more than usual? What color is it? What does it look like? Is it foul-smelling? When did it begin? Have you noted any connection with vaginal itching, rash, or pain with intercourse?

◀ *Normal discharge is minimal, clear or cloudy, and nonirritating. A change may suggest a vaginal infection (vaginitis), and the specific appearance of the discharge may indicate the causative organism. Irritation from the discharge can cause itching, rash, or pain on intercourse.*

- Are you currently taking any medications? If so, what are you taking and for what?

◀ *Medications that can cause problems include oral contraceptives, which increase the glycogen content of the vaginal epithelium and provide a fertile ground for organisms, and broad-spectrum antibiotics, which alter the balance of the normal vaginal flora.*

CHANGES IN URINATION

- Do you have problems with urination? Pain or burning? Do you have to urinate frequently? Do you feel that you cannot wait to urinate? Do you awaken during the night to urinate? Do you urinate small amounts frequently? Is there ever any blood in your urine? Is it dark, cloudy, or foul-smelling?
- Do you have difficulty controlling your bladder, wetting yourself? Do you urinate when you laugh, sneeze, bear down, or pick up a heavy load?
- What have you done to treat the incontinence? Have you used medications? Done exercises? Had surgery? Have any of these methods been effective?

◀ *Urinary tract problems or problems with voiding, such as urinary incontinence, are common problems for many women, especially as they get older. Women at highest risk for problems with urinary incontinence are those who have had children, who are overweight, and who have weak musculature of the pelvic floor.*

BIRTH CONTROL

- Are you currently sexually active? If so, are you currently using any birth control measures? If so, what type? How long have you been using this product? How effective do you feel this has been? Has it affected your general physical or mental health? Do you use this product every time you have intercourse? Do you have any difficulty using it (problems with inserting it, remembering it, retaining it)?

◀ *All women who are in heterosexual relationships, who are premenopausal, who have not been sterilized, and who are sexually active should be questioned about contraceptive practices. Information should be gathered about appropriate use of the contraception, length of use, and satisfaction with the product.*

PREGNANCY

- Have you ever been pregnant? If so, how many times? How many babies have you had? Have you had any miscarriages, abortions, or babies that died before they were born? If so, how many?
- For each pregnancy, describe its outcome, complications, labor and delivery, and the baby's sex, birth weight, and condition.
- Do you think you may be pregnant now? What symptoms have you noted?

◀ *This forms the obstetric history.*

◀ *Symptoms may include missed or abnormal periods; history of sexual activity; nausea or vomiting; breast changes or tenderness; tiredness.*

■ Have you ever had difficulty becoming pregnant? If so, have you seen a health care practitioner? What have you tried to do to become pregnant? How do you feel about not being able to become pregnant?

◀ *It is equally as important to inquire about difficulty becoming pregnant as it is to inquire about actual pregnancy. It is often quite distressing for a couple in which the woman is trying unsuccessfully to become pregnant.*

MENOPAUSE

■ Have your menstrual periods slowed down or stopped? Do you have any of the following symptoms: hot flashes, numbness or tingling, back pain, palpitations, headaches, painful intercourse, changes in sexual desire, excessive sweating, mood swings, or vaginal dryness or itching?

◀ *The perimenopausal period occurs from ages 40 to 55 years. Changes occur in hormonal control, and these cause vasomotor instability.*

■ Are you being treated for any symptoms associated with menopause? Are you taking estrogen replacements? If so, how much? Is this helping? Have you noted any side effects?

◀ *The side effects of estrogen replacement therapy include fluid retention, breast pain or enlargement, and vaginal bleeding.*

■ How do you feel about going through menopause? Do you recall your mother going through menopause? Did she describe her experiences to you? How old was she?

◀ *Although this is a normal life stage, psychologic reactions range from a sense of loss to positive acceptance.*

PAPANICOLAOU (PAP) SMEAR

■ How often do you have a gynecologic examination? When was your last Pap smear? What were the results?

◀ *Assess self-care behaviors.*

■ Has your mother ever mentioned taking hormones while she was pregnant with you?

◀ *DES ingested by the mother has produced vaginal and cervical abnormalities in female offspring.*

■ Has any woman in your family ever had cancer of the cervix, ovary, uterus, or breast? Colon? If so, who? When? How was it treated?

◀ *It is important to determine the woman's risk for cancer.*

Risk Factors for Cancer

Cervical cancer
- Onset of intercourse before the age of 20
- Multiple sex partners
- Infections with human papilloma virus (HPV)
- Cigarette smoking
- Lower socioeconomic status
- Age between 40 and 50 years

Ovarian cancer
- Age 50 or older
- Family history of ovarian cancer
- More than 40 years of active ovulation
- Nulliparity or first pregnancy after age 30
- High-fat, low-fiber diet; vitamin A–deficient diet

- Prolonged exposure to asbestos and talc

Endometrial cancer
- Large body frame and obesity
- High-fat diet
- Nulliparity
- Infertility
- Menstrual irregularities
- Late onset of menopause
- Dysfunctional uterine bleeding during menopause
- Adenomatous hyperplasia of the endometrium
- Family history of breast, colon, or ovarian cancer
- History of diabetes or hypertension
- Family history of endocrine cancers

QUESTIONS	RATIONALE

SEXUALLY TRANSMITTED DISEASES: LESIONS AND DISCHARGES

■ Do you have any other problems in the genital area, such as sores or lesions, or have you had these in the past? If so, how were these treated? Do you currently have any vaginal discharge? If so, describe its odor, consistency, changes in characteristics. Has the onset of the vaginal discharge been sudden or gradual? Does your sexual partner have any discharge? Do you have any associated symptoms, such as itching; tender, inflamed, or bleeding external tissues; a rash; dysuria or burning on urination; abdominal pain; or pelvic fullness. Do you have any abdominal pain?

◀ *It is important to determine if the client has any signs of any sexually transmitted diseases. Common problems include herpes, genital warts, molluscum contagiosum, gonorrhea, syphilis, chlamydia, monilial vaginitis, and trichomoniasis (see the Common Problems section at the end of this chapter).*

■ Have you had a sexual relationship with someone who has a sexually transmitted disease, such as gonorrhea, herpes, AIDS, chlamydial infection, venereal warts, or syphilis? If so, when? Have you ever been treated for any of these problems? If so, was the treatment successful? Were there any complications? Do you use any precautions to prevent the transmission of AIDS or other sexually transmitted diseases? Do you have any questions or concerns about these diseases?

◀ *If the client has a sexually transmitted disease and the client's partner has not been treated, steps should be taken to obtain permission to contact the partner and to initiate treatment.*

SURGERY

■ Have you ever had surgery on the uterus, vagina, or ovaries? If so, what was done? When? Why? How do you feel about having the surgery? How has it affected you?

◀ *If the client has had surgery, determine what surgery was done, when, and why. Then determine her feelings about the procedure. If it was a hysterectomy, the client may fear a loss of sexual response.*

SEXUALITY

■ Are you currently in a relationship that involves sexual intercourse? Do you have one or multiple partners? How frequently do you engage in sexual activities? Are you and your partner(s) satisfied with the sexual relationship? Do you communicate comfortably about sex? Do you and your partner(s) use a contraceptive/protective method? Which one? Is it satisfactory to you? Do you have any questions about the method?

◀ *It is important to determine the type of sexual activity the individual has, as well as the client's satisfaction regarding that activity. The rationale for the type of questioning is to determine if the client has one or numerous sexual partners and what type of contraception is used. This information may be used to determine the client's risk for sexually transmitted disease. The rationale for asking about client satisfaction is to determine if the client is satisfied with her sexuality and the sexual practices she is engaging in.*

■ How many sexual partners have you had in the past 6 months? Do you prefer relationships with men, women, or both? (If the client is a lesbian, inquire if she is in a significant relationship and has a partner.)

◀ *Lesbians need to feel acceptance to discuss their health concerns. If the examiner seems genuinely interested and concerned, the client may appreciate the opportunity to discuss sexuality issues or problems.*

INFANTS

The areas that should be assessed for the female infant include the following questions:

■ When the child was born, did anyone tell you that there was anything wrong with the infant's genitalia? Does the infant have any congenital problems?

◄ *Baseline information.*

■ Since birth, has the baby had any difficulty with urination or any crying when attempting to urinate?

◄ *Baseline information to establish that the child has normal urination.*

■ Does the child ever have a diaper rash? If so, what does it look like and what do you do to treat it? Do you use cloth or disposable diapers? If you use cloth diapers, what type of detergent and fabric softeners are used?

◄ *Diaper rashes are common. Some infants are sensitive to certain brands of disposable diapers. Many times they may be improved with proper cleaning, frequent diaper change, and using a diaper that is not irritating to the infant.*

CHILDREN

The history questions focus on toilet training, urinary function, vaginal itching or discharge, and bleeding. Ask the following questions:

■ Has toilet training begun yet? If so, at what age did you begin to toilet-train? Has it been successful? If not, describe. How is it going?

◄ *Most parents begin to toilet-train children by age 2 or 2½.*

■ Does the child ever wet the bed at night? If so, does it occur frequently or on rare occasions? What have you done about this? How does the child feel about wetting the bed?

◄ *Almost all children wet the bed at some time. What is important to assess is whether the bed wetting occurs frequently, whether it occurs because of physiologic dysfunction, psychosocial dysfunction, or a too-full bladder before the child goes to bed.*

■ Does the child have any sores, rashes, or complaints of itching on the genitalia? Does she ever cry when she urinates? Do you ever put bubble bath in the bath tub when the child is bathing?

■ *To child:* Do you have trouble cleaning yourself after you go the bathroom? *To parent:* Has the child ever placed foreign objects into her vagina?

◄ *Vaginal discharge, itching, and rash may be caused by poor hygiene or the presence of a foreign body. If any of these are present, explore the history of similar problems or past urinary tract infections or the use of bubble bath. Bubble bath frequently is an irritant for little girls.*

■ Does the child frequently play with her own genitalia? If so, is she able to stop when you tell her to? Does her playing with herself bother you?

◄ *Exploration of the genitalia is a normal developmental phenomenon. It is important to assess how the parent feels about this and how they interact with the child regarding the self-play.*

■ For preschool or young school-age children, ask the following: Have you ever been touched on your vagina or between your legs by someone when you did not want them to? If so, when did this happen? Who did it? Did you tell anyone?

◄ *Screen for sexual abuse or genitalia touching by anyone.*

Talking with Children Who Reveal Abuse

- Provide a private time and place to talk.
- Do not promise not to tell; tell the child that you are required to report the abuse.
- Do not express shock or criticize the family.
- Use the child's vocabulary to discuss the body part.
- Avoid using any leading statements that can distort the child's story.
- Reassure the child that he or she has done the right thing by telling.
- Tell the child that the touching or abuse is not his or her fault; he or she is not bad or to blame.
- Determine the child's immediate need for safety.
- Let the child know when you report the situation.

(From Wong, 1995.)

OLDER CHILDREN

Many of the assessment questions previously asked in either the younger child or the adult sections also apply to the older child. Refer to the adolescent section to locate the questions that should be asked of the older female child if and when that child demonstrates the maturational changes of the preadolescent. As the child matures, the history assessment should change to include more assessment about maturational development and sexuality. When asking questions, ask the question in a matter-of-fact manner. Questions about developmental changes, sexuality, and self-esteem related to these changes should be targeted to the child's level. Do not add judgment or shame. Use simple language and speak to the child's developmental level.

ADOLESCENTS

In addition to the questions asked of adults, ask the following of girls showing sexual maturity, such as signs of breast and pubic hair development. Use the following guidelines when asking questions: (1) Ask questions appropriate for the girl's age but be aware that "normal" varies widely; it is better to ask too many questions than to omit anything. (2) Ask questions that are direct and professional; avoid judgmental phrases. Consider beginning by establishing that it is normal to feel or think a certain thing, for example, "Girls your age often feel. . . ." (3) Ask questions that assume rather than ask for an admission. You may say, "When you . . . " rather than "Do you . . . ." This implies that the individual is normal.

- What changes have you noticed in your body over the last 2 years? What do you like about the changes? What don't you like?
- Often around age 11, girls begin to develop breasts and pubic hair. Have you seen pictures of normal breast and hair development? Let's look at these now.

- Have you started having periods? How did you feel about this? Were you ready or was it a surprise?

Note the adolescent's attitude toward changes taking place.

This assesses the adolescent's level of information about the changes that are taking place and provides an opportunity for education.

This establishes menarche, as well as the adolescent's feelings about the event. Her level of information is also noted.

QUESTIONS

■ Who do you usually talk to about body changes and sex information? Are you comfortable in these talks? Do you think you get enough information? Have you taken sex education classes in school? Is there someone outside of the family, maybe at school or church, with whom you can discuss these issues?

■ Often girls your age have questions about sexual activity. Do you? Have you ever had sex? Are you dating someone now? Do you and your partner have sex? If you do, do you use some type of protection? If so, what method of birth control are you using? Do you always use this method of protection every time you have sex or just once in a while? What questions do you have about sex?

■ Have you ever had an infection on your genitalia? If so, what kind? How was it treated? If not, has anyone ever discussed information about sexually transmitted diseases or how you get AIDS or other infections? Tell me about what you know about how these infections or diseases are spread. Do you know what you can do to keep from getting these diseases?

■ Sometimes someone touches a girl in a way she does not want to be touched or sometimes has sex with her when the girl does not want to. Has this happened to you? If that happens, remember that it is not your fault and you need to tell an adult about it immediately.

OLDER ADULTS

Because sexuality is a lifelong activity, the elderly woman should be asked all of the questions for adults, especially the questions related to menopause and urinary incontinence. Additional questions dealing with issues specific to her age include the following:

■ Do you have any problems with urination or vaginal itching or dryness?

■ Have you had any vaginal bleeding since menopause?

■ Are you in a relationship where you have sexual intercourse? If so, is it satisfying to you? Does it ever hurt when you have intercourse? If so, what have you done to decrease the discomfort? Do you have difficulty with urinary frequency or urgency during sexual stimulation?

RATIONALE

◄ *It is important to assess where and how the client gets her information. In addition, it is important to assess how accurate and complete the information is.*

◄ *It is important to establish a history of sexual activity, as well as to assess methods of contraception used.*

◄ *It is important to establish a baseline about knowledge that the adolescent either has or does not have, as well as to assess the accuracy of that information. This will provide the platform for health promotion education.*

◄ *A screening assessment should always be made for child abuse, sexual assault, or incest.*

◄ *Physiologic changes may cause a decrease in vaginal fluids, which may lead to vaginal itching and dryness. In addition, a relaxation of the pelvic floor and decreased sphincter tone may lead to urinary incontinence or a feeling of urgency.*

◄ *Postmenopausal bleeding may result from numerous causes, from friable vaginal tissue to cancer of the uterus. If the client has postmenopausal bleeding, she should be referred to a medical practitioner for further evaluation.*

◄ *Sexual activity is normal at any adult age. As the client becomes older, it is most important to assess if the client is satisfied with her sexual activity and if it occurs in a manner that feels satisfying to her. If the client has vaginal dryness secondary to hormonal changes, intercourse may be painful for her. It is important to assess if this is the case and, if so, determine what she is doing to treat the problem.*

QUESTIONS

RATIONALE

■ Do you have other physical problems that interfere with sexual behavior (for example, painful joints, fatigue, dyspnea, or fear of injuring yourself or causing illness)?

Sexual activity for the older adult should be pleasurable. If the client has physical difficulties that interfere, it is important to assess what these are, how much they interfere, and what the client or her partner has done about them.

PREGNANT WOMEN

In addition to all previously described questions for the adult female, ask the following:

■ How many times have you been pregnant? Have you had any abortions? If so, how many? Did you have any complications following the abortions?

■ When did you become pregnant with this child? What is the exact date of your last menstrual period? When did you last have sexual intercourse? Have you felt the baby move? If so, when did the movement start? Are you aware of any previous or current childbearing risks you have?

■ If you have had other pregnancies, did you have any problems? How many babies have you given birth to? Did all of these babies live? Did any have problems at birth?

■ Are you excited about this baby? Was it a planned pregnancy? How many other children do you have at home?

■ Have you had any problems with this pregnancy, such as vomiting that won't stop, bleeding, premature contractions, leakage of fluid from your vagina, or odor from your vagina?

■ Do you currently smoke or drink alcohol? If so, how much each day? Do you know how alcohol or tobacco may affect your baby? Have you thought about quitting while you are pregnant? If not, for what reason do you continue either smoking or drinking?

■ Do you take any medications? If so, what?

Baseline information about past pregnancies, abortions, and problems.

Determine the EDC (the expected date of conception).

Determine baseline information about successful or unsuccessful pregnancies and the history of any special problems, such as a tubal pregnancy or fetal demise.

It is important to determine if this is a wanted pregnancy and if the woman is happy to be pregnant.

Baseline information about the health of the pregnancy and the mother.

Fetal alcohol syndrome (FAS) secondary to the mother drinking while pregnant, and premature and small babies secondary to smoking during pregnancy, are major public health problems. All pregnant women should be questioned about alcohol and tobacco use and, if needed, educated about how these behaviors may harm the baby.

🌐 Cultural Note

A number of maternal and neonatal differences are noted across cultural groupings. Prenatal care is sought earlier and in greater numbers by white and Asian-American women. Over 80% of white women seek health care contact in the first trimester. First-trimester health care is 75% for Asian Americans, 65% for African Americans, 60% for Hispanics, and 58% for American Indians. Maternal mortality is three times greater than the general population's rate in African Americans and 13% higher in American Indians. Neonatal mortality is also increased in African Americans and in Alaskan Natives. The birth rate for African Americans is three times the national average. The birth rate for Hispanics and American Indians is twice the national average. Teenage births are also above the national average in African Americans and American Indians. Teen births are less than half the national average in Asian Americans.

EXAMINATION Procedures and Findings

Guidelines Before beginning the examination, ask the client if she has emptied her bladder recently. If not, instruct her to do so. Also ask if the client has had a pelvic examination before and if she knows what to expect. During the examination, ensure privacy for the client by providing a drape over the lower abdomen and upper legs, which may be pushed back in the middle to provide adequate visualization of the genitalia. Before you begin, ensure that all equipment is within easy reach and arrange the light for good visualization of the external genitalia. As instructed below, help the client into position, and tell her that you will tell her what you plan to do before you actually do it.

EQUIPMENT

Disposable gloves
Vaginal speculum of appropriate size
  Graves' speculum (used for most adult women;
    available in varying lengths and widths)
  Pederson speculum (has narrow blades and is
    used for virginal or postmenopausal women with
    a narrowed introitus)
Sterile cotton swabs or large cotton-tipped
  applicators (rectal swabs)

Materials for cytologic study:
  Glass slides
  Sterile cotton-tipped applicator
  Ayre's spatula
  Cytologic fixative spray
  Small bottle of normal saline solution
  Small bottle of potassium hydroxide (KOH)
  Bottle of acetic acid (white vinegar)
  Water-soluble lubricant
  Examination lamp (goose-necked, with a strong light)

TECHNIQUES and NORMAL FINDINGS

ABNORMAL FINDINGS

Start by helping the woman into the lithotomy position, with body supine, feet in the stirrups, and knees apart. Provide adequate draping with a sheet. Position the client with her buttocks at the edge of the examination table. Her socks and shoes may be left on. Ask the woman to place her arms at her sides or across her chest, but not over her head (this tightens the abdominal muscles). Position the drape completely over the client's lower abdomen and upper legs, exposing only the vulva for your examination. Push the drape down so that you can see the woman's face as you proceed. Sit on a stool at the end of the table between the client's legs.

Help the woman to relax. The lithotomy position may make the woman feel embarrassed and vulnerable. If the client seems uncomfortable or embarrassed you may (1) ask her if she would like her head elevated so that she can see you better; (2) readjust the stirrups either outward or inward to reduce the stress on the pelvis and legs; (3) make sure that the client is adequately draped and that you are in a private location where others may not walk in during the examination; (4) reassure her that you will tell her everything that you are going to do before you actually do it; (5) assure her that if she becomes too uncomfortable that you will stop what you are doing and reassess what is happening; (6) always remember to touch the inner aspect of her thigh before you actually touch the external genitalia; and (7) talk to the woman throughout the examination to tell her what you are doing, what you are seeing or feeling, and how long it will be until you are finished. Before you actually begin the examination, make sure that the client is adequately positioned, comfortable, informed, and make sure that you have within easy reach all of the necessary equipment and supplies that you need to perform and complete the examination.

Clinical Note

It may be uncomfortable for both the client and the examiner if they are of the opposite sex. If there is no objection by the client, proceed in a professional manner. Also remember that it is always best to have an escort in the examination room during the assessment.

| 2INDINGS | ABNORMAL FINDINGS |

EXTERNAL GENITALIA

The client should be positioned and draped as shown in Fig. 18-6.

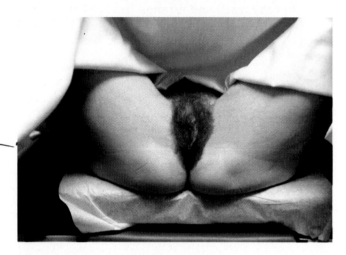

Fig. 18-6 Draped client in dorsal lithotomy position. *(From Seidel et al, 1995.)*

INSPECT the pubic hair for Distribution. Hair distribution varies but usually covers an inverse triangle with the base over the mons pubis; some hair may extend up midline toward the umbilicus.

INSPECT the skin over the mons pubis and inguinal area for Characteristics. No parasites or skin lesions should be apparent. The skin should be smooth and clear.

■ Note any male hair distribution (diamond-shaped pattern), patchy loss of hair, absence of hair in any client over 16 years of age, or presence of lesions or skin infestations.

🌐 Racial Variation

The consistency, color, and amount of pubic hair at sexual maturity is variable across racial groups. African Americans tend to have black pubic hair that is shorter and more tightly coiled than other races. Pubic hair color is dark in darker-skinned individuals but often matches or is slightly darker than the head hair color in whites. Pubic hair is generally sparser in Asian Americans and American Indians/Alaskan Natives. The labia majora vary in color, with darker-skinned individuals having darker pigmentation.

INSPECT and PALPATE the labia majora for Pigmentation and Surface Characteristics. Pigmentation should be darker than the client's general skin tone, and the tissues should appear shriveled or full, gaping or closed, usually symmetric, with a smooth skin surface and a dry or moist texture.

Begin palpation by gently touching the client on the inner thigh and telling her that you are going to touch her external genitalia and that you are going to spread the labia apart to visualize the skin characteristics.

■ Observe for signs of inflammation, ulceration, lesions, nodules, or marked asymmetry.
■ Note inflammation, leukoplakia (white patches), lesions, nodules, varicosities, marked asymmetry, swelling, or excoriation.

TECHNIQUES and NORMAL FINDINGS

ABNORMAL FINDINGS

Note: **Remember to wear gloves.**

Spread the labia majora with the fingers of one hand to view the inner surface of the labia majora and the labia minora and surface of the vestibule (Fig. 18-7). Pigmentation should be dark pink. The area should appear moist, and the tissue should appear symmetric and without lesions or sores.

■ Look for areas of inflammation, irritation, excoriation, or vaginal discharge. Discoloration or tenderness may be the result of traumatic bruising.

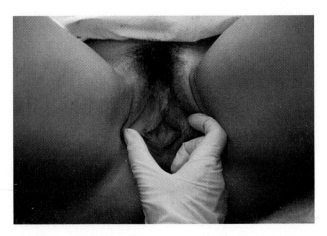

Fig. 18-7 Inspection of the labia. *(From Edge and Miller, 1994.)*

INSPECT and PALPATE the labia minora for Pigmentation and Surface Characteristics.
Palpate the labia minora between your thumb and second fingers of your other hand. The tissue should feel smooth and soft, without nodules, masses or statements of discomfort from the client.

INSPECT the clitoris for Size and Length.
The clitoris should be approximately 0.75 inch (2 cm) or less in length (visible length) and 0.5 cm in diameter.

■ Note any enlargement, atrophy, or inflammation.

INSPECT the urethral meatus, vaginal introitus, perineum, and anus for Positioning and Surface Characteristics.
Inspect the urethral meatus and the tissues immediately surrounding it. There should be a midline location of an irregular opening or slit close to or slightly within the vaginal introitus.

Inspect the vaginal introitus and the tissues immediately surrounding it. The introitus may appear as a thin vertical slit or a large orifice with irregular edges from the hymenal remnants (hymenal carbuncles); the tissues should appear moist.

■ Note any discharge from the surrounding (Skene) glands or the urethral opening, polyps, inflammation, urethral caruncle, or a lateral position of the meatus.
■ Note any surrounding inflammation, discolored or foul-smelling vaginal discharge, bleeding or blood clots, swelling, skin discoloration indicative of tissue bruising, or lesions.
■ Record any inflammation, fistulas, lesions, or masses.

Inspect the posterior skin surface of the perineum between the vaginal introitus and the anus. The skin should appear smooth and without lesions or discoloration. If the client has had an episiotomy, a scar (midline or mediolateral) may be visible.

Inspect the anus skin surface, which should exhibit increased pigmentation and coarse skin.

■ Note scars, skin tags, lesions, inflammation, fissures, lumps, or excoriation.

PALPATE the Skene and Bartholin glands for Surface Characteristics, Discharge, and Pain or Discomfort.
With the labia still spread apart, insert the index finger of your other hand (palm surface up) into the vagina as far as possible. Exert upward pressure on the anterior vaginal wall surface and milk the Skene glands by moving your finger outward toward the vaginal opening (Fig. 18-8).

The glands area should be nontender and without discharge.

■ Note any tenderness or discharge; prepare a culture of any discharge that is present. Discharge from the Skene and Bartholin glands is usually indicative of an infection.

TECHNIQUES and NORMAL FINDINGS   **ABNORMAL FINDINGS**

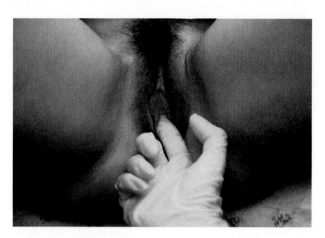

Fig. 18-8 Palpation of Skene gland. *(From Edge and Miller, 1994.)*

Next, palpate bilaterally the lateral tissue of the vagina. Use your thumb and index finger to palpate the entire area, paying attention to the posterolateral portion of the labia majora where the Bartholin glands are located (Fig. 18-9). The surface should be homogeneous, nontender, and without discharge.

■ Swelling in the area of the Bartholin glands that is painful and "hot to the touch" may indicate an abscess of the Bartholin gland. The abscess is generally pus-filled and is gonococcal or staphylococcal in origin. A nontender mass, which is the result of chronic inflammation of the gland, is usually indicative of a Bartholin cyst.

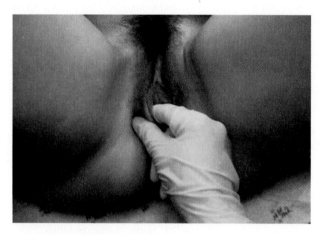

Fig. 18-9 Palpation of Bartholin gland. *(From Edge and Miller, 1994.)*

INSPECT and PALPATE muscle tone for Vaginal Wall Tone, Rectal Muscle Tone, and Urinary Incontinence. With your examining finger still in the vagina, instruct the client to squeeze the vaginal orifice around your finger. The nulliparous client (has had no children) usually squeezes tightly, so that you will feel the vaginal wall tissue firmly around your examining finger (Fig. 18-10). If the woman is multiparous (has had a baby) the tightness of the tissue will be much less.

■ Note inability of client to constrict the vaginal orifice around your finger.

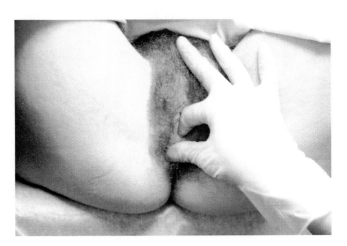

Fig. 18-10　Palpating the perineum.　*(From Seidel et al, 1995.)*

Remove your finger from the vagina. Next, ask the client to bear down as you watch for vaginal wall bulging and urinary incontinence. Ask the client to cough and again inspect for bulging and incontinence.

■ Bulging of the anterior wall may indicate a *cystocele.*

■ Bulging of the posterior vaginal wall may indicate a *rectocele.*

■ If the cervix is visible at the opening of the vagina, it may indicate signs of a *uterine prolapse.*

■ The presence of urine during either bearing down or coughing may be indicative of *stress incontinence.*

INTERNAL GENITALIA: SPECULUM EXAMINATION

Tell the client that you will now use a speculum to do the internal examination.

Clinical Notes

■ Make sure that you know how to use the speculum before you start. Especially know how to lock the blades open in place and know how to release the lock.

■ Make sure that the speculum is warm (especially if it is metal). If necessary, run it under warm water to warm it up. Or the speculum may be kept warm by wrapping it in a heating pad or placing it under a warming light.

■ Pick the correct size speculum for the client. Do not assume that a wide-blade Graves' speculum will be comfortable for all women. If the client is not sexually active, she will most likely need a narrower blade speculum.

■ Lubricate the speculum with warm water. Do not use lubricant. This will interfere with cytologic analysis.

■ Make sure that you have all of the necessary supplies within handy reach before you start (e.g., slides, applicators, test tubes with KOH and saline).

Using a speculum of appropriate size, follow these steps:

- ■ Place two fingers just inside the vaginal introitus and apply pressure downward against the posterior wall; wait for the vaginal wall muscles to relax.
- ■ Gently insert the closed speculum (holding the closed blades at an oblique angle) over your fingers (Fig. 18-11).
- ■ Continue to insert the speculum and direct it at a 45°-angle downward into the vagina (Fig. 18-12).
- ■ Insert the speculum further, rotating the speculum downward toward the rectal wall (Fig. 18-13).
- ■ With speculum fully inserted and blades horizontal, open the blades of the speculum and lock blades in open position (Fig. 18-14). The cervix should be visible.

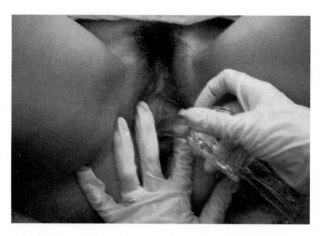

Fig. 18-11 Gently insert the closed speculum blades into the vagina. *(From Edge and Miller, 1994.)*

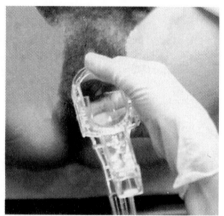

Fig. 18-12 Direct the speculum downward at 45° angle. *(From Seidel et al, 1995.)*

A

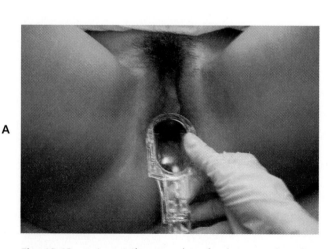

B

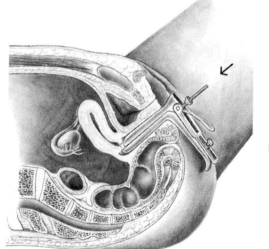

Fig. 18-13 **A,** Insert the speculum further, rotating the speculum downward toward the rectal wall. **B,** Internal view.   *(**A,** From Edge and Miller, 1994; **B,** from Seidel et al, 1995.)*

A

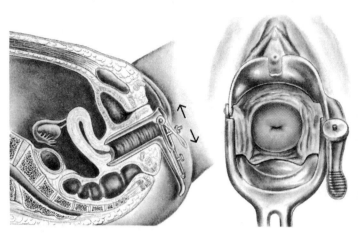

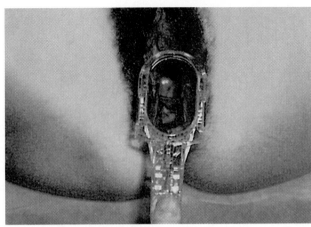

B

Fig. 18-14 Speculum in place, locked, and stabilized. Note cervix in full view. *(From Seidel et al, 1995.)*

INSPECT the cervix for Color. The cervix should be an evenly distributed pink color or, in pregnancy, a blue color secondary to increased vascularity. A symmetric, circumscribed erythema surrounding the os (the opening) may indicate the normal condition of exposed columnar epithelium.

INSPECT the cervix for Surface Characteristics. Inspect the surface of the cervix. It should appear smooth, with an occasional squamocolumnar junction (symmetric reddened circle around the os) visible. You may see nabothian cysts, which appear as smooth, round, small, yellow raised areas.

INSPECT the cervix for Position. It should be midline and point in a direction that is related to the position of the uterus. An anterior-pointing cervix indicates a retroverted uterus. A posterior-pointing cervix indicates an anteverted uterus. A cervix in the midline indicates a midposition uterus. The cervix should be midline and may project into the vagina 1 to 3 cm (0.4 to 1.2 inches), causing 1- to 3-cm (0.4 to 1.2 inches) fornices surrounding the cervix.

INSPECT the cervix for Size and Shape. The cervix is usually about 1 inch (2.5 cm) in diameter. The os of a nulliparous client is small, round, and oval. The os of a multiparous client is generally slit-shaped and may be irregular (Fig. 18-15).

■ Note any reddened granular area around the os (especially if asymmetric), friable tissue, red patches or lesions, strawberry spots, or white patches.

■ Reddened, irregular color or patchy appearance with irregular borders is an abnormal finding and requires further investigation.

■ Report if the cervix is situated laterally or if there is a projection of more than 3 cm (1.2 inches) into the vaginal tube.
■ A cervix deviating to either the right or left from a midline position may indicate a pelvic mass, uterine adhesions, or pregnancy.
■ If the cervix projects into the vagina more than 3 cm (1.2 inches), it may indicate a pelvic or uterine mass.

■ Note if the cervix is over 1.5 inches (4 cm) in diameter.
■ Injury secondary to childbirth, abortion, or removal of an intrauterine device may cause a change in the shape of the cervical os.

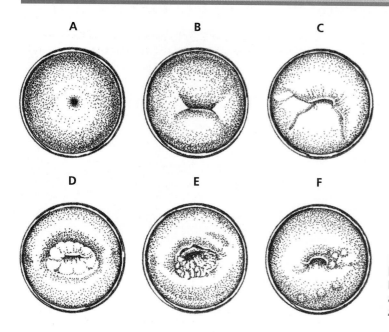

Fig. 18-15   Common appearances of the cervix. **A,** Nulliparous cervix. Note rounded os. **B,** Parous cervix. Note slit appearance of os. **C,** Multigravidous, lacerated. **D,** Everted. **E,** Eroded. **F,** Nabothian cysts.   *(From Seidel et al, 1995.)*

INSPECT the cervical os for Discharge. First, if a discharge is present, determine whether it is coming from the cervix itself or whether it is from the vagina and has only pooled near the cervix. A mucous plug may be present at the os of the cervix. If a discharge is present, it should be odorless, creamy or clear, thin, thick, or stringy. At the midcycle of the menstrual cycle or immediately after menstruation, the discharge may be heavier.

OBTAIN Vaginal Smears and Cultures. Often during the speculum examination, a culture or smear is indicated. If specimens are collected, follow the guidelines as indicated in Table 18-4, and obtain the specimens in the following sequence.

- Pap smear first.
- All other cultures and smears *after* the Pap smear.

Label all specimens.

■ A discharge with an odor or a discharge that is colored, such as yellow, green, or gray, most probably indicates a bacterial or fungal infection.

Clinical Note

The Papanicolaou (Pap) smear is recommended as a routine part of an annual pelvic examination for women over the age of 18. It is used to detect neoplastic cell secretions from the cervix and vagina. The test can detect early cellular changes in premalignant or existing malignant conditions. It has been found to be 95% accurate in detecting cervical carcinoma and 40% accurate in detecting endometrial carcinoma. If a Pap smear is found to be abnormal, the client should have further gynecologic evaluation.

(From Edge and Miller, 1994.)

TABLE 18-4   Procedures for Collecting Cervical and Vaginal Specimens

First, always remember to follow the Centers for Disease Control and Prevention's guidelines for the safe collection and transport of human secretions by wearing gloves and properly packaging all collected specimens, so that those handling and transporting the specimens may be protected from contamination.

Papanicolaou (Pap) Smear

Brushes are now being used in conjunction with or instead of the conventional spatula to improve the quality of cells obtained. The cytobrush (a cylindric type brush) collects endocervical cells only. Use the following steps to collect a Pap smear.

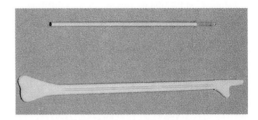

Cytobrush and spatula.   *(From Seidel et al., 1995.)*

1. Use the broad, bifid end of the spatula to collect a sample from the ectocervix. Insert the longer projection tip of the spatula into the cervical os.
2. Rotate the tip of the spatula 360°, keeping it flush against the cervical tissue.
3. Remove the spatula and, using a single light stroke, spread a thin layer of the specimen across the slide.
4. Immediately spray the specimen on the slide with cytologic fixative and label the slide as the ectocervical specimen.
5. Insert the cytobrush into the cervical os until only the bristles closest to the handle are exposed.
6. Carefully and slowly rotate the brush one half to one full turn.
7. Remove the brush and place an endocervical specimen on a glass slide, using a rolling and twisting motion with moderate pressure across the glass slide.
8. Immediately spray the specimen on the slide with cytologic fixative, and label the slide as the endocervical specimen.
9. Inform the client that she may experience a slight amount of bleeding following this procedure.

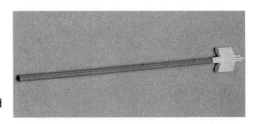

Cervex-brush.   *(From Seidel et al., 1995.)*

Gonococcal Culture Specimen

This specimen may be collected after the Pap smear specimen has been collected.

1. Using a long-stemmed sterile cotton swab, insert the swab into the vagina and into the cervical os.
2. Hold the swab in the os for 20 to 30 seconds.
3. Then withdraw the swab and, using a Z-type motion, rotate the swab over the culture medium, leaving a streak of specimen on the culture plate.
4. Immediately label the culture plate with the client's name and indicate that the specimen is a gonococcal culture specimen collected from the os of the cervix.
5. If indicated, a rectal swab inserted approximately 1 inch (2.5 cm) into the rectum may be used to collect a gonococcal culture specimen from the rectum.

Chlamydial Enzyme Immunoassay Specimen

If indicated, this specimen should be collected after the gonococcal specimen using the following procedure.

1. Use a clean swab to remove as much excess mucus from the ectocervix as possible. Discard this swab.
2. Use the swab that comes with the special kit for this specimen and place the swab into the vagina and into the cervical os.
3. Rotate the swab in the os for 20 to 30 seconds to absorb the fluids from the os.
4. Without touching the walls of the vagina with the swab, remove the swab and place it in the transport tube containing the specimen reagent.
5. The tip of the swab with the specimen must be below the level of the solution in the transport tube.
6. Label the tube appropriately and send for analysis.

Dry Smear, Wet Mount, and Potassium Hydroxide (KOH) Procedures

Before obtaining these specimens, prepare the glass slides and make them ready to receive the specimens.
For Gardnerella (Haemophilus) vaginalis: Prepare a dry glass slide.
For Trichomonas vaginalis: Mix the secretions with one or two drops of saline and place on a glass slide. This is commonly called a "wet prep."
For Candida albicans: Mix the secretions with one or two drops of potassium hydroxide (KOH) and place on a glass slide. To collect the specimens:

1. Introduce the wooden end of a sterile cotton swab applicator into the vagina, and roll it in the vaginal secretions.
2. Remove the applicator from the vagina and prepare the appropriate slides.
3. Cover the glass slides with cover slips, and label the slides according to the examination to be performed.
4. The slides should be microscopically examined immediately following the examination.

TECHNIQUES and NORMAL FINDINGS

ABNORMAL FINDINGS

INSPECT the vaginal walls for Color and Surface Characteristics. Following the specimen collection, carefully unlock the speculum and, while the blades are still partially open, gently begin to remove the speculum from the vagina. The blades of the speculum tend to close by themselves. As the speculum is being removed, slowly rotate the blades of the speculum and inspect the walls of the vagina. The walls should be pink, with transverse rugae (which diminish after vaginal deliveries), moist and smooth, and homogeneous in consistency.

Inspect any vaginal secretions. They should be thin, clear or cloudy, odorless, and minimal to moderate in amount.

■ Note if the wall is reddened or pale; if there are lesions, leukoplakia, cracks, a dried surface, or bleeding; or if it appears nodular or swollen.

■ Report any secretions that are thick, curdy, frothy, gray, green, yellow, foul-smelling, or profuse.

INTERNAL GENITALIA: BIMANUAL EXAMINATION

PALPATE the vagina, cervix, uterus, and ovaries for Position, Size and Shape, Tissue Characteristics, Mobility, and Pain or Discomfort. Use a bimanual technique. First, tell the client that you are going to perform an internal examination with your fingers and hand. Next, move to a standing position at the end of the examination table between the client's legs. If your gloves have become soiled or contaminated, put on a clean pair of gloves. Lubricate the index and middle fingers of the hand that will be placed internally.

■ Abnormalities of the vaginal wall include nodules, cysts, discomfort, or unusual tissue growths.

> **Clinical Note**
>
> You must decide which hand will be the internal examination hand and which one will be used for the external manual palpation. Most examiners find it helpful to use the nondominant hand as the internal hand because its primary function is to immobilize the cervix. The more sensitive dominant hand may then be used to palpate and differentiate abdominal characteristics. **What is important is deciding how you will position your hands *before* you approach the client.**

Gently insert the middle and index fingers of the internal examination hand into the vaginal opening. Insert downward pressure on the posterior vaginal wall. Wait for a moment for the vaginal opening to relax. Then gradually insert your fingers their full length into the vagina (Fig. 18-16).

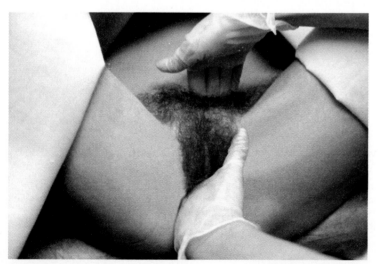

Fig. 18-16 Bimanual palpation of the uterus.
(From Seidel et al, 1995.)

PALPATE the vagina. Palpate the vaginal wall as you insert your fingers. The wall should feel smooth, homogeneous, and nontender. Once your fingers are fully extended into the vaginal wall, position your thumb (which is outside the vagina and near *but not on* the urethra and clitoris) out of the way so that it is not uncomfortable for the client.

Place the palmar surface of the fingers of your other hand on the lower abdomen midway between the umbilicus and the pubis.

PALPATE the cervix. Locate the cervix with the fingers of your internal hand. The hand on the abdomen should be used to gently hold the uterus downward against the internal examination hand so that the cervix can be evaluated. Palpate the cervix and fornices with the palmar surfaces of the fingers of your internal hand. The cervix should measure 2.5 to 4 cm (1 to 1.6 inches), be evenly rounded or slightly ovoid, feel firm (like the tip of a nose) and smooth, and move 1 to 2 cm (0.4 to 0.78 inches) in each direction without causing the woman discomfort. It should be located in the midline position.

- Note if the cervix is enlarged, irregular, soft or nodular, hard, immobile or associated with discomfort as it moves, and laterally displaced (not in the midline).
- Painful cervical movement suggests a pelvic inflammatory process such as acute pelvic inflammatory disease (PID) or a ruptured tubal pregnancy.

PALPATE the cervical os. Insert one finger gently into the cervical os. The os should admit the fingertip 0.5 cm, the fornices (pockets surrounding the cervical protrusion) should be pliable and smooth, and there should be no tenderness.

- Note any stenosis of the os (narrowing); a hardened, nodular, or irregular surface; and tenderness on palpation.

PALPATE the uterus Position. Move the fingers of your internal examination hand from the cervical os into the anterior fornix of the vagina. Slowly slide the hand that is on the abdomen toward the pubis with the palmar surface of your fingers pressing downward. First, palpate the uterus with the abdominal hand to determine the location of the fundus.

- Report any irregular contour; soft, nodular consistency; or masses.

- If *anteverted*, the fundus will be palpated at the level of the pubis between the abdominal and internal hands; the cervix will be aimed posteriorly and the uterus anteriorly. Most women have an anteverted uterus (Fig. 18-17).

- An enlarged uterus in a nonpregnant woman, or a uterus that feels irregular or nonsmooth, is abnormal and requires further evaluation.

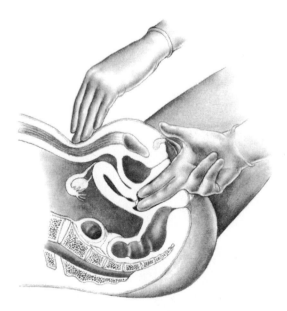

Fig. 18-17 Anteverted uterus. *(From Seidel et al, 1995.)*

- If *mid-positioned,* the fundus may not be palpable. It will depend on the amount of abdominal adipose tissue and the degree of abdominal muscle relaxation; the cervix is pointed along the axis of the vaginal canal (Fig. 18-18).

- If *anteflexed,* the fundus is palpable at the pubis between the abdominal and the internal hands; the cervix points along the axis of the vaginal canal (Fig. 18-19).

- If *retroflexed,* the fundus is positioned posteriorly and is not palpable, and the cervix is directed along the axis of the vaginal canal (Fig. 18-20).

- If *retroverted,* the fundus is positioned posteriorly and is not palpable, and the cervix is aimed anteriorly (Fig. 18-21).

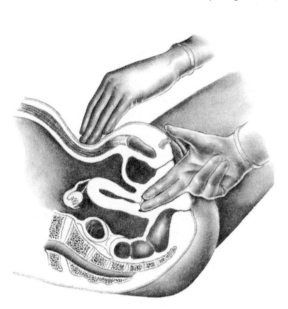

Fig. 18-18   Uterus at midposition.   *(From Seidel et al, 1995.)*

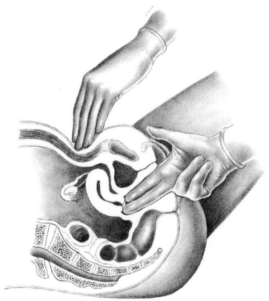

Fig. 18-19   Anteflexed uterus.   *(From Seidel et al, 1995.)*

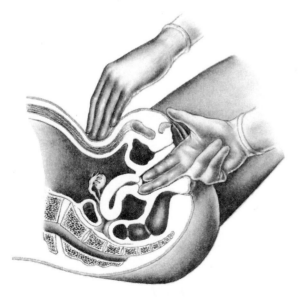

Fig. 18-20   Retroflexed uterus.   *(From Seidel et al, 1995.)*

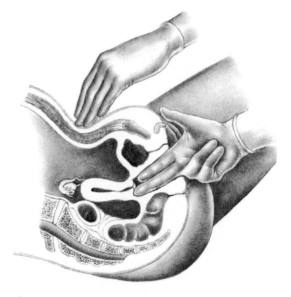

Fig. 18-21   Retroverted uterus.   *(From Seidel et al, 1995.)*

TECHNIQUES and NORMAL FINDINGS

ABNORMAL FINDINGS

Clinical Note

If you are unable to feel the uterus and cannot determine the position of the fundus, move the fingers of your intravaginal hand into the posterior fornix. Place your abdominal hand immediately above the symphysis pubis and press downward with the abdominal hand; if the uterus is retroverted or retroflexed, you should be able to feel the uterus with this maneuver.

If you still cannot feel the uterus, try repositioning your intravaginal hand fingers on either side of the cervix (top and bottom) and again press downward with your abdominal hand. If the uterus is in a midposition, it may now be felt.

PALPATE the uterus for Size, Shape, and Contour. Continuing to stabilize the cervix with your internal hand, use the abdominal hand to palpate the uterus. The uterus should be pear-shaped and approximately 6 to 8 cm (2.4 to 3.1 inches) in length. If the client has had children (is multiparous), the uterus may feel larger. The contour of the fundus should be rounded, and the consistency should feel firm and smooth.

Mobility. Gently bounce the uterus between the intravaginal hand and the hand over the abdomen. It should be freely movable and nontender.

■ Note if the uterus is fixed or tender during this maneuver. A fixed uterus may indicate adhesions. Tenderness may indicate pelvic inflammation or a ruptured tubal pregnancy.

PALPATE the adnexa and ovaries. Place the abdominal hand on the left lower abdominal quadrant and the intravaginal hand in the left fornix of the vagina. Using a sweeping motion of the palmar surfaces of the fingers of the abdominal hand, palpate the left ovary. You will know if you have located the ovary when you reach a slight bulging area in the lower quadrant and when the client complains of a "twinge" sensation of slight tenderness. The ovary may not always be palpable, but if it is, it should feel smooth, firm, and ovoid. The ovaries are approximately walnut-sized (about 4 cm [1.6 inches]) and should be mobile. Continue to palpate the left lower quadrant adnexa for masses or tenderness. In thin women, the only other structure that may be palpable is the round ligament. Reverse the position of the hands to the right side and use the same techniques to evaluate the right ovary and adnexa.

■ Note marked tenderness, nodularity, enlargement, and masses that seem immobile. All of these findings should be considered abnormal.

■ If any masses are noted in the adnexa, evaluate their characteristics: size, shape, location, tenderness, and consistency.

Withdraw the fingers from the vagina and examine the secretions on the fingers. Secretions should be odorless, clear or creamy, and minimal to moderate in amount.

■ Note any foul odor; gray, yellow, or frothy color; and profuse quantity.

RECTOVAGINAL EXAMINATION

PALPATE the pelvic region for Surface Characteristics, Position of Uterus and Adnexa, and Anal Sphincter Tone. Use the rectovaginal examination technique. If the glove is soiled, replace the intravaginal hand glove with a clean examination glove. Tell the client what you will be doing and that the procedure will be uncomfortable; she may feel the urgency of a bowel movement. Lubricate the first two fingers of the newly gloved hand. Insert your index finger into the vagina and middle finger into the anus. Place your other hand on the lower abdomen.

TECHNIQUES and NORMAL FINDINGS

ABNORMAL FINDINGS

PALPATE the rectal wall. With the index and middle fingers inserted as far as possible, instruct the client to bear down. This will bring more rectal wall into the range of palpation. Gently rotate the finger in the rectum (middle finger) to evaluate the characteristics of the rectal wall. The wall should feel smooth and be without any areas of tenderness.

The septum between the vagina and the rectum should be thin and smooth.

- Note any areas of masses, polyps, nodules, strictures, irregularities, and tenderness.

PALPATE the uterus and adnexa. With one hand positioned in the vagina and rectum and the other hand on the abdomen, use the same downward sweeping motion of the abdominal hand to again assess the uterus and adnexa areas. The findings should be the same as previously described in the bimanual examination procedure section.

- Note marked tenderness, nodularity, enlargement, and masses that seem immobile. All of these findings should be considered abnormal.
- If any masses are noted in the adnexa, evaluate their characteristics: size, shape, location, tenderness, and consistency.

PALPATE the anal sphincter. Withdraw your fingers slowly and evaluate the characteristics of the anal tone with the middle finger. The anus should tighten evenly around the examination finger. Examine the characteristics of the stool on the examination finger. For techniques and findings of the anus and stool characteristics, see Chapter 20.

Following the examination, assist the client in scooting back on the examination table. Offer her a tissue or cloth to clean herself and provide her with privacy so that she may regain her position and composure.

AGE-RELATED VARIATIONS

INFANTS

■ APPROACH

During infancy and childhood the examination is limited to an evaluation of the external genitalia to determine if the structures are intact, the vagina is present, and the hymen is patent. The infant is placed on the examination table in frog-leg position (hips flexed with the soles of the feet together and up to the buttocks). Using gloved hands, place both thumbs on either side of the labia major and gently push the tissue laterally while pushing the perineum down. This should permit visualization of the perineal area, the urethra, the clitoris, the hymen, and possibly the vaginal opening.

■ FINDINGS

Secondary to maternal hormones, the newborn's genitalia generally appear somewhat engorged, with swollen labia majora and prominent and protruding labia minora. The clitoris also looks relatively enlarged and the hymen may appear thick. It may be difficult to see the vaginal opening. A mucoid, whitish vaginal discharge may be observed during the early period following birth. This should disappear by one month. Vaginal discharges noted after the child is a month old may occur secondary to diaper or powder irritation.

CHILDREN

■ APPROACH

The extent of the genitalia examination in children depends on their age and the presence of problems. If the child is healthy and has no problems that need investiga-

tion, an external assessment of the genitalia is all that is usually needed. If, on the other hand, the child has a history of urinary tract problems, vaginal discharge or irritation, or complaints of itching, rash, or pain, then a more complete examination is necessary. A complete examination is also necessary if there is any indication of sexual abuse or mishandling of the child.

Regardless of what level of examination is necessary, the nurse must take the time to gain the cooperation and understanding of the child. By the time a child is 4 to 6 years of age, you will need to spend considerable time reassuring the child that the procedure involves looking at her genitalia and touching her on the outside only. It is often quite difficult to get the child to understand that it is okay for you to perform a genitalia examination but that if someone else touches her in a way that she should not be touched, that it is not okay. It is often important to include the parent in the discussion of the necessity for the examination and to actually be with the child and help to position the child during the examination. During the examination, you may actually enlist the child's help by taking her hand and having her first touch herself, then you proceed with palpation. In all cases, ensure privacy for the child. Positioning for the examination is best performed by having the child lie on her back and place the legs in a frog-leg position (hips flexed with the soles of the feet together and up to her buttocks).

School-age girls will dislike the examination even more than younger children. It is best to approach the child in a matter-of-fact manner and to tell her what you are going to do. If you take your time and tell the child that you need her cooperation, the examination will usually occur without incident. The child should participate in the decision about whether the parent is present in the room or not during the examination. Some girls may want a parent present and some may not. Confer with the child before the examination and, if appropriate, ask the parent to wait outside.

Older, more mature girls may be even shier about their bodies and want as much privacy as possible. It is important to respect their wishes. Because many are becoming very interested in their own bodies and the changes that may be taking place, they may want to actually take part in the examination. This may be a perfect time to teach the child about her own anatomy and the changes that she will experience. A mirror may be used during the examination for instruction.

■ FINDINGS

The techniques of the external genitalia examination are the same as for the infant. Using gloved hands, gently spread the labia so that the genitalia may be inspected. Until approximately age 7, the labia majora are flat, the labia minora are thin, the clitoris is relatively small, and the hymen is tissue-paper thin. Following that time, the mons pubis thickens, the labia majora thicken, and the labia minora become slightly rounded. By the time the child reaches preadolescence, usually between the ages of 8 and 11, pubic hair will begin to develop (see the anatomy and physiology section for adolescent development). There should be no vaginal discharge, vaginal odor, or evidence of bruising. Just before menarche, there is a physiologic increase in the amount of vaginal secretions. If any abnormal findings are present, further investigation is warranted. A rectal examination is necessary if there is any expected history of fondling, abuse, or the possibility of a foreign body in the rectum.

ADOLESCENTS

■ APPROACH

The adolescent should be given a choice to be examined alone, and she should be assured of privacy and confidentiality. Fully discuss with her the progress of puberty, including any questions she may have, and health concerns. Assess her growth, menstrual history, and sexual maturity rating using the charts referred to in the anatomy and physiology and history sections of this chapter. Reassure the client of the normal aspects of the changes her body is undergoing. The adolescent's first pelvic examination is probably the most important of her entire life. Time and care should be taken to explain the procedures, show the equipment, and tell the client exactly what she may expect. Always remember to assess the size and sexual history of the client in choosing the correct size and type of vaginal speculum. The speculum most commonly used that does not cause discomfort is a pediatric speculum with blades that are 1.0 to 1.5 cm wide. If the client is sexually active, a larger speculum may be used.

■ FINDINGS

The positioning and techniques for examination of the external genitalia and possibly pelvic examination are the same as for the adult. A pelvic examination should be performed if the adolescent desires contraception, if she is sexually active and has sexual intercourse, or if she is 18 years of age or older. Additionally, a pelvic examination is warranted any time the client has any signs of genitalia or vaginal irritation, infection, or related problems. This will include periodic Pap tests when intercourse begins. The procedures to be followed are the same as for an adult woman, but additional time must be allowed for the counseling and support needed with an adolescent client. All findings for the genitalia examination of the adolescent are the same as for the adult.

■ APPROACH

The examination procedures for the older adult are the same as for the younger adult. Often there is a temptation to defer the routine pelvic examination of the older woman because it may be difficult for her to be positioned in stirrups, she is postmenopausal, or she is no longer sexually active. None of these are reasons to defer the examination. Instead, older women have different problems, such as urinary incontinence, pelvic relaxation, vaginal irritation, dryness, or rectal problems that warrant evaluation. What is important to remember when examining an older adult is that she may need assistance to help hold her legs if she is unable to tolerate their positioning in the stirrups. In addition, she may need more assistance in assuming a modified lithotomy position and may not be able to stay in the position as long as a younger woman. If the client is no longer sexually active, a smaller speculum with narrower blades may be necessary to prevent discomfort from the introital constriction. Also, because of the decrease in the amount of natural lubrication in the vagina, it becomes necessary to lubricate the speculum and the fingers of the examining hand adequately to avoid causing discomfort during the examination.

■ FINDINGS

The labia of the older woman become flatter and smaller. The skin may appear dry and have a shiny appearance. The pubic hair often appears sparse and fine. There may be patchy loss of pubic hair or, in some cases, total absence. The clitoris also becomes smaller. During the bimanual examination the examiner may find that the client's introitus is smaller and may admit only one finger, or, in multiparous women, the introitus may be gaping, with vaginal walls rolling toward the opening. Either should be noted and evaluated accordingly.

The examiner may also find that the client's vagina is narrower and shorter and that there is an absence of rugation of the vaginal wall. Likewise, the cervix may appear smaller and paler, and the fornices may be smaller or absent. Following menopause, the uterus also diminishes in size and may actually not be palpable upon examination. If the uterus is palpable, it should be smooth, firm, freely movable, and nontender. Any uterine enlargement; nodular, irregular, hardened, or indurated areas; areas that are tender on palpation; and fixed, nonmovable areas in the pelvis should be further evaluated. Ovaries atrophy with age and are rarely palpable in aging women.

During the rectovaginal examination, you will most likely feel the rectovaginal septum to be thin, smooth, and pliable. The anal sphincter tone may be somewhat diminished, and because of pelvic musculature relaxation, the client may have stress incontinence and prolapse of the vaginal walls or uterus. All should be carefully assessed.

CLIENTS WITH SITUATIONAL VARIATIONS

■ APPROACH

The gynecologic examination of the pregnant woman is the same as for all other adult clients. What is different is the evaluation of the physiologic changes during pregnancy, the evaluation of the growing fetus, and the assessment of the pelvic structures that will permit vaginal delivery of the infant.

■ FINDINGS

Physiologic Changes

In early pregnancy, the isthmus will soften but the cervix remains firm. By the second month, the cervix, vagina, and vulva take on a bluish color, and there will be increased vaginal secretions secondary to increased vascularity in the pelvis. The cervix also becomes much softer and may feel like lips instead of the tip of a nose. See other signs of early pregnancy in the anatomy and physiology section of this chapter.

Uterine Size

The uterine size during pregnancy may be used to estimate the gestational age of the fetus. While there is a lack of consensus about the accuracy of the size of the uterus at various weeks, it still may provide an estimate. To measure the uterine size, centimeters of height should be used to measure the fundal height

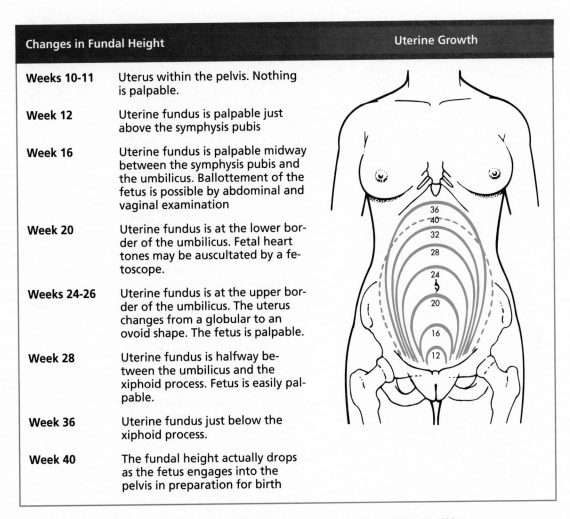

Changes in Fundal Height		Uterine Growth

Weeks 10-11 Uterus within the pelvis. Nothing is palpable.

Week 12 Uterine fundus is palpable just above the symphysis pubis

Week 16 Uterine fundus is palpable midway between the symphysis pubis and the umbilicus. Ballottement of the fetus is possible by abdominal and vaginal examination

Week 20 Uterine fundus is at the lower border of the umbilicus. Fetal heart tones may be auscultated by a fetoscope.

Weeks 24-26 Uterine fundus is at the upper border of the umbilicus. The uterus changes from a globular to an ovoid shape. The fetus is palpable.

Week 28 Uterine fundus is halfway between the umbilicus and the xiphoid process. Fetus is easily palpable.

Week 36 Uterine fundus just below the xiphoid process.

Week 40 The fundal height actually drops as the fetus engages into the pelvis in preparation for birth

Fig. 18-22 Changes in fundal height with pregnancy. *(Modified from Seidel et al, 1995.)*

from the symphysis pubis. Fig. 18-22 shows the stages of uterine growth and fetal development. Also refer to Chapter 7 for a more detailed discussion of measuring uterine and fetal growth.

Pelvis Size

During one of the prenatal visits, usually at the beginning of the third trimester, it is important to estimate the client's pelvis size to determine its adequacy for vaginal delivery of the infant. If there are any questions about the adequacy of the pelvis size, the measurements may be confirmed by computed tomography or ultrasound. Use the following steps for measurement:

1. Determine the *pelvic inlet* by measuring the *diagonal conjugate.* To do this, insert your first two fingers into the vagina until the tips of the fingers reach the sacral promontory (Fig. 18-23). With the index finger of your other hand, mark the area on the intravaginal hand where the symphysis meets the hand. Remove the intravaginal hand and measure with a ruler the diameter of the diagonal conjugate. A normal distance is 12.5 to 13 cm (4.9 to 5.1 inches).

2. Next, estimate the *obstetric conjugate,* which is the anteroposterior (A:P) diameter of the pelvic inlet, by taking the *diagonal conjugate* and subtracting 1.5 to 2 cm (0.6 to 0.8 inches) (Fig. 18-24). An adequate obstetric conjugate should be estimated at about 11 cm (4.3 inches). If necessary, this measurement may be accurately calculated by x-ray.

3. The *midplane* of the pelvis is measured by estimating the *transverse diameter* or the *interspinous diameter.* To do this, insert your first two examining fingers into the vagina and locate the ischial spines (Fig. 18-25). Estimate the distance between the ischial spines by moving your fingers from side to side. An expected measurement is approximately 10 to 11 cm (3.9 to 4.3 inches).

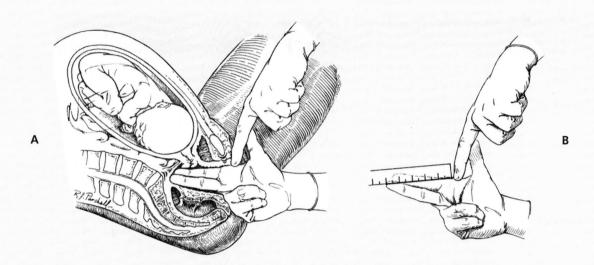

Fig. 18-23 Measuring the diagonal conjugate. **A,** Insert the fingers until the tips reach the sacral promontory. With a finger of the other hand against the inferior border of the symphysis, mark where the symphysis pubis meets the hand. **B,** Compare the hand distance with a ruler to determine the diameter of the diagonal conjugate. *(From Seidel et al, 1995.)*

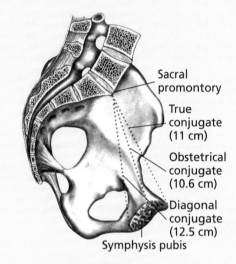

Sacral promontory

True conjugate (11 cm)

Obstetrical conjugate (10.6 cm)

Diagonal conjugate (12.5 cm)

Symphysis pubis

Fig. 18-24 Estimate the obstetric conjugate using the diagonal conjugate. The diagonal conjugate varies in length depending on the height and inclination of the symphysis pubis. *(From Seidel et al, 1995.)*

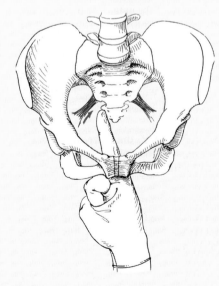

Fig. 18-25 Estimating the transverse (interspinous) diameter. Insert the two examining fingers into the vagina and locate the ischial spines. If the spines are prominent, they may project into the pelvis similar to spikes. If they are flush with the pelvic walls, you might locate them by identifying the sacrospinous ligament and following it anteriorly to the spines. Estimate the distance between the ischial spines by moving your fingers from side to side. *(From Seidel et al, 1995.)*

4. Measure the *outlet* of the pelvis by estimating the *biischial diameter,* the *intertuberous diameter,* or the *transverse diameter.* The biischial diameter is estimated by using a Thompelvimeter to measure the external surface distance between the tuberosities (Fig. 18-26). Place the Thompelvimeter centrally below the vagina and extend the tips of the crossbar laterally until they touch the ischial tuberosities. If a Thompelvimeter is not available, the distance may also be estimated by placing your closed fist against the perineum between the ischial tuberosities, then measuring the width of your fist and any additional distance to the tuberosities (Fig. 18-27).

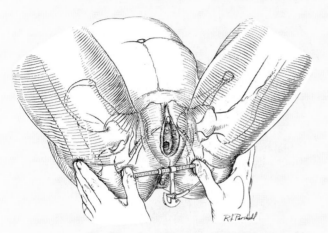

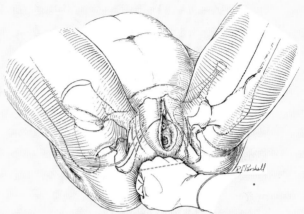

Fig. 18-26 Determining the biischial diameter. Measure the distance between the tuberosities using the Thompelvimeter; position it centrally and extend the tips of the crossbar until they touch the ischial tuberosities. *(From Seidel et al, 1995.)*

Fig. 18-27 Alternate technique for determining the biischial diameter. First, measure your closed fist to determine its width; then, place your fist against the perineum between the ischial tuberosities. Determine the distance between the tuberosities compared with your fist. *(From Seidel et al, 1995.)*

Preparation for Infant Delivery

Several changes occur in preparation for the delivery of the infant. Each of these should be evaluated every time the client is assessed.

1. *Cervical Dilation and Length.* The nonpregnant cervical os is closed. In the pregnant client, the cervix dilates to a diameter of 10 cm (4 inches) to permit the delivery of the child. At 10 cm (4 inches) the cervix is said to be completely dilated. The actual time of the beginning of cervical dilation depends many times on the parity of the client, the weeks of gestation, and the progression of labor.

2. *Stations of the Infant's Presenting Part.* The *station* is the relationship of the presenting part to the ischial spines in the mother's pelvis. The station measurement is an estimate of the position of the child in relation to the location of the mother's ischial spines. The range of measurements goes from −5 to +5 cm (Fig. 18-28).

3. *Fetal Head Position.* When cervical os dilation has begun, the examiner may assess for the infant's fetal head position. To do this, insert your two examining fingers, palmar surface up, into the posterior aspect of client's vagina and move your fingers forward over the fetal head as you slowly turn your fingers downward (Fig. 18-29, *A*). During this maneuver, locate the sagittal sutures of the fetus and then, using a circular motion, move alongside the fetal head until the other fontanel is located and differentiated (Fig. 18-29, *B*).

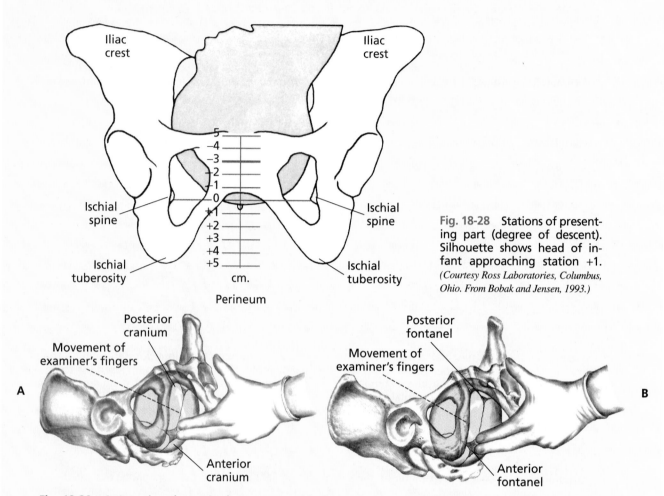

Fig. 18-28 Stations of presenting part (degree of descent). Silhouette shows head of infant approaching station +1. *(Courtesy Ross Laboratories, Columbus, Ohio. From Bobak and Jensen, 1993.)*

Fig. 18-29 **A,** Locating the sagittal suture on vaginal examination. **B,** Differentiating the fontanels on vaginal examination. *(From Seidel et al, 1995.)*

CLIENTS WHO HAVE HAD A HYSTERECTOMY

■ APPROACH

Performing a pelvic examination on a client who has had a hysterectomy is essentially no different than examining any other client. Before the examination, it is important to assess if the client had the hysterectomy by the abdominal or vaginal approach, and to determine if she has had a *total* (fallopian tubes and ovaries removed) or a *partial* (tubes and ovaries not removed) hysterectomy. In addition, it is important to find out why she had the hysterectomy, when it was performed, if she had any accompanying bowel or bladder repairs, and what problems or concerns she has had since the surgery.

■ FINDINGS

Probably the most obvious finding during the assessment will be the absence of a cervix and uterus. Despite this, a thorough vaginal examination should be performed and a routine Pap smear should be collected from along the suture line, using the blunt end of a spatula. Be sure to label the specimen as vaginal cells taken from the suture line. If the client has had her ovaries removed, the findings on examination may show many of the findings that are present in older, postmenopausal women.

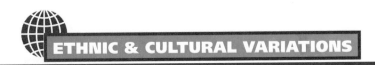

ETHNIC & CULTURAL VARIATIONS

■ **FINDINGS**

Some documented differences do exist across ethnic groups in female genitalia. Pubic hair color, consistency, and amount vary, as does the color of external genitalia. Incidence and mortality of various gynecologic cancers is also varied by ethnic grouping. Risk for endometrial cancer is higher for Hawaiian Natives and whites, while risk for cervical cancer is greater for African Americans, Hispanics, and American Indians. Reproductive health statistics also vary by cultural group. African Americans are less likely to seek early prenatal care, have higher birth rates, especially among teenagers, and have higher incidences of maternal and infant mortality. The same pattern is seen in American Indians and Alaskan Natives.

EXAMINATION **S U M M A R Y**
Female Genitalia

External Genitalia *(pp. 498-501)*
- Inspect the pubic hair for:
  Distribution
- Inspect the skin of the mons pubis and inguinal area for:
  Surface characteristics
- Inspect and palpate the labia majora for:
  Pigmentation
  Surface characteristics
- Inspect and palpate the labia minora for:
  Pigmentation
  Surface characteristics
- Inspect the clitoris for:
  Size and length
- Inspect the urethral meatus, vaginal introitus, perineum, and anus for:
  Positioning
  Surface characteristics
- Palpate the Skene and Bartholin glands for:
  Surface characteristics
  Discharge
  Pain or discomfort
- Inspect and palpate muscle tone for:
  Vaginal wall tone
  Rectal muscle tone
  Urinary incontinence

Internal Genitalia: Speculum Examination *(pp. 501-506)*
- Inspect the cervix for:
  Color
  Surface characteristics
  Position
  Size and shape
- Inspect the cervical os for:
  Discharge
- Obtain all cervical and vaginal cultures and smears
- Inspect the vaginal walls for:
  Color
  Surface characteristics

Internal Genitalia: Bimanual Examination *(pp. 506-510)*
- Palpate the vagina, cervix, uterus, and ovaries for:
  Position
  Size and shape
  Tissue characteristics
  Mobility
  Pain or discomfort
- Palpate the pelvic region using the rectovaginal examination technique for:
  Surface characteristics
  Position of the uterus and adnexa
  Rectal wall characteristics
  Anal sphincter tone

COMMON PROBLEMS/CONDITIONS
associated with the Female Genitalia

■ **Premenstrual syndrome (PMS):** A combination of affective (emotional) and somatic (physical) symptoms that begins shortly after ovulation (about 14 to 16 days) and diminishes after menstruation begins. PMS is most prevalent in women over 30 years of age. It has been estimated that 50% of all women will experience PMS at some time during their lives.

CERVIX

■ **Cervical cancer:** Begins as a neoplastic change in the junction between the exocervix (the outer surface of the cervix), which is covered with squamous epithelium, and the endocervix (the inside of the cervical canal), which is covered with columnar epithelium (Fig. 18-30). Cervical cancer is now generally considered to be a sexually transmitted disease.

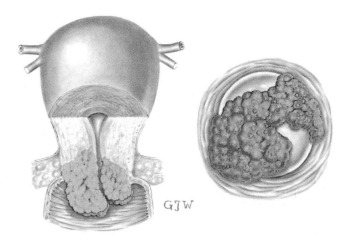

Fig. 18-30   Advanced cervical cancer.   *(From Belcher, 1992.)*

■ **Nabothian cysts:** Enlarged, fluid-filled retention cysts, often distorting the shape of the cervix.

UTERUS

■ **Endometriosis:** The development of stroma (connective tissue) and endometrial glands (identical to uterine tissue) outside the uterus (Fig. 18-31). It has been estimated that as many as 20% to 25% of all women have some degree of endometriosis during their lives. The most common sites of endometriosis are the uterosacral ligaments, round ligaments, sigmoid colon, rectovaginal septum, pelvic peritoneum, ovaries, cul-de-sac, and urinary bladder.

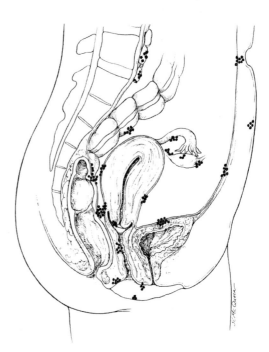

Fig. 18-31   Common sites of endometriosis.   *(From Droege-mueller, 1987.)*

■ *Fibroids (myomas):* Common, benign uterine tumors that are firm and irregular in shape (Fig. 18-32). The tumor nodules usually appear in the vulva or the uterus. The prevalence in women over the age of 35 is 20% to 25%.

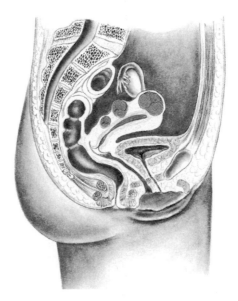

Fig. 18-32 Myomas of the uterus (fibroids). *(From Seidel et al, 1995.)*

■ *Uterine prolapse:* May result from the weakening of the supporting structures of the floor of the pelvis. There is often a concurrent cystocele and rectocele. When there is a prolapse, the uterus becomes progressively retroverted and descends into the vagina. In *first degree* prolapse the cervix remains within the vagina (Fig. 18-33, *A*). In *second degree* prolapse the cervix is in the introitus (Fig. 18-33, *B*). In *third degree* prolapse the cervix and vagina drop outside the introitus (Fig. 18-33, *C*).

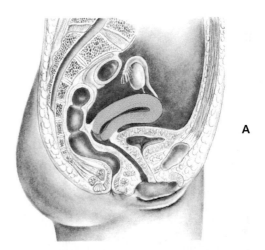

A

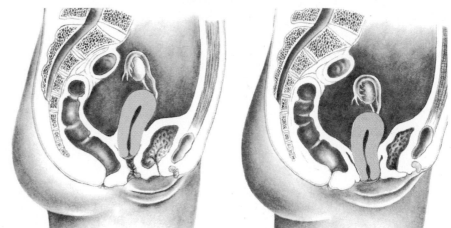

B

C

Fig. 18-33 Uterine prolapse. **A,** Expected uterine position. **B,** First-degree prolapse of the uterus. **C,** Second-degree prolapse of the uterus. *(From Seidel et al, 1995.)*

■ *Endometrial cancer:* The most common gynecologic malignancy; one of the six leading causes of death in women attributed to cancer (Fig. 18-34). Because the tumor is usually well-differentiated and localized, the cure rate is about 87%.

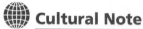 Cultural Note

Endometrial cancer is the most common gynecologic cancer, and incidence does vary by cultural group. Hawaiian Native women are at highest risk (1 in 3500) followed closely by whites (1 in 3800). The risk is much less for African Americans, Hispanics, Asian Americans, and American Indians/Alaskan Natives, ranging from 1 in 6000 to 1 in 15,000. Cervical cancer rates for African Americans, American Indians/Alaskan Natives, and Hispanics are over twice those of whites.

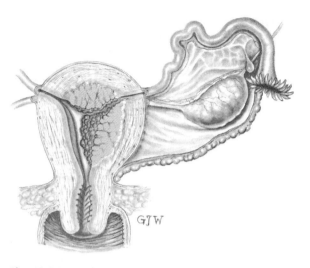

Fig. 18-34   Endometrial cancer.   *(From Belcher, 1992.)*

OVARIES

■ *Ovarian cancer:* Develops from cells present during embryonic ovarian development (Fig. 18-35). It is the fourth leading cause of cancer-related deaths in women. The incidence of ovarian cancer, which is rising, is highest among western, industrialized, white women over the age of 50. Ovarian cancer is very difficult to cure because it usually has either no symptoms or very mild symptoms until it reaches stage III, which means that it involves one or both ovaries and has peritoneal metastasis outside the pelvis or regional lymph node metastasis.

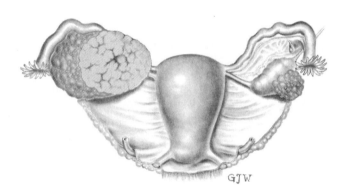

Fig. 18-35   Cancer of the ovaries.   *(From Belcher, 1992.)*

VULVA AND VAGINA

■ *Inflamed Bartholin glands:* Commonly but not always caused by gonococcal infection. It may be acute or chronic. The acute inflammation causes a red, hot, and tender swelling of the gland that may drain pus (Fig. 18-36). Nonacute or chronic inflammation causes a nontender cyst on the labia.

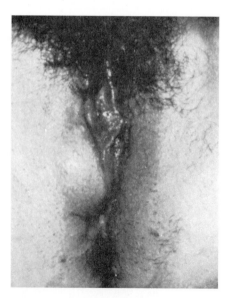

Fig. 18-36   Inflammation of Bartholin glands.   *(From Gardner and Kaufman, 1969.)*

■ *Cystocele:* A hernia type protrusion of the urinary bladder through the anterior wall of the vagina (Fig. 18-37). The bulging is usually seen and felt as the woman bears down. If the cystocele is severe, it may be accompanied by stress incontinence.

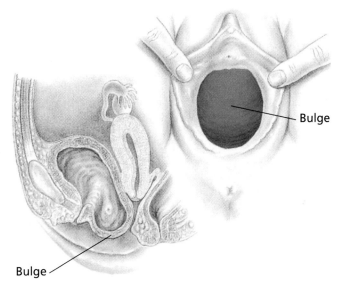

Fig. 18-37 Cystocele. *(From Seidel et al, 1995.)*

■ *Rectocele:* A hernia-type protrusion of the rectum through the posterior wall of the vagina (Fig. 18-38). Bulging of the posterior vaginal wall may be seen as the woman bears down.

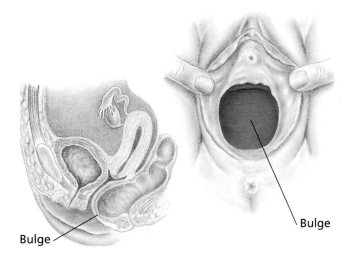

Fig. 18-38 Rectocele. *(From Seidel et al, 1995.)*

SEXUALLY TRANSMITTED DISEASE (STD)

■ *Herpes simplex virus (HSV):* May be one of five major types. Type I (HSV-1) is usually found above the waist; Type 2 (HSV-2) is usually found below the waist, although orogenital sex may result in cross-contamination of these locations. Types 3, 4, and 5 are generally not associated with sexual contact. The initial infection may manifest as a single vesicle or multiple vesicles that rupture and form small, painful ulcers, which heal without scarring in about 14 to 21 days (Fig. 18-39). Other symptoms may involve fever and flulike symptoms. Subsequent infections are usually less severe and are shorter in duration.

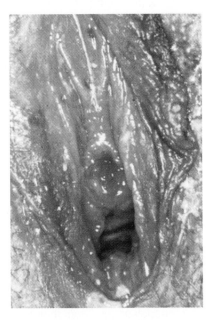

Fig. 18-39 Herpes infection of the labia. *(From Edge and Miller, 1994.)*

■ *Genital warts (condylomata):* Wart- or fig-like growths that are referred to as condylomata acuminata, which occur secondary to a sexually transmitted infection by the human papilloma virus (HPV) (Fig. 18-40). The warts are pink to brown, elongated lesions that cluster and resemble a cauliflower. The incubation period for HPV is 1 to 6 months.

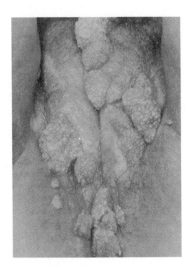

Fig. 18-40 Condyloma acuminatum. *(From Grimes, 1991.)*

■ *Chlamydia:* An intracellular pathogen that is the leading cause of blindness when eyes are infected at birth or through poor hygiene. The initial vaginal infection may be asymptomatic or may have a yellow mucopurulent discharge from the cervical os. The vaginal tissue may be edematous and friable. If this very common STD is untreated, it may lead to infertility.

■ *Monilia vaginitis (Candidiasis):* A fungal or yeast infection. It is caused by *Candida albicans*. It has been estimated that 75% of all women have a yeast infection sometime during their lifetime. Yeast infections are more prevalent in women in tropical climates and occur most frequently before menstruation and during pregnancy. Some women are asymptomatic, whereas others may have a thick, cheesy, white vaginal discharge.

■ *Molluscum contagiosum:* A benign condition that affects the mucous membranes and skin, producing genital lesions or papules (Fig. 18-41). This sexually transmitted disease is most frequently seen in girls and young women ages 10 to 16.

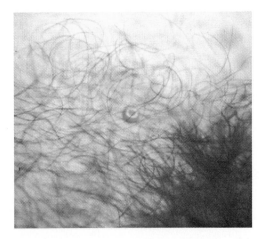

Fig. 18-41 Papule caused by molluscum contagiosum virus (MCV). *(From Seidel et al, 1995.)*

■ *Gonorrhea:* Currently the most frequently reported sexually transmitted disease in the United States. If left untreated, gonorrhea may lead to pelvic inflammatory disease (PID). Gonorrhea most commonly causes a yellow or green vaginal discharge, dysuria, pelvic or abdominal pain, and abnormal menses. The vaginal itching and burning may be severe.

■ *Syphilis:* A chronic systemic disease characterized by a primary lesion. The first symptom of this STD is a single, firm, painless open sore or chancre at the site of entry on the genitals or mouth (Fig. 18-42). The incubation period is 10 to 90 days, with an average of about 3 weeks. Syphilis has additional stages beyond the primary lesion. Stage 2, developing 6 to 12 weeks after the initial lesion, involves a skin rash, condylomata and lymphadenopathy, and round, flat, or oval grayish papules. Stage 3 is neurosyphilis, which involves the neurologic system and includes symptoms such as ataxia and confusion. If left untreated, confusion and insanity may result.

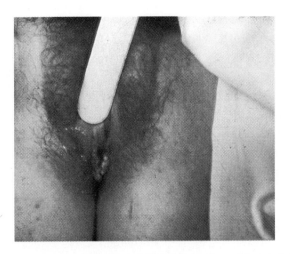

Fig. 18-42 Primary syphilis of the vulva with condyloma at bottom of labia near rectum. *(From Edge and Miller, 1994.)*

■ *Trichomoniasis:* A vaginal inflammation that may involve the labia and vulva. It is caused by the *Trichomonas* organism, which is a one-celled, flagellated protozoa. Trichomoniasis produces a frothy or bubbly, heavy greenish-gray discharge that has a foul "fishy" smell. The genitalia may be red with scratch marks or edema, and vaginal bleeding may be present. The walls of the vagina and the cervix may have petechial "strawberry patches." Some women may be asymptomatic.

Signs and Symptoms of Sexually Transmitted Diseases (STDs)

There are over 50 STDs. It is impossible to describe the symptoms for all of them. The most common signs and symptoms are the following:

- *Chlamydia*

  At first, the woman has no symptoms. When symptoms do appear, usually within 1 to 3 weeks after infection, they include pain on urination, vaginal discharge, or abdominal pain. If left untreated, chlamydia may lead to pelvic inflammatory disease (PID).

- *Genital herpes*

  Early symptoms include burning or pain with urination; pain in the buttocks, legs, or genital area; vaginal discharge; or a feeling of pressure in the pelvic area. In a few days, small red bumps appear in the genital area; later the bumps develop into blisters, which open, crust, and then heal. Even after the sores disappear, the herpes virus remains in the body and can reactivate at any time.

- *Gonorrhea*

  Often there are no signs. The woman may experience pain or burning when urinating. There may be a yellowish vaginal discharge. Advanced symptoms include bleeding between menstrual periods, swollen joints, fever, or pain in the pelvic area.

- *Genital warts*

  These warts are painless small, bumpy warts that appear on or near the sex organs, usually 3 weeks to 3 months after sex with an infected partner. The warts, which are flesh-colored single or cauliflower-like masses, sometimes develop inside the vagina, on the lips of the vagina, or around the anus.

- *Syphilis*

  The first symptom of syphilis, which usually occurs 1 to 12 weeks after sex with an infected partner, often is a painless sore on the genitals. The sore disappears within a few weeks, but the disease progresses. In the second stage, a skin rash appears, along with flulike symptoms. Left untreated, syphilis can lead to blindness, heart disease, brain damage, and even death.

- *Human immuno-deficiency virus (HIV) infection and AIDS*

  HIV infection and AIDS may produce no symptoms for months or years. As the immune system weakens, the symptoms include swollen lymph glands, fever, night sweats, fatigue, and weight loss.

- *Vaginitis*

  The most common symptom is an unusual vaginal discharge. *Trichomoniasis* produces a frothy yellow discharge with a persistent itching or burning and an unpleasant odor. *Yeast infection* produces a discharge that looks like cottage cheese and possibly an intense itch.

- *Gardnerella*

  Gardnerella infection causes a grayish-white, watery, strong-smelling discharge.

Sample Documentation & Nursing Diagnosis

CASE 1 48-year-old African-American woman with complaints of "hot flashes."

Subjective

Client thinks she is "going through the change"; states periods have become very irregular, sometimes lasting only 1 day; time between periods is 3 to 7 weeks. Last period was 4½ weeks ago; awakens frequently during the night "in a sweat" with increased perspiration. Sexually active and wants to know if she can still get pregnant now that she is entering menopause. Concerned about the effect of "the change" on the way she looks and on her sexuality. Last Pap smear was 10 months ago during routine examination.

Objective

External genitalia unremarkable; no lesions or discoloration; cervix pink, midline, without lesions; parous os; vaginal discharge clear, odorless, and scant. Vaginal walls smooth and rugated; no masses, discoloration, or lesions noted. Slight discomfort to palpation of the ovaries. Ovaries smooth and not enlarged. Rectovaginal examination not remarkable; slight cystocele noted when client bears down; no evidence of stress incontinence.

• •

Nursing Diagnosis #1

Knowledge deficit related to lack of information about self-care management.

Defining Characteristics Hot flashes, irregular periods, age 48. Concerned about getting pregnant with onset of menopause.

Nursing Diagnosis #2

Body image disturbance related to body change.

Defining Characteristics Concerned about appearance and sexuality.

*&*Nursing Diagnosis

CASE 2   77-year-old white woman stating that her abdomen is getting bigger as if she is pregnant and she thinks that she has cancer.

Subjective

Anxious-appearing client states she went through menopause between 53 and 55 years of age. Since then she has been healthy until her abdomen started getting bigger. Approximately 10 months ago she noticed it was more difficult to button her skirt button. Since then her abdomen has continued to grow. Client cannot wear any clothing with a limiting waistband. Reports no discomfort or pain, no vaginal bleeding, and no vaginal discharge. Last Pap smear approximately 5 years ago. Takes no medications; has no other complaints. Reports 15-lb weight gain in past 6 months. States has not sought medical care for her abdominal enlargement because of belief that she "is sure that she has cancer and that she is going to die."

Objective

Well-nourished, healthy-appearing, white woman with obvious enlargement of the abdomen.

Abdomen appears enlarged from symphis pubis to umbilicus. External genitalia unremarkable; pubic hair distribution is thinning and has fine texture. Approximately 1 cm (0.5 inch) of posterior vaginal wall bulging noted when client bears down. Cervix is pink and slightly anteverted; no evidence of cervical nodules, discoloration, or lesions; walls of vagina are smooth and dark pink; no evidence of dryness and irritation along both lateral walls. Uterus firm, irregular, and enlarged; uterus is slightly mobile with palpation. No discomfort in region of uterus; client does report slight discomfort in the vulva. Ovaries are not palpable due to enlarged uterus. Client complains of slight discomfort in both right and left adnexa regions. Rectovaginal examination is unremarkable.

• •

Nursing Diagnosis #1

Fear related to possible diagnosis of cancer.

Defining Characteristics   Weight gain, enlarged abdomen, states "sure that she has cancer and that she is going to die."

Nursing Diagnosis #2

Body image disturbance related to body change.

Defining Characteristics   Enlarged abdomen, 15-lb weight gain, clothes not fitting, enlarged uterus on examination.

HEALTH PROMOTION

■ **Rape Prevention Guidelines** Every woman may become a victim of sexual assault. Use the following principles to reduce your risk.

1. Never assume that you are an unlikely candidate for personal assault.
2. Think carefully about your patterns of movement to and from class or work. Alter your routes frequently.
3. Walk briskly with a sense of purpose. Try not to walk alone at night.
4. Dress so that the clothes you wear do not unnecessarily restrict your movement or make you more vulnerable.
5. Always be sure of your surroundings. Look over your shoulder occasionally. Know where you are so that you won't get lost.
6. If you think you are being followed, look for a safe retreat. This might be a store, a fire or police station, or a group of people.
7. Be especially cautious of first dates, blind dates, or people you meet at a party or bar who push to be alone with you.
8. Let trusted friends know where you are and when you plan to return.
9. Keep your car in good working order. Think beforehand how you would handle the situation should your car break down.
10. Trust your best instincts if you are assaulted. Each situation is different. Do what you can to protect your life.

(Payne and Hahn, 1992)

■ **Premenstrual Syndrome (PMS)** Because PMS is a progesterone-deficiency illness, taking synthetic progesterone, or a natural progesterone such as wild yams, may help, but by itself this will not control PMS. Treatment involves relieving the symptoms and, when possible, correcting the cause. Things that you can do to control your body's response include:

1. Reduce your salt intake to reduce bloating and fluid retention.
2. Do some form of moderate, enjoyable exercise at least four times each week.
3. Reduce your intake of caffeine and sugar.

4. Keep your weight at a proper level. If you are 15 pounds or more over your desirable weight, consider a gradual weight-loss program.
5. Reduce your stress level whenever possible. Don't schedule too many activities on the days you expect your symptoms to be severe.

■ **Vulvar Self-Examination** A vulvar self-examination includes inspection of all of the external genital organs, including the pubic mound, clitoris, urinary opening, vaginal opening, and anus (Fig. 18-43, A).
To perform a self-examination, use a flashlight and a hand mirror and follow these steps:

1. Sit on the edge of a toilet seat, your bed, or the bathtub. Sit with your legs spread apart and inspect the entire vulvar region (Fig. 18-43, B).
2. Examine both sides of the labia and see if they are similar. With your fingers, separate the inner lips of the vulva, and check the clitoris, the urinary opening, the vagina, and the skin between the vagina and the anus (Fig. 18-43, C).
3. Press down on all areas of the vulva, feeling for any lumps or masses (Fig. 18-43, D).
4. Gently squeeze the vaginal opening between your thumb and forefinger. It should feel soft and moist (Fig. 18-43, E).
5. If you notice any lumps, masses, growths, or changes in skin color, see your health care professional.

■ **Pelvic Muscle Exercises** *Kegel* exercises are perineal exercises that help to decrease stress incontinence by strengthening the perineal floor muscles. To perform the exercises, do the following:

1. During urination, tighten the muscles and stop the flow of urine in midstream. You should feel a sensation of pulling upward into the vagina, and the buttocks will be squeezed together.
2. Repeat the procedure by stopping and starting the urine flow. Stop urination for 3 to 5 seconds, then relax and start the flow again.
3. Repeat this sequence 12 to 24 times during urination.

To be effective, Kegel exercises should be performed at least four times each day.

A B C D E

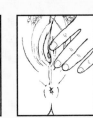
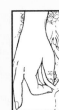

Pubic mound
Clitoris
Urinary opening
Vaginal opening
Anus
Rectal opening

Fig. 18-43 Vulvar self-examination. (See text for details.) *(From Edge and Miller, 1994.)*

HEALTH PROMOTION—cont'd

■ **Safe Sex** The term "safe sex" refers to the practice of protecting yourself against sexually transmitted diseases (STDs), HIV/AIDS, and pregnancy. This may range from teaching abstinence to using contraceptives. Fig. 18-44 shows many of the common protective devices that are currently available.

■ **Menopause and Osteoporosis** A woman is considered to have reached menopause when she has gone without a period for 1 year. At the time of menopause, ovarian function diminishes and there is a decrease of estrogen in the tissues. Current research indicates that osteoporosis and heart disease increase after menopause, because estrogen has a protective effect in preventing these disorders. Osteoporosis usually occurs after age 50 without any prior symptoms or warning. Prevention of osteoporosis focuses on stimulating bone formation and preventing reabsorption of bone. Treatment includes early education for the production of healthy bones, exercise, calcium supplements, and possibly estrogen therapy.

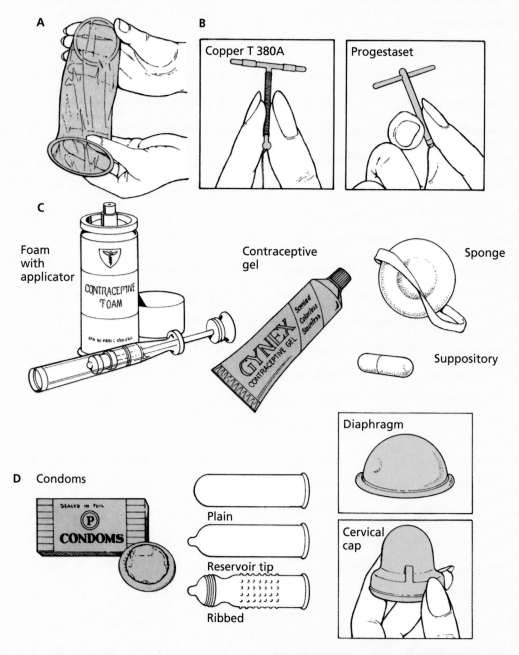

Fig. 18-44   Contraceptives. **A,** Female condom. **B,** Intrauterine devices (IUDs). **C,** Vaginal spermicides. **D,** Mechanical barriers.   *(From Edge and Miller, 1994.)*

???????STUDY QUESTIONS???????

1. Identify the center of sexual excitement in the female. Where is it located anatomically?

2. Identify and describe the two major parts of the uterus. List two functions of the uterus.

3. Describe the five phases of the menstrual cycle.

4. Describe the changes that occur in the female during puberty. When does puberty begin?

5. What is the first indicator that a woman might be pregnant? List four other changes that occur during pregnancy.

6. List two changes in the external genitalia that occur with aging. List three changes in the internal genitalia that occur with aging.

7. A woman comes in with tender breasts and says she is depressed and weepy. What other information do you need to collect?

8. A 35-year-old woman confides confidentially that she "wets on herself" sometimes and finds it embarrassing. What additional information should you collect?

9. What information are you seeking when you gather an obstetric history?

10. A 50-year-old woman reports that she has irregular periods that occur every 17 to 21 days, and she is more irritable than usual. Further questions reveal that she has suddenly started to sweat all of the time and she is no longer interested in intercourse because it hurts. What do you think may be happening to this woman? What other signs and symptoms do you want to inquire about?

11. Identify three types of gynecologic cancer and the risk factors for each. Which of the risk factors are modifiable?

12. What information are you seeking when you take a history on sexual activity? Why is a history of an individual's sexual activity important to a health care provider?

13. List at least one area in history-taking that is specific to the following female age groups: (a) 6-month-old, (b) 3-year-old, (c) 9-year-old, (d) 14-year-old, (e) 85-year-old.

14. As you place a 20-year-old woman in the lithotomy position for examination, you notice her discomfort. What do you need to do next?

15. Describe how you would palpate the Skene and Bartholin glands. What are you looking for? What could be considered an abnormal finding?

16. Describe how to insert and position a speculum.

17. What are you looking for as you inspect the cervix? What does it mean if the cervix is an inch in diameter? What does it mean if the cervix is covered with a creamy, odorless discharge?

18. Describe the steps needed to perform a Pap smear. How do you take a specimen for gonococcal culture? How do you take a specimen for chlamydial immunoassay? If you need all three specimens from one individual, is the order of collection important?

19. When you perform a bimanual exam, what structures are you palpating? What are you looking for?

20. When performing a rectovaginal exam, you notice that the septum between the vagina and rectum is thin and smooth and there is no tenderness or bleeding. Is this an expected finding?

21. Is an internal pelvic exam ever warranted on an infant or small child? At what age is a pelvic exam usually started?

22. Describe how you measure the pelvis of a pregnant woman to determine whether it is adequate in size for a vaginal delivery.

23. When a woman is in labor, what three things are changing as labor progresses and need to be assessed on a frequent basis?

24. Why is ovarian cancer hard to cure?

25. Distinguish a cystocele from a rectocele.

26. Discuss the differences and similarities of chlamydia, candidiasis, and trichomoniasis.

27. Describe things a woman may do to decrease her chances of being raped.

28. Describe how to perform a vulvar self-examination.

29. What are Kegel exercises? What are they used for? How are they performed? How often should they be performed? Who might you teach Kegel exercises to?

30. What two problems increase in women once they cease to ovulate? What can be done to prevent these problems?

CHAPTER 19

Male Genitalia

ANATOMY AND PHYSIOLOGY

The male reproductive system can be divided into two types of structures, internal and external. The external genitalia are largely made up of the penis and the scrotum; the scrotum contains the testes and the epididymides, where sperm are produced and transported through the vas deferens into the penis. The internal structures consist of two vas deferens, two seminal vesicles, the ejaculatory duct, and the prostate gland (Fig. 19-1). In addition, the urethra, the duct that serves the dual functions of conveying urine and ejaculating semen, extends from the urinary bladder to the urethral meatus at the tip of the penis.

EXTERNAL STRUCTURES

Penis. The penis serves two functions: it is the final excretory organ in urination, and during intercourse it introduces sperm into the vagina. The body of the penis contains three layers; the two outer layers of spongy tissue, the *corpora cavernosa* and the *corpus spongiosum,* encase the urethra (Fig. 19-2). This smooth, semifirm, spongy tissue becomes firm when engorged with blood on erection. The corpus spongiosum expands at its distal end to form the glans penis.

The *glans penis,* the end of the penis, is a lighter pink than the rest of the penis. It is only exposed when the *prepuce* (the foreskin) is either pulled back or surgically removed (circumcision). The *corona* is the ridge that separates the glans from the shaft of the penis. The skin covering the penis is thin, hairless, and a little darker than the rest of the body; it adheres loosely to the shaft to allow for expansion with erection.

Erection is a neurovascular reflex that occurs when the two corpora cavernosa become engorged with blood, a phenomenon caused by increased arterial dilation and decreased venous outflow. This reflex can be induced by psychogenic and local reflex mechanisms, both under the control of the autonomic nervous system. The psychogenic erection can be initiated by any type of sensory input—auditory, visual, tactile, or imaginative—whereas the local reflex mechanisms are initiated by tactile stimuli. Cortical input can also suppress erection. Ejaculation—the emission of secretions from the vas deferens, epididymides, prostate, and seminal vesicles—is followed by constriction of the vessels supplying blood to the corpora cavernosa and gradual return of the penis to its relaxed, flaccid state.

Urethra. The innermost tube of the penis, the urethra, is usually about 7 to 7.9 inches (18 to 20 cm) from bladder to meatus. It extends out of the base of the bladder, traveling through the prostate gland into the pelvic floor and through the penile shaft (Fig. 19-3). The urethral orifice is a small slit approximately 2 mm ventral to the tip of the glans.

Scrotum. The scrotum is a pouch covered with thin, darkly pigmented, rugous (wrinkled) skin. A septum divides the scrotum into two pendulous compartments, or sacs. Each sac contains a testis and an epididymis, which is suspended by the spermatic cord—a network of nerves, blood vessels, and the vas deferens (Fig. 19-4). Because sperm production requires a temperature slightly below body temperature, the testes are suspended outside the body cavity; its temperature is controlled by a layer of muscle under the scrotal skin that contracts when the outside temperature is cold and retracts the pouch and its contents upward toward the body. Conversely, when body heat rises, the wrinkled sac allows it to relax, expand, and drop downward. The left side of the scrotum is usually slightly lower than the right side.

 Racial Variation

Skin color of the external male genitalia ranges from a light beige to deep brownish-black. Darker-skinned individuals have darker skin covering the penis and scrotum. Red-headed whites may have a reddish cast to the genital skin, which would be otherwise considered an abnormal finding.

Testes and epididymides. The testes each contain a series of coiled ducts (seminiferous tubules), where sperm production (spermatogenesis) occurs. Each testis is approximately 1.8 × 1.2 × 0.8 inches (4.5 × 3 × 2 cm), ovoid, rubbery in texture, and smooth on the surface. On production, the sperm move toward the center of the testis, traveling into the efferent tubules adjacent to the comma-shaped epididymis on the posterolateral surface of each testis. The epididymis is about 2 inches (5 cm) long. The sperm receive nutrients and mature in an elaborate, coiled duct within the epididymis. They are stored in the ductus epididymis and eventually travel through the vas deferens into the penis.

INTERNAL STRUCTURES

Vas deferens. The vas deferens begins at the tail of the epididymis. It ascends from the scrotum through the external

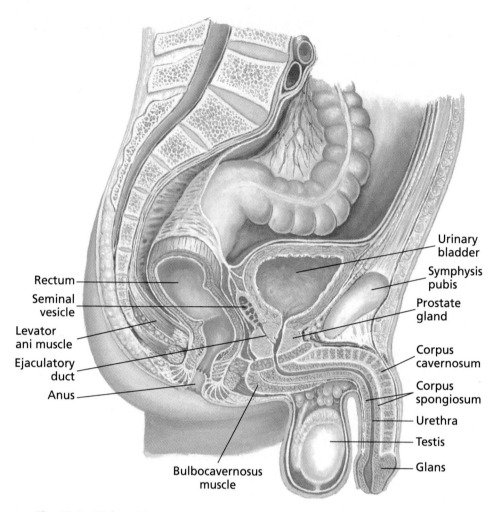

Fig. 19-1 **Male pelvic organs.** *(From Seidel et al, 1995.)*

Rectum

Seminal
vesicle

Levator
ani muscle

Ejaculatory
duct

Anus

Bulbocavernosus
muscle

Urinary
bladder

Symphysis
pubis

Prostate
gland

Corpus
cavernosum

Corpus
spongiosum

Urethra

Testis

Glans

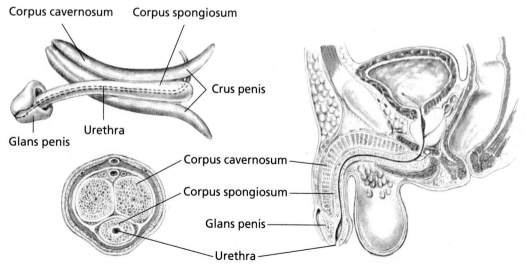

Corpus cavernosum   Corpus spongiosum

Crus penis

Glans penis

Urethra

Corpus cavernosum

Corpus spongiosum

Glans penis

Urethra

Fig. 19-2 Anatomy of the penis. *(From Seidel et al, 1995.)*

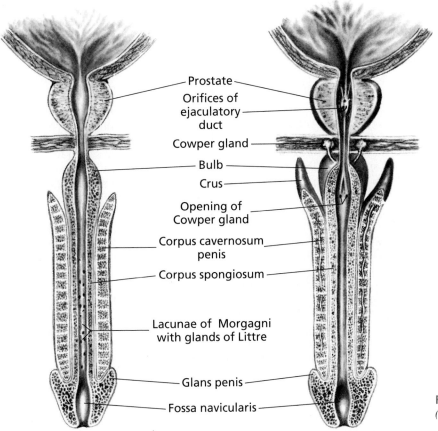

Fig. 19-3　Anatomy of urethra and penis.
(From Bobak and Jensen, 1993.)

Prostate
Orifices of ejaculatory duct
Cowper gland
Bulb
Crus
Opening of Cowper gland
Corpus cavernosum penis
Corpus spongiosum
Lacunae of Morgagni with glands of Littre
Glans penis
Fossa navicularis

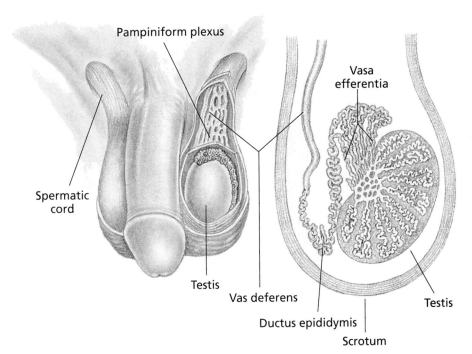

Pampiniform plexus
Vasa efferentia
Spermatic cord
Testis
Vas deferens
Ductus epididymis
Scrotum
Testis

Fig. 19-4　Scrotum and its contents.　*(From Seidel et al, 1995.)*

inguinal ring to the posterior aspect of the bladder. It unites with the seminal vesicle, forming the ejaculatory duct.

Seminal vesicles.   The seminal vesicles, small pouches lying between the rectum and the posterior bladder wall, join the ejaculatory duct at the base of the prostate. These vesicles, along with the vas deferens, the prostate, and the bulbourethral glands, produce all secretions and nutrients needed within the semen to maximize the health, lifespan, and motility of the sperm.

Prostate gland.   The prostate gland, at the base of the bladder, is approximately the same size as a testis. Its function is not completely understood, but it is assumed to aid sperm motility by producing most of the ejaculatory fluid. The prostate is more thoroughly discussed in Chapter 20.

THE INGUINAL AREA

As the vas deferens passes from the scrotum through the abdominal muscles into the penis, it is encased by the inguinal canal, a 1.6- to 2.4-inch (4- to 6-cm) tube that runs parallel to the inguinal ligament (Poupart's ligament). This ligament connects the pubic tubercle and the superior iliac spine. The area of the external ring is palpable; the internal ring is not. The external inguinal ring is vulnerable to hernias in cases of protrusion of the abdominal contents. These hernias may be of two types: a direct hernia (emerging from behind the external ring and through the ring to the surface) or an indirect hernia (entering the internal ring and descending through the canal, sometimes down into the scrotal sac). It is sometimes possible to feel a bulge if a finger is inserted into the inguinal area at the point of the external ring as the client holds his breath and bears down. Hernias can occur also at the fossa ovalis, an opening from the abdominal area that admits the femoral artery and vein to pass through to the leg. The site of a femoral hernia is just medial to the femoral artery.

DEVELOPMENTAL CONSIDERATIONS

INFANTS AND CHILDREN

Fetal development.   Until the eighth week of gestation, male and female genitalia are indistinguishable; fetal insult during the eighth or ninth gestational week may lead to anomalies of the external genitalia. By 12 weeks' gestation, differentiation is notable.

Testes descend from the retroperitoneal space into the scrotum during the third trimester. Separation of the glans and inner preputial epithelium also begins during the third trimester.

Neonates.   At birth, one or both testes may still lie in the inguinal canal; final descent may not occur until the early

postnatal period and may be arrested at any point. The scrotum is sometimes edematous, but this is considered normal. The infant should void within 24 hours of birth. Completed separation of the glans and inner preputial epithelium will usually not be complete until the age of 3 to 6 years.

PREADOLESCENTS AND ADOLESCENTS

Puberty begins at some time between ages 9½ and 13½ years. The first sign is an enlargement of the testes, followed by pubic hair development, and finally, an increase in penis size. See Fig. 19-5 for Tanner's classical sexual maturity rating chart for males (Tanner, 1962). Sparse, downy hair appears at the base of the penis, and the scrotal skin reddens, thins, and expands at the onset of puberty. At the same time, the testes and penis enlarge. Later, pubic hair darkens and extends until it is dense, coarse, and curly, forming a diamond-shaped pattern from the umbilicus to the anus. The prostate gland also enlarges in later adolescence (Table 19-1).

OLDER ADULTS

Although sperm production time will not change and ejaculatory volume is suspected of actually increasing with age, sperm viability is assumed to decrease, since the rate of conception has been observed to decline with age. Externally, pubic hair becomes finer and less abundant, sometimes leading to pubic alopecia. In addition, the scrotum becomes more pendulous.

Sexual activity tends to decline in frequency, correlating, as a rule, with the individual's frequency of sexual activity in youth. Erection may develop more slowly, and ejaculation may be less intense.

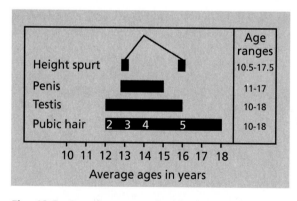

Fig. 19-5 Development of male genitalia and pubic hair. *(From Tanner, 1962.)*

TABLE 19-1	Tanner's Sex Maturity Development		
STAGES	**PUBIC HAIR**	**PENIS**	**SCROTUM**
1	No pubic hair.	Appears like smaller child's penis.	Testes begins to enlarge, but scrotum remains small and undeveloped.
2	Pubic hair starting to develop. Appears as straight, long, and downy texture.	Little enlargement.	Both testes and scrotum enlarge. The scrotum begins to acquire darker skin tone and change in texture.
3	Increasing hair growth over entire pubic region. Hair is darker, curly, and beginning to become coarse.	Penis begins to enlarge. Enlargement is more in length than general size.	Growth and skin texture continue to develop.
4	Hair is thick and coarse over entire pubic area.	Penis grows in both length and diameter. The glans also develops.	The scrotum is like the adult, darker tone and the testes are almost adult size.
5	Mature pubic hair distribution, including on upper medial thighs.	Adult appearance of penis.	Full development and adult-appearing testes.

Photographs from Van Wieringen, 1971. Reprinted by permission of Kluwer Academic Publishers.

HEALTH HISTORY | Male Genitalia

Significant history questions about the male genitalia include urinary symptoms (frequency, urgency, nocturia, and dysuria, as well as hesitancy and straining); past genitourinary problems, including infections and disorders of the penis (pain, lesions, discharge) and scrotum (pain or lumps); self-care and self-examination behaviors; and sexual concerns (relationships and sexually transmitted diseases).

QUESTIONS

RATIONALE

PAIN

■ Describe exactly where the pain is and if it travels. Is the pain in your lower back? Bladder? Testicle? Groin? When did it begin? Has it become worse over the past 24 hours? If so, what seems to make it worse? Is the pain constant or just at certain times? Is it associated with movement or lifting? Is the pain associated with nausea or vomiting? Abdominal distention? Fever or chills?

◀ *Sudden onset of pain may signal a serious problem. If it occurs in the lower back along the costovertebral angle, it may be related to pyelonephritis. If it is a spasmodic, colicky pain from upper ureteral dilation, it may cause referred pain to the testis on the same side. If it is pain from lower ureteral dilation, the client may feel pain referred to the scrotum. Either of these ureteral pains are very severe, and the client will usually appear very restless and uncomfortable.*

■ Have you noticed any pain, lumps, or swelling in your groin, testes, or scrotum? Does the scrotum seem to have changed in size? Any bulges? How long has the bulge been there? Have you ever been diagnosed with a hernia? Have you noticed a dragging or heavy feeling in the scrotum? Do you perform testicular self-examination?

◀ *Pain in the groin may occur from a number of causes, including problems in the spermatic cord, testicles, prostate gland, or lymph nodes; hernia; herpes zoster; or a number of neurologic problems.*

◀ *Testicular pain can occur secondary to almost any problem of the testis or epididymis. Such problems include: epididymitis; orchitis; hydrocele; spermatic cord torsion; and tumor, such as testicular cancer.*

◀ Priapism *(a persistent erection of the penis that does not occur secondary to sexual excitement) causes pain secondary to a thrombosis of the corpora cavernosa.*

CHANGES IN URINATION

■ Do you think you are urinating more frequently than you consider normal? Do you ever feel that you cannot wait to urinate? Do you awaken at night because you have to urinate? How often? For how long has this been occurring?

◀ *The normal adult male urinates 5 to 6 times each day, with variations depending on fluid intake and activity, as well as individual habits. When the client has a urinary tract disorder or*

QUESTIONS

RATIONALE

prostate problem, there is usually an increase in nocturia (awakening at night to urinate), urinary frequency, and urgency. Medications, especially those for cardiovascular problems, diuretics, and antihistamines, may also cause changes in urination.

■ Have you experienced any pain or burning with urination? Is the urine clear or cloudy? Discolored? Bloody? Foul-smelling? (A more detailed history of the possibility of urinary tract infection is found in Chapter 17.)

◄ *These symptoms may accompany problems such as infection, acute cystitis, prostatitis, and urethritis.*

■ Do you have any trouble initiating a urine stream? Do you strain to get started or maintain the stream? Is the stream narrower or weaker than usual? Have you noticed that you must stand closer to the toilet because there is dribbling of urine? Do you have to press on your abdomen to start your urine flow? Afterward, do you feel that you still have to urinate? (See Chapter 20 for a complete discussion of prostate problems.)

◄ *Hesitancy, straining, loss of force or decreased caliber of the stream, terminal dribbling, sensation of residual urine, and recurrent episodes of acute cystitis may be symptoms of a progressive prostatic obstruction.*

■ Are you passing large amounts of urine? If so, has it been a slow or sudden onset? Are you drinking large amounts of water or do you have excessive thirst? Have you had any other signs such as weight gain or loss? Weakness? Blurred vision?

◄ *It is always important to consider metabolic diseases such as diabetes mellitus and diabetes insipidus because polyuria is associated with diabetes.*

LESIONS ON PENIS OR DISCHARGE

■ Do you have any pain in your penis? Any lesions on it? Have you noticed any discharge from the penis? Do you notice any staining in the front of your underwear? If so, how much? Is it increasing or decreasing? What color is it? Does it have a particular odor? Do you notice it when you are urinating? Is there pain?

◄ *Lesions on the shaft or head of the penis or discharge from the penis may indicate an infection or sexually transmitted disease.*

■ Have you had any sexual contact with a partner who has a sexually transmitted disease (for example, gonorrhea, AIDS, syphilis, herpes, chlamydia, or venereal warts)? When? Were you infected? How has it been treated? Have there been any complications? Do you use condoms to prevent sexual transmission of diseases? Do you have any questions about these diseases?

◄ *Questions concerning sexual activity should be professional and a routine part of the examination. Allow the client to feel comfortable discussing sexual issues by beginning with an open-ended question, showing your acceptance of him. Then ask questions that seem appropriate in light of what he communicates to you. Remember that your comfort with the topics being discussed will prompt the client's comfort in responding.*

DIFFICULTY WITH ERECTION OR EJACULATION

■ Do you ever have difficulty maintaining an erection or, if you have a prolonged erection, is it painful? If so, describe details. Does your penis ever erect at times when there is no sexual stimulation? Does your penis curve in any direction when you have an erection?

◄ *Erection impotence is an important but delicate topic. Impotence may be a sign of a sexual dissatisfaction or deep-seated emotional problems. If the nurse identifies that a client has difficulty with erection or ejaculation, it is generally best to refer the client to a health care professional who is a specialist in those areas.*

QUESTIONS

RATIONALE

Incidence of Male Sexual Dysfunction

■ Sexual dysfunction in the male may be noted any-time after the onset of puberty. The incidence of men who seek treatment for erectile dysfunction increases with age.

- By age 40, 1.5% of all men have sought treatment for sexual dysfunction.
- By age 70, 25% of all men have sought treatment for sexual dysfunction.

■ The relative incidence of impotence from psychogenic versus organic causes has received great attention. Some investigators have reported that 90% to 95% of the cases of impotence result from psychogenic causes (Smith, 1981; Libertino, 1982).

■ More recent data using more sophisticated diagnostic techniques reveal an increased percentage of men whose erectile dysfunction has organic as well as psychogenic components (Libertino, 1991).

■ *If the client is having difficulty with having or maintaining an erection, ask:* Do you currently take medications? If so, what kinds, and how long have you been taking them?

■ Do you have painful or premature ejaculation? What have you done to deal with this problem? Has it helped? When you do ejaculate, what is the color, consistency, and amount of fluid?

◀ *Medications that may lead to difficulty with sexual function include diuretics, sedatives, antihypertensives, tranquilizers, and inhibitors of androgen synthesis.*

SEXUALITY

■ Are you currently in a relationship that involves sexual intercourse? Do you have one or multiple partners? How frequently do you engage in sexual activities? Are you and your partner(s) satisfied with the sexual relationship? Do you communicate comfortably about sex? Do you and your partner(s) use a contraceptive or protective method? Which one? Is it satisfactory to you? Do you have any questions about the method?

◀ *It is important to determine the type of sexual activity the individual has, as well as the client's satisfaction regarding that activity. The rationale for the type of activity is to determine if the client has one or numerous sexual partners, as well as what type of contraception is used. This may, in turn, lead to more information about the client's risk for sexually transmitted diseases. The rationale for asking about client satisfaction is to determine whether the client is satisfied with his sexuality and the sexual practices he is engaging in.*

■ How many sexual partners have you had in the last 6 months? Do you prefer relationships with men, women, or both? (If the client is gay, inquire if he is in a significant relationship and has a partner.)

◀ *Gay men need to feel acceptance to discuss their health concerns. If the examiner seems genuinely interested and concerned, the client may appreciate the opportunity to discuss sexuality issues or problems.*

QUESTIONS

RATIONALE

INFANTS

Several areas should be assessed. These include any congenital abnormalities, current urinary functioning, and care of the penis. Questions include:

- Has the infant been diagnosed with any problems, such as malpositioning of the opening at the end of the penis (*hypospadias* or *epispadias*), edema of the scrotum, undescended testes, or difficulty telling the child's sex by looking at the genitalia (ambiguous genitalia)?

  ◄ *It is important to identify congenital problems that may have been corrected following birth or problems that may still remain.*

- Have you noticed the child having any difficulty with urinating? Does the infant cry or hold his genitals? Does the urinary stream seem straight? Has he had any urinary tract infections?

  ◄ *It is important to ask screening questions that may provide information about possible infection or urinary tract problems.*

- Does the baby's scrotum ever swell when he cries?

  ◄ *Scrotal swelling, with or without crying, may indicate the presence of a hydrocele.*

- Has the child been circumcised? Were there any problems following the circumcision?

  ◄ *Identification of problems that may have occurred either during or following the circumcision may provide information related to current problems or parent concerns.*

- *If the child has not been circumcised, ask:* How do you clean the end of the child's penis? Are you able to retract the foreskin? Does the foreskin ever seem to interfere with the infant's ability to urinate?

  ◄ *If the infant is not circumcised, it is important to assess how the parent cleans under the foreskin. If the foreskin is not retracted routinely for cleaning, the skin may retract down around the end of the penis and may make it difficult to adequately clean the penis.*

- Does the child ever have a diaper rash? If so, what does it look like and what do you do to treat it? Do you use cloth or disposable diapers? If you use cloth diapers, what type of detergent and fabric softener is used?

  ◄ *Diaper rashes are common. Many times they may be improved with proper cleaning, frequent diaper change, and using a diaper that is not irritating to the infant.*

CHILDREN

YOUNG CHILDREN

First, continue to assess those areas that were assessed for the infant, including difficulty urinating, circumcision, genitalia cleaning if the child has not been circumcised, and genitalia rashes if the child is not toilet-trained. Additional questions are focused on developmental maturation and exploration. These questions include:

- Has toilet training begun yet? If so, at what age did you begin to toilet-train? Has it been successful? If not, describe how it is going.

  ◄ *Most parents begin to toilet-train their child by age 2 or 2½ years of age.*

- Does the child ever wet the bed at night? If so, does it occur frequently or on rare occasion? What have you done about this? How does the child feel about wetting the bed?

  ◄ *Almost all children wet the bed at some time. What is important to assess is whether the bed wetting occurs frequently, whether it occurs because of physiologic dysfunction, psychosocial dysfunction, or a too-full bladder before the child goes to bed.*

QUESTIONS

■ Does the child have any lesions, swelling, or discoloration on the penis or scrotum? Does he ever cry when he urinates?

■ Does the child frequently play with his own genitalia? If so, is he able to stop when you tell him to? Does his playing with himself bother you?

■ *For preschool or young school-age children, ask the following:* Have you ever been touched on your penis or between your legs by someone when you did not want them to? If so, when did this happen? Who did it? Did you tell anyone?

RATIONALE

◄ *Assessment for infection, hydrocele, hernia, or injury/abuse.*

◄ *Exploration of the genitalia is a normal developmental phenomenon. It is important to assess how the parents feel about it and how they interact with the child regarding the self-play.*

◄ *Screen for sexual abuse or genitalia-touching by anyone.*

Talking with Children Who Reveal Abuse

■ Provide a private time and place to talk.

■ Do not promise not to tell; tell the child that you are required to report the abuse.

■ Do not express shock or criticize the family.

■ Use the child's vocabulary to discuss the body part.

■ Avoid using any leading statements that can distort the child's story.

■ Reassure the child that he or she has done the right thing by telling.

■ Tell the child that the touching or abuse is not his or her fault, that he or she is not bad or to blame.

■ Determine the child's immediate need for safety.

■ Let the child know when you report the situation.

(From Wong, 1995.)

OLDER CHILDREN

Many of the assessment questions previously asked in either the younger child or the adult sections also apply to the older child. Refer to the adolescent section to locate the questions that should be asked of the older male child if and when that child demonstrates the maturational changes of the preadolescent. As the child matures, the history assessment should change to include more assessment of maturational development and sexuality. When asking questions, use a matter-of-fact manner. Questions about developmental changes, sexuality, and self-esteem related to these changes should be targeted to the child's developmental level. Do not add judgment or shame.

ADOLESCENTS

These questions should be asked of preadolescents and adolescents (depending on the degree of maturation present). It is important to bear in mind the following cautions: (1) Ask questions appropriate for the boy's age, but be aware that "normal" varies widely; it is better to ask too many questions than to omit anything. (2) Ask questions that are direct and professional; avoid judgmental phrases. Consider beginning by establishing that it is normal to feel or think a certain thing, for example, "Young men your age often feel . . . ." (3) Ask questions that assume rather than ask for an admission. Include the following questions:

QUESTIONS

- Have you noticed changes in your body over the last 2 years? What do you like about the changes? What don't you like?
- Often a young man about your age (usually 12 or 13) will begin to notice that his penis and scrotum has begun to change and grow. What changes have you noticed? Have you ever seen charts of normal growth patterns for boys? Let's look at these now.
- Also, young men about your age (age 12 or 13) experience fluid coming out of the penis at night, called nocturnal emissions, or "wet dreams." Have you had this?
- Other things guys your age often experience are having an erection at embarrassing times, masturbating, or having sexual fantasies. Do you have any questions about these things? Would you like to talk about any of these concerns?
- Who do you usually talk to about body changes and sexual information? Are you comfortable in these talks? Do you think you get enough information? Have you taken sex education classes in school? Is there someone either in or outside of the family, maybe at school or church, with whom you can discuss these issues?

- Often young men your age have questions about sexual activity. Do you? Do you have questions about birth control or sexually transmitted diseases like AIDS or gonorrhea? Are you dating someone?

- Do you and your partner have sex? If so, what method of protection did you use the last time you had sex? What questions do you have?
- Have you been taught by a doctor or nurse how to examine your own testicles to make sure they are healthy?

RATIONALE

◀ *Note the adolescent's attitude toward developmental changes taking place.*

◀ *This assesses the adolescent's level of information about the changes that are taking place and provides an opportunity for education.*

◀ *Occasionally boys believe that this indicates a sexually transmitted disease or feel guilty about it.*

◀ *Boys may feel guilty about these things and should be reassured that they are normal.*

◀ *Adolescents need accurate information about their changing body and sexuality issues. It is important to identify where the client gets his current information and how complete that information may be.*

◀ *Assess the adolescent's level of knowledge. It is common for boys not to admit that they need more information.*

◀ *Assess if birth control or protection is being used.*

◀ *Assess the level of knowledge about self-care.*

OLDER ADULTS

The older adult should be asked all of the same questions as for adult. In addition, ask the following questions that deal with issues specific to his age.

- Do you need to get up at night to urinate? What medications are you taking? What do you drink, and how much fluid do you drink in the evening before you go to bed?
- Have you noticed any difficulty when beginning to urinate? Do you have to strain? Do you have any dribbling or feel like your bladder does not empty? (See Chapter 20 for further questions.)
- As men get older, they may notice a change in sexual relationships or sexual response. It is normal for an erection to develop more slowly. It is not a sign of impotence. Have you noticed any changes you would like to discuss?

◀ *Medications or drinking too many fluids or diuretic fluids at night may produce nocturia.*

◀ *"Yes" answers to these questions may indicate a prostate problem.*

◀ *Sexual function continues throughout life, although aging and illness may produce changes. Most men welcome the opportunity to discuss sexual issues; this can be a time of education and encouragement. Some drugs depress sexual function—for example, antihypertensives, sedatives, tranquilizers, and alcohol.*

EXAMINATION Procedures and Findings

Guidelines Men usually feel apprehensive about having their genitalia examined, especially if the examiner is female. This may be seen as an invasion of privacy rather than accepted as a part of the physical examination. Concerns may center around modesty, fear of pain or negative judgments, or a memory of a previous unpleasant experience. In addition, the client may be afraid he will experience an erection that would be misinterpreted by the examiner. Men may hide their apprehension by becoming uncooperative and insisting on a male examiner; by acting resigned or embarrassed, and adopting an avoidance posture; or by laughing and making jokes.

As the examiner, you must be aware of these concerns and any of your own apprehension in the situation. It is normal for you to feel embarrassment, lack confidence, fear causing pain, or worry about "causing" an erection. You must deal with these feelings and approach the examination of a male patient in a professional, matter-of-fact way. The client's history should be taken before, not during, the examination. Use a firm, deliberate touch. If an erection occurs, reassure the client that this is a normal physiologic response to touch and that he could not have prevented it. Do not stop the evaluation or leave the room; this will focus further on the erection and reinforce the client's embarrassment.

EQUIPMENT	**Gloves**
	Penlight or transilluminator
	Glass slide for urethral specimen (if needed)

TECHNIQUES and NORMAL FINDINGS

ABNORMAL FINDINGS

Start by positioning the client. He may be positioned in one of two ways, either standing with his underwear pulled down or lying down. If the client is lying down, he will need to stand later for adequate evaluation of possible hernia. In either case the examiner should be seated.

Clinical Note

It may be uncomfortable for both the client and the examiner if they are of opposite sexes. If the client makes no objection, proceed in a professional manner.
Also remember that it is always best to have an escort in the examination room during the assessment.

PUBIC HAIR

INSPECT client's pubic hair for Distribution and General Characteristics. Hair distribution varies widely but is normally in a diamond-shaped pattern that may extend to the umbilicus. The hair should appear coarser than scalp hair. The hair should be free of parasites, and the skin should be smooth and clear.

 Racial Variation

The consistency, color, and amount of pubic hair at sexual maturity is variable across racial groups. African Americans tend to have black pubic hair that is shorter and more tightly coiled than other races. Pubic hair color is dark in darker-skinned individuals, but often matches or is slightly darker than the hair color of the head in whites. Pubic hair is generally sparser in Asian Americans and American Indians/Alaskan Natives.

- Note patchy growth, loss, or absence of hair; distribution of hair in a female pattern (triangular, with the base over the pubis); nits or pubic lice; scars; lower abdominal or inguinal lesions; or a rash.
- *Tinea cruris* ("jock itch") is a common fungal infection found in the groin that appears as large, clearly marginated, reddened patches that are pruritic and often associated with "athlete's foot."
- *Monilial* infections are red, eroded patches with scaling and pustules, and are associated with immobility and disability, systemic antibiotics, and immunologic deficits.

TECHNIQUES and NORMAL FINDINGS

ABNORMAL FINDINGS

PENIS

Remember to wear gloves.

INSPECT the penis for General Characteristics, Color, and Discharge.
The dorsal vein should be apparent on the dorsal surface of the shaft of the penis. The skin is usually dark and hairless, with a wrinkled surface and frequently apparent vascularity. Ask the client to retract the foreskin, if present. It should retract easily to reveal the glans and return to the original position easily.

 Cultural Note

Circumcision has been a common practice of the dominant American culture. However, that practice is changing, and fewer male infants currently undergo circumcision than 15 years ago. When circumcision is performed it is often culturally based. Jews and Muslims incorporate circumcision as part of their belief systems. Most American Indians/Alaskan Natives and Hispanics are uncircumcised, as it does not conform to their belief system. Other groups are circumcised in varying degrees.

In uncircumcised men, the prepuce is present and folded over the glans; in circumcised men the prepuce is often absent (Fig. 19-6), or small flaps may remain at the corona. If the client has not been circumcised, ask him to retract the foreskin. The foreskin should retract easily and completely over the glans.

Inspect the glans and under the fold of the prepuce. The glans should be smooth, pink, and bulbous. Note any redness, lesions, swellings, nodules, or presence of discharge. (If discharge or smegma is present, obtain a specimen on a slide for microscopic examination). The prepuce fold is wrinkled and loosely attached to the underlying glans; it is darker than the glans. *Note:* Circumcised penises have a varying length of foreskin remaining; some have multiple folds and others have none.

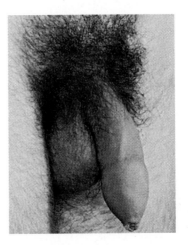

Fig. 19-7   Phimosis.   *(From* 400 Self-assessment picture tests in clinical medicine, *1984.)*

■ Failure of the ability to retract the foreskin, discomfort on retraction, or difficulty of returning the foreskin to the original position should be considered abnormal.

■ *Phimosis* is a very tight foreskin that cannot be retracted over the glans (Fig. 19-7). This condition is usually congenital but may occur during early childhood, either because of the foreskin not being routinely retracted during bathing or because of repeated infection.

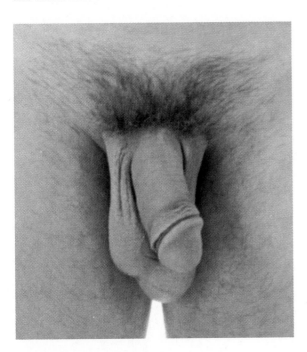

Fig. 19-6   Circumcised penis.

TECHNIQUES and NORMAL FINDINGS

ABNORMAL FINDINGS

■ *Paraphimosis* is the inability to return the foreskin over the glans.
■ *Balanitis* is inflammation of the glans that commonly occurs in clients with phimosis (Fig. 19-8).

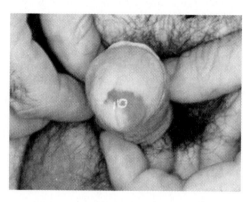

Fig. 19-8　**Balantitis.**　*(From Lloyd-Davies et al, 1983.)*

Inspect the urethral meatus. It should be located centrally at the distal tip of the glans, and no discharge should be present. The meatus should appear as a slit-like opening.

■ Note if the meatus is located either on the upper surface of the penis *(epispadias)* or on the bottom of the penis *(hypospadias)* and if there is a discharge present. The discharge may be yellow-green or milky-white, or have a foul odor.
■ Report any reddening, swelling, discharge, or crusting.

Palpate or ask the client to compress the glans anteroposteriorly to open the distal end of the urethra (Fig. 19-9). The surface should be pink and smooth, and no discharge should be present.

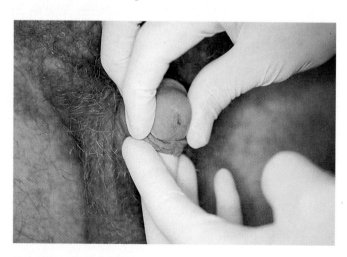

Fig. 19-9　Examination of urethral meatus.

PALPATE the penis for Tenderness and Induration. Palpate the entire shaft of the penis between the thumb and first two fingers. The penis shaft should be nontender and smooth, with a semifirm consistency.

■ Note tenderness, swelling, nodules, or induration.

TECHNIQUES and NORMAL FINDINGS

ABNORMAL FINDINGS

SCROTUM AND TESTES

INSPECT the scrotum for Texture and General Characteristics, Color, and Asymmetry. Ask the client to hold the penis out of the way while you inspect the scrotum (Fig. 19-10). The sac should be divided in half by the septum; the left sac may be larger than the right. Size varies, and the scrotum may appear pendulous. It should appear more deeply pigmented than the body skin. The surface should feel coarse and free of lesions.

- Temperature affects the position of the testes in the scrotum. When the environmental temperature is very cold, the testes slightly retract upward. Likewise, when the temperature is hot or if the client has a fever, the testes will extend more downward.

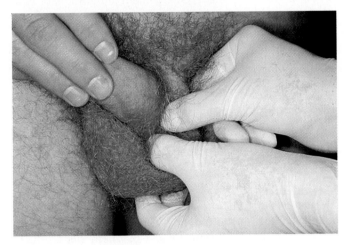

Fig. 19-10 Inspection of scrotum and ventral surface of penis as client positions his penis.

The thickness of the skin of the scrotum changes with temperature and age. In cold or cool temperatures, the scrotal skin feels thickened. As the individual ages, the skin thins.

Lift the scrotum to examine its underside (be sure to spread the rugated surface for a better view). This area is deeply pigmented, hairless, and has a rugous surface.

PALPATE the scrotum for Presence of Testes. Palpate each half of the scrotum (Fig. 19-11). It should be nontender with thin, loose skin over a muscular layer.

- Scrotal lesions or either generalized or isolated redness are considered abnormal and may indicate an infection. Sebaceous cysts are common findings.
- Report any redness, edema, absence of rugae, rash, or lesions.
- Note any marked tenderness or swelling.

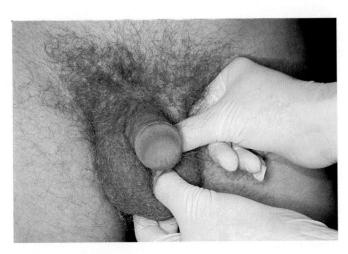

Fig. 19-11 Palpating contents of scrotum and testes.

TECHNIQUES and NORMAL FINDINGS

PALPATE the testes, epididymides, and vas deferens for Location, Consistency, Tenderness, and Nodules. Palpate the testes simultaneously with both hands, using the thumb and the first two fingers. Note that the testes are present in each sac and measure about 1.5 × 1 × 0.75 inch (4 × 3 × 2 cm); they should be equal in size, mildly sensitive but nontender to moderate compression, smooth and ovoid, and movable.

PALPATE the epididymides. This area should be nontender, usually on the posterolateral surface of each testis, discretely palpable, comma-shaped, and smooth.

PALPATE the vas deferens. This should be nontender, discretely palpable from the epididymis to the external inguinal ring, smooth and cord-like, and movable.

TRANSILLUMINATE the scrotum for evidence of Fluid and Masses. Transilluminate each scrotal sac if a mass, fluid, or irregularity is suspected. There should be no additional contents or fluid. The testes and epididymides do not transilluminate.

HERNIA ASSESSMENT

Evaluate the inguinal region for hernia. *Note:* The client should stand and the examiner sit if possible.

INSPECT both inguinal regions for Bulges. There should be none. Ask the client to strain while you continue to inspect the area.

PALPATE the inguinal canal for evidence of Indirect Hernia or Direct Hernia. Palpate both right and left inguinal rings. Use your index finger or little finger of the hand corresponding to the client's side (Fig. 19-12) (e.g., right hand for right side). Ask the client to strain down. The finger should follow the spermatic cord upward to the triangular, slit-like opening, which may or may not admit the finger. If it does admit your finger, insert it gently into the canal and again ask the client to bear down. You should not feel any bulging against your finger tip.

Palpate each femoral area (fossa ovalis) for bulges while the client strains.

For assessment of the anus, rectum, and prostate areas, see Chapter 20.

ABNORMAL FINDINGS

■ Note if the testes are not distended into the sac, enlarged (unilaterally or bilaterally), atrophied, markedly tender, nodular or irregular, or fixed.

■ Report any tenderness, irregular placement, enlargement, induration, or nodules.

■ If a problem is noted, determine its position in relation to the testes (i.e., proximal or distal); whether it can be moved with your fingers; if it disappears when the client lies down; and whether you hear any sounds if you auscultate it (e.g., bowel sounds).

■ Report any tenderness, tortuosity, thickened or beaded area, or induration.

■ Note any mass that is distal or proximal to the testis. It may or may not be tender. *Hydroceles* and *spermatoceles* are fluid-filled and therefore transilluminate; tumors, hernias, and epididymitis do not.

■ Note any bulges in the area of the external ring, the Hesselbach triangle, or the femoral area.

■ Note any palpable mass that touches your fingertip or pushes against the side of your finger (see Table 19-3).

■ A soft bulge that emerges at the fossa should be noted.

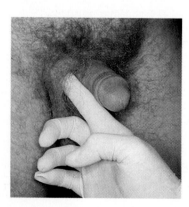

Fig. 19-12 Checking for inguinal hernia; gloved finger inserted through inguinal canal.

AGE-RELATED VARIATIONS

INFANTS

■ APPROACH

The examination of the male infant's genitalia is straightforward. The child should be undressed so that the genitalia are completely exposed. When the infant is not actually being examined, he should have his genitalia covered in case of unexpected urination.

■ FINDINGS

The full-term infant has testes that are pendulous with deep rugae; the scrotum may be edematous. Note that the scrotum appears pink in white infants and dark brown in dark-skinned infants. The urethra should be at the tip of the penis. The penis should measure 1.2 to 1.6 inches (3 to 4 cm) in length and 0.4 to 0.5 inch (1 to 1.3 cm) in width. If possible, observe the infant's urine stream. It should be full and strong. A weak stream with dribbling may be an indication of urethral meatus stenosis.

If the infant is uncircumcised, the foreskin (prepuce) should cover the glans. The foreskin should retract enough to permit a good urinary stream and general cleaning. Do not attempt to retract the foreskin more than necessary to see the urethra. Force may actually cause a tear the prepuce from the glans, which in turn could cause binding adhesions to form between the prepuce and the glans. As the infant becomes older, the foreskin will have more mobility. By age 3 to 4 years, the foreskin should be completely retractable.

The size of the scrotum in the infant usually appears large when compared to the penis. Palpation of the scrotum should indicate the presence of one or both testes (Fig. 19-13). If either or both testicles are not palpable, gently

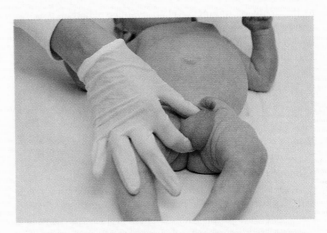

Fig. 19-13   Palpation of the scrotum in an infant.

place a finger over the upper inguinal ring and gently push downward toward the scrotum. If the testicle can be pushed into the scrotum, it is considered descended even though it retracts into the inguinal canal.

Finally, the presence of fluid (hydrocele) or mass (possible hernia) in the testicle should be evaluated by using transillumination. This technique is performed by using a bright penlight or transilluminator and pressing the light source up against the scrotal sac. A hydrocele will transilluminate and will most likely become bigger as the child cries or becomes stressed. Hydroceles are commonly found in boys less than 2 years of age; they usually disappear on their own as the child matures. A mass that does not transilluminate is most probably a hernia.

CHILDREN

■ APPROACH

The techniques of examining the male child's genitalia are the same as for the infant. The major difference in the examination is the approach. In this culture, children are taught at a very early age that the genitalia should not be exposed or touched. In the presence of the child's parent, reassure him that you must examine his genitalia just as you have examined all of his other body areas. Whenever possible, reassure the child that he is growing up just like he should. Because children are now taught that the touching of the genitalia by strangers is not an "okay" thing, it is important that the parent reassure the child that you need to examine him to make sure that he is healthy.

The examination is easiest to perform if the child is sitting in either a slightly reclining position with his knees flexed and heels near the buttock (Fig. 19-14), or sitting Indian-style with his knees spread and ankles crossed.

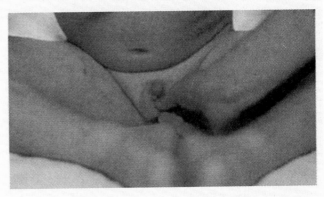

Fig. 19-14   Position of young child for examination of genitalia.   *(From Wong, 1995.)*

■ FINDINGS

The basic findings are the same as for the infant. Remember, if the child has not been circumcised, do not force the foreskin to be retracted. Retract the foreskin only to the point of tightness. Then evaluate whether it is retracted far enough to permit adequate urination and cleaning. Evaluate to determine if the child has any discharge, crusting, or lesions around or under the foreskin. By age 6, the foreskin should be easily retracted.

In addition to examining the scrotum for shape, size, and color, it should specifically be examined to determine the presence of testicles in the scrotum. If the scrotum has well-formed rugae, it indicates that the testes have descended into the scrotum, even if the testes are not apparent in the scrotum. When palpated, the testes should be about 0.4 inch (1 cm) in diameter. If the scrotum remains small, flat, and underdeveloped, it may well indicate *cryptorchidism* (undescended testes).

ADOLESCENTS

■ APPROACH

Genitalia assessment of the adolescent male is very important to ensure that the maturational development is progressing according to schedule. This is also the time when teen modesty is at its peak. The examiner must take time to develop a relationship with the client and reassure him in a matter-of-fact manner that the examination of the genitalia is an essential part of a complete examination. It is also vitally important to ensure privacy and adequate draping when the genitalia are not being examined. It is usually best to defer the examination of the genitalia to the last procedure of the examination.

To actually examine the genitalia and assess the inguinal area for a hernia, the client should be standing as instructed for the adult.

■ FINDINGS

The normal findings are dependent on the maturational stage of the client. Review Table 19-1 for the expected and normal findings of the maturing male.

OLDER ADULTS

■ APPROACH

The approach to examining the male genitalia of the older adult is the same as for the younger adult.

■ FINDINGS

The scrotal sac of the client may appear elongated or pendulous. The client may actually have injury or excoriation of the scrotal sac surface secondary to sitting on the scrotum. The testes may feel slightly smaller and softer than in the younger client.

CLIENTS WITH SITUATIONAL VARIATIONS

CLIENTS WITH PARALYSIS

■ APPROACH

The examination of the genitalia of a client with paralysis is the same as for all other male clients. The differences in the approach to clients with paralysis relate to the questions asked when taking the history—specifically regarding urination, sexuality, and sexual function.

■ FINDINGS

The findings of the genitalia examination are the same as for all other adult clients.

GAY MEN

■ APPROACH

Gay men may be at high risk for sexually transmitted diseases. If the client is currently or has been in gay sexual relationships, assess the client for specific problems such as exposure to hepatitis B and HIV/AIDS; use of sexual protective devices, and sexual expression, including high-risk sexual practices (e.g., fisting, rimming, etc.).

■ FINDINGS

Perform a careful genitalia examination, including assessment for STDs and anal/rectal intactness.

ETHNIC & CULTURAL VARIATIONS

■ FINDINGS

Stereotypes abound about the sexual prowess and size of the male genitalia in certain ethnic groups. However, there is no documentation to support these stereotypes. Variations in size are largely individual, as is sexual appetite. There are documented ethnic differences in the color of external male genitalia and in the amount, consistency, and color of pubic hair. Cultural differences exist in the practice of circumcision. Once a practice of the dominant American culture, the incidence of circumcision is declining except in Jewish and Muslim groups. The practice is almost nonexistent among American Indians and Alaskan Natives, and is seldom seen in Hispanics.

E X A M I N A T I O N   S U M M A R Y
Male Genitalia

Pubic hair *(p. 542)*
- Inspect the pubic hair for:
  Distribution
  General characteristics

Penis *(pp. 543-544)*
- Inspect the penis for:
  General characteristics
  Color
  Discharge
- Palpate the penis for:
  Tenderness
  Induration

Scrotum and Testes *(pp. 545-546)*
- Inspect the scrotum for:
  Texture and general characteristics
  Color
  Asymmetry

- Palpate the scrotum for:
  Presence of testes
- Palpate the testes, epididymides, and vas deferens for:
  Location
  Consistency
  Tenderness
  Nodules
- Transilluminate the scrotum for evidence of:
  Fluid
  Masses

Hernia Assessment *(p. 546)*
- Inspect both inguinal regions for:
  Bulges
- Palpate the inguinal canal for evidence of:
  Direct hernia
  Indirect hernia

COMMON PROBLEMS/CONDITIONS
associated with the Male Genitalia

HERNIA

Three common types of hernias are commonly found when examining the inguinal area of the genitalia. These are the indirect inguinal hernia, the direct inguinal hernia, and the femoral hernia. See Table 19-2 for comparison of the common types of hernias.

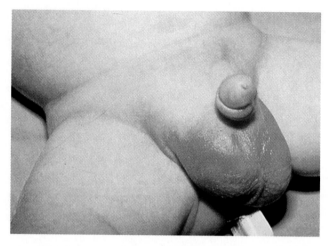

Fig. 19-15 Incarceration and strangulation of an inguinal hernia appears as redness and erythema overlying a firm groin mass. *(From Zitelli and Davis, 1992.)*

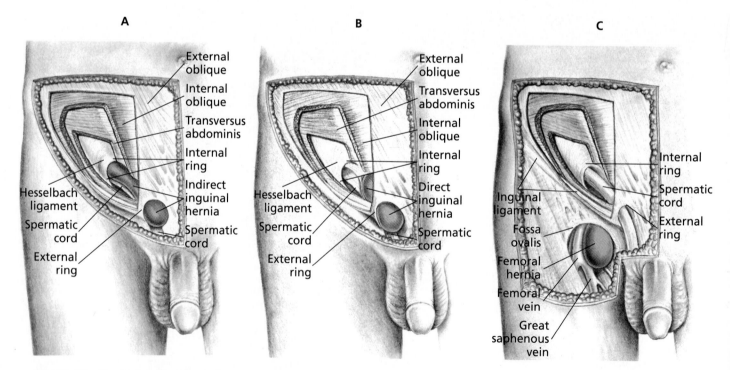

Fig. 19-16 Anatomy of region of common pelvic hernias. **A,** Indirect inguinal hernia. **B,** Direct inguinal hernia. **C,** Femoral hernia. *(From Seidel et al, 1995.)*

TABLE 19-2	Hernia Evaluation		
	INDIRECT HERNIA	**DIRECT HERNIA**	**FEMORAL HERNIA**
Description	The sac herniates through the internal inguinal ring. It can remain in the inguinal canal, exit through the external canal, or actually pass into the scrotum.	The sac herniates through the external inguinal ring. Hernia is located in the Hesselbach triangle region. It rarely enters the scrotum.	The sac extends through the femoral ring, canal, and below the inguinal ligament.
Clinical Signs	Hernia comes down to meet examiner's fingertip with feeling of soft swelling. Client complains of pain on straining. May decrease when client lies down.	Client has a bulge in the Hesselbach triangle area. Usually feels no pain. Hernia pushes against examiner's fingertip when client bears down. May decrease when client lies down.	Pain in inguinal area. Right side more likely to have hernia than left. Pain may be severe.
Occurrence	The most frequent type of hernia. May occur in both sexes and in children (mostly males).	Less common. Occurs most frequently in males over 40 years of age. Uncommon in women.	The least common type of hernia. Occurs most frequently in women.

PENIS

■ *Paraphimosis:* A condition in which the foreskin of the penis is retracted at the base of the glans and it cannot be relaxed into its normal position (Fig. 19-17).

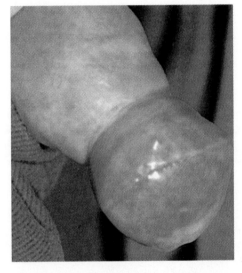

Fig. 19-17   Paraphimosis.   *(From Lloyd-Davies et al, 1994.)*

■ *Carcinoma:* Cancer of the penis is frequently squamous cell carcinoma (Fig. 19-18). It occurs most often in uncircumcised males who have had poor hygiene habits.

Risk Factors for Cancer of the Penis
■ Not circumcised
■ Chronic poor hygiene care
■ Repeated infections, including condyloma acuminatum (genital warts)

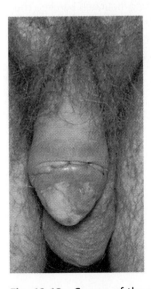

Fig. 19-18   Cancer of the penis.   *(From Lloyd-Davies et al, 1994.)*

SEXUALLY TRANSMITTED DISEASES

■ *Genital herpes:* A viral infection that may appear anywhere along the shaft of the penis or near the glans (Fig. 19-19). The lesion is identified because of the red superficial vesicles that are frequently quite painful. At the time of an acute exacerbation, the client may also have a fever and swollen inguinal lymph nodes. This is a chronic condition with exacerbation and re-lapses.

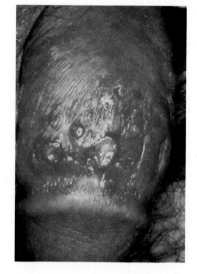

Fig. 19-19   Genital herpes on the penis.   *(From Grimes, 1991.)*

■ *Condyloma acuminatum (genital warts):* Lesions caused by a papillovirus and commonly found on the glans, the shaft of the penis, or within the urethra itself (Fig. 19-20). The individual may go on to acquire carcinoma of the penis as a secondary change of these lesions.

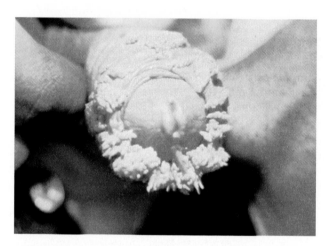

Fig. 19-20   Condyloma acuminatum (genital warts).   *(From Grimes, 1991.)*

■ *Syphilis:* The primary syphilis lesion is called a "chancre" (Fig. 19-21). It occurs about 2 weeks after exposure and ap-pears as a painless ulcerated lesion with indurated borders. The most frequent location for the lesion is on the glans of the penis.

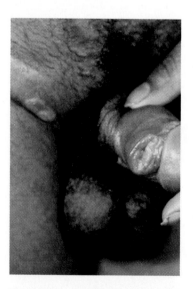

Fig. 19-21 Syphilis chancre on the penis.   *(From Grimes, 1991.)*

■ *Lymphogranuloma venereum:* Disease caused by the chlamydial organism (Fig. 19-22). The initial lesion appears as a painless erosion near the border between the shaft of the penis and the glans. There may be inguinal area lymph node enlargement which, if left untreated, may cause systemic symptoms.

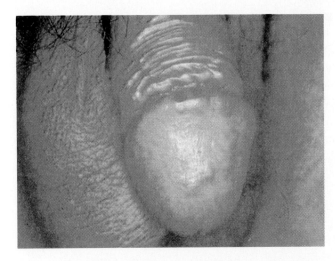

Fig. 19-22 **Lymphogranuloma venereum.** *(From Seidel et al, 1991.)*

SCROTUM/TESTES

■ *Testicular torsion:* Occurs most frequently in children and adolescents. This rapid-onset condition, which is a twisting of the testis on the spermatic cord, is a surgical emergency. The testicle becomes very tender, and the scrotum becomes swollen and often slightly discolored.

■ *Hydrocele:* Results from fluid accumulation in the tunica vaginalis (Fig. 19-23). The scrotum appears enlarged and, when transilluminated, will have a light red glow that indicates the presence of fluid. The condition is most frequent during early infancy and will usually resolve on its own. If not, it may need to be surgically corrected.

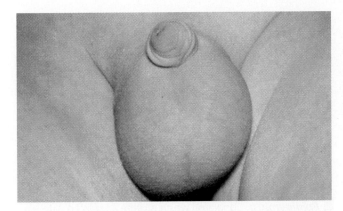

Fig. 19-23 **Bilateral congenital hydroceles. Groin swellings are absent, distinguishing them from hernias.** *(From Zitelli and Davis, 1992.)*

▪ **Spermatocele:** A cystic swelling that occurs in the epididymis (Fig. 19-24). Because the lesion is a cyst, it will transilluminate.

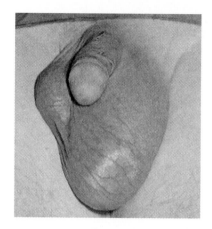

Fig. 19-24 Spermatocele. *(From Seidel et al, 1995.)*

▪ **Varicocele (bag of worms):** An abnormal dilation and tortuosity of the veins along the spermatic cord (Fig. 19-25). The client may have pain and, if the condition is left untreated, reduced fertility secondary to increased testicular pressure.

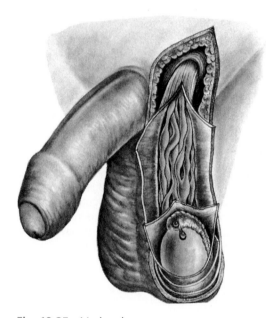

Fig. 19-25 Variocele. *(From Seidel et al, 1995.)*

▪ **Epididymitis:** Condition, which is often associated with a urinary tract infection (UTI), that causes the scrotum to become erythematous and the epididymis to become very swollen and tender (Fig. 19-26). The client may also have systemic signs such as fever and bacteria and white cells in his urine.

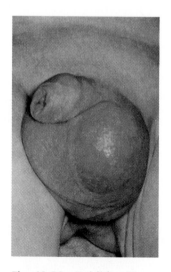

Fig. 19-26 Epididymitis. *(From Seidel et al, 1995.)*

&Nursing Diagnosis

CASE 1 6-month-old Hispanic male infant with swollen scrotum.

Subjective

Mother is concerned that child's scrotum swells when he cries. Symptom present off and on since child was 1 month old. Mother states when child is not crying, scrotum is not swollen. Reported that child has no problems with urination and does not seem bothered by swollen scrotum. There is no history of injury.

Objective

Weight 14 lb (6 kg).

Temperature 98.4° F (36.9° C).

Pulse 112.

Respiration rate 32.

General appearance External genitalia appear normal for age of child. Uncircumcised penis without lesions or discoloration. Urethral opening centered. Foreskin retracts slightly over glans without difficulty. Good hygiene. Scrotum small, with slight rugation of skin.

Transillumination of scrotum Scrotal sac has small amount of illumination around shadowing of testes. There does not appear to be excess fluid present at this time.

Palpation Penis and scrotum nontender to palpation. Testicles present in scrotal sac bilaterally. No evidence of masses.

• •

Nursing Diagnosis #1

Knowledge deficit related to treatment for inguinal hernia.

Defining characteristics Painless scrotal swelling that appears when infant crying and disappears at rest.

Nursing Diagnosis #2

Potential for altered growth and development related to unknown cause.

Defining characteristics 6-month-old weighing 14 lb (10th percentile) (additional data needed).

Sample Documentation &Nursing Diagnosis

CASE 2   42-year-old white man with complaint of discharge from penis.

Subjective

Client states that 3 days ago he noticed a small amount of yellow staining in his undershorts, then noted a small amount of discharge from penis just before urination. One area of the penis at the uretheral opening also has a sore on it. Client states that 1 week ago he had sexual intercourse with a woman on a blind date. He did not use any personal protection during intercourse. States he has never had any previous infections or problems associated with the genitalia.

Objective

General characteristics   Pubic hair distribution is diamond-shaped with hair extension to umbilicus. Skin intact and without lesions.

Penis   Normal circumcised penis with uretheral opening centered at distal tip. Penis without lesions except for small 0.2 to 0.4 inch (0.5 × 1 cm) area of erosion on left lateral surface of the glans near the urethra. Small amount milky discharge noted when tip of penis was compressed. (Specimen sent for serology examination.) No masses or tenderness identified with penis shaft palpation.

Scrotum/Testes   Scrotum well-shaped; left side slightly lower than right. Skin is even, dark rose color without lesions. Scrotum and testes are smooth and without tenderness, swelling, or masses.

Inguinal region   No lymph nodes are palpable. Inguinal canals without bulges, or tenderness bilaterally.

Nursing Diagnosis #1

High risk for infection related to presence of pathogens in exudate from urethra.

Defining characteristics   Discharge from penis reported and observed, sore at urethral opening, no lesions noted.

Nursing Diagnosis #2

Noncompliance versus knowledge deficit related to preventing sexually transmitted diseases.

Defining characteristics   Unprotected sexual intercourse with woman on blind date 1 week before penile discharge.

HEALTH PROMOTION

■ **Genital Self Examination (GSE):** There are two main reasons for teaching GSE. The first is that testicular cancer is the most common type of cancer in young men. The second is that it is an excellent way to identify sexually transmitted diseases, especially for clients who are frequently sexually active or who have multiple sexual partners. Every man from puberty onward should be asked if he routinely examines his own genitalia and, if so, what he actually does and how he does it. Following are the guidelines:

1. Instruct the client to take his penis in his hand and examine the tip for any evidence of swelling, sores, blisters, or discharge from the tip. If the client is not circumcised, instruct him to retract the foreskin so that the glans may be adequately examined. Uncircumcised males should also be instructed to especially examine the area of the junction between the foreskin and the glans.

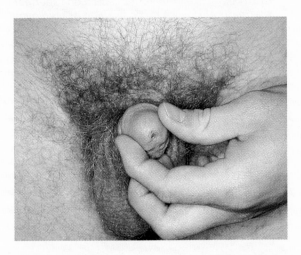

2. Next, instruct the client to palpate the entire shaft of the penis. Instruct him to examine all areas and all surfaces around the entire shaft from the base to the tip. He should feel for lumps, tenderness, and swelling.

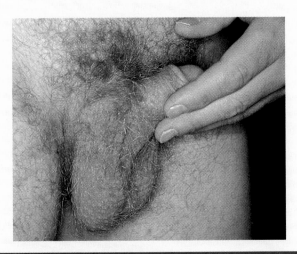

3. Finally, instruct the client to examine his scrotum and testes. To do this, tell him to use the hand on the opposite side from the testicle being examined to lift his penis up and out of the way. First inspect the scrotum for color, texture, and evidence of swelling. Then, with the available hand, gently palpate the scrotum for evidence of lumps, tenderness, or swelling.

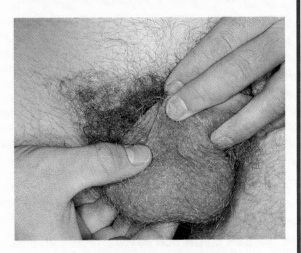

4. Instruct the client to change hands and palpate the other side of the scrotum with the other hand.

Instruct the client to examine himself when he is in the shower or in front of a mirror. The frequency of examination should be at least monthly. If the client is sexually active and is at high risk for infection, he should examine himself more frequently.

■ **Personal Protection for Sexually Active Males** Personal protection for men is just as important as it is for women. First, a condom will function as a barrier to prevent the transmission of semen and seminal fluid to the client's sexual partner. Second, it will protect the client, as well as the client's partner, from direct tissue-to-tissue contact, thus decreasing the chance of the exposure of sexually transmitted diseases, including AIDS (acquired immunodeficiency syndrome).

The client should be educated about the transmission of sexually transmitted diseases and the risk of acquiring such a disease if no personal protection is used. All sexually active males, especially young men, should be taught of their equal responsibility during sexual relations to prevent an unwanted pregnancy.

Assess the client's knowledge about how to apply a condom and, if necessary, use a penis model to actually demonstrate the method of putting a condom on the erect penis. In addition, teach the client that the condom is a single-use item that should be discarded after use.

???????STUDY QUESTIONS???????

1. Describe the process by which the penis introduces sperm into the vagina.
2. What is the function of the scrotum? Testes?
3. What problem is common with the external inguinal ring?
4. At what point in fetal development is differentiation of gender possible?
5. Describe the genital changes that occur during puberty.
6. Describe the genital changes that occur during the aging process.
7. A man reports pain in the lower back. What else do you need to know about the pain? What related possibilities do you want to explore?
8. A male reports urinating 5 to 6 times a day. Is this cause for concern? What else do you need to know about his urinary habits?
9. A man tells you, sort of ashamedly, that he's having trouble "getting it up." What additional information do you need to collect?
10. Describe at least one area that you want to explore with the following male individuals: (a) 6-month-old, (b) 3-year-old, (c) 8-year-old, (d) 13-year-old, (e) 75-year-old.
11. If you are female, how do you proceed with a genital exam of a male who is uncooperative?

12. Describe how you palpate the penis and scrotum. What are you looking for? List four abnormalities that you might encounter.
13. What is the transillumination process used for when examining an infant?
14. What approach should you use when examining the genitalia of a 3-year-old child?
15. What is the primary focus when examining the genitalia of an adolescent boy?
16. What changes might you expect to see when examining the genitalia of a 70-year-old man?
17. Match the STD with the appropriate signs/symptoms:

    Herpes　　　　　　　*Single painless ulcerated lesion*
    Warts　　　　　　　*Small multiple lesions on the glans*
    Syphilis　　　　　　*Erosion between shaft and glans*
    Lymphogranuloma　*Painful red vesicles on the shaft*

18. Match the scrotal condition with the appropriate description:

    Hydrocele　　　　*Tortuous veins along spermatic cord*
    Spermatocele　　*A cystic swelling of epididymis*
    Varicocele　　　　*Tender epididymis after UTI*
    Epididymitis　　　*Fluid in tunica vaginalis*

19. Outline a teaching plan for genital self-examination.
20. Why should you address the topic of personal protection with sexually active males?

CHAPTER 20

Anus, Rectum, and Prostate

ANATOMY AND PHYSIOLOGY

The anus, rectum, and prostate are dealt with as a unit in this chapter, since their examination often occurs simultaneously. The anus and rectum serve together as the terminal instruments of the alimentary tract's excretory functions. In males, the prostate gland is also examined in conjunction with the anus and rectum since it is accessible while the rectum is being examined.

ANUS

As the final segment of the colon, the anal canal opens into the perineum (Fig. 20-1). It is approximately 1 to 1.6 inches (2.5 to 4 cm) long, slanting forward toward the umbilicus and forming a right angle with the rectum. It is kept securely closed by concentric rings of muscle, called the internal and external sphincters. The internal ring, a smooth muscle, is under involuntary, or autonomic, control; sympathetic stimulation contracts it, and parasympathetic stimulation relaxes it. The external, striated muscle is under voluntary control. This external sphincter controls defecation. Just as control mechanisms differ for internal and external sphincters, variable degrees of sensitivity are related to these neurologic mechanisms. The lower anus is sensitive to painful stimuli through its somatic sensory nerves, while the upper half, under autonomic control, is relatively insensitive.

The internal canal is lined with the columns of Morgagni, mucosal tissue columns that fuse, forming the anorectal junction. The anal glands empty into small crypts between these columns. Near these columns are a series of veins. When dilated, these veins are referred to as internal hemorrhoids. The lower segment of the anal canal contains a venous plexus; this drains into the inferior rectal veins. Varicose veins of this plexus are called external hemorrhoids.

RECTUM

Superior to the anal canal lies the rectum. This 4.7-inch (12-cm) column is continuous, at its proximal end, with the sigmoid colon. It is lined with columnar epithelium. The distal end, above the anorectal junction, dilates and turns posteriorly, forming the rectal ampulla, which stores flatus and feces. Four semilunar transverse folds, called the valves of Houston, extend across half the circumference of the rectal lumen, apparently to support feces while allowing flatus to pass.

In females, the anterior rectum lies in contact with the vagina and is separated from it by the rectovaginal septum. In males, the anterior rectum is in close contact with the prostate, discussed below.

PROSTATE GLAND

The prostate gland, a trilobed, fibromuscular organ at the base of the bladder, is approximately $1.6 \times 1.2 \times 0.8$ inches ($4 \times 3 \times 2$ cm). It surrounds the urethra as it emerges from the bladder. Its posterior surface is adjacent to the anterior rectal wall, so it can be palpated during a rectal examination (Fig. 20-2). The three lobes are not well defined, but the palpable portion manifests right and left vertical lobes divided by a sulcus (a slight groove). The function of the prostate and the prostatic secretions is not completely understood, with the exception that it is known to produce most of the fibrinolysin-rich ejaculatory fluid. Fibrinolysin is an enzyme that liquefies coagulated semen, which is suspected to aid sperm motility. If the prostate gland enlarges, it may cause mechanical obstruction of urination by causing constriction of the urethra.

559

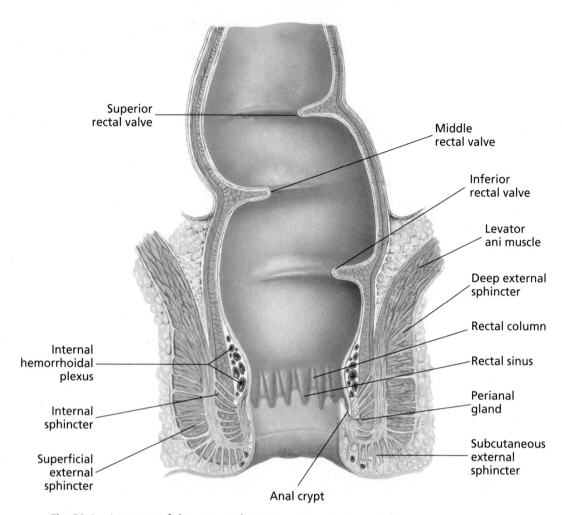

Superior rectal valve

Middle rectal valve

Inferior rectal valve

Levator ani muscle

Deep external sphincter

Rectal column

Rectal sinus

Perianal gland

Subcutaneous external sphincter

Internal hemorrhoidal plexus

Internal sphincter

Superficial external sphincter

Anal crypt

Fig. 20-1   Anatomy of the anus and rectum.   *(From Seidel et al, 1995.)*

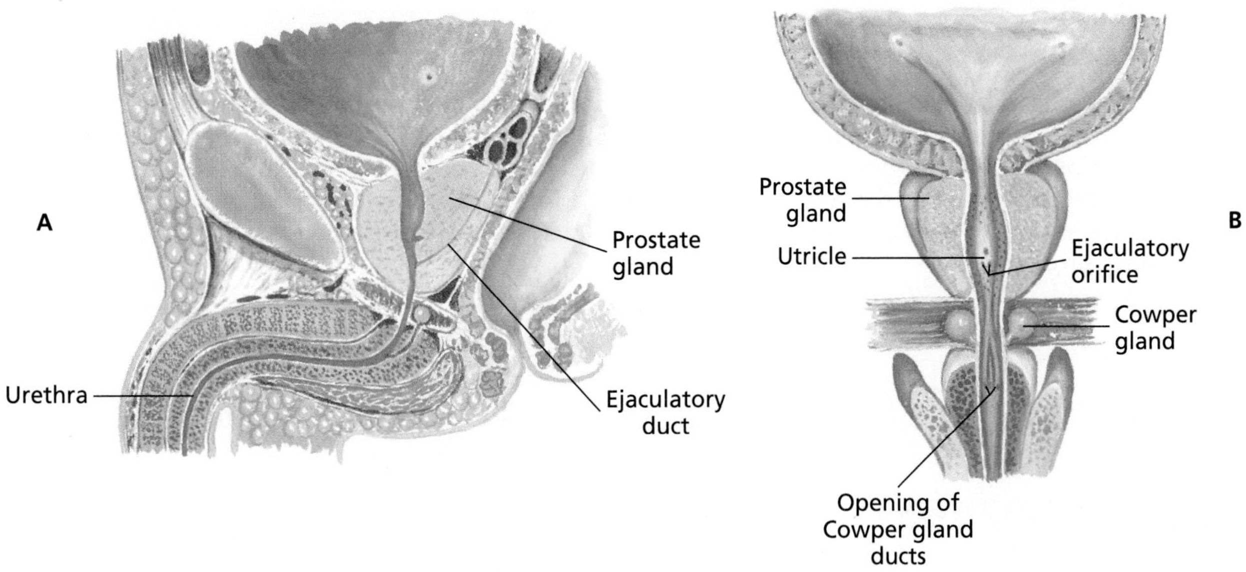

Fig. 20-2 Anatomy of the prostate gland and seminal vesicles. **A,** Lateral view. **B,** Cross section. *(From Seidel et al, 1995.)*

DEVELOPMENTAL CONSIDERATIONS

INFANTS AND CHILDREN

At 7 weeks gestation, a urogenital sinus, a rectum, and an anorectal septum are all detectable. By 8 weeks gestation, a membrane covering the urogenital sinus develops into the anal opening. This partitioning process is the origin of most anorectal malformations.

At birth, meconium stool is passed within 24 to 48 hours; this indicates anal patency. After this first step, newborns commonly experience the gastrocolic reflex, causing a stool production after each feeding. At this age, because myelination of the spinal cord is incomplete, both the internal and external sphincters are under involuntary reflexive control; control of the external anal sphincter will not be achieved until sometime between the ages of 18 and 24 months. By the end of the first year, bowel movements will drop to one or two per day.

In males, the prostate will be undeveloped, unpalpable, and inactive until the androgenic influences of puberty initiate its functions.

PREGNANT WOMEN

Pregnant women become susceptible to constipation and, ultimately, hemorrhoids for a variety of reasons, including in-creased blood flow and pressure in the veins below the enlarged uterus; dietary and hormonal changes that decrease gastrointestinal (GI) tract tone and motility; and, finally, increased pressure on the pelvic floor during labor, which may cause protrusion and inflammation of hemorrhoids during the puerperium.

OLDER ADULTS

With increasing age, the rectal wall's afferent neurons degenerate, interfering with pressure sensitivity and internal sphincter relaxation in response to rectal distention. Because of this, the older adult may experience stool retention. At the same time, as the internal sphincter loses tone, the external sphincter is not able to control the bowels on its own, so the older adult may experience fecal incontinence instead of retention. Fecal incontinence is not a normal finding.

In men, with loss of secretory alveolar function, the prostate gland atrophies. This is often obscured, however, by benign hyperplasia of the glandular tissue. Collagen progressively replaces the muscular component of the prostate.

HEALTH HISTORY | Anus, Rectum, and Prostate

The questions to be asked of the client in compiling the history concern usual bowel routines, such as frequency and stool color; changes in bowel habits, including diarrhea and constipation; rectal conditions, for example, pruritus, hemorrhoids, fissures, and fistulas; medications being taken; dietary factors, specifically focusing on high-fiber foods; and, for males, difficulty with urination, pressure in the rectal area, and risk factors related to prostate problems.

QUESTIONS

RATIONALE

CHANGE IN BOWEL FUNCTION

- Have you noticed a change in your bowel movements? *If so:* When did it start? Did it start suddenly or gradually? Have you had a dietary change? Activity change? Stressful life change?
- Describe the change in your bowel function. Has it been a change in number of stools per day? Consistency? Presence of mucus or blood? Odor? Color? Pain associated with your bowel movements?

These questions will establish a baseline for the client or a deviation from normal for that client. Deviations in bowel function may be caused by a number of variables, from lack of adequate fluid or bulk in the diet to an ulcerative or polyp condition in the bowel to emotional stress or medications. In all cases, it is important to sort out the variables involved in the bowel habit changes.

- Have you had other symptoms such as increased gas (flatus), pain, fever, nausea, vomiting, abdominal pain or cramping, or discomfort after eating? Have you noted any connection with specific foods? Does anyone else in your family have the same symptoms?

Gastroenteritis, colitis, and irritable colon syndrome may cause diarrhea. The symptoms listed could also indicate food poisoning.

Colorectal Cancer Risk Factors

- Over 40 years of age (peak ages 65-74)
- Family history of colon cancer, familial polyposis, Gardner syndrome, Peutz-Jeghers syndrome
- Personal history of colon polyps; Crohn's disease; Gardner syndrome; ovarian, breast, or endometrial cancer; ulcerative colitis of more than 10 years duration
- Diet high in beef and animal fats, low in fiber
- Exposure to asbestos, acrylics, and other carcinogens

From Seidel et al, 1995.

QUESTIONS

RATIONALE

■ Are you taking any medications? Which ones? Do you use laxatives or stool softeners? How often? Which ones? Do you take iron supplements? Do you need to use enemas to move your bowels? How often? What kind of enema do you use? What is in it?

◀ *The use of bowel-related medications or preparations is very common. As part of a comprehensive assessment, especially for clients with bowel problems, carefully assess the use of bowel-related medications or laxatives, as well as routine bowel practices, such as the use of enemas.*

■ Briefly describe your diet. Do you routinely eat high-fiber foods such as apples or other fruits, cereals and whole-grain breads, and vegetables? How many glasses of water do you drink each day?

◀ *Note that high-fiber foods should be encouraged to lower cholesterol levels, fight obesity, stabilize blood sugar levels, and ameliorate certain gastrointestinal disturbances. Insoluble-fiber foods (e.g., cereals and wheat germ) reduce the risk of colon cancer.*

RECTAL BLEEDING

■ Have you ever had black or bloody stools? If so, what is the color of the blood? Bright red? Dark red? Black and tarry? When did you first notice this?
■ How much blood have you noticed? Just a spot? A great deal? Did it fill the toilet bowl with red? Have you noticed a smell accompanying the bloody stool?

◀ *Bleeding from high in the intestinal tract will produce black, tarry stools, whereas bleeding near the rectum will produce bright red bleeding. Black stools may result from occult blood or melena caused by gastrointestinal bleeding; these stools are generally tarry. Black, nontarry stools may occur with certain medications. Red blood in stools usually occurs with gastrointestinal bleeding or bleeding in the area around the rectum and anus.*

■ If you are having rectal bleeding, have you also noticed the presence of mucus in the stools? Have you had accompanying abdominal cramping or pain?

◀ *Gastrointestinal problems such as ulcerative colitis may cause rectal bleeding accompanied by increased mucus production and abdominal cramping.*

■ Have you ever noticed clay-colored stools, mucus in the stools, or frothiness of the stool?

◀ *Clay-colored stools result from a lack of bile pigment. Excessive fat in the stool results from malabsorption of fat.*

RECTAL PAIN

■ Do you ever experience pain while having a bowel movement? Is the pain related to body position or straining to have a bowel movement?
■ Do you have hemorrhoids? *If so:* Do they ever bleed? If they bother you, how do you treat them?
■ Does the rectal pain interfere with your activities of daily living?

◀ *Rectal pain may be caused by hemorrhoids, fissures, constipation, or a higher gastrointestinal problem.*

RECTAL ITCHING, BURNING, STINGING

■ Do you currently have any rectal burning, itching, or stinging? If so, what is it associated with? Bowel movements? Hemorrhoids? Bathing? Use of medications such as hemorrhoid preparations? Do you ever notice that there is bleeding associated with the problem?

◀ *Rectal burning, itching, or stinging may also be associated with a number of factors, from poor hygiene to hemorrhoids to a parasite such as pinworms.*

QUESTIONS	RATIONALE

■ What have you done to decrease the problem? Has it helped?

◄ *Most clients will attempt self-treatment before seeking professional care.*

■ Have you ever had a fissure or a fistula? *If so:* How was this treated? Have you ever experienced difficulty controlling bowel movements?

◄ *Prolapsed hemorrhoids may cause the patient to have mucoid discharge and soiled underwear.*

FECAL INCONTINENCE

■ Do you ever soil your underwear? If so, how often does this occur? When did it begin? Why do you think that it is happening? Is it that you cannot make it to the restroom in time, or is it that you are unaware that you are becoming incontinent of stool? What have you done about it? Does it interfere with your activities of daily living?

◄ *Incontinence of stool may be associated with neurologic dysfunction, or it may be due to poor sphincter control or a gastrointestinal bowel problem.*

PROSTATE-RELATED DISCOMFORT (MALE CLIENTS)

■ Have you recently noticed a change in your urinary function? Is it difficult for you to begin to urinate? Is your urine stream weak? Do you dribble urine? Do you feel like you have to urinate but can't? Do you have to get up in the middle of the night to urinate? Do you have a urethral discharge?

◄ *Prostate problems are common in men, especially as they become older.*

■ Have you ever been told that you have a problem with your prostate, such as an enlarged prostate, infection of the prostate (prostatitis), or cancer?

🌐 Cultural Note

Prostate cancer is the most common cancer in men, and incidence does vary by cultural group. African American men are at highest risk (1 in 800), followed by whites and Hispanics (1 in 1250). The risk is much less for Pacific Islanders, Asian Americans, and American Indians/Alaskan Natives, ranging from 1 in 2000 to 1 in 3000. It is, however, the most common cancer in American Indian men.

Prostate Cancer Risk Factors

- Males over 50 years old
- Residence in the United States
- Diet high in animal fats
- Use of alcohol
- Family history of prostate cancer
- Occupational exposure to cadmium, fertilizer, exhaust fumes, and rubber
- Prostate-specific antigen (PSA) level >4 mg/ml

From Seidel et al, 1995.

INFANTS

Serious rectal and anal problems, such as an imperforate anus, should have been identified following the child's birth. Later-identified problems that should be recognized in the infant include such things as structural problems—fissure or megacolon—and stool characteristics that may be a significant sign of a more serious problem. Ask the following questions.

■ When the infant was born did he or she have any problem having a bowel movement? Did anyone at the hospital tell you that they were concerned about the infant's rectum or ability to defecate?

◄ *Baseline information.*

■ Describe the infant's stool characteristics. Color? General texture: diarrhea; formed and soft; formed and hard? Does the baby cry or strain during a bowel movement? How frequently does the infant have a stool?

◄ *It is important to correlate the infant's stool characteristics with the type of diet and fluid intake. Often, crying or straining with a bowel movement may be indicative of hard stools or constipation.*

QUESTIONS

RATIONALE

■ Describe the infant's diet. Breast-feeding? Bottle? If bottle-feeding, what type of formula? Plus iron? Does the baby drink fluids other than formula, such as juices or water? *If so:* How much?

◄ *Diet will affect the stool composition and color.*

Infant Stool Characteristics
Breast-Fed
Stool will be mushy, loose, golden color; frequency varies from after each feeding to every few days. The stool is generally not irritating to the skin.
Formula-Fed
Stool is light-colored, with a foul odor; frequency varies from several times a day to every few days. The stool is frequently irritating to the skin.

CHILDREN

In addition to the questions asked for the infant, inquire about toilet training, anal or rectal itching, and general bowel functioning. Ask the following questions.

YOUNG CHILDREN

■ Have you started to toilet-train the child? *If so:* How old was the child when you started? Has it been successful? *If so:* When did the child successfully complete bowel training?

◄ *There is a wide range of professional opinions about when toilet training should begin and how it should be done. It is most important to learn how the parent is doing the training and how successful it has been. This will provide baseline information should additional education or assistance become necessary.*

ALL CHILDREN

■ What are the child's normal bowel habits?

◄ *Baseline information.*

■ Have you noticed that the child has had any problems with his or her bowels? Constipation? Diarrhea? Cramping? *If any of these are present:* How long has the problem existed? When did it start?
■ Is there a family history of similar problems or diseases affecting the bowels?
■ Are there any current stresses in the family? Please describe them.
■ Describe the child's diet for a day. How much food, juice, and water is consumed in a 24-hour period?

◄ *These symptoms may be indications of problems from inadequate diet to parental punishment if the child has an "accident" to a more serious problem such as megacolon. If any are present, it is important to try to identify the causative factors.*

PREGNANT WOMEN

Bowel problems that pregnant women have are most generally related to the growing fetus and pressure on the colon and rectum. Prenatal vitamins containing iron may also commonly cause constipation. In addition to the questions in the adult section, ask the following questions.

- Do you have any problems with your bowels, such as constipation? *If so:* Describe. What have you done to treat the problem?
- Are you having any problem with actually having a bowel movement? *If so:* Are you having to strain to have a bowel movement? Do you have hemorrhoids? *If so:* Are they bothering you? Do they bleed?
- Describe your current diet, including daily fluid intake.
- Are you taking prenatal vitamins? Do they contain iron?

◄ *Constipation and hemorrhoids are common problems for women who are pregnant. It is important to assess whether these problems are present and to determine their severity.*

◄ *Prenatal vitamins containing iron may cause constipation and tarry-appearing stools.*

OLDER ADULTS

Elderly clients frequently express numerous problems associated with elimination, and individuals may be preoccupied with bowel movement regularity to the extent that it can alter daily living functions. Clarification of symptoms is needed. If the symptoms are long-standing, ask carefully about the client's method of self-treatment. The questions to be asked are the same as for adults, but care should be taken to pay attention to the client's responses concerning constipation, gas in the stomach, diarrhea, or abdominal cramping. Medications are often more likely to produce changes in bowel motility in older clients and should be carefully evaluated. Additional specific questions to ask include the following.

- Have you noticed a change in your bowel function? *If so:* Describe. Has the change been gradual or sudden? What have you done to treat the problem?
- *If the client has bowel changes, ask:* Have you noticed a recent weight loss? Rectal or abdominal pain? Abdominal distention? Rectal bleeding? *If so:* Describe.
- Describe your diet. Do any specific foods bother you? *If so:* Which ones and how?

◄ *Changes in bowel function may be associated with diet changes such as lack of bulk or roughage in the diet, decreased fluid intake, decreased exercise, or more serious problems such as a bowel obstruction secondary to cancer.*

The older male adult is most likely to have prostate problems. It is important to ask all of the questions presented in the adult history section related to the prostate.

EXAMINATION Procedures and Findings

Guidelines Rectal examination with testing of the stool for blood should be performed at least annually for the adult, starting at age 18. If the client has a specific problem, the examination should be performed as frequently as necessary. Children and infants do not routinely have a rectal examination performed unless there is a problem.

Positioning the client for the rectal examination usually depends on the client's gender and age.

Males: Lying on left side with the hips and knees flexed; knee-chest position; or, most commonly, standing with the hips flexed and the client bending over the examination table.

Females: Lying on left side with hips and knees flexed; knee-chest position; or, most commonly, in the lithotomy position if the examination is being done in conjunction with the genitalia examination. The rectal examination will most usually be performed with the client in the lithotomy position.

EQUIPMENT	Gloves
	Penlight
	Water-soluble lubricant
	Guaiac test reagents
	Goose-neck floor lamp

TECHNIQUES and NORMAL FINDINGS

ABNORMAL FINDINGS

The examination of the rectum and anus is the same for males and females with the exception of the prostate, which should also be examined in the male client. The techniques of the examination include inspection and palpation.

Examination gloves should be worn throughout the entire examination procedure.

Clinical Note

It may be uncomfortable for both the client and the examiner if they are of opposite genders. If it is not possible for an examiner of the client's gender to perform the procedure, proceed in a professional manner.

Also remember that it is always best to have an escort in the examination room with the examiner during the assessment.

ANUS AND RECTUM

INSPECT the sacrococcygeal and perianal areas for Color and Surface Characteristics. The skin surface should be smooth and clear.

■ Lesions or infections in the sacrococcygeal or perianal area may be indicative of a localized infection or parasite, or they may be signs of a systemic disease such as diabetes.

INSPECT for Lesions, Dimpling, and Tufts of Hair. Note any lumps, rash, inflammation, scars, or lesions. Also inspect the area for pilonidal dimpling or tufts of hair at the pilonidal area.

■ Other abnormalities include perianal and perirectal abscesses; pilonidal cyst; or pilonidal sinus (see the Common Problems section, later in this chapter).

TECHNIQUES and NORMAL FINDINGS

ABNORMAL FINDINGS

PALPATE the coccygeal area for Tenderness. None should be present.

Spread the buttocks with both hands. INSPECT the anus for Surface Characteristics. (Adequate client positioning and a bright gooseneck floor light are necessary to perform a thorough assessment). (*Note:* It is important to always tell the client what is about to happen, especially as the buttock is spread and then when a gloved finger is inserted for the internal examination. If the client is extremely tense or uncomfortable with the examination, take the time to explain the purpose and the importance of adequately examining the rectum and prostate.) Pigmentation of the skin near the anal opening should be increased and the skin more coarse. Note any areas of inflammation, lesions, scars, skin tags, fissures, lumps, swelling, excoriation, hemorrhoids, or mucosal bulging. Ask the client to bear down and repeat the inspection of the anal area for presence of hemorrhoids or areas of discoloration or lesions. None should be present.

■ Hemorrhoids are the most common abnormality found near the anus. There are two types of hemorrhoids: internal (Fig. 20-3, *A*) and external (prolapsed) (Fig. 20-3, *B*). Hemorrhoids may range from one single hemorrhoid that may only appear when the client strains during a bowel movement to multiple hemorrhoids that may cause continuous pain and may frequently bleed with any straining.

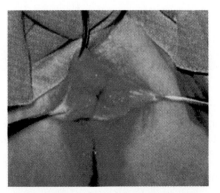

A

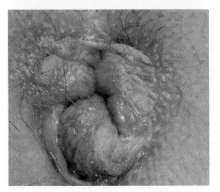

B

Fig. 20-3 A, Primary internal hemorrhoids. **B,** Prolapsed hemorrhoids. *(From Seidel et al, 1995; courtesy Gershon Efron, MD, Sinai Hospital of Baltimore.)*

TECHNIQUES and NORMAL FINDINGS

ABNORMAL FINDINGS

PALPATE the anus for Sphincter Tone. Ask the client to bear down again. Place the finger pad surface of a gloved and lubricated index finger at the anal opening; as the sphincter relaxes, slowly insert the finger, pointing toward the client's umbilicus. The sphincter should tighten evenly around your finger with minimum discomfort to the client. *To perform an adequate internal rectal examination, the client's hips should be in a flexed position* (Fig. 20-4).

■ Report if the client is unable to tighten the sphincter around your finger or experiences discomfort with sphincter tightening.

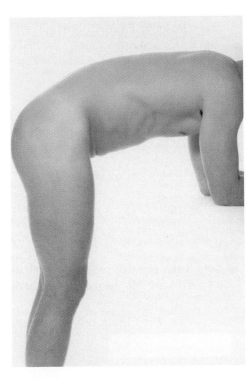

Fig. 20-4 Male client in hips-flexed position for prostate examination.

Rotate the finger around the musculature of the anal ring to palpate the surface characteristics (Fig. 20-5). The area should be smooth, with even pressure on your finger.

Insert the finger as far as possible into the rectum (2.4 to 3.9 inches, or 6 to 10 cm) to palpate all four rectal walls. There should be a continuous smooth surface, and the client should experience only minimal discomfort.

■ Note any nodules or irregularities.

■ Note nodules or masses. (*Note:* In females, occasionally the cervix may be palpable on the anterior wall; do not mistake this for a mass.) Note any tenderness, irregularities, or polyps.

TECHNIQUES and NORMAL FINDINGS

ABNORMAL FINDINGS

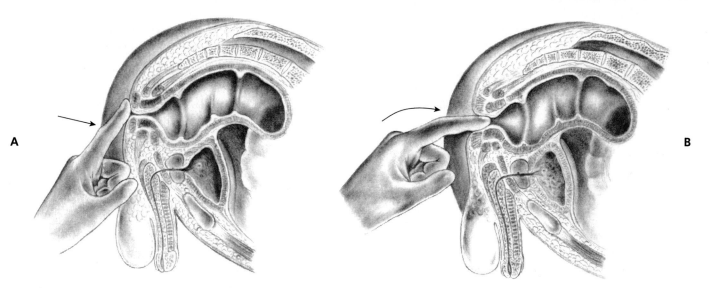

A   B

Fig. 20-5 Correct procedure for introducing finger into rectum. **A,** Press pad of finger against the anal opening. **B,** As external sphincter relaxes, slip the fingertip into the anal canal. Note that client is in the hips-flexed position. *(From Seidel et al, 1995.)*

PROSTATE GLAND (FOR MALE CLIENTS)

PALPATE the anterior rectal surface to Evaluate the prostate. Palpate the posterior surface of the prostate gland by palpating the anterior surface of the rectum (Fig. 20-6). (*Note:* The client may state that he has the urge to urinate during the prostate examination. Reassure him that this is only a sensation and that he will not urinate.) Note the size, contour, consistency, and mobility of the gland. It should be about 1.5 inches (3.8 cm) in diameter and project less than 0.4 inch (1 cm) into the rectum. The contour is symmetric and bilobed, with a palpable sulcus. There should be a firm, smooth consistency and no tenderness.

■ Note if the prostate projects more than 0.4 inch (1 cm) into the rectum (Fig. 20-6).

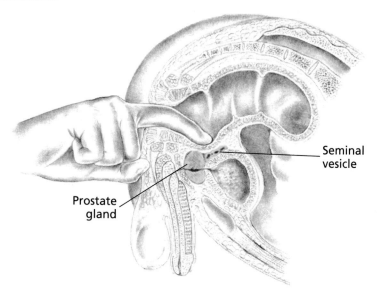

Seminal vesicle

Prostate gland

Fig. 20-6 Palpation of the anterior surface of the prostate gland. Feel for the lateral lobes and median sulcus. *(From Seidel et al, 1995.)*

TECHNIQUES and NORMAL FINDINGS

ABNORMAL FINDINGS

Classifications of Prostate Enlargement	
GRADE	**PROTRUSION INTO RECTUM**
Grade I	0.4 to 0.8 inch (1 to 2 cm)
Grade II	0.8 to 1.2 inches (2 to 3 cm)
Grade III	1.2 to 1.6 inches (3 to 4 cm)
Grade IV	greater than 1.6 inches (4 cm)

■ Note if there is asymmetry or if the median sulcus is obliterated; also note any tenderness, a boggy feeling, irregularity, or nodules. A *rubbery or boggy consistency* may be indicative of *benign hypertrophy*. A *stony-hard or nodular* prostate may indicate *carcinoma, prostate calculi, or fibrosis.*

STOOL EXAMINATION

INSPECT any fecal material for Characteristics. Do this as the gloved finger is slowly removed from the client's rectum. Inspect the color and consistency of any stool. It should be brown and soft.

■ Note the presence of blood, either bright red or tarry black; pus; pale yellow or light tan or gray stool.

Stool Colors and Significance	
COLOR	**SIGNIFICANCE**
Bright red	Hemorrhoidal or lower rectal bleeding
Tarry black	Upper intestinal tract bleeding or excessive iron or bismuth ingestion
Light tan or gray	Obstruction of the biliary tract (obstructive jaundice)
Pale yellow	Malabsorption syndrome

EXAMINE fecal material for Presence of Occult Blood. Use a guaiac test to evaluate for occult blood on all stool specimens. A negative response is normal.

■ Report any positive guaiac test, which indicates the presence of occult blood.

AGE-RELATED VARIATIONS

NEWBORNS/INFANTS/CHILDREN

■ APPROACH

The external perianal examination is routinely performed during a comprehensive assessment. The internal rectal examination is generally not performed in children unless there are specific symptoms such as abdominal pain, constipation, or diarrhea or the child is ill. If the examination is performed, the examiner should respect the child's modesty and apprehension and should take the time to explain what is going to happen and what the child can expect.

If an examination is performed, the infant is generally placed on his or her back with the feet held in the examiner's hand and the infant's knees flexed upward toward the abdomen. Older children should be positioned so that the perianal area is adequately exposed and so that the child is comfortable. Most often, the child should be positioned on the left side with the hips and knees flexed toward the abdomen (the same positioning as for the adult).

■ FINDINGS

The basic findings are the same for the infant and child as for the adult. Variations are based on developmental maturity. For the infant, first observe the lower back and buttocks. The pilonidal area should be observed for Mongolian spots, birthmarks, sinuses, tufts of hair, and dimpling, which may indicate a lower spinal deformity. Buttocks should be firm and rounded. Asymmetry of the buttocks may indicate hip dislocation. The color around the anus should be slightly deeper than the child's general skin tone. Gently stroke the anal area and note a quick contraction of the sphincter. If the quick contraction is not present, it may indicate a lower spinal cord lesion. Verify by parent history that the infant has a patent anus and that stool is passed with no difficulty. If stool is present when the diaper is removed, note the characteristics, color, odor, and consistency. Check the perianal skin and entire diaper area for color and smoothness. Redness or irritation may be indication of a bacterial or fungal infection or pinworms. If any pustules or signs of physical or sexual abuse are noted during the examination, such as bruising, anal tearing, or extreme or inappropriate apprehension from the child, assess the finding further with the family. If there is suspicion of child abuse or assault, report the findings to the appropriate local health authorities.

If an internal rectal examination is warranted, the examiner should use the little finger to actually perform the examination. Even when this is done, there may occasionally be slight rectal bleeding. The parent should be told about this possibility before the examination. The procedures and findings for the internal examination are the same as for the adult. The prostate in the small child is not palpable.

ADOLESCENTS

■ APPROACH

The rectal and prostate examination should be part of a comprehensive assessment for the older adolescent. It is recommended that males have a baseline rectal and prostate examination by age 18. It will provide baseline information and, for males, will provide an opportunity to discuss the importance of a periodic prostate examination. Because many adolescents may never have had a rectal examination before, it is important to take the time to explain what will be done and what you are trying to assess.

■ FINDINGS

The procedures and findings are the same as for the adult.

OLDER ADULTS

■ APPROACH

The examiner may need to assist the client into an adequate position for the examination. If the client is lying on his or her back on the examination table, care should be taken to assist the client into a left lateral lying position.

■ FINDINGS

The examination procedures and findings for the older adult are the same as for the adult. Because older male clients are at highest risk for developing prostatic hypertrophy, the prostate gland should be carefully examined. The older adult's prostate is more likely to feel smooth and rubbery. The median sulcus may or may not be palpable. The examiner may also note a relaxation of the client's perianal muscles and decreased sphincter control when the older adult bears down. Because the older adult is also more likely to develop polyps and carcinoma, the rectal examination becomes an important part of the client's overall examination.

CLIENTS WITH SITUATIONAL VARIATIONS

PREGNANT WOMEN

■ APPROACH

The perianal and rectal examination for the pregnant woman is just as important as for all other adults. In fact, because pregnancy often causes hemorrhoids to appear, the rectal examination is vital. Early during pregnancy, the client should have minimal difficulty attaining and maintaining the position for the examination. Later in pregnancy, however, a large fetus may cause client positioning for the rectal examination to become a major problem. The rectum and anus are most commonly examined while the client is in the lithotomy position with her legs up in stirrups.

■ FINDINGS

During pregnancy, the client's stools may become either more solid and constipated or softer with the possibility of diarrhea. The color of the stool may range from normal to dark green to black, depending on the iron content in the prenatal vitamins. The presence of hemorrhoids is the most common variation usually considered normal with pregnancy. The client may not have hemorrhoids during the early phase of pregnancy, but toward the last trimester the hemorrhoids may appear secondary to pressure on the pelvic floor or possible constipation with straining when having a bowel movement. The hemorrhoids may be either internal in the lower segment of the rectum or prolapsed as external hemorrhoids.

CLIENTS WITH ILEOSTOMY OR COLOSTOMY

■ APPROACH

Clients who have had either an ileostomy or colostomy have had to deal with many issues ranging from altered body functioning to body image changes to concern about "accidents and odors" to possibly dealing with a serious disease such as cancer. Each individual will adjust to the alteration differently. It is important to assess the client individually and to determine his or her knowledge and coping skills in dealing with the colostomy or ileostomy. Because the client is usually quite skilled in caring for their ostomy, the examiner should encourage the client to be a participant in the examination by having him or her remove the external pouch bag (if present) and actually have the client describe if the ostomy appears healthy and "normal."

■ FINDINGS

The stoma of either the ileostomy or the colostomy should appear red and moist. Because the stoma is actually inverted bowel, it has no sensory nerve endings. The area where the ostomy attaches to the skin should appear well-healed and without lesions, irritation, or areas of excoriation. Observe the skin characteristics around the ostomy to note areas of irritation or excoriation. If skin irritation is noted, inquire about cleaning techniques and use of preparations that will help prevent skin breakdown.

The stool characteristics of an individual with an ostomy will depend upon the level of the ostomy. Clients with an ileostomy (small-bowel area) will have uncontrollable drainage of stool that is of a thick liquid or mushy consistency. If the client has had a transverse (upper colon) level colostomy, the stool will be mushy and uncontrollable. If the client's colostomy is in the area of the descending or sigmoid (lower) colon, the stool will be more solid and may actually become predictable, so that some clients may elect to not wear a pouch.

Types of Ostomies

Colostomy
A surgical procedure that creates an opening, or stoma, between the colon and the abdominal wall. A colostomy is performed when a portion of the large bowel, including the colon, rectum, or anus, is diseased and must be bypassed or removed. The most common reasons for a colostomy are diverticulitis, tumors, injury, or birth injury.

Ileostomy
A surgical procedure in which an opening, or stoma, is created by bringing the ileum of the small intestine through the abdominal wall.

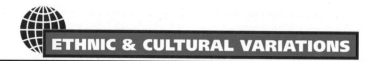

ETHNIC & CULTURAL VARIATIONS

■ **FINDINGS**

Differences across racial groups in the anatomy and physiology of the rectum, anus, and prostate are not apparent. There is a difference in the incidence of prostate cancer across cultural groups, with African-American men having the highest risk and American Indians the lowest risk. However, age remains the most predictable determinant of prostate cancer risk. The incidence rate for those over age 85 is a striking 90%.

E X A M I N A T I O N S U M M A R Y
Anus, Rectum, and Prostate

Anus and Rectum *(pp. 567-570)*
- Inspect the sacrococcygeal and perianal areas for:
   Color
   Surface characteristics
   Lesions
   Pilonidal dimpling or tufts of hair
- Palpate the coccygeal area for:
   Tenderness
- Inspect the anus for:
   Surface characteristics
- Palpate the anus for:
   Sphincter tone

Prostate Gland *(pp. 570-571)*
- In males: Palpate the anterior rectal surface to evelute the prostate for:
   Size
   Contour
   Consistency
   Mobility

Stool Evaluation *(p. 571)*
- Inspect and examine the fecal material for:
   Color
   Consistency
   Presence of occult blood by guaiac test

COMMON PROBLEMS/CONDITIONS

associated with the Anus, Rectum, and Prostate

ANUS AND RECTUM

■ *Pilonidal cyst or sinus:* A dimpled, open area that many times contains a tuft of hair. It is located in the midline of the back in the lower sacrum area and may appear erythematous. Many times the cyst or sinus may not be identified until the client is a young adult. Unless the cyst becomes infected or abscessed, the client will be asymptomatic.

■ *Anorectal fissure:* A painful tear of the anal mucosa that occurs most frequently secondary to trauma, such as passing a hard large stool or irritating diarrhea stools (Fig. 20-7). Most frequently the fissure is located midline in the posterior wall of the rectum. The client complains of rectal pain, itching, and often bleeding.

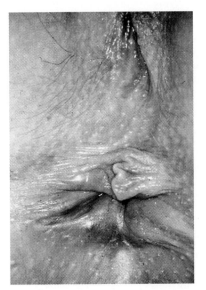

Fig. 20-7 Lateral anal fissure in adult. *(From Seidel et al, 1995; courtesy Gershon Efron, MD, Sinai Hospital of Baltimore.)*

■ *External hemorrhoids:* Usually painless varicose veins that originate below the anorectal line and appear as flaps of tissue or skin (see Fig. 20-3). If they become irritated by defecation, standing, or walking, they may cause localized itching and perhaps bleeding. If bleeding occurs, the hemorrhoids have most likely become thrombosed. If the hemorrhoids become severe, they may require surgical resection.

■ *Internal hemorrhoids:* Varicose veins that originate above the anorectal junction. Although they may be present in the rectum, they may not be identified clinically unless they become thrombosed, prolapsed, or infected.

■ *Polyps:* Common protruding growths that may occur anywhere in the intestinal tract. If irritated, they may cause rectal bleeding. Biopsy is necessary to distinguish the polyp from carcinoma.

■ *Carcinoma:* Feels like a multisided, irregular mass with nodular raised edges when palpated. Cancer of the rectum is often asymptomatic. In the center of the mass is an area of depression.

■ **Rectal prolapse:** An actual "inside out" falling of the rectum through the anal ring and outside the individual (Fig. 20-8). The prolapse appears as pink mucosal bulge that is described as a "doughnut" or "rosette."

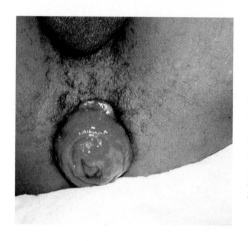

Fig. 20-8 Prolapse of the rectum. *(From Seidel et al, 1995; courtesy Gershon Efron, MD, Sinai Hospital of Baltimore.)*

PROSTATE

■ **Benign prostatic hypertrophy (BPH):** An asymptomatic enlargement of the prostate gland that frequently occurs in older men (Fig. 20-9). When palpated, the prostate feels smooth, firm, and rubbery. The client often presents with difficulty starting to urinate or maintaining a steady urine stream.

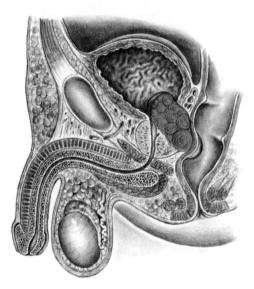

Fig. 20-9 Benign prostatic hypertrophy. *(From Seidel et al, 1995.)*

■ **Prostatitis:** Symptomatic and asymmetric enlargement of the prostate (Fig. 20-10) if acute. There is acute tenderness, a ureteral discharge, and a fever. If the prostate is chronically inflamed, it may feel boggy and enlarged. There may or may not be pain.

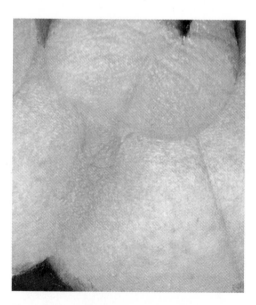

Fig. 20-10 Prostatitis. *(From Seidel et al, 1995.)*

■ **Prostate cancer:** Occurs mostly in men over the age of 50. Urinary obstruction with difficulty urinating may be the first sign of a problem. On palpation, the prostate feels hard and irregular. The median sulcus is obliterated as the prostate tumor grows (Fig. 20-11). Surgery with biopsy is the only method to confirm a diagnosis.

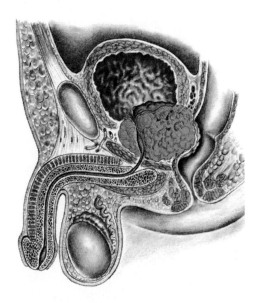

Fig. 20-11 **Carcinoma of prostate.** *(From Seidel et al, 1995.)*

&Nursing Diagnosis

CASE 1   81-year-old white woman with complaint of rectal bleeding.

Subjective

Client states during the past 2 weeks she has noted bright red blood on toilet tissue and in her underwear. States she has had no previous episodes of rectal bleeding or any problems with her bowels. Frequently has constipation and the past couple of weeks have been worse than usual. Reports her stools have been hard and dark brown. Frequency of elimination is once per day. Because of her bad teeth she eats mainly soft vegetables, fruits, and breads. Her arthritic knees keep her from exercising like she used to. Denies any other health care problems.

Objective

Height 5'1".

Weight 172 lb (78.2 kg).

Well-nourished, healthy, obese white woman. Perianal area appears intact, with no evidence of active bleeding, lesions, or excoriation. Multiple external, pale hemorrhoids noted around anus. One hemorrhoid at 9 o'clock position from symphysis pubis is thrombosed and appears dark purple in color. Upon palpation, the hemorrhoid is painful and feels full. Anal sphincter tone is strong around examiner's finger. No evidence of internal rectal wall lesions, masses, nodules, or discomfort to digital palpation. Guaiac testing of fecal material showed trace of blood present.

• •

Nursing Diagnosis #1

Pain related to hemorrhoids.

Defining Characteristics   Reports of rectal bleeding; hemorrhoids observed, one thrombosed, dark and purple; pain on palpation on hemorrhoids.

Nursing Diagnosis #2

Constipation related to inadequate dietary bulk and exercise.

Defining Characteristics   History of constipation, report of hard stools, eating soft vegetables and fruits, inability to exercise because of arthritis in knee.

Sample Documentation & Nursing Diagnosis

CASE 2   62-year-old Asian man with a history of difficult urinating.

Subjective

Client states that over past 6 months he has had increasing difficulty with urination, especially starting to urinate. Urine stream is not as strong as it used to be and following urination his urine continues to dribble. Reports frequency of urination has increased and he usually gets up at least one or two times during the night to urinate. Urination does not cause pain or discomfort. No difficulty with bowel movements nor any change in bowel movement pattern. No pain or discomfort, no weight change, no dietary changes. Client has not had a physical examination or prostate examination for 4 years.

Objective

Height   5'6".

Weight   142 lb (64.5 kg).

Well-nourished, healthy Asian man. Sacrococcygeal and perianal areas are without lesions, dimpling, or skin discoloration. Anus intact, with dark even pigment, and without lesions, hemorrhoids, polyps, or fissures. Strong anal sphincter tone around examiner's finger. Rectal walls are smooth and without evidence of masses, swelling, or tenderness. Prostate palpated on the posterior wall of the rectum extends into the rectum approximately 3 cm. Prostate is symmetric and feels smooth, rubbery, and enlarged. The median sulcus is not evident. Guaiac testing of fecal material is negative.

Nursing Diagnosis #1

Altered patterns of elimination related to bladder outlet obstruction.

Defining Characteristics   Difficulty initiating urine stream; decreased urinary stream; frequency of urination, nocturia; enlarged prostate palpated.

Nursing Diagnosis #2

Urinary retention related to bladder outlet obstruction.

Defining Characteristics   Postvoiding dribbling, frequency of urination, nocturia, enlarged prostate palpated.

HEALTH PROMOTION

■ **Constipation** Constipation is a very difficult term to define. It should be more related to the consistency of the stool than the frequency of stool evacuation. The normal frequency of stool evacuation ranges from once or twice a day to once or twice each week. Either may be normal. The normal stool should be soft and easily eliminated. When the stool is hard and difficult to evacuate, constipation exists. To promote healthy bowel function and to prevent constipation, the client should do the following:

• Eat a diet high in fiber (the skins of fresh vegetables and fruits, whole-grain breads, bran cereals, nuts, beans, and peas). This is necessary because these foods provide the bulk the large intestine needs to carry away body wastes.
• Drink a minimum of 8 to 10 8-oz. glasses of fluid a day.
• Increase your activity.
• Establish regular bowel habits and respond promptly to the urge to defecate.

■ **Colon and Rectal Cancer** Much can be done to reduce the risk of colon and rectal cancer or to improve its identification should it occur. Follow these dietary guidelines:

• Reduce the amount of fat in your diet to 30% of your total daily calorie intake.
• Limit the amount of alcohol you drink to one or two drinks a day.
• Limit the amount of charbroiled, smoked, and salted foods you eat.

• Eat foods high in:
  • *Vitamin A* (apricots, peaches, carrots, spinach, asparagus, squash, and sweet potatoes)
  • *Vitamin C* (oranges, lemons, grapefruit, strawberries, tomatoes, cabbage, and walnuts)
  • *Vitamin E* (lettuce, alfalfa, and vegetable oils)
  • *Fiber* (fresh vegetables and fruits, whole-grain breads and cereals, nuts, beans, and peas).
• Have all colorectal polyps removed.
• Know the cancer warning signs:
  • Rectal bleeding.
  • Change in your stools.
  • Pain in the abdomen.
  • Pressure in the rectum.
• Have an annual digital rectal examination starting at age 40.
• Have annual guaiac testing of fecal matter starting at age 50.
• Have an annual inspection of the colon with a special instrument (sigmoidoscopy) starting at age 50.

■ **Prostate Cancer** There are no prevention guidelines for prostate cancer. All men should have an annual prostate examination after age 40.

• Know the warning signs of prostate cancer:
  • Difficulty urinating.
  • Painful and frequent urination.
  • Blood in the urine.
  • Nocturia.

??????? STUDY QUESTIONS ???????

1. Describe the function of the internal and external anal sphincters. Which is more sensitive? What is the difference between internal and external hemorrhoids?

2. What is the function of the rectum? Prostate? What happens if the prostate gland enlarges?

3. How long after birth should a neonate produce a stool? When should an infant have control of the anal sphincters?

4. When is the prostate fully developed in males?

5. What two common problems of the rectum and anus are women susceptible to when pregnant? What causes these problems?

6. What are two common problems with the anus experienced by older adults?

7. An individual reports a two-day history of diarrhea. What additional information about this problem do you need to collect when taking a history?

8. A young man reports having hard, infrequent stools streaked with bright red blood. What additional information do you need to know?

9. An 8-year-old is having itching and burning of the rectum. What additional information do you need to know?

10. A 70-year-old man is complaining of difficulty in urinating at night. What additional information do you need to know?

11. List the risk factors for prostate cancer. What cultural group is at highest risk?

12. Describe how you would position a client for a rectal exam.

13. Describe how you would inspect the anus. What are you looking for? What common abnormality might you encounter?

14. Describe how you would perform an internal rectal exam. What are you looking for?

15. How would you palpate the prostate gland? When is the prostate considered enlarged? What might you palpate that would be indicative of benign prostatic hypertrophy?

16. How can you tell whether stool contains occult blood?

17. When is a rectal exam of a small child warranted? Should a rectal and prostate exam be a part of a comprehensive physical in an adolescent?

18. What exam position works best when examining the rectum of a woman who is 7 months pregnant?

19. Distinguish between an ileostomy and a colostomy. Describe the character of normal stool for an individual with a colostomy.

20. Match the common problem with the appropriate characteristic:

Pilonidal cyst	Pink mucosal bulge of rectum
Anorectal fissure	Dimpled, open area of sacrum
Polyps	Protruding intestinal growths
Rectal prolapse	Tear in rectal mucosa

21. When palpating the prostate, what do you expect to find in an individual with prostatitis? BPH? Prostate cancer?

22. Devise a teaching plan to help an individual prevent constipation.

23. What alterations in the diet can an individual make to decrease the risk of colorectal cancer?

24. What are the warning signs for colorectal cancer? What are the warning signs for prostate cancer?

CHAPTER 21

Musculoskeletal System

ANATOMY AND PHYSIOLOGY

The musculoskeletal system provides both support and mobility for the body and protection for internal organs. This system also provides red blood cell production and mineral storage.

SKELETON

The human skeleton can be divided into two separate structures. The axial skeleton comprises the skull, facial bones, auditory ossicles, vertebrae, ribs, sternum, and hyoid bone; the appendicular skeleton comprises bones of the upper and lower extremities. Each of the skeleton's 206 bones is shaped to facilitate its functioning. Major bones of the body are shown in Figs. 21-1, 21-2, 21-3, and 21-4.

SKELETAL MUSCLES

Skeletal muscles are composed of muscle fibers that attach to bones to facilitate movement. Muscles interact with nerves, minerals, blood vessels, skin, and connective tissue to initiate muscle contractions. While some skeletal muscles move by reflex, most are under voluntary control. Skeletal muscle fibers may be arranged parallel to the long axis of bones to which they attach, or they may be obliquely attached. Muscles attach at each end to a bone, ligament, tendon, or fascia. Muscles of the arms, legs, trunk, and pelvis are shown in Figs. 21-5, 21-6, and 21-7.

🌐 Racial Variation

Muscle mass is greater in both male and female African Americans than in the general population.

JOINTS

Joints are articulations where two or more bones are joined one to another or where two bone surfaces come together. Joints help hold the bones firmly together while allowing movement between them.

Joints are classified in two ways. First, they are classified by the type of material between the bones: fibrous, cartilagi-

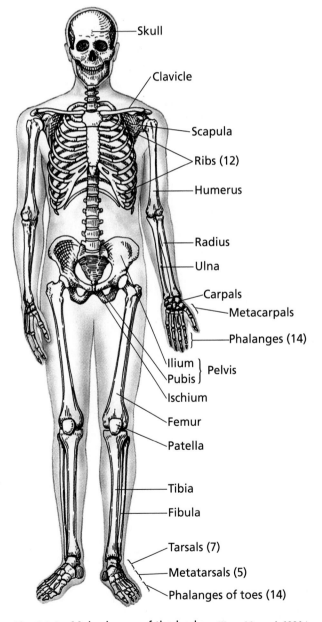

Fig. 21-1 Major bones of the body. *(From Mourad, 1991.)*

Labels on figure: Skull, Clavicle, Scapula, Ribs (12), Humerus, Radius, Ulna, Carpals, Metacarpals, Phalanges (14), Ilium, Pubis, Pelvis, Ischium, Femur, Patella, Tibia, Fibula, Tarsals (7), Metatarsals (5), Phalanges of toes (14)

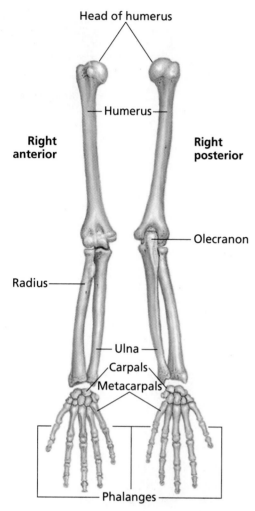

Fig. 21-2   Bones of the arm.   *(From Mourad, 1991.)*

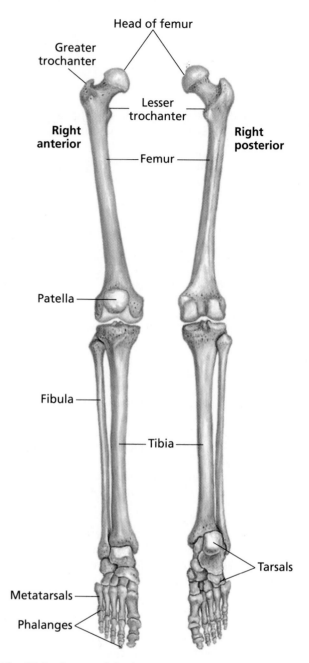

Fig. 21-3   Bones of the leg.   *(From Mourad, 1991.)*

nous, or synovial. Joints also are classified by their degree of movement: immovable joints are synarthrotic, slightly movable joints are amphiarthrotic, and freely movable joints are diarthrotic.

Diarthrotic joints are further classified by their type of movement. Hinge joints permit back and forth extension and flexion; examples are the knee, elbow, and fingers. Pivot joints permit movement of one bone articulating with a ring or notch of another bone, such as the head of the radius, which articulates with the radial notch of the ulna. The ends of saddle-shaped bone articulate with each other; the base of the thumb is the only example. Condyloid or ellipsoidal joints consist of the condyle of one bone that fits into the elliptically shaped portion of its articulating bone; for instance, the distal

Anterior

Posterior

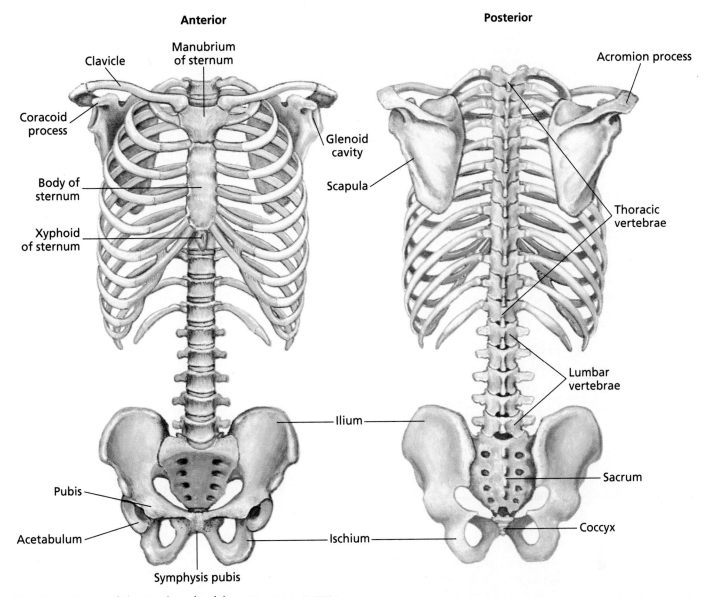

Fig. 21-4　Bones of the trunk and pelvis.　*(From Mourad, 1991.)*

end of the radius articulates with three wrist bones. Ball and socket joints are made of a ball-shaped bone that fits into a concave area of its articulating bone, such as the hip and shoulder joints. Gliding joints permit movement along various axes through relatively flat articulating surfaces, such as joints between two vertebrae.

JOINT MOVEMENT AND RANGE OF MOTION

Only the diarthrotic joints have one or more ranges of motion (Fig. 21-8). These are as follows:

- *Flexion:* A forward bend that decreases the angle between connected bones.
- *Extension:* Straightening a limb, increasing the joint angle.

- *Abduction:* Moving a limb away from the body's midline.
- *Adduction:* Moving a limb toward the body's central axis or beyond it.
- *Internal rotation:* Turning a body part toward midline (the central axis).
- *External rotation:* Turning a body part away from midline.
- *Circumduction:* Circular movement of a body part, accomplished by combining several motions.
- *Supination:* Turning the palm upward.
- *Pronation:* Turning the hand so that the palm faces downward.
- *Inversion:* Turning a hand or foot inward.
- *Eversion:* Turning a hand or foot outward.

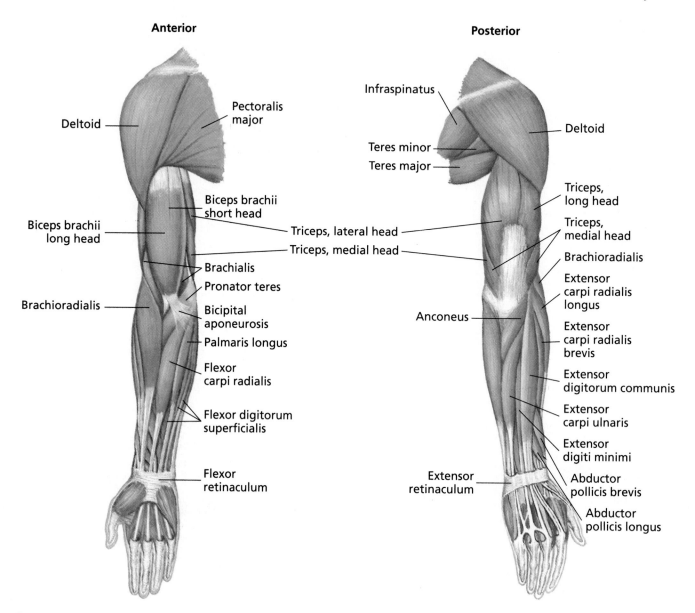

Fig. 21-5 Muscles of the arm. *(From Mourad, 1991.)*

Diarthrotic joints are also called *synovial joints* because they are lined with synovial fluid. Some synovial joints such as the knee also have a disk called the *meniscus,* which is a pad of cartilage that cushions the joint (Fig. 21-9). Synovial joints have a covering surrounding them, called the *joint capsule,* which is an extension of the periosteum of the articulating bone. Ligaments also encase the capsule to add strength.

LIGAMENTS AND TENDONS

The difference between tendons and ligaments is more functional than structural. Ligaments are strong, dense, flexi-

ble bands of connective tissue that hold bones to bones, encircling the joints to add strength and stability. They can provide support in several ways: by encircling the joint, by gripping it obliquely, or by lying parallel to the bone ends, across the joint. They can simultaneously allow some movements while restricting others.

Conversely, tendons are strong, nonelastic cords of collagen located at the ends of muscles to attach them to bones. Tendons support bone movement in response to skeletal muscle contractions, transmitting remarkable force at times from the contracting muscles to the bone without sustaining injury

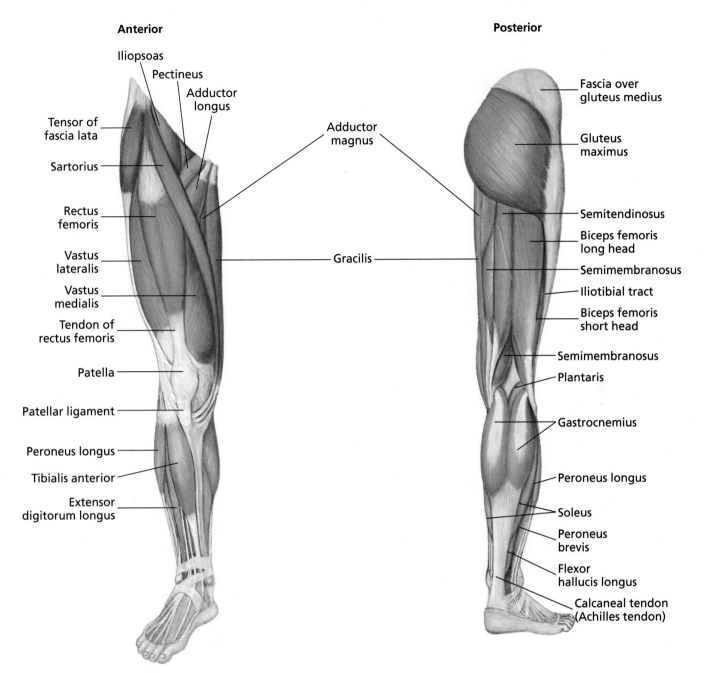

Fig. 21-6 Muscles of the leg. *(From Mourad, 1991.)*

themselves. Ligaments and tendons of the knee joint are shown in Fig. 21-10.

CARTILAGE AND BURSAE

Cartilage is a semismooth, gel-like supporting tissue that forms a cap over the ends of bones, providing a smooth surface for articulation. Cartilage absorbs weight and stress. Because it contains no blood vessels, cartilage receives its nutrition from the synovial fluids forced into it during movement and weight-

bearing activities. For this reason, weight-bearing activity and joint movement are essential to maintaining cartilage health.

Bursae are small sacs or cavities in the connective tissues (usually the tendons) surrounding or near a joint. Each bursa is lined with synovial membrane and contains synovial fluid. Even though bursae are normally part of the musculoskeletal tissues, they can form spontaneously as a result of pressure or friction over a prominent part (see Fig. 21-9).

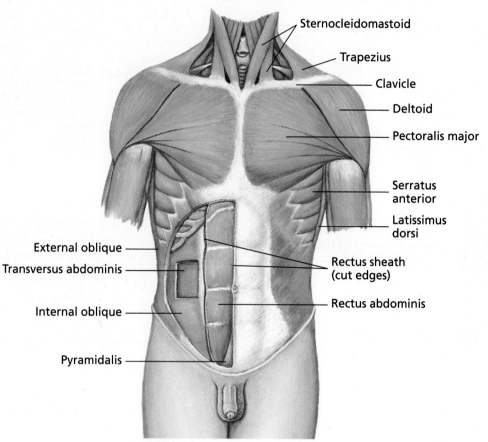

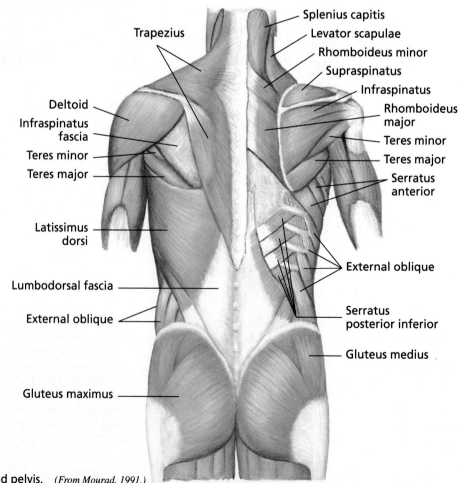

Fig. 21-7   **Muscles of the trunk and pelvis.**   *(From Mourad, 1991.)*

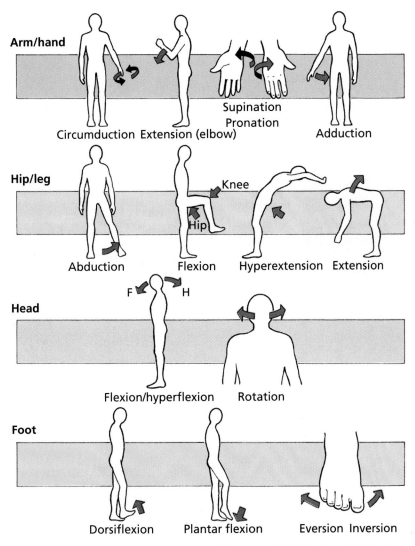

Fig. 21-8 Body movements provided by synovial (diarthrodial) joints. *(From Mourad, 1991.)*

AXIAL SKELETON AND SUPPORTING STRUCTURES

Skull and neck.   The seven bones of the cranium—two frontal, two parietal, two temporal, and one occipital—are fused together. The face consists of eight bones—the nasal, frontal, lacrimal, sphenoid, zygomatic, ethmoid, and maxillary bones and the movable mandible. The neck is supported by the cervical vertebrae, ligaments, and the sternocleidomastoid and trapezius muscles, with its greatest mobility at the level of C4-5 or C5-6. The sternocleidomastoid muscle stretches from the upper sternum and anterior clavicle to the mastoid process; the trapezius links the scapula, the lateral third of the clavicle, and the vertebrae, extending to the occipital prominence.

These muscle and joint connections form triangles that can be used as anatomic landmarks. They are particularly helpful in locating specific lymph nodes.

Spine.   The spine is composed of seven cervical, twelve thoracic, five lumbar, and five sacral vertebrae, which are all sep-arated from each other by fibrocartilaginous disks. The one exception to this is the sacral vertebrae, which are fused. The vertebral joints glide slightly over one another's surfaces, permitting more than one type of movement by creating several axes at each joint. Of all of these, the cervical joints are most active.

APPENDICULAR SKELETON AND SUPPORTING STRUCTURES

Upper extremities.

Shoulder and arm.   The shoulder joint—also called the glenohumeral joint—consists of the point where the humerus and the glenoid fossa of the scapula meet and articulate. The acromion and coracoid processes and surrounding ligaments protect the joint, and contribute to the wide movements possible with this ball-and-socket–type joint. Besides the glenohumeral joint, two other joints contribute to shoulder movement: the acromioclavicular joint (between the acromion process and the clavicle) and the sternoclavicular joint (between the sternal manubrium and the clavicle).

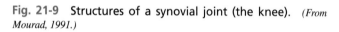

Fig. 21-9   Structures of a synovial joint (the knee).   *(From Mourad, 1991.)*

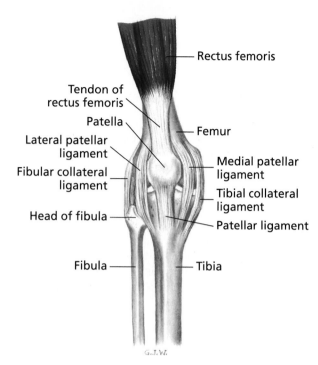

Fig. 21-10   Ligaments and tendons of the knee joint.   *(From Mourad, 1991.)*

Elbow and wrist. The elbow joint consists of the humerus, radius, and ulna enclosed in a single synovial cavity protected by ligaments and a bursa between the olecranon and the skin. The elbow is a hinge joint, permitting movement on one plane. The wrist joins the radius and the carpal bones with articular disks, ligaments, and a fibrous capsule to form a condyloid joint, permitting movement in two planes.

Hand. There are small, subtle movements or articulations within the hand between the carpals and metacarpals, the metacarpals and proximal phalanges, and between the middle and distal phalanges. Ligaments protect the diarthrotic joints, which allow flexion and extension.

Lower extremities.

Hip and thigh. Together the acetabulum and femur form the hip joint, protected by a fibrous capsule and three bursae. Like the shoulder, this is a ball-and-socket joint.

Knee and lower leg. The knee, a hinge joint, is a more complex joint than some. It serves as the point of articulation between the femur, tibia, and patella, making use of fibrocartilaginous disks (medial and lateral menisci), which cushion the tibia and femur and connect to the articulated capsule. Ligaments join the bursae in lending stability, while the bursae reduce friction on movement between the femur and tibia.

Ankle and foot. The ankle joint, or tibiotalar joint, forms a hinge joint, permitting flexion and extension in one plane. It joins the tibia, fibula, and talus with protective medial and lateral ligaments. Smaller joints within the ankle permit a pivot or rotation movement. These are the talocalcaneal (subtalar) joint and the transverse tarsal joint. Like the hand, the foot has several smaller articulations occurring between the tarsals and metatarsals, the metatarsal and proximal phalanges, and the middle and distal phalanges.

⊕ Racial Variation

The following skeletal variations have been documented:
Skull—Frontal bones are thickest in African-American males; parietal bones are thickest in white males.
Face—Protuberances along the suture line of the hard palate and on the lingual surface of the mandible occur in Asian Americans and American Indians and Alaskan Natives as frequently as 50% of the time. They are seen in Hispanics, whites, and African Americans less than 25% of the time.
Long bones—The long bones are longer, narrower, and denser in African Americans than in whites. Bone density is lowest in Asian Americans and Alaskan Natives. Bone density is lower in females than in males across all racial groups.
Femur—Curvature of the femur tends to be straight in African Americans, convex anterior in American Indians and Alaskan Natives, and intermediate in whites.
Humerus—Humeral torsion is more pronounced and one-sided in whites than in African Americans.
Vertebrae—The general population has 24 vertebrae; 11% of African-American females have 23 vertebrae, and 12% of American Indian and Alaskan Natives have 25 vertebrae.
Pelvis—Width of pelvis is largest in white females and smallest in Asian-American females. African-American females have smaller pelvic structure than whites.
Tarsals—Second toe is greater in length than great toe in up to one third of whites and one half of all Asian Americans.

DEVELOPMENTAL CONSIDERATIONS

INFANTS

At birth the cranial bones are soft; they are separated by the sagittal, coronal, and lambdoid sutures. During vaginal births, the skull is molded or shaped by the vaginal canal, causing the cranial bones to overlap or shift. The skull resumes its appropriate size and shape within several days. Membranous spaces where four cranial bones meet and intersect form anterior and posterior fontanels. These fontanels ossify at variable rates, with the posterior fontanel usually closing by 2 months of age and the anterior fontanel closing by 24 months. Brain growth is accommodated by intercranial spaces that permit expansion of the skull. At about 6 years of age, when brain growth declines, these sutures will begin to ossify, a process completed by adulthood.

The infant's spine is flexible, with convex dorsal and sacral curves; extremities have full range of motion at birth. Posture, fine-motor skills, and gross-motor skills develop at a remarkable pace over the first two years of life and beyond.

Proliferation of cartilage at the growth plates increases the length of long bones, while in smaller bones ossification centers form in calcified cartilage. Until adolescence, ligaments will be stronger than bone.

CHILDREN

Throughout childhood long bones increase in diameter and length. There is a specific sequence and timing of bone growth and ossification during this time. Ligaments are stronger than bones until adolescence, increasing the risk of fracture. Muscle fibers lengthen during childhood as the skeletal system grows.

ADOLESCENTS

Facial structure and appearance undergo a variety of subtle changes throughout adolescence. Adolescence is a period of decreased strength and flexibility, enhancing the potential for injury. This is due to the rapid bone growth during this period. Bone growth is completed at about age 20, but bone mass peaks, in both genders, at around age 35.

PREGNANT WOMEN

During pregnancy, lordosis—curvature of the spine—is not uncommon, caused by the weight of the uterus, which usually weighs, at full term, about 12 pounds. This posture may cause backache or aching, numbness, or weakness in the extremities. In addition, ligaments and joints of the spine and pelvis soften under hormonal influence, causing more strain and pelvic instability. In the second half of pregnancy, temporary blood shunting and hypocalcemia may cause muscle cramps, usually in the gastrocnemius, thigh, or gluteal muscles, especially at night or after awakening and initiating movement. After delivery, posture and comfort should soon return to the prepregnancy state.

OLDER ADULTS

The aging process may be accompanied by a number of musculoskeletal changes such as a decrease in bone mass, making the client increasingly vulnerable to stress in weight-bearing areas and resultant fractures. Intervertebral disks become thin and sometimes collapse, while cartilage and ligaments are prone to calcification.

Tendons and muscles decrease in elasticity and tone, with the muscles losing both mass and strength, although this decrease usually does not exceed a 10% to 20% loss at 60 years of age. This alteration in muscle tone and strength means the individual will be less able to perform sudden, intense exercise or to endure exercise for extended periods of time; there will also be a loss of agility.

HEALTH HISTORY | Musculoskeletal System

The history gathered by the examiner in dealing with musculoskeletal areas should focus on the following: pain, weakness, deformity, limitation of motion, stiffness, joint clicking, and self-care behaviors.

QUESTIONS

RATIONALE

PAIN

- When did you first notice the pain? Where do you feel the pain? Describe how the pain feels. How severe is the pain on a scale of 1 to 10, with 10 being the worst pain possible?

◀ Joint pain *is the most common musculoskeletal symptom for which clients seek help. Pain is felt in and around the joint and may be accompanied by edema and erythema. Movement usually makes joint pain worse except in rheumatoid arthritis, in which movement often reduces pain.*

Bone pain is typically described as "deep," "dull," "boring," or "intense." Bone pain frequently is not related to movement unless the bone is fractured, in which case the pain is described as "sharp."

Muscle pain is described as "crampy." Muscle pain that occurs while walking but is relieved by rest is associated with peripheral vascular ischemia. Muscle pain associated with weakness suggests a primary muscular disorder.

- Did the pain occur suddenly? When during the day do you feel the pain? Were you ill before the onset of pain?

◀ *Sudden onset of pain in a joint of the feet suggests gout. Severe pain often awakens clients from sleep. Pain from rheumatoid arthritis and tendinitis may awaken the client, especially when the client is lying on the affected limb.*

- What makes the pain worse? What do you do to relieve the pain? Does the pain change according to the weather? Does the pain shoot to another part of your body?
- Does the pain move from one joint to another? Has there been any injury, overuse, or strain?

◀ *Pain caused by compression of nerves may cause a radiating pain (e.g., spinal nerve roots compressed by a herniated disk may cause radiating pain along the sciatic nerve in the leg). Some disorders cause migratory arthritis in which pain moves among joints (e.g., acute rheumatic fever, leukemia, or juvenile arthritis). Viral illnesses can cause muscle aches and pain (myalgia).*

- Do you have joint stiffness? Is it worse during a particular time of the day?

◀ *Clients with rheumatoid arthritis often have stiff joints after periods of joint rest, especially in the morning.*

QUESTIONS	RATIONALE

■ Have you had a recent sore throat?

◄ *Joint pain that occurs 10 to 14 days after a sore throat may be rheumatic fever.*

■ Are your joints swollen, red, or hot to the touch? Is your range of motion limited?

◄ *Acute inflammation produces redness, warmth, and swelling. Decreased range of motion occurs in injury to the cartilage or capsule or with muscle contractures.*

WEAKNESS AND DEFORMITY

■ Do you feel any weakness in your muscles? Where? How long have you had this? Do the muscles appear smaller in that area?

■ Does the weakness affect your ability to perform daily activities? Do you have trouble standing up after sitting in a chair?

◄ *Proximal muscle weakness is usually a myopathy, while distal weakness is usually a neuropathy.*

◄ *Distinguish muscle weakness from fatigue by asking which activities of daily living the client is unable to perform because of the "weakness"; fatigue usually does not interfere with specific activities.*

■ Does the weakness become worse as the day progresses? Do you have trouble with double vision, swallowing, or chewing?

◄ *Myasthenia gravis, a neurologic disorder, causes muscle weakness with difficulty seeing, swallowing, and chewing. The weakness is relieved by rest.*

■ Do you have any joint or bone deformities? What caused this? Have you noticed a change in the deformity over time? Is your range of motion limited in this area?

◄ *Determine whether the deformity resulted from a congenital malformation or an acquired condition.*

■ Have you ever had any accidents or trauma that affected the bones or joints? This includes fractures, strains of the joints, sprains, and dislocations. When? What was done for the problem? Have you noticed any continuing problems or difficulties that seem related to this previous incident?

◄ *Scar tissue formed after previous injuries may contribute to weakness.*

JOINT CLICKING

■ Do you ever hear a clicking sound when moving joints, for example, extremities, fingers?

◄ *Joint clicking may be associated with the presence of dislocations of the humerus, degenerative joint disease, damaged knee meniscus, or temporomandibular joint problems.*

LIMITATIONS OF SELF-CARE BEHAVIORS

■ What activities are limited by your musculoskeletal problems? Bathing (getting in and out of the tub, turning on or off faucets)? Toileting (urinating, defecating, ability to raise or lower yourself onto or off of the toilet)? Dressing (buttoning, zipping, fastening openings behind your neck, pulling a dress or shirt over your head, pulling up your pants, tying shoes, having shoes fit your feet)? Grooming (shaving, brushing teeth, brushing or fixing hair, applying makeup)? Eating (holding utensils, preparing meals, pouring, cutting up foods, bringing food to your mouth, drinking)? Moving around (walking, going up or down stairs, getting in or out of bed, getting out of the house)? Communicating (writing, talking, using the telephone)?

◄ *Note any impaired mobility or function as a measure of self-care deficit.*

■ Does your job involve heavy lifting, repetitive movements, or chronic stress on the joints?

◄ *These activities may cause weakness or pain from repeated stress and strain on bones, muscles, ligaments, and tendons.*

QUESTIONS

■ *For clients who have chronic disability or a crippling disease:* How has your illness affected your interactions with your family? How has it affected your relationships with friends? How do you feel about yourself?

INFANTS

■ Did the infant suffer any trauma during labor and delivery? Was the baby born head first? Were forceps used? Did the infant need resuscitation?

■ Did the infant achieve developmental milestones at about the same time as other children his or her age or siblings did?

CHILDREN

■ Has the child ever broken or dislocated any bones? Which ones? What treatment was given?
■ Have your ever noticed any bone deformity? Does the child's spine seem curved abnormally? Are the toes or feet abnormally shaped? When did you notice this? Have you ever come for treatment of these problems? What was done?

ADOLESCENTS

■ Are you taking part in any sports at school or after school? Which ones? How frequently?

■ Is any special equipment used? Did you have to undergo a training program before you could participate?

■ Describe your daily warm-up.

■ What do you do if you are hurt during the sport?
■ How does your participation in this sport fit into the rest of your schedule of activities, specifically schoolwork?

OLDER ADULTS

Assess older adult's level of self-care. Assess safety and loss of function, and determine how long the situation has been in existence.

■ Have you had any falls lately? How often? How long has this been a problem?

■ Do you use any mobility aids to help you get around (examples include canes and walkers)?
■ Have you noticed any weaknesses or progression of previous weakness over the last few months or years?

RATIONALE

Assess for disturbance of self-esteem, body image, or role performance; loss of independence; or social isolation.

Trauma during delivery increases the risk for fractures and other injuries to the musculoskeletal system. A period of anoxia can cause hypotonia of the muscles (floppy infant syndrome).
Developmental delays may indicate musculoskeletal disorders.

Trauma to bones may affect growth or create scar tissue that interferes with motion.

Assess safety of this sport, noting specifically the appropriateness of the client's weight and height.
Safe equipment and adequate adult supervision can reduce the risk of injuries during sports activities.
Lack of adequate warm-up, particularly stretching and flexibility training, can increase the risk of injury.
Determine if the adolescent is failing to report injury in order to maintain his or her level of participation.

Falls injure the musculoskeletal system by straining ligaments and tendons and bruising tissues, but they also may cause fractures.
Mobility aids can prevent falls and improve independence.
Decreased muscle mass or a neurologic disorder may cause weakness and increase risk of injuries.

EXAMINATION Procedures and Findings

Guidelines Objective data collection about the client's musculoskeletal system begins when the examiner first meets the client. For example, the examiner observes client's gait and posture; how he or she sits in and rises from a chair; takes off or puts on a coat or jacket; manipulates small objects such as a pen; and rises from a supine position. This will add information to or confirm data collected during the history.

Use a drape to cover the areas not being examined. The client needs to disrobe to undergarments for this examination so that the examiner can examine the muscles, bones, and joints. Adequate light is needed to visualize structures.

Use a cephalocaudal organization with a side-to-side comparison for examining bones, muscles, and joints. This organization provides an inclusive order so that nothing will be overlooked. Examining the musculoskeletal system begins with a general inspection and palpation of the muscles, bones, and joints, followed by a more detailed examination of each body region. The following description begins with the general examination using inspection and palpation, followed by assessment of range of motion and muscle strength. The description then continues by depicting how specific body regions are assessed.

EQUIPMENT Tape measure to record length or circumference of extremities
Goniometer to measure joint motion

TECHNIQUES and NORMAL FINDINGS

ABNORMAL FINDINGS

ROUTINE EXAMINATION

INSPECT skeleton and extremities for Alignment, Contour, Symmetry, Size, and Gross Deformities. Observe the client standing upright and straight from the front, back and sides (Fig. 21-11). He or she should stand erect, with body parts symmetric. The spine should be straight with normal curvatures (cervical concave, thoracic convex, lumbar concave). The knees should be in a straight line between the hips and ankles, and the feet should be flat on the floor and pointing directly forward.

■ Note any inability to maintain straight posture or asymmetry of body parts.

INSPECT the skin and subcutaneous tissues covering muscles, cartilage, bones, and joints for Color, Edema, and Masses.

■ Abnormalities found indicate injuries to underlying tissues.

INSPECT muscles for Symmetry, Size, Fasciculations, or Spasms. Muscle size should appear relatively symmetric bilaterally. (No person has exact symmetry side-to-side.) Muscle circumference can be measured with a cloth or paper tape measure to provide a baseline for future comparisons and to make side-to-side comparisons. Remember that the dominant side usually is slightly larger than the nondominant side. Areas for measurement are found in Table 21-1. To ensure consistency of measurement, record the number of centimeters above or below the joint of the muscle measured or include a diagram like the one shown in Fig. 21-12. Measurement differences less than 1 cm usually are not significant.

■ Atrophy of muscle mass may indicate disuse from lack of neuronal stimulation, such as a spinal cord injury, or from pain on movement. Muscular atrophy also can occur with malnutrition or lipodystrophy.

OBSERVE gait for Conformity, Symmetry, and Rhythm. Ask the client to walk across the room and back. Note conformity (ability to follow gait sequencing of both stance and swing), regular smooth rhythm, symmetry in length of leg swing, smooth swaying related to the gait phase, and smooth, symmetric arm swing.

■ Report any pain or discomfort, unsteadiness, jerky motions, asymmetry or irregularity of stride length, irregular trunk posture, or arm swing that is jerky, asymmetric, or unrelated to gait.

PALPATE bones, joints, and muscles for Tenderness, Heat, Edema, and Crepitus. Muscles should feel firm, not hard or soft. No discomfort, heat, edema, or crepitus should be noted.

■ Tenderness, heat, or edema over bones may indicate tumor or inflammation. Trauma to a bone may also result in nerve damage. Crepitus indicates bone fragments or articular surfaces rubbing together.

A   **B**   **C**

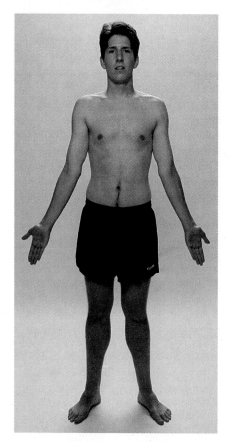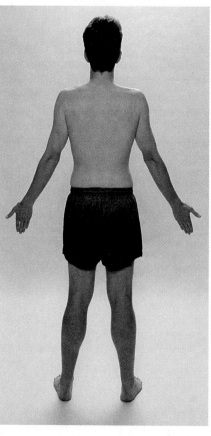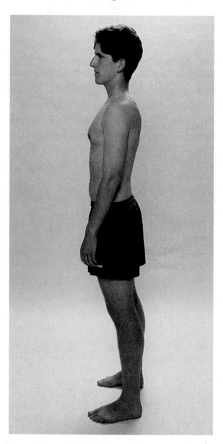

Fig. 21-11   Inspection of overall body posture. Note the even contour of the shoulders, level scapulae and iliac crests, alignment of the head over the gluteal folds, and symmetry and alignment of extremities. **A,** Anterior view. **B,** Posterior view. **C,** Lateral view.

A
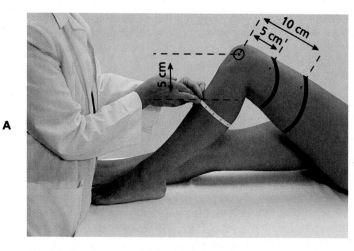
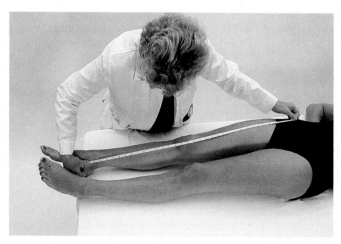
B

Fig. 21-12   Sites at which a limb is measured. Exact location of measurement should be noted for future comparison. **A,** Measurement of midgastrocnemius at 5 cm below patella. **B,** Measurement of limb length.

TECHNIQUES and NORMAL FINDINGS

ABNORMAL FINDINGS

TABLE 21-1	Anatomic Guideposts for Measuring Extremities	
AREA	**FROM**	**TO**
Entire upper extremity	Tip of acromion process	Tip of middle finger
Upper arm	Tip of acromion process	Tip of olecranon process
Forearm	Tip of olecranon process	Styloid process of ulna
Entire lower extremity	Lower edge of anterosuperior iliac spine	Tibial malleolus
Thigh	Lower edge of anterosuperior iliac spine	Medial aspect of knee joint
Lower leg	Medial aspect of knee	Tibial malleolus

Modified from Barkauskas VH et al: Health and physical assessment, *St. Louis, 1994, Mosby.*

ASSESS each major joint and adjacent muscles for Range of Motion, Tenderness of Movement, Joint Stability, Deformity, and Contracture. The client relaxes as the examiner moves the client's joints passively through the full range of motion. Do not force movement of a joint when it is painful or spastic. Then ask the client to perform range of motion actively.

No crepitus should be reported on joint movement.

When a joint seems to have increased or decreased range of motion, use a goniometer to measure the angle (Fig. 21-13). With the joint in neutral position or fully extended, flex the joint as far as possible and measure the angles of greatest flexion and extension.

ASSESS muscle strength and compare contralateral sides. Testing muscle strength may be performed as part of the musculoskeletal or neurologic system examinations. Ask the client to flex the muscle being evaluated and then to resist when you apply opposing force against that flexion. Compare the muscle strength bilaterally. (Descriptions of muscle testing are shown in Table 21-2.) Expect muscle strength to be bilaterally symmetric, with full resistance to opposition. Full muscle strength requires full, active range of motion. Muscle strength is graded on a scale of 0-5, as described in Table 21-3.

■ Limited range of motion may indicate inflammation such as arthritis; fluid in the joint; altered nerve supply; or contracture of muscle, ligament, or capsule. By contrast, increased mobility of a joint may indicate connective tissue disruption, tear of a ligament, or an interarticular fracture.

■ Crepitus is a crackling sound produced by movement of a joint that has irregularities in the articulating surfaces (e.g., osteoarthritis).

■ Differences between active and passive range of motion may indicate an actual muscle weakness or a joint disorder.

■ Muscle weakness may indicate a neurologic, muscular, or joint disease.

TECHNIQUES and NORMAL FINDINGS

ABNORMAL FINDINGS

TABLE 21-2   Screening Tests for Muscle Strength

MUSCLES TESTED	CLIENT ACTIVITY	EXAMINER ACTIVITY
Ocular musculature		
Lids	Close eyes tightly	Attempt to resist closure
Eye muscles	Track object in six cardinal positions	
Facial musculature	Blow out cheeks	Assess pressure in cheeks with fingertips
	Place tongue in cheek	Assess pressure in cheek with fingertips
	Stick out tongue, move it to right and left	Observe strength and coordination of thrust and extension
Neck muscles	Extend head backward	Push head forward
	Flex head forward	Push head backward
	Rotate head in full circle	Observe mobility, coordination
	Touch shoulders with head	Observe range of motion
Deltoid	Hold arms upward	Push down on arms
Biceps	Flex arm	Pull to extend arm
Triceps	Extend arm	Push to flex arm
Wrist musculature	Extend hand	Push to flex
	Flex hand	Push to extend
Finger muscles	Extend fingers	Push dorsal surface of fingers
	Flex fingers	Push ventral surface of fingers
	Spread fingers	Hold fingers together
Hip musculature	In supine position raise extended leg	Push down on leg above knee
Hamstring, gluteal, abductor, and adductor muscles of leg	Sit and perform alternate leg crossing	Push in opposite direction of crossing limb
Quadriceps	Extend leg	Push to flex leg
Hamstring	Bend knees to flex leg	Push to extend leg
Ankle and foot muscles	Bend foot up (dorsiflexion)	Push to plantar flexion
	Bend foot down (plantar flexion)	Push to dorsiflexion
Antigravity muscles	Walk on toes	
	Walk on heels	

From Barkauskas VH et al: Health and physical assessment, *St. Louis, 1994,*
Mosby.

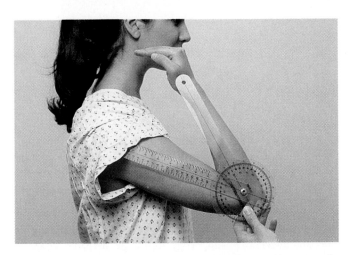

Fig. 21-13   Use of goniometer to measure joint range of motion.

TABLE 21-3	Criteria for Grading and Recording Muscle Strength		
FUNCTIONAL LEVEL	**LOVETT SCALE**	**GRADE**	**PERCENT OF NORMAL**
No evidence of contractility	Zero (0)	0	0
Evidence of slight contractility	Trace (T)	1	10
Complete range of motion with gravity eliminated	Poor (P)	2	25
Complete range of motion with gravity	Fair (F)	3	50
Complete range of motion against gravity with some resistance	Good (G)	4	75
Complete range of motion against gravity with full resistance	Normal (N)	5	100

From Barkauskas VH et al: Health and physical assessment, *St. Louis, 1994, Mosby.*

TECHNIQUES and NORMAL FINDINGS

ABNORMAL FINDINGS

EXAMINATION OF SPECIFIC MUSCULOSKELETAL REGIONS

Have the client sit on the examination table while you observe the musculature of the face and neck for symmetry.

■ Asymmetry, atrophy, or hypertrophy are all abnormal findings.

Ask the client to open and close his or her mouth.

PALPATE each temporomandibular joint in front of the tragus of each ear for Movement, Sounds, and Tenderness. The mandible should move smoothly and painlessly. An audible or palpable snapping or clicking is not unusual. (See Fig. 11-14.)

■ Note any pain, limited range of motion, or crepitus of the temporomandibular joint (TMJ). Pain, crepitus, locking or popping indicate a temporomandibular joint disorder.

ASSESS range of motion. Ask the client to open and close the mouth. It should open between 3 and 6 cm (1.5 and 2.5 inches) between upper and lower teeth (Fig. 21-14, *A*). Ask the client to move the jaw side to side; the mandible should move 1 to 2 cm (0.375 to 0.75 inch) in each direction (Fig. 21-14, *B*). Finally, the client should be able to protrude and retract the chin without difficulty or pain.

■ Difficulty opening the mouth may result from injury or arthritic changes. Pain in the TMJ may indicate malocclusion of teeth or arthritic changes. Muscle spasms secondary to trigeminal neuralgia may occur.

Test Muscle Strength. Muscle strength of the temporalis muscle is assessed by asking the client to clench the teeth while the examiner palpates the contracted muscle and applies opposing force. This procedure also tests the trigeminal nerve (cranial nerve V).

A
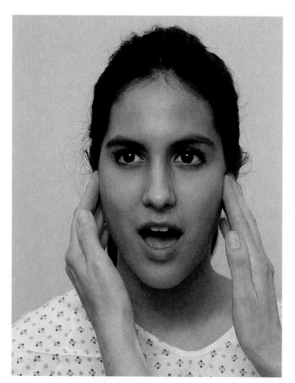

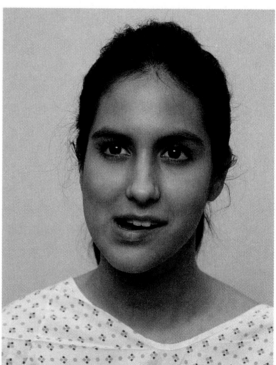
B

Fig. 21-14   **A,** Palpation of temporomandibular joint. **B,** Lateral range of motion in the temporomandibular joint.

TECHNIQUES and NORMAL FINDINGS

ABNORMAL FINDINGS

INSPECT cervical spine for Alignment and Symmetry; PALPATE the posterior neck, cervical spine, paravertebral muscles, and trapezius muscle for Tenderness. Note the position of C7 and T1. The cervical spine should show no evidence of pain.

PALPATE neck for Masses, Enlarged Lymph Nodes, Sensation, and Range of Motion. The neck is soft, firm without numbness or tingling, spasms, or palpable lymph nodes and masses.

ASSESS neck for Range of Motion. Ask the client to flex chin to the chest. It should move to a point 45° from midline.

Ask the client to hyperextend the head; it should reach 55° from midline (Fig. 21-15, *A*).

Have the client laterally bend his or her head to the right and the left. Range should be 40° from midline each way (Fig. 21-15, *B*).

Have the client rotate the chin to the shoulders first to the right and then to the left. It should reach 70° from midline (Fig. 21-15, *C*).

■ Tenderness, nodules, or muscular spasms should be noted. Hyperextension and flexion may be limited because of cervical vertebral disk or osteoarthritic changes.

■ Note limited or painful range of motion.
■ Changes in sensation may indicate compression of cervical spinal root nerves. Lymph node assessment is in Chapter 9. Enlargement may indicate inflammation or lymphoma.

■ Note any crepitus of the cervical spine.

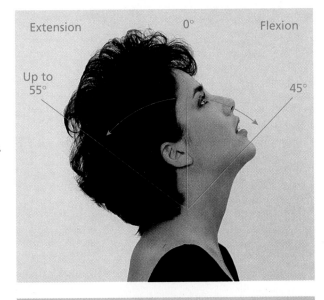

A

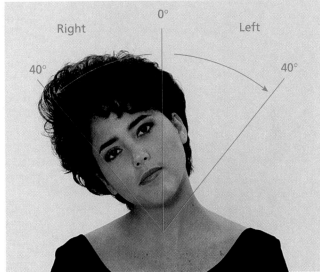

B

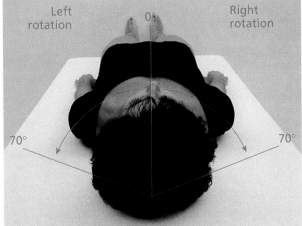

C

Fig. 21-15 Range of motion of the cervical spine. **A,** Flexion and hyperextension. **B,** Lateral bending. **C,** Rotation.

TECHNIQUES and NORMAL FINDINGS

ABNORMAL FINDINGS

ASSESS neck muscles for Strength. To assess muscle strength of the neck, ask client to repeat the rotation of the head against resistance of your hand to test strength of the sternocleidomastoid muscle (Fig. 21-16, *A*). Ask client to flex chin to the chest and maintain the position while the examiner palpates the sternocleidomastoid muscle and tries to manually force the head upright. If reasonable muscle strength is present, you should be unable to force the head upright (Fig. 21-16, *B*).

Have the client hyperextend the head and maintain position while you try to manually force the head upright to assess the trapezius muscle strength (Fig. 21-16, *C*). If reasonable muscle strength is present, you should be unable to force the head upright.

■ Note if you can break the muscular flexion before the anticipated point.

■ Note if you are able to break muscular flexion before the anticipated point.

A
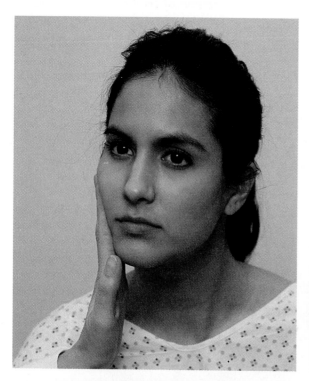

B
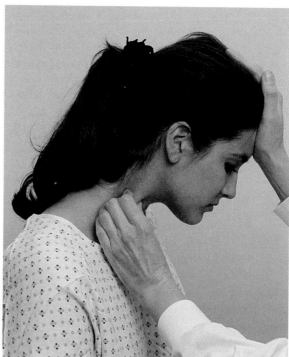

C
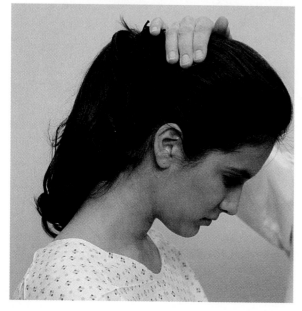

Fig. 21-16 Examining the strength of the sternocleidomastoid and trapezius muscles. **A,** Rotation against resistance. **B,** Flexion with palpation of the sternocleidomastoid muscle. **C,** Extension against resistance.

TECHNIQUES and NORMAL FINDINGS

ABNORMAL FINDINGS

INSPECT the spine, iliac crests, and shoulders for Alignment and Symmetry. Ask the client to move from a standing position to a straight bend to touching the toes. Spine should be straight, iliac crests and shoulders at equal height, and thoracic spine convex (Fig. 21-17).

■ Note any lateral deviation of the spine or asymmetry of shoulder or iliac height. Scoliosis is a lateral curvature of the spine; lordosis is an anterior curvature (concavity) of the spine; kyphosis is a posterior curvature (convexity) of the thoracic spine.

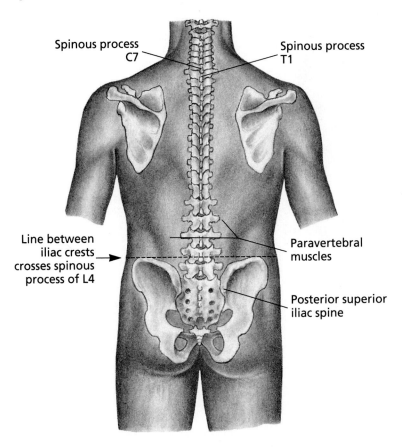

Spinous process C7

Spinous process T1

Line between iliac crests crosses spinous process of L4

Paravertebral muscles

Posterior superior iliac spine

Fig. 21-17   Landmarks of the back.   *(From Seidel et al, 1995.)*

TEST Range of Motion. Observe range of motion as client slowly bends forward and touches toes; should be able to reach 75° flexion (Fig. 21-18, *A*).

Observe for range of motion as client *hyperextends* the spine; it should reach 30° back from the neutral position (Fig. 21-18, *B*).

Ask the client to *bend* laterally right and left. *Note:* It may be necessary to stabilize the client's hips. He or she should be able to reach 35° of flexion both ways from midline (Fig. 21-18, *C*).

Have the client *rotate* the upper trunk (you may need to stabilize pelvis) to the right and left; he or she should achieve 30° of rotation in both directions from a directly forward position (Fig. 21-18, *D*).

■ Note inability to hyperextend without losing balance or pain.
■ Note any decreased ability to flex to 35° or pain on flexion.

■ Note any decreased ability to rotate or discomfort rotating.

TECHNIQUES and NORMAL FINDINGS

ABNORMAL FINDINGS

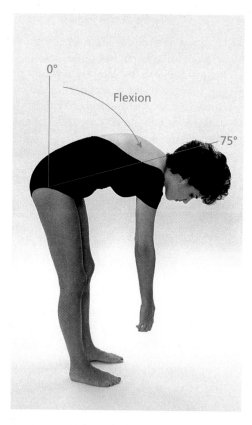

A

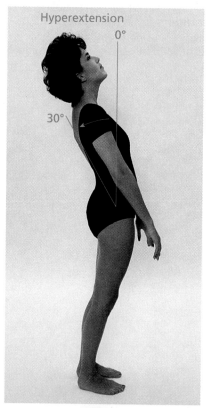

B

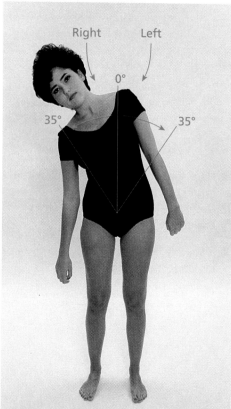

C

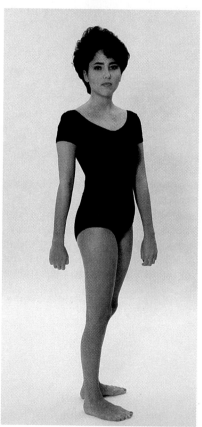

D

Fig. 21-18   Range of motion of the thoracic and lumbar spine. **A,** Flexion. **B,** Hyperextension. **C,** Lateral bending. **D,** Rotation of the upper trunk.

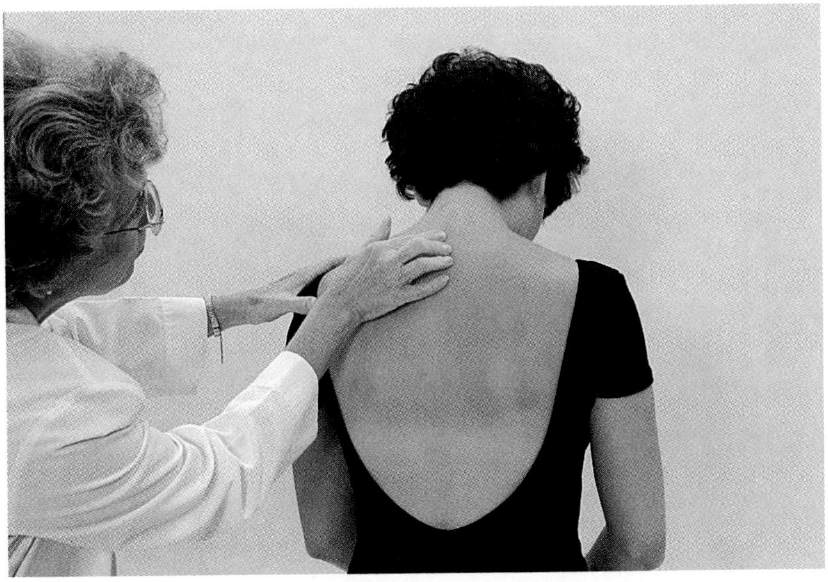

Fig. 21-19 Palpation of the spinal processes of the vertebrae.

PALPATE spinal processes and paravertebral muscles for Alignment and Tenderness. The spine should be straight and nontender. (*Note:* It may be helpful to have the client hunch his or her shoulders forward and slightly flex the neck [Fig. 21-19].)

PERCUSS spinal processes for Tenderness. First tap each process with one finger, and then lightly tap each side of the spine with the ulnar surface of your fist. No muscle spasm or tenderness should be noted to palpation or percussion.

INSPECT the shoulders and shoulder girdle for Equality of Height and Contour. Inspect both scapulae and clavicles and the acromioclavicular junction for equality of height and symmetry. Observe the trapezius muscle for shape and size. All structures should be smooth, regular, and bilaterally symmetric. Shoulders should be rounded and firm, with smooth contour and no bony prominences. Each shoulder should be equidistant from the vertebral column and located over thoracic ribs two through seven. Trapezius muscles are firm, full, and supple.

PALPATE the shoulders for Firmness, Fullness, Tenderness, and Masses. This includes the acromioclavicular joint, trapezius muscle, humerus, and biceps, triceps, and deltoid. These areas should be nontender, smooth, firm and full without masses, and bilaterally symmetric. The muscles of the dominant arm may be slightly larger.

TEST trapezius muscles for Strength. Ask the client to shrug shoulders while you attempt to push them down (Fig. 21-20).

■ Curvature of the spine, tenderness, and spasm of paravertebral muscles should be reported.

■ Tenderness or pain along spinous processes may indicate arthritis or diskitis. Radicular pain down the leg may indicate herniation of a disk.

■ Note any redness, swelling, or nodules. Shoulder joints may have some deformity from trauma or arthritic changes. Pain or functional changes may be noted from cervical arthropathy or secondary cerebrovascular accident involving paralysis of one arm.

■ Note any tenderness, pain, or edema.

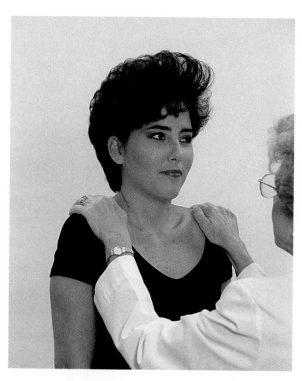

Fig. 21-20   Test strength of the trapezius muscle with the shrugged shoulder movement.

ASSESS the shoulders for Range of Motion. Ask the client to extend arms straight up beside the head. Arms should reach 180 degrees from resting neutral position, be bilaterally equal, and show no discomfort (Fig. 21-21, *A*).

Ask the client to hyperextend the arms backward. They should reach 50° and be bilaterally equal and without discomfort.

Ask client to lift both arms laterally over head. Expected shoulder abduction is 180°. Then ask client to swing each arm across the front of the body. Expected adduction is 50° (Fig. 21-21, *B*).

To test external rotation, have the client start in an abducted location with the arms extended directly forward from the shoulder. Then have client place the hands behind the head with elbows out. A range of 90° is normal, and should be bilaterally equal and without discomfort (Fig. 21-21, *C*).

To test internal rotation, ask the client to start with the forearms extended in abducted location, then place the hands behind the small of back. Range should be 90°, with movements bilaterally equal and without discomfort (Fig. 21-21, *D*).

■ Limited range of motion, pain with movement, crepitations, and asymmetry are abnormal findings.
■ Note limited range of motion, pain with movement, crepitations, and asymmetry.

■ Note any limitation of movement, pain, crepitations or asymmetry.

■ Note limited range of motion, pain, crepitations, or asymmetry.

TECHNIQUES and NORMAL FINDINGS

ABNORMAL FINDINGS

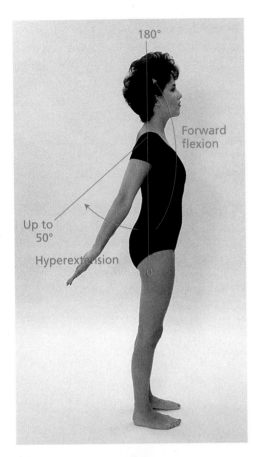

A

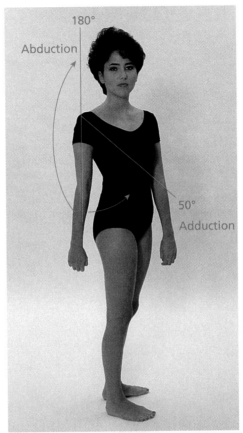

B

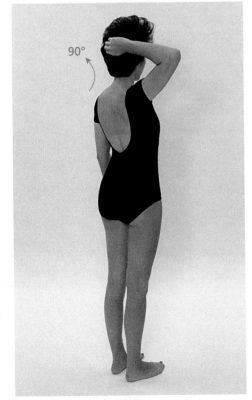

C

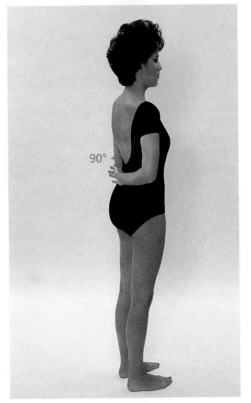

D

Fig. 21-21　Range of motion of the shoulders. **A,** Forward flexion and hyperextension. **B,** Abduction and adduction. **C,** External rotation. **D,** Internal rotation.

TECHNIQUES and NORMAL FINDINGS

ABNORMAL FINDINGS

ASSESS arms for Muscle Strength. Have the client hold arms up while you try to push them down. They should be bilaterally strong and you should not be able to move them out of position.

To test triceps muscle strength, ask client to extend arm while you resist by pushing arm to a flexed position (Fig. 21-22, *A*).

To test biceps strength, have client try to flex the arm into a fighting position while you try to extend his or her forearm. The examiner should be unable to move the arm out of position, and strength should be equal bilaterally (Fig. 21-22, *B*).

INSPECT the elbows in flexed and extended position for Contour and Carrying Angle. Expected carrying angle is between 5° and 15° laterally. They should have smooth, firm contour.

PALPATE the elbow for Tenderness. Note intact skin over the extensor surface of the ulna; smooth olecranon process (Fig. 21-23); nontender area without nodules or discomfort over groove on either side of olecranon; and painless, nontender lateral epicondyle.

■ Abnormal findings include symmetrically unequal response, weak response, pain during testing, or muscular spasm.

■ Note any areas of swelling, inflammation, general tenderness, subcutaneous nodules, point tenderness, or palpable nodes. Subcutaneous nodules at pressure points of the ulnar surface may indicate rheumatoid arthritis.

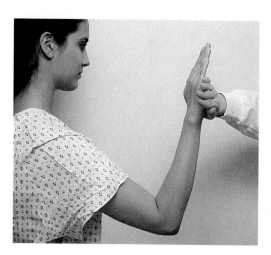

A

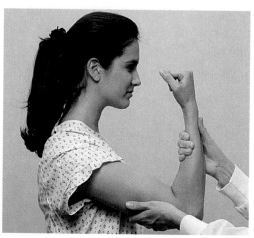

B

Fig. 21-22　Testing muscle strength of arms. **A,** Testing triceps muscle strength. **B,** Testing biceps muscle strenth.

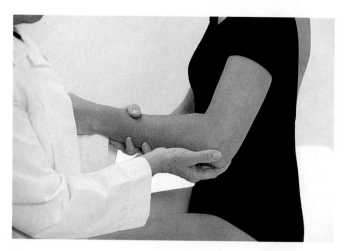

Fig. 21-23　Palpation of the olecranon process grooves.

TECHNIQUES and NORMAL FINDINGS

Ask the client to flex and extend the elbow; 160° of full movement should be present bilaterally without discomfort (Fig. 21-24, *A*).

Assess pronation and supination of elbow by having client rotate hands palms up and palms down (pronate and supinate). Ninety degrees should be achieved in each direction, and the movements should be bilaterally equal and without discomfort (Fig. 21-24, *B*).

ABNORMAL FINDINGS

■ Note any limitation to the movement, asymmetry of movement, or pain at the elbow.

■ Note any limitation of motion, asymmetry of movement, or pain at the elbow. Subcutaneous nodules just inferior to olecranon process (elbow joint) may indicate rheumatoid arthritis. Tenderness or pain with pronation and supination of the elbow and point tenderness on the lateral epicondyle may indicate tendinitis or epicondylitis (tennis elbow), while point tenderness on the medial epicondyle may indicate golfer's elbow.

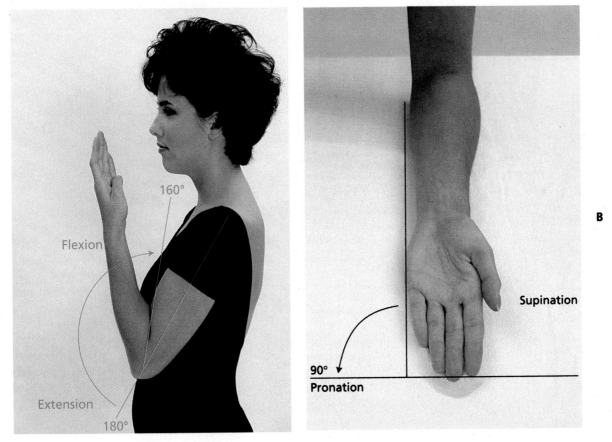

A **B**

Fig. 21-24 **Range of motion of the elbow. A,** Flexion and extension. **B,** Palm up, supination; palm down, pronation.

TECHNIQUES and NORMAL FINDINGS

ABNORMAL FINDINGS

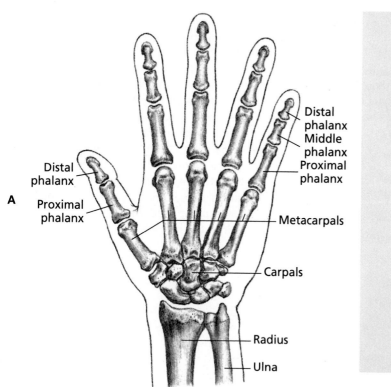

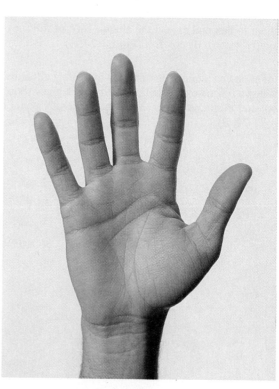

Fig. 21-25 **A,** Bony structures of the right hand and wrist. Note alignment of fingers with the radius. **B,** Palmar aspect of right hand. *(A From Seidel et al, 1995.)*

INSPECT joints of both wrists and hands for Position, Contour, and Number of Digits. They should be smooth, firm, and symmetric, with no edema or deformities. The hand with five digits is aligned with the wrist, and fingers are aligned with wrist and forearm (Fig. 21-25, *A* and *B*).

■ Edema of the wrist joint usually appears on the dorsal surface distal to the ulnar tip. Rheumatoid arthritis may cause wrists and interphalangeal joints to appear hot, tender, painful, deformed, and edematous. Swan neck and boutonniere deformities of interphalangeal joints may be related to rheumatoid arthritis. Osteoarthritis may cause Bouchard nodes in proximal interphalangeal (PIP) joints, while Heberden nodes (Fig. 21-26) form in the distal interphalangeal (DIP) joints.

PALPATE each joint of the hand and wrist for Surface Characteristics and Tenderness. Palpate interphalangeal joints with your thumb and index finger. Palpate metacarpophalangeal joints with both thumbs. Palpate wrist and radiocarpal groove with your thumbs on the dorsal surface and your fingers on the palmar surface. Joint surfaces should be smooth without nodules, edema or tenderness (Fig. 21-27, *A, B, C*).

■ Painful, edematous joints are found in osteoarthritis. A firm mass over the dorsum of the wrist may be a ganglion. Note asymmetric responses or pain on movement.

TECHNIQUES and NORMAL FINDINGS

ABNORMAL FINDINGS

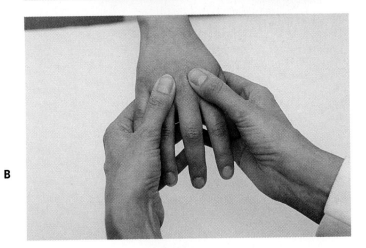

A

B

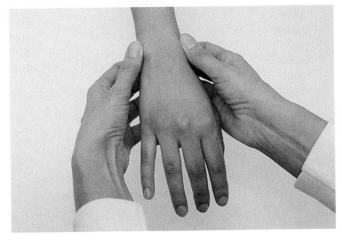

C

Fig. 21-27   Palpation of joints of the hand and wrist. **A,** Interphalangeal joints. **B,** Metacarpophalangeal joints. **C,** Radiocarpal groove and wrist.

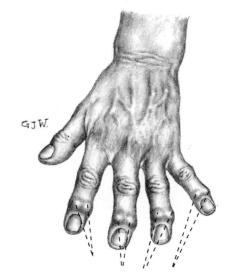

Heberden's nodes

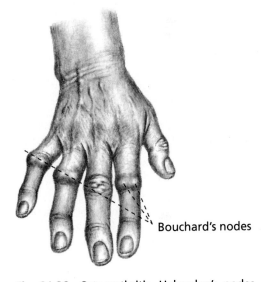

Bouchard's nodes

Fig. 21-26   Osteoarthritis. Heberden's nodes and Bouchard's nodes.   *(From Mourad, 1991.)*

TECHNIQUES and NORMAL FINDINGS

ABNORMAL FINDINGS

A

B

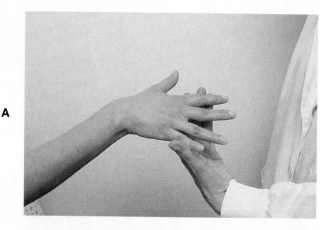

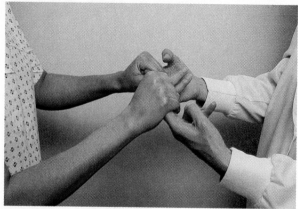

Fig. 21-28   **A,** Assessment of finger strength. **B,** Assessment of grip strength.

ASSESS hands and fingers for Muscle Strength and Range of Motion.

First, ask client to extend and spread fingers (both hands) while you attempt to push fingers together (Fig. 21-28, *A*). The response should be symmetric, to full flexion and extension, without discomfort and with sufficient muscle strength to overcome resistance applied by examiner.

Next, have the client grip your first two fingers on each hand. The response should be bilaterally equal, and the grip tight (Fig. 21-28, *B*).

Observe the range of motion of both hands and wrists as the client bends the hand up at the wrist (hyperextension to 70°), flexes the hand down at the wrist (palmar flexion of 90°) (Fig. 21-29, *A*), and flexes the fingers up and down at the metacarpophalangeal joints (flexion of 90°, hyperextension of 30°) (Fig. 21-29, *B*).

Then, with the client's palms flat on the table, ask the client to turn them outward and in (ulnar deviation of 50° to 60°, radial deviation of 20°) (Fig. 21-29, *C*), spread the fingers apart (Fig. 21-29, *D*), and then make a fist (abduction of 20°, fist tight) (Fig. 21-29, *E*), and touch the thumb to each finger (opposition) and to the base of the fifth finger (able to perform all motions) (Fig. 21-29, *F*). These findings should be bilaterally equal.

■ Note any inequality of response or decreased response.

■ Note any limitation of movement or pain or discomfort with movements.

🌐 Racial Variation

The palmaris longus muscle, responsible for wrist flexion, is absent in up to 20% of whites and 12% of American Indians. Its absence is a rare finding in African Americans and Asian Americans.

TECHNIQUES and NORMAL FINDINGS

ABNORMAL FINDINGS

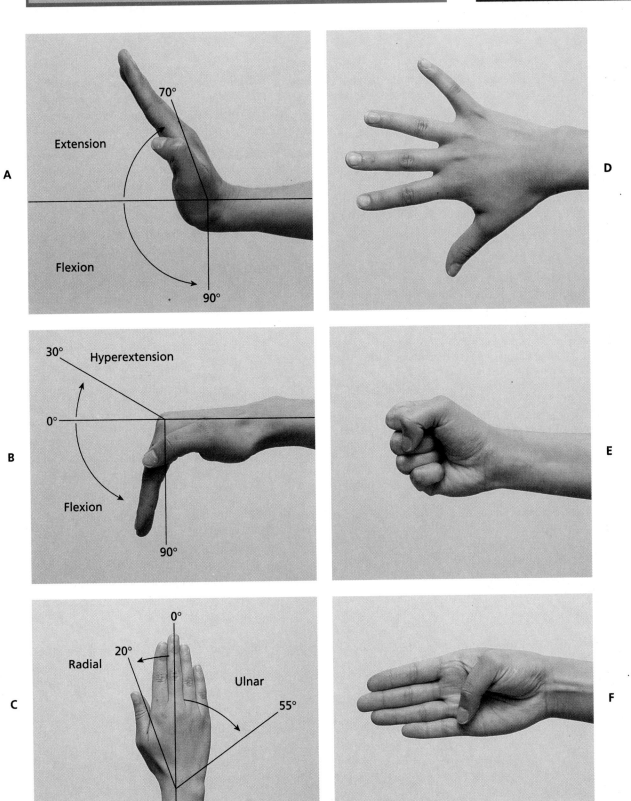

Fig. 21-29   Range of motion of hand and wrist. **A,** Wrist flexion and hyperextension. **B,** Metacarpophalangeal flexion and hyperextension. **C,** Wrist radial and ulnar movement. **D,** Finger abduction. **E,** Finger flexion: fist formation. **F,** Finger flexion: thumb to each fingertip and to base of little finger.

TECHNIQUES and NORMAL FINDINGS	ABNORMAL FINDINGS

Have client lie supine.

INSPECT both hips for Symmetry. PALPATE hips for Stability and Tenderness. Use the iliac crests and greater trochanter of the femur as landmarks. Findings should be bilaterally symmetric with stable, painless hip areas.

- ■ Note any painful area as to whether it is diffuse or pinpoint tenderness and report any crepitations. Bursae are not palpable unless they are edematous.

TEST hips for Range of Motion. To evaluate hip range of motion, ask client to alternately pull each knee up to the chest. Client should achieve 120° flexion from the straight, extended position. (Fig. 21-30, *A*)

Next, have the client raise the leg to flex the hip as far as possible without bending the knee. Results should be 90° from the straight extended position (Fig. 21-30, *B*).

- ■ Note any limitation of motion, pain or discomfort with movement, flexion of the opposite thigh, and crepitations.
- ■ Note limited range of motion, pain or discomfort with motion, and crepitations. Back pain caused by straight leg raises may indicate compression of spinal nerve roots.

Ask the client to place the lateral aspect of one foot on the opposite patella to test external hip rotation (Patrick test). Rotation should reach 45° from the straight midline position (Fig. 21-30, *C*).

To test hip for internal rotation, ask client to flex the knee and turn medially (inward) as you pull the heel laterally (outward) to test internal hip rotation. Rotation should reach 40° from the straight midline position (Fig. 21-30, *D*).

Ask client to move leg with knee straight laterally to test abduction and medially to test adduction. Expected range for abduction is up to 45°, and for adduction up to 30° (Fig. 21-30, *E*).

With client standing or prone, test hyperextension of hip by swinging leg with knee straight behind body. Expected range of movement is up to 30° (Fig. 21-30, *F*).

- ■ Report limited range of motion, pain or discomfort with movement, or crepitations.
- ■ Note limited range of motion, pain or discomfort with movement, or crepitation.

TEST hips for Muscle Strength. Have the client lie supine. Ask him or her to attempt to raise the legs while you try to hold them down. Evaluate one leg at a time, noting if the response is bilaterally strong and if you are unable to deter the movement.

- ■ Note symmetric unequal responses, weak responses, and pain during testing.

To test the quadriceps, have the client extend the legs at the knee while you attempt to flex the knee. Strength should be bilaterally equal, and you should be unable to flex the knee.

To evaluate the hamstrings, have the client attempt to bend his or her knee while you attempt to straighten it. Strength should be bilaterally equal, and you should be unable to flex the knee.

- ■ Note if responses are asymmetric or weak or if there is pain during the testing.
- ■ Note asymmetric or weak responses, or pain during the evaluation.

Client should be supine or sitting.

INSPECT both knees for Symmetric Alignment, Edema, or Erythema.

- ■ Report if the knee appears edematous, bowlegged (genu valgum), knock-kneed (genu varum), thick, boggy, or inflamed.

TECHNIQUES and NORMAL FINDINGS

ABNORMAL FINDINGS

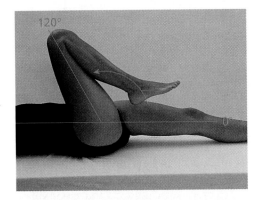

A

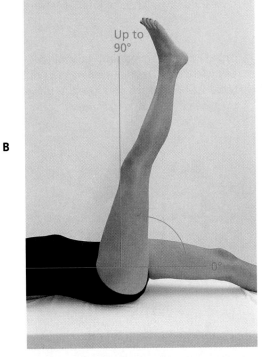

B

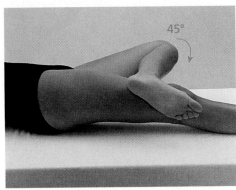

C

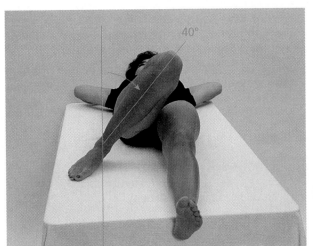

D

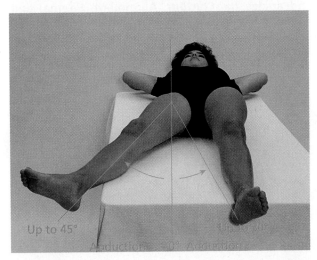

E

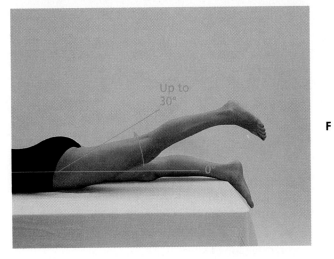

F

Fig. 21-30 Range of motion of hips. **A,** Hip flexion, knee flexed. **B,** Hip flexion, leg extended. **C,** External rotation of hip. **D,** Internal rotation of hip. **E,** Abduction and adduction of hip. **F,** Hyperextension of hip, leg extended.

TECHNIQUES and NORMAL FINDINGS

PALPATE knees for Contour and Tenderness. First, palpate the suprapatellar pouch on each side of the quadriceps with the thumb and fingers of one or both hands; it should feel smooth and nontender.

Next, compress the suprapatellar pouch with one hand; then palpate each side of the patella and over the tibiofemoral joint space. These areas should be smooth and nontender.

Palpate the popliteal space for contour, tenderness, and edema. It should be smooth and nontender.

TEST knees for Range of Motion. Evaluate the knees' range of motion by having the client flex the knees (Fig. 21-31). Flexion should reach 130° from the straight extended position without discomfort or difficulty.

ASSESS knee muscles for Strength. Apply opposing force while client tries to maintain flexion and extension.

INSPECT the feet and ankles for Contour, Alignment, Edema, and Number of Toes. They should be smooth, with no edema or deformity; five toes maintain extended and straight position on each foot, and feet maintain straight position aligned with long axis of lower leg.

ABNORMAL FINDINGS

- Note bogginess, thickening, tenderness, or pain. Edema of the suprapatellar pouch may indicate synovitis.
- Note any bogginess, thickening, tenderness, or pain.

- Note tenderness, redness, nodules, or edema. Popliteal edema is more noticeable when the knee is extended.

- Note any decreased range of motion, pain with movement, or crepitation.

- Note muscle weakness or joint instability.

- Note any inflammation, edema over any joint, gout, medial deviation of the toes, hallux valgus (Fig. 21-32), clawtoes, hammer toes, or calluses.

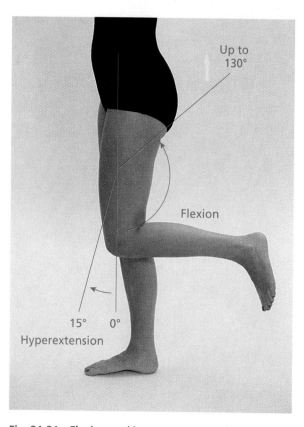

Fig. 21-31   Flexion and hyperextension of knee.

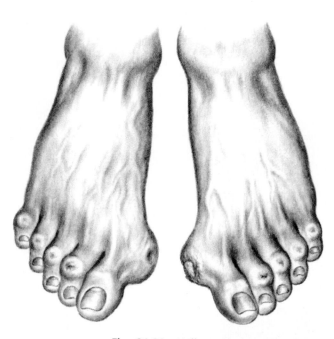

Fig. 21-32   Hallux valgus with bunions and hammer toes. *(From Mourad, 1991.)*

TECHNIQUES and NORMAL FINDINGS	**ABNORMAL FINDINGS**

PALPATE the feet and ankles for Contour and Tenderness. These structures should be smooth and nontender.

■ Note tenderness (diffuse versus pinpoint), edema, inflammation, ulcerations, or nodules.

TEST the feet and ankles for Range of Motion. To evaluate the range of motion of both feet and ankles, have the client dorsiflex and plantar flex the foot. Dorsiflexion should reach 20° from midline, and plantar flexion 45° from midline (Fig. 21-33, *A*). Then have the client invert and evert the foot. (*Note:* You may need to stabilize the heel during these maneuvers.) Inversion is 30° and eversion 20° from midline position (Fig. 21-33, *B*). Next, ask the client to rotate the ankle, turning the foot away from and then toward the other foot while the examiner stabilizes the leg. Expect abduction of 10° and adduction of 20° (Fig. 21-33, *C*). Finally, have the client flex and extend the toes. These should be active movements. All movements should be bilaterally equal and without discomfort.

■ Note limitations in the range of motion, pain, crepitations, and asymmetry.

TEST the feet and ankle muscles for Strength. Ask the client to maintain dorsiflexion and plantar flexion while you apply opposing force to evaluate strength of ankle muscles. Abduction and adduction of the ankle and flexion and extension of the great toe may also be used to assess muscle strength.

■ Note responses that are unequal, weak, or produce pain.

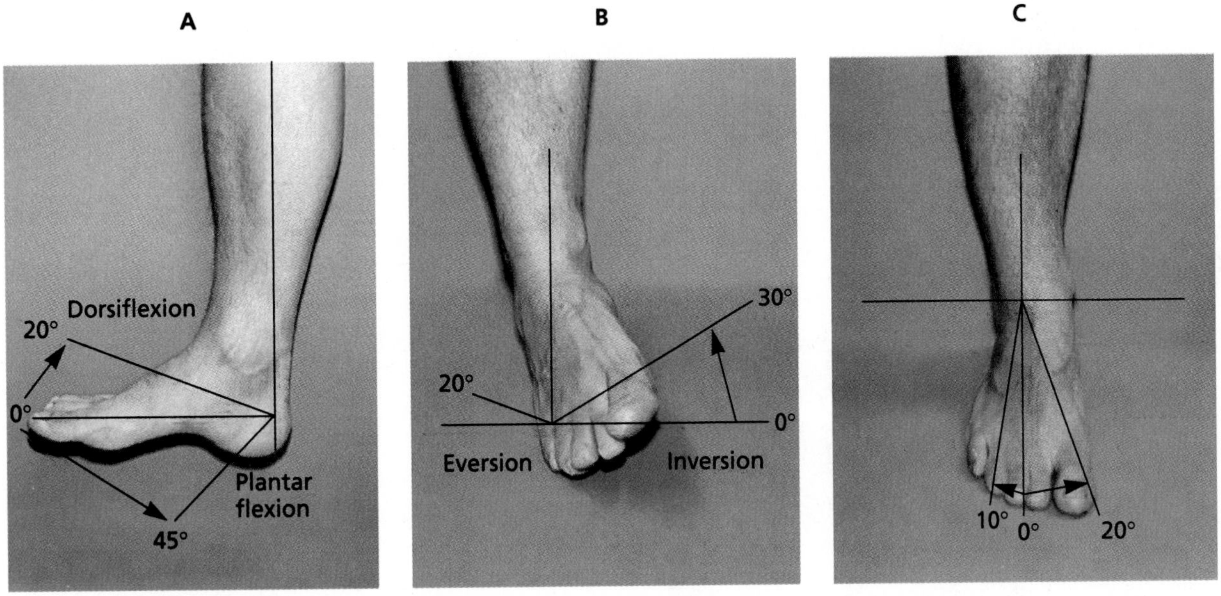

🌐 Racial Variation

The peroneus tertius muscle responsible for dorsiflexion of the foot is absent in 15% of African Americans and 10% of Asian Americans and American Indians/Alaskan Natives.

A   **B**   **C**

Fig. 21-33 **Range of motion of the ankle. A,** Dorsiflexion and plantar flexion. **B,** Inversion and eversion. **C,** Abduction and adduction. *(From Seidel et al, 1995.)*

TECHNIQUES and NORMAL FINDINGS   **ABNORMAL FINDINGS**

ADDITIONAL ASSESSMENT TECHNIQUES FOR SPECIAL CASES

There are two tests for carpal tunnel syndrome (see Common Problems/Conditions section later in this chapter). *Phalen's sign* is performed by asking the client to flex both wrists and press the dorsum of the hands against each other (Fig. 21-34).

■ A positive Phalen's sign occurs if the client complains of numbness or paresthesia over the palmar surface of the hand and the first three fingers and part of the fourth.

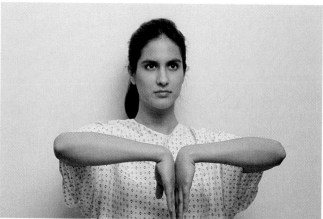

Fig. 21-34   Phalen's test for carpal tunnel syndrome.

Tinel's sign is performed by tapping on the median nerve where it passes through the carpal tunnel under the flexor retinaculum and volar carpal ligament. No report of tingling sensation is a negative Tinel's sign (Fig. 21-35).

■ A positive Tinel's sign occurs when the client reports a tingling sensation radiating from the wrist to the hand along the median nerve.

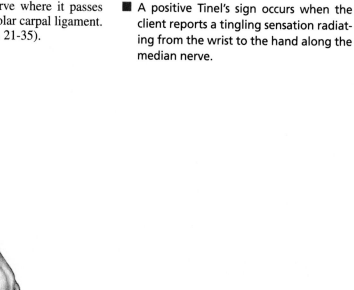

Flexor
retinaculum

Carpal canal
(sulcus carpi)

Median nerve

Fig. 21-35   Tinel's sign for carpal tunnel syndrome. *(From Seidel et al, 1995.)*

TECHNIQUES and NORMAL FINDINGS

Two tests evaluate presence of fluid in the knee joint. The *bulge sign* tests for small effusion of the knee. Elicit the bulge sign by extending the knee and milking the medial aspect upward two or three times. Then tap on the lateral side of the patella. No fluid waves or bulging should be seen on the opposite side of the joint (Fig. 21-36, *A* and *B*). The second test, *ballottement,* is used for larger effusion. With knee extended, apply downward pressure on the suprapatellar pouch with the thumb and fingers of one hand, and with the other hand push the patella firmly against the femur. Release the pressure from the patella, but leave fingers in contact with the knee to detect any fluid wave (Fig. 21-37).

ABNORMAL FINDINGS

■ If fluid is present, fluid waves are palpable on the opposite side of the joint.

■ Palpation of a fluid wave after release of pressure against the patella is *ballottement,* indicating excess fluid in the knee joint.

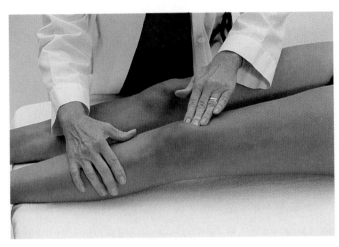
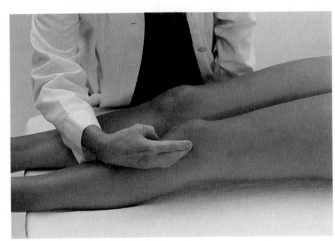

Fig. 21-36 Bulge sign to detect small effusion in knee joint. **A,** Milk the medial aspect of the knee two or three times. **B,** Then tap the lateral side of the patella.

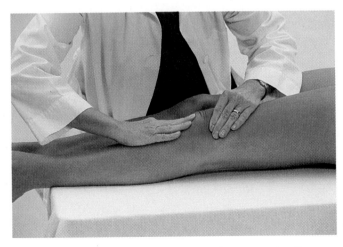

Fig. 21-37 Ballottement procedure to detect large effusion in knee joint.

TECHNIQUES and NORMAL FINDINGS

ABNORMAL FINDINGS

Perform the *Drawer test* to evaluate intactness of the cruciate ligaments. Have the client in supine position with the knee flexed at a right angle. Sit on the client's foot to stabilize it. Instruct the client to relax the muscles in the flexed leg. Then press the head of the tibia forward or backward with both hands. You should not be able to displace the knee from its position (Fig. 21-38).

■ Note if the tibia can be pulled anteriorly from under the femur, which indicates injury to the anterior cruciate ligament. Report if the tibia can be pushed posteriorly from under the femur, indicating injury to the posterior cruciate ligament.

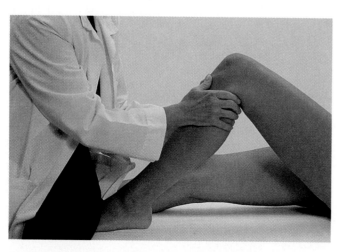

Fig. 21-38   Drawer test for assessment of anterior and posterior stability.

Perform the *McMurray test* to evaluate the presence of a damaged or torn meniscus. Have the client sitting or supine with hips and knees flexed 90°. Stabilize one hand on the client's knee, with the thumb and index finger on either side of the joint space. With the other hand, grasp the client's heel and externally rotate the knee and apply resistance to the lateral aspect of the knee at the same time (Fig. 21-39). This tests the lateral meniscus. The medial meniscus is tested by using the same flexed position, but internally rotating the knee and applying pressure to the medial aspect of the knee. The knee should remain stable, and no discomfort should be present.

■ Findings considered positive for the presence of meniscal damage are pain on lateral surfaces of knee, clicking on movement, or inability to extend the knee.

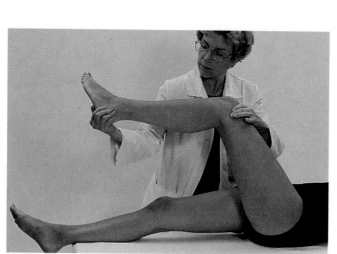

Fig. 21-39   Examination of the knee with the McMurray test. Knee is flexed after lower leg is rotated to medial position.

TECHNIQUES and NORMAL FINDINGS

ABNORMAL FINDINGS

When the client complains of knee locking, perform the *Apley test* to detect meniscal tear. With the client in prone position, flex the knee to 90°. Press down on the client's foot so that the tibia is firmly opposed to the femur; then rotate the knee internally and externally. No pain or locking is a negative test (Fig. 21-40).

■ Pain, locking of the knee, or clicking during rotation of the knee is a positive Apley test, indicating meniscal tear.

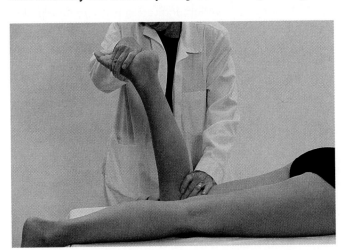

Fig. 21-40 Examination of the knee with the Apley test.

Perform the *Thomas test* to evaluate for flexion contractures of the hip. Have the client lie supine and ask him or her to fully extend one leg on the table and flex the other knee up toward the chest as far as possible. Observe if extended leg remains flat on the table when other leg is flexed. The extended leg should remain flat on the table (Fig. 21-41).

■ Lifting of extended leg off the table in response to other leg being flexed indicates a hip flexion contracture. Note the degree of flexion.

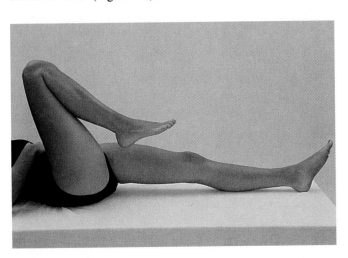

Fig. 21-41 Examination of the hip with the Thomas test. Response is negative in this client.

TECHNIQUES and NORMAL FINDINGS

ABNORMAL FINDINGS

To evaluate the presence of nerve root irritation (e.g., sciatic neuritis), perform the *LaSègue's test*. With the client supine, flex the client's hip. Holding the hip flexed and leg straight, dorsiflex the ankle. No pain should be felt (Fig. 21-42).

To evaluate for lumbar disk injury, perform *straight leg raises*. With the client supine, raise one leg, keeping the knee straight. Tightness may be felt, but there should be no pain present.

■ Pain felt in thigh of client with sciatic neuritis indicates inflammation of a peripheral nerve.

■ Note pain felt in leg with 30° to 60° elevation, indicating pressure on a peripheral nerve by a disc.

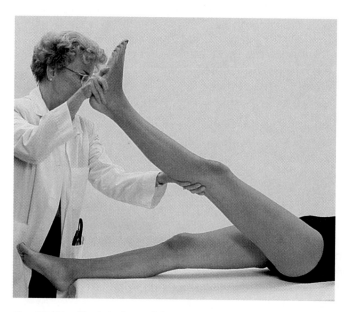

Fig. 21-42   Straight leg raising test.

AGE-RELATED VARIATIONS

INFANTS

■ APPROACH

Assessment of the infant's musculoskeletal system should focus on normal development and identification of congenital anomalies. Examine the infant fully undressed and lying on his or her back. Place the newborn on a warming table to maintain body temperature.

■ FINDINGS

A newborn's feet are often held in varus or valgus position. They should be flexible and not fixed. Scratch the outside of the bottom of the foot, or immobilize the heel with one hand and gently push the forefoot to neutral position with the other hand. If deformity is self-correctable, the foot assumes a normal right angle to the lower leg (moves into neutral position). Note the relationship of the forefoot to the hindfoot. The hindfoot aligns with the lower leg and the forefoot turns inward slightly. This usually resolves spontaneously by age 3. Place both of the infant's feet flat on the table and push to flex up the knees. With the patella and tibial tubercle in a straight line, place your fingers on the malleoli. The line connecting the four malleoli should be parallel to the table. Note if more than 20° of deviation is present or if the lateral malleolus is anterior to the medial malleolus (tibial torsion).

Check the hips for congenital dislocation using the Barlow-Ortolani maneuver (Fig. 21-43, A and B). With the infant supine, flex the knees, holding your thumbs on the inner mid-thighs and your fingers outside on the hips touching the greater trochanters. Adduct the legs until your thumbs touch. Then abduct, moving the knees apart and down to touch the table with their lateral aspects. This maneuver should feel smooth and be soundless. Note any click that occurs when you perform external rotation. This is a positive Barlow-Ortolani's sign and should be reported (Fig. 21-44).

Palpate the length of the clavicles, which should feel smooth, regular, and without crepitus. Note if there is equal range of motion during the Moro (startle) reflex (Chapter 22). Range of motion will be limited if a fractured clavicle is present.

Observe the back and spine. The spine should be flexible with convex dorsal and sacral curves, no masses, and easy movement in and out of fetal position. Note asymmetric back curve, masses (hair tufts, dimples), and abnormal posturing.

Evaluate the extremities. Normally extremities are bilaterally symmetric and equal. The arms and legs remain flexed but have a full range of motion. There should be five digits on each hand and foot; the feet should not have lon-

A

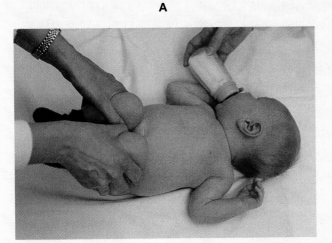

B

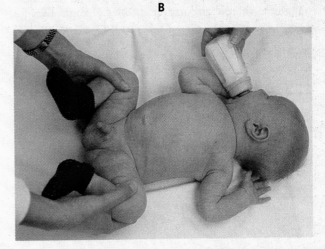

Fig. 21-43 Barlow-Ortolani maneuver to detect hip dislocation. **A,** Phase I, adduction. **B,** Phase II, abduction.

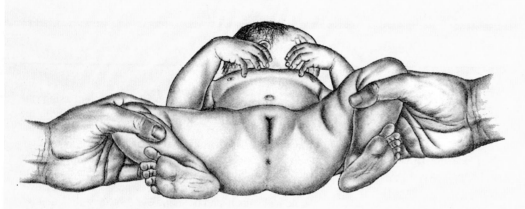

Fig. 21-44 Sign of hip dislocation: limitation of abduction and asymmetric gluteal folds. *(From Seidel et al, 1995.)*

gitudinal arches. The positional foot curves straighten under gentle pressure. Hip and back creases are even, as are arm and leg lengths. Abduction is achieved without difficulty. Abnormal findings include no or few heel creases (occurs in preterm infants), asymmetry, limited movement, syndactyly (fused digits), polydactyly (extra digits), metatarsus varus (toeing in or pigeon toed), talipes equinovarus (clubfoot), Erb's palsy (paralysis of shoulder and upper arm muscles), uneven gluteal folds, and hip clicks with abduction.

CHILDREN

■ APPROACH

When evaluating children, compare data obtained with tables of normal age and sequence of motor development. (Chapter 2 discusses expected motor development for children.) Next the child should be weighed and measured, with these values compared with tables of percentiles for growth and weight. (See Chapter 7 for height and weight tables.) Areas that change with growth and maturation form the bulk of the examination that differs in children from the procedures used in adults.

■ FINDINGS

Observe the spine. It should be straight, with curves varying according to age, as follows: 3 to 4 months—cervical curve develops as child holds head up; 12 to 18 months—lumbar curve develops as child learns to walk; lumbar lordosis is common in toddlers; after 18 months, cervical spine is concave, thoracic spine convex (although less than that of adults), and lumbar spine is concave like an adult's. There should be no bulges or dimpling along the spine. Lordosis is seen more frequently in African-American children, but should not be seen in children over the age of 6 years. Note if the spine is curved either in the standing or the bent-over position.

Note the child's gait. Newly walking babies and toddlers have a wide stance and a wide-waddle gait pattern, which tends to disappear by age 2 to 2½ years. The gait should become progressively stronger, steadier, and smoother as the child matures. Any deviation from the pattern or a history of increasing falls or balance problems should be considered abnormal.

Examine the knees. Knees should be in a direct straight line between the hip, the ankle, and the great toe. Valgus rotation (medial malleolus greater than 1 inch [2.5 cm] apart with knees touching) is normal in children 2 to 3½ years of age, and may be present and normal in children as old as 12 years of age. Varus rotation (medial malleolus touching, with knees greater than 1 inch [2.5 cm] apart) requires further evaluation for tibial torsion; it may be normal until 18 to 24 months of age.

ADOLESCENTS

■ APPROACH

It is extremely important to pay attention to the posture of the spine in adolescents, particularly females. Chronic poor posture can cause kyphosis, and scoliosis can become severe. Also, be aware of sports injuries that occur in adolescents, and evaluate complaints of pain or limitation of movement.

■ FINDINGS

Seat yourself behind the standing client and ask him or her to bend forward to touch the toes. There should be a straight vertical spine while standing and while bending forward. The posterior ribs should be symmetric, and the shoulders, scapulae, and iliac crests symmetrically elevated. Mark the tips of the spinous processes and line them up to reveal whether there is even a slight curve. Any curve should be evaluated further.

OLDER ADULTS

■ APPROACH

Examination of the older adult is the same as the adult. They may be slower at performing range of motion and muscle strength assessments. Remember to distinguish normal changes of aging described in the beginning of this chapter from musculoskeletal disorders.

 Cultural Note

Osteoporosis is lowest in African-American males and highest in white females. Asian Americans and American Indians also have higher incidences of osteoporosis as they age.

■ FINDINGS

Mobility of joints may be affected by osteoarthritic changes; muscle strength may be reduced by muscle atrophy. Many joints may not have the expected degree of movement. Assessment of the client's ability to perform activities of daily living is important. Guidelines for this assessment are found in Chapter 4.

CLIENTS WITH SITUATIONAL VARIATIONS

PREGNANT WOMEN

■ FINDINGS

Changes that are expected during pregnancy include progressive lordosis, anterior cervical flexion, kyphosis, and slumped shoulders. A characteristic "waddling" gait develops at the end of pregnancy due to the enlarged abdomen and relaxed joint mobility. Muscle strains can be caused by exaggerated posture or excessive activity. Preexisting conditions may become worse both during the pregnancy and after delivery.

Common complaints include backache; softening of the ligaments and joints of the spinal column and pelvis; aching, numbness, or weakness of the extremities; pulling on the ulnar and median nerves; and muscle cramps. Posture and comfort return to prepregnant status soon after delivery.

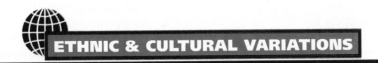 **ETHNIC & CULTURAL VARIATIONS**

■ FINDINGS

A number of racial variations have been noted in the anatomy of the skeleton and of the skeletal muscles and some do have clinical significance. Long bones are generally longer, narrower, and denser in African Americans, particularly African-American males. They are thus less subject to osteoporosis and other diseases involving the loss of bone density. Protuberances on the mandible and hard palate found frequently in Asian Americans and American Indians/Alaskan Natives make dentures difficult to fit and maintain. The number of vertebrae varies from 23 to 25. The increased number, most frequently found in American Indian/Alaskan Natives, can aggravate low back pain and contribute to lordosis. Asian and African-American women with smaller pelvic structures may have increased difficulty in vaginal delivery of children. The longer second toe length seen most frequently in Asian Americans and whites may increase foot problems, particularly in athletes.

Muscle mass is greater in African Americans, contributing to a greater strength potential. The palmaris longus and peroneus tertius may be absent in various racial groups. However, this has little functional significance, as there are other muscles that also control flexion of the wrist and foot.

E X A M I N A T I O N S U M M A R Y
Musculoskeletal System

Routine Examination *(pp. 595-599)*
- Inspect skeleton and extremities for:
  Alignment
  Contour
  Symmetry
  Size
  Gross deformities
- Inspect skin and subcutaneous tissues for:
  Color
  Edema
  Masses
- Inspect muscles for:
  Symmetry
  Size
  Fasciculations
  Spasms
- Observe gait for:
  Conformity
  Symmetry
  Rhythm
- Palpate bones, joints, and muscles for:
  Tenderness
  Heat
  Edema
  Crepitus
- Assess joints for active and passive range of motion comparing contralateral sides for:
  Tenderness on motion
  Joint stability
  Deformity
  Contracture
- Assess muscles for strength and compare contralateral sides

Specific Musculoskeletal Regions *(pp. 600-617)*
Temporomandibular joint *(p. 600)*
- Palpate for:
  Movement
  Sounds (clicking or popping)
  Tenderness
- Assess range of motion
- Assess muscle strength
Cervical Spine *(pp. 601-602)*
- Inspect for:
  Alignment
  Symmetry
- Palpate for:
  Tenderness
- Assess range of motion of neck:
  Forward flexion
  Hyperextension
  Lateral bending
  Rotation
- Assess strength of sternocleidomastoid and trapezius muscles

Thoracic and Lumbar Spine *(pp. 603-605)*
- Inspect spine, iliac crest, and shoulders for:
  Alignment
  Symmetry
- Assess range of motion:
  Forward flexion and hyperextension
  Lateral bending
  Rotation
- Palpate spinal processes and paravertebral muscles for:
  Alignment
  Tenderness
- Percuss spinal processes for:
  Tenderness
Shoulders *(pp. 605-607)*
- Inspect shoulders and shoulder girdle for:
  Equality of height
  Contour
- Palpate shoulders for:
  Firmness and fullness
  Tenderness
  Masses
- Assess muscle strength of trapezius muscles
- Assess range of motion:
  Forward flexion and hyperextension
  Abduction and adduction
  External and internal rotation
Arms *(p. 608)*
- Assess muscle strength and compare contralateral side of triceps and biceps muscles
Elbows *(pp. 608-609)*
- Inspect elbows in flexed and extended position for:
  Contour
  Carrying angle
- Palpate elbows for:
  Tenderness
- Assess range of motion:
  Flexion and extension
  Pronation and supination
Hands and Wrists *(pp. 610-613)*
- Inspect joints for:
  Position
  Contour
  Number of digits
- Palpate each joint for:
  Surface characteristics
  Tenderness
- Assess muscles for strength
- Assess range of motion:
  Wrist hyperextension and flexion
  Metacarpophalangeal flexion and hyperextension

Ulnar and radial motion
Abduction and adduction of fingers
Finger flexion (forming fist)
Thumb opposition

Hips *(p. 614)*
- Inspect for symmetry
- Palpate for stability and tenderness
- Assess range of motion:
  Flexion and hyperextension
  Internal and external rotation
  Abduction and adduction
- Assess muscle strength

Knees *(pp. 614-616)*
- Inspect knees for:
  Alignment
  Edema
  Erythema
- Palpate knees for:
  Contour
  Tenderness
- Assess range of motion for:

Flexion
Extension
- Assess muscle strength around the knee

Feet and ankles *(pp. 616-617)*
- Inspect feet and ankles for:
  Contour
  Alignment
  Edema
  Number of toes
- Palpate feet and ankles for:
  Contour
  Tenderness
- Assess range of motion:
  Dorsiflexion and plantar flexion
  Inversion and eversion
  Abduction and adduction
  Flexion and extension of toes
- Assess muscles for strength

Additional Assessment Techniques for Special Cases
(pp. 618-622)

COMMON PROBLEMS/CONDITIONS
associated with the Musculoskeletal System

■ *Temporomandibular joint syndrome:* Painful jaw movement due to congenital anomalies, malocclusion, trauma, arthritis, and other joint diseases. Unilateral jaw pain is worse with jaw movement. Pain may be referred to the face or neck. Clients complain of muscle spasm and clicking; popping or crepitus can be palpated.

■ *Carpal tunnel syndrome:* A common painful disorder of the wrist and hand induced by compression of the median nerve between the inelastic carpal ligament and other structures within the carpal tunnel. Symptoms include burning, numbness, and tingling in the hands, often at night. The hands become weak, and the thenar eminence in the palm flattens. It is associated with repetitive movement of the hands and arms, rheumatoid arthritis, gout, hypothyroidism, and hormonal changes of pregnancy and menopause. Use Phalen's sign or Tinel's sign to assess for this disorder.

■ *Gout:* A hereditary disease involving an overproduction or decreased excretion of uric acid and urate salts, leading to high serum uric acid levels. The disease is thought to be caused by lack of an enzyme needed to completely metabolize purines for renal excretion. Uric acids accumulate commonly in the great toe, but also in other joints such as wrists, hands, ankles, and knees. The symptoms include erythema and edema of joints that are very painful to move and thus limited in the range of motion. Tophi are a sign of gout; these are round, pealike deposits of uric acid in ear cartilage or large, irregularly shaped deposits in other joints. This disorder primarily affects men over 40 years of age.

■ *Osteomyelitis:* An infection of the bone and its marrow, often due to systemic infection or an open wound (Fig. 21-45). It is usually caused by bacteria introduced by trauma or surgery, by direct extension from a nearby infection, or via bloodstream. Purulent exudate spreads through the cortex of the bone and into the soft tissues. Assessment findings include signs of localized inflammation (edema, erythema, warmth at the site of infection, pain on movement) as well as signs of systemic inflammation (fever).

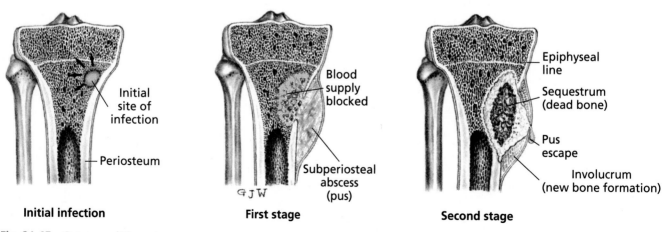

Initial infection — Initial site of infection; Periosteum

First stage — Blood supply blocked; Subperiosteal abscess (pus)

Second stage — Epiphyseal line; Sequestrum (dead bone); Pus escape; Involucrum (new bone formation)

Fig. 21-45 Osteomyelitis. *(From Mourad, 1991.)*

■ **Bursitis:** An inflammation of a bursa, the connective tissue structure surrounding a joint, caused by constant friction around joints (Fig. 21-46). It may be precipitated by arthritis, infection, injury, or excessive exercise. Common sites of bursitis are the shoulder, elbow, hip, and knee. Assessment findings include limited and painful range of motion, edema, point tenderness, and erythema.

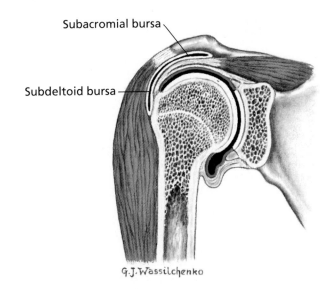

Subacromial bursa

Subdeltoid bursa

G.J. Wassilchenko

Fig. 21-46 Bursitis. *(From Mourad, 1991.)*

■ **Rheumatoid arthritis:** A chronic, systemic autoimmune inflammatory disease of the connective tissue of the body. Even though this is a systemic disease, the synovial lining of joints is one of the major tissues initially inflamed. Joint pain, edema and stiffness of the fingers, wrists, ankles, feet, and knees are common symptoms. Joints are symmetrically and bilaterally inflamed. Inflammation leads to deterioration of cartilage and erosion of surfaces, causing bone fissures, cysts, and bone spurs. Ligaments and tendons around inflamed joints become fibrotic and shortened, causing contractures and subluxation (partial dislocation) of joints. Women have rheumatoid arthritis three times more often than men. The incidence is lower in Asians and Hispanics than in whites and African Americans.

■ **Injuries:** Overuse of the musculoskeletal system resulting from sports, exercise, or repetitive trauma. Such injuries can result in the following disorders.

Muscle strain develops from stretching, tearing, or forceful contraction of a muscle beyond its functional capacity. Severity ranges from a mild intrafibrinous tear to a total rupture of a single muscle. Signs include temporary weakness, numbness, and contusion.

Sprain is a stretching or tearing of a ligament by forced movement beyond its normal range, characterized by pain, edema, discoloration of the skin over the joint, and loss of function. The duration and severity of symptoms vary with the extent of damage to supporting tissue. Severe sprains may rupture ligaments, causing joint instability if not treated.

Dislocation is a displacement of a bone from its normal articulation, often caused by pressure or force pushing the bone out of the joint. Signs and symptoms include deformity, edema, pain, and loss of function.

Fracture is a traumatic injury in which there is a partial or complete break in the continuity of a bone. This injury results in muscle spasm and shortening of tissue around the bone, causing deformity. Additional signs and symptoms are edema, pain, loss of function, skin color changes, and paresthesia.

INFANTS AND CHILDREN

■ *Myelomeningocele/spina bifida:* A developmental defect of the central nervous system in which a hernial sac containing a portion of the spinal cord, its meninges, and cerebrospinal fluid protrudes through a congenital cleft in the vertebral column (Fig. 21-47). The defect of the vertebra (spina bifida) may range from displacement of a lamina to complete absence of lamina. The condition is primarily caused by failure of the neural tube to close during embryonic development. Signs vary, depending on the damage to the spinal cord, and may include paralysis, anesthesia, and loss of bowel and bladder function.

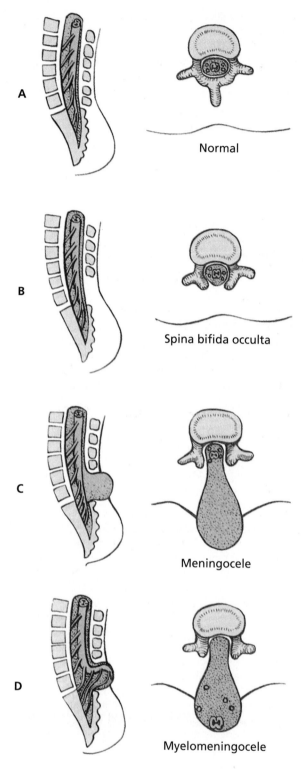

Fig. 21-47 Midline defects of osseous spine with varying degrees of neural herniations. **A,** Normal. **B,** Spina bifida occulta. **C,** Meningocele. **D,** Myelomeningocele. *(From Wong, 1995.)*

■ *Congenital dislocation of the hip:* (Also called developmental dysplasia.) A congenital defect in which the head of the femur does not articulate with the acetabulum because of an abnormal shallowness of the acetabulum. This dislocation is assessed using the Barlow-Ortolani maneuver.

■ **Talipes equinovarus (clubfoot):** A fixed congenital deformity of the ankle and foot caused by intrauterine constriction (Fig. 21-48). It is characterized by unilateral or bilateral deviation of the metatarsal bones of the forefoot. Most deformities are *equinovarus*, in which there is a medial deviation and plantar flexion of the forefoot, but a few cases may be *calcaneovarus,* in which there is lateral deviation and dorsiflexion of the forefoot.

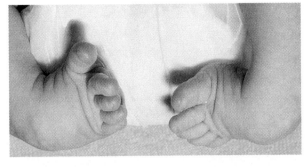

Fig. 21-48 Bilateral deviation. *(From Zitelli and Davis, 1992.)*

■ **Metatarsus adductus (metatarsus varus):** The most common foot deformity; involves medial adduction of the toes and forefoot from angulation at the tarsometatarsal joint (Fig. 21-49). This deformity is also called pigeon-toed or toeing in.

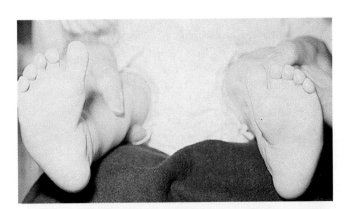

A

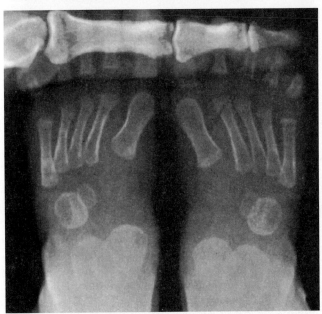

B

Fig. 21-49 Bilateral metatarsus adductus. **A,** When viewed from the planar aspect, rounding of the lateral border of the feet can be appreciated. **B,** The metatarsals are deviated medially with respect to the remainder of the foot; otherwise, the bony structures are normal. *(From Zitelli and Davis, 1992.)*

■ **Muscular dystrophy:** A group of genetically transmitted diseases characterized by progressive atrophy of symmetric groups of skeletal muscle fibers without evidence of degeneration of neural tissue. In all forms of muscular dystrophy there is a progressive weakness and muscle atrophy or pseudohypertrophy from fatty infiltration. Each type differs in the group of muscles affected, age of onset, rate of progression, and mode of genetic inheritance.

■ *Scoliosis:* A skeletal deformity with a concave curvature of the anterior vertebral bodies, convex posterior curves, and lateral rotation of the thoracic spine (Fig. 21-50). Causes include congenital malformations of the spine, poliomyelitis, skeletal dysplasia, spastic paralysis, and unequal leg length. Scoliosis produces uneven shoulders and hip levels. Rotation deformity also may cause a rib hump and flank asymmetry on forward flexion. Depending on the severity of the curve, physiologic function of lungs, spine, and pelvis may be compromised. Structural scoliosis affects girls more often than boys and progresses during early adolescence.

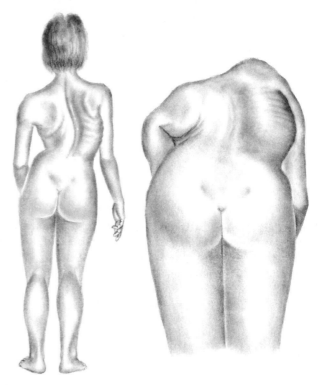

Fig. 21-50   Scoliosis.   *(From Mourad, 1991.)*

OLDER ADULTS

■ *Osteoporosis:* A systemic condition of overall reduction in bone mass or density when bone reabsorption is greater than bone deposition (Fig. 21-51). Lack of bone density increases risk of fractures. An increase in the thoracic kyphotic curve and lumbar lordotic curve develops, which decreases height. It occurs in about 30% of all women over the age of 45.

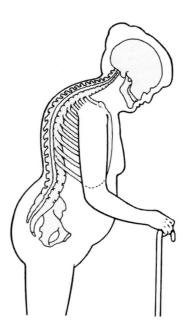

Fig. 21-51 Hallmark of osteoporosis: dowager hump.
(From Seidel et al, 1995.)

■ *Osteoarthritis:* A condition characterized by degenerative changes in articular cartilage, mainly in the major weight-bearing joints, although other joints may be affected. Symptoms include sore, aching joint pain that becomes sharp on weight-bearing. Joint deformities of fingers develop (Heberden's nodes in distal interphangeal joints and Bouchard's nodes in proximal interphangeal joints) (see Fig. 21-26). The incidence increases with age, affecting about 90% of people over 60 years of age.

Nursing Diagnosis

Sample Documentation &

CASE 1   33-year-old Native American man complaining of right wrist pain.

Subjective

Pain in right wrist noticed 1 week ago; slowly getting worse; hand swollen; painful on movement, 6 on a scale of 10. Some pain relief after taking ibuprofen. No history of trauma to wrist. Does not participate in sports. Unable to perform job as computer programmer; painful to tie necktie, shave face, and button shirt.

Objective

Alert, cooperative client in no apparent distress.

Right wrist   Edema over right distal radius and medial carpals; no redness or heat noted. Pain on flexion and hyperextension of radiocarpal joint; grip strength ⅗ with pain on contraction; able to perform thumb opposition, but slowly and with pain; negative Tinel sign; sensation present in all fingers.

Left wrist   No pain on range of motion, grip strength ⅘, thumb opposition brisk without pain; negative Tinel's sign; sensation present in all fingers.

Nursing Diagnosis #1

Pain related to inflammation of tendons.

Defining characteristics   Report of 6/10 pain, right wrist edema, pain on range of motion of right wrist.

Nursing Diagnosis #2

Impaired physical mobility related to limitation of joint function and pain.

Defining characteristics   Unable to perform job as computer programmer due to pain and edema; painful to tie necktie, shave face, and button shirt.

Sample Documentation & Nursing Diagnosis

CASE 2   76-year-old white woman with osteoarthritis.

Subjective

Stiffness of left hip and knee getting worse, gradual change over the past several months; stiff when arising in morning, lasts 15 to 20 minutes; joints painful when walking, cleaning, or ironing, but relieved by rest; pain is an ache, cannot localize pain precisely. No fatigue reported. Unable to walk in evening with husband because of pain.

Objective

Temperature   98.2° F (36.7° C).

Pulse   88.

Rate   16.

Blood pressure   148/88.

Height   5'5" (165 cm).

Weight   175 lb (79 kg).

Ambulates independently, slowing, symmetrically.

Left hip and knee   Pain on palpation, no heat or edema; crepitus on movement, positive ballottement and bulge signs.

Range of motion   Hip flexion, knee extended 75°; hip flexion, knee flexed 90°, internal rotation 30°, abduction 35°, peripheral pulses 2+; sensation to sharp, dull, and vibratory sense present.

Right hip and knee   No pain on palpation, no heat, edema, or crepitus.

Range of motion   Hip flexion, knee extended 85°; hip flexion, knee flexed 100°, internal rotation 35°, abduction 45°, peripheral pulses 2+; sensation to sharp, dull, and vibratory sense present.

• •

Nursing Diagnosis #1

Impaired physical mobility related to joint degeneration.

Defining characteristics   Left knee and hip joints painful when walking, cleaning, or ironing, relieved by rest; reduced range of motion of affected joints.

Nursing Diagnosis #2

Pain related to joint degeneration.

Defining characteristics   Client complains of pain relieved by rest, painful left hip and knee joint on palpation, unable to walk because of pain.

Nursing Diagnosis #3

Altered nutrition: more than body requirements related to lack of exercise.

Defining characteristics   Height is 5'5" (165 cm); weight 175 lb (79 kg); unable to walk due to joint pain and stiffness.

HEALTH PROMOTION

◼ **Risk Factors for Osteoporosis** There are several risk factors for developing osteoporosis.

1. White, American Indian, and Asian women are at higher risk, for unknown reasons.
2. Women who exert minimal stress on their bones, such as thin women.
3. Women who have decreased estrogen blood levels, such as those who have had total hysterectomies or completed menopause and chose not to take hormone replacement therapy, and those who smoke cigarettes.
4. Women who consume alcohol daily, because it suppresses synthesis of new bone. More than two drinks daily increases the chance of hip fracture by 25% to 50%, and more than 4 drinks daily increases risk of vertebral fracture by 50% (Dorbrand et al, 1993).

Osteoporosis can be prevented by regular exercise to stress bones, which maintains deposition of calcium in the bones, and adequate intake of calcium. The daily amount of calcium recommended is 1 gram for premenopausal woman and 1.5 grams for postmenopausal women. Also, based on the risk factors listed above, limiting alcohol consumption, stopping smoking, and using estrogen replacement therapy are other preventive strategies for osteoporosis.

◼ **Maintaining Healthy Body Weight and Exercising Regularly** Obesity strains bones, muscles, and joints. While weight-bearing on bones is needed to maintain calcium deposition, excessive weight can exert too much stress on bones, as well as on ligaments, tendons, and muscles. Regular exercise (at least walking) for 20 minutes three times a week is recommended to provide sufficient stress on bones and to help maintain weight. The other side of the equation to maintaining body weight is a sensible diet following recommendations from the food pyramid (see Chapter 7).

◼ **Preventing Injuries** Injuries related to exercise can be prevented by stretching muscle, tendons, and ligaments before exercising. Starting an exercise program gradually is also recommended; for example, begin with 5 minutes of walking and increase the exercise time by 5 minutes each week. Using proper body mechanics when pushing, pulling, or lifting prevents strain of back muscles. By using the longest and strongest muscles, those in the legs, rather than those in the back, individuals can prevent back injuries. Falls can be prevented by maintaining a safe environment, for example, using handrails and night lights, removing throw rugs, and applying nonslip mats in the bathtub.

??????? STUDY QUESTIONS ???????

1. Identify and describe the two major skeletal structures.
2. Identify the seven ranges of motion that can occur with diarthrotic joints. Which specific joints can perform each of these ranges?
3. Identify differences in the skeleton in infants. What skeletal changes occur in childhood? What skeletal changes occur in adolescence? What musculoskeletal changes can be attributed to the aging process?
4. What musculoskeletal changes occur in pregnancy?
5. What anatomic racial variations are present in the skeleton? Do these make any difference in health concerns? If so, what?
6. An individual reports morning pain and stiffness in the knees. What additional information do you need to collect related to this complaint?
7. A 37-year-old man comes to you with a chief complaint of tiredness and feeling weak all the time. What additional information do you need to collect?
8. What additional areas do you need to address when taking a history for an (a) infant; (b) child; (c) adolescent; (d) older adult?
9. What general approach should you take to examining the musculoskeletal system? What preliminary things are important to inspect when first meeting the client?
10. What are you looking for when you palpate the bones, joints, and muscles?
11. What may a limited range of motion in the knee joint indicate? How do you confirm a limited range?
12. Describe how to test muscle strength for each major muscle group.
13. When inspecting and palpating the spine, what are you looking for? What findings would be cause for concern?
14. As you pronate the elbow, you notice a range of 45°. Is this a normal finding? Hip flexion is 90°, internal rotation is 40°, and external rotation is 45°. Are these normal?
15. What two structures of the knee should be palpated? Describe where they are located. What are you looking for?
16. Describe how to assess someone for the presence of carpal tunnel syndrome. What results would you expect if carpal tunnel syndrome is present?
17. Describe what tests to use to determine whether an individual has fluid on the knee. What results do you expect if fluid is present?
18. How can you assess damage to the cruciate ligament? How can you determine whether there is a possible torn meniscus?
19. What procedure do you use to assess an infant for hip dislocation? Describe how to perform the procedure.

20. Who is most likely to present with osteoporosis? Why?

21. What changes on physical examination are expected during pregnancy?

22. Match the disease or condition with the appropriate characteristic:

Osteomyelitis	Edematous, painful big toe
Bursitis	Infection of cortex of bone
Gout	Inflammation of the bursa
Arthritis	Inflammation of the synovial lining

23. List and describe three congenital deformities of the musculoskeletal system.

24. What is the difference between osteoporosis and osteoarthritis? What is the difference between rheumatoid arthritis and osteoarthritis?

25. Describe health promotion activities that women can engage in to prevent osteoporosis.

CHAPTER 22

Neurologic System and Mental Status

ANATOMY AND PHYSIOLOGY REVIEW

The nervous system controls all body functions through voluntary and autonomic responses of the body to both external and internal stimuli. Two distinct structural categories of the nervous system are the central nervous system, which consists of the brain and spinal cord, and the peripheral nervous system, made up of 12 pairs of cranial nerves, 31 pairs of spinal nerves, and the autonomic nervous system. The autonomic nervous system is further divided into sympathetic and parasympathetic subdivisions.

CENTRAL NERVOUS SYSTEM

Protective structures. The brain is protected by the bony structure of the skull. At the base of the skull in the occipital bone is a large oval opening called the foramen magnum, where the brain and spinal cord become continuous. Also at the base of the skull are a series of openings (foramina) for the entrance and exit of paired cranial nerves and cerebral blood vessels.

Between the skull and brain lie three connective tissues layers called meninges. The outer layer is a fibrous, double layer called the dura mater. The falx cerebri is a vertical fold of dura mater that separates the two cerebral hemispheres. The tentorium cerebelli is a horizontal double fold of dura that supports the temporal and occipital lobes and separates the cerebral hemispheres from the brainstem and cerebellum. Structures above the tentorium are referred to as supratentorial and those below as infratentorial (Fig. 22-1).

The middle meningeal layer is called the arachnoid. It is a two-layer, fibrous, elastic membrane that covers the folds and fissures of the brain. Between the arachnoid and the inner meningeal layer is the subarachnoid space, where the cerebrospinal fluid (CSF) circulates.

The inner meningeal layer is called the pia mater. It is rich in small blood vessels, which supply the brain.

Cerebral ventricular system and cerebrospinal fluid. The cerebral ventricular system consists of four interconnecting chambers or ventricles that produce and circulate CSF (Fig. 22-2). There is one lateral ventricle in each hemisphere, with a third ventricle adjacent to the thalamus and a fourth adjacent to the brainstem.

Cerebrospinal fluid is a colorless, odorless fluid containing glucose, electrolytes, oxygen, water, and carbon dioxide, a small amount of protein, and a few leukocytes. CSF is produced in the choroid plexus of the ventricles. It circulates around the brain and spinal cord to provide a cushion, as well as to remove metabolic wastes, provide nutrition, and maintain normal intracranial pressure.

Brain. The brain, consisting of the cerebrum, cerebellum, and brainstem, is made up of gray matter (cell bodies) and white matter (myelinated nerve fibers). Blood flows to the brain from two internal carotid arteries, two vertebral arteries, and the basilar artery, and drains away from the brain through venous sinuses that empty into the jugular veins (Fig. 22-3). At the base of the brain the cerebral arteries are connected by their communicating branches into an arterial circle called the circle of Willis. The purpose of the circle of Willis is to provide circulation if one of the four main blood vessels is interrupted (Fig. 22-4).

Cerebrum. The cerebrum is the largest part of the brain and is composed of two hemispheres. Each hemisphere is divided into four lobes: frontal lobe, parietal lobe, temporal lobe, and occipital lobe. Each lobe controls its respective function for the opposite (contralateral) side of the body (Fig. 22-5).

The frontal lobe contains the primary motor cortex and is responsible for functions related to motor activity. The location in the frontal lobe motor strip that provides motor nerves to specific parts of the body is shown in Fig. 22-6, *A*. The left frontal lobe contains Broca's area (see Fig. 22-5), which controls the ability to produce spoken words. The frontal lobe also controls higher intellectual function, awareness of self, and autonomic responses related to emotion.

The parietal lobe contains the primary sensory cortex. One of its major functions is to process sensory input such as position sense, touch, shape, and consistency of objects. The location in the parietal lobe sensory strip that receives sensory nerves from specific parts of the body is shown in Fig. 22-6, *B*.

The temporal lobe contains the primary auditory cortex. Wernicke's area (see Fig. 22-5), located in the left temporal lobe, is responsible for comprehension of spoken and written language. The temporal lobe also contains the interpretative area where auditory, visual, and somatic input are integrated into thought and memory.

Text continued on p. 642

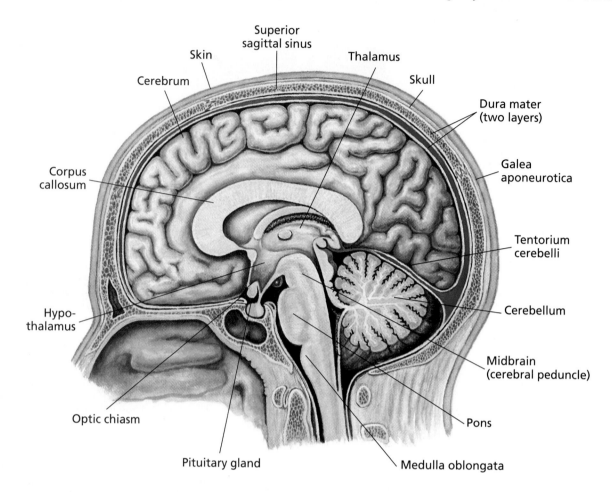

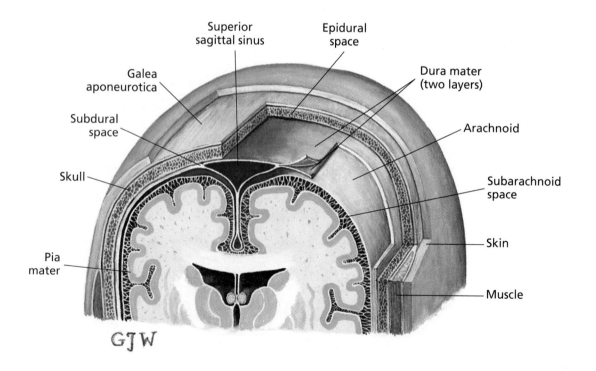

Fig. 22-1 Meningeal layers of the brain. *(From Chipps, Clanin, Campbell, 1992.)*

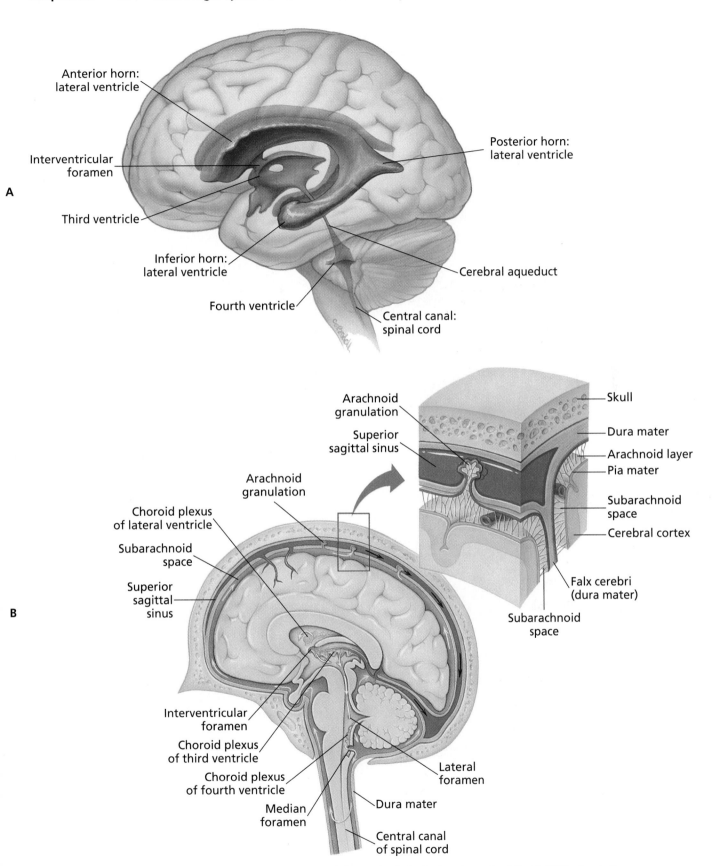

Fig. 22-2 **A,** Ventricles of the brain viewed from the left. **B,** Cerebrospinal fluid (CSF) circulation. *White arrows* represent the route of the CSF. *Black arrows* represent the route of blood flow. CSF is produced in the ventricles, exits the fourth ventricle, and returns to the venous circulation in the superior sagittal sinus. The inset depicts the arachnoid granulations in the superior sagittal sinus, where the CSF enters the circulation. *(From Seeley, Stephens, Tate, 1995.)*

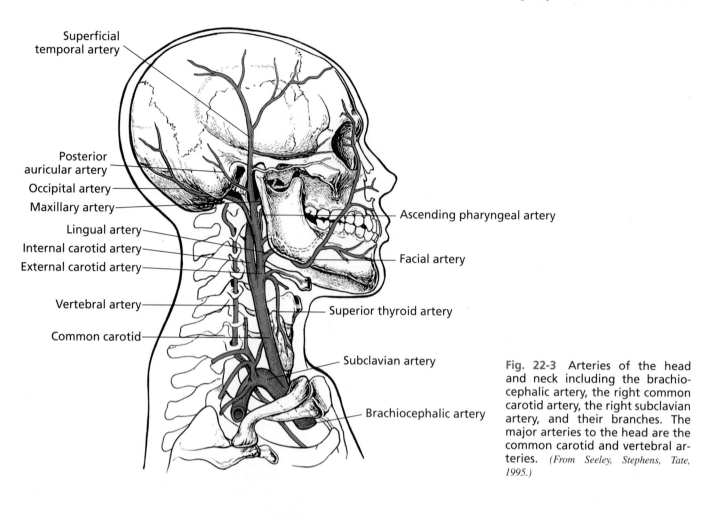

Fig. 22-3 Arteries of the head and neck including the brachiocephalic artery, the right common carotid artery, the right subclavian artery, and their branches. The major arteries to the head are the common carotid and vertebral arteries. *(From Seeley, Stephens, Tate, 1995.)*

Superficial temporal artery

Posterior auricular artery

Occipital artery

Maxillary artery

Lingual artery

Internal carotid artery

External carotid artery

Vertebral artery

Common carotid

Ascending pharyngeal artery

Facial artery

Superior thyroid artery

Subclavian artery

Brachiocephalic artery

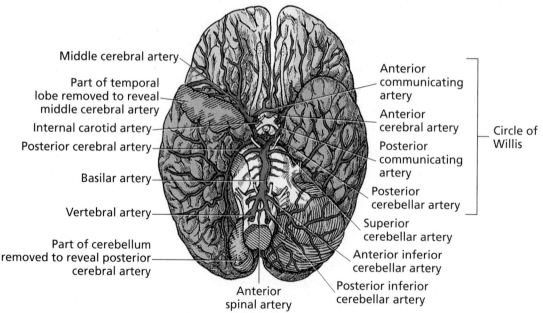

Middle cerebral artery

Part of temporal lobe removed to reveal middle cerebral artery

Internal carotid artery

Posterior cerebral artery

Basilar artery

Vertebral artery

Part of cerebellum removed to reveal posterior cerebral artery

Anterior spinal artery

Anterior communicating artery

Anterior cerebral artery

Posterior communicating artery

Posterior cerebellar artery

Circle of Willis

Superior cerebellar artery

Anterior inferior cerebellar artery

Posterior inferior cerebellar artery

Fig. 22-4 Circle of Willis. Inferior view of the brain showing the vertebral, basilar, and internal carotid arteries. *(From Seeley, Stephens, Tate, 1995.)*

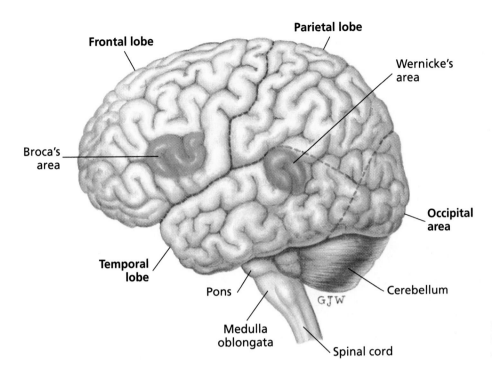

Fig. 22-5 Cerebral hemispheres. Lateral view of the brain. *(From Chipps, Clanin, Campbell, 1992.)*

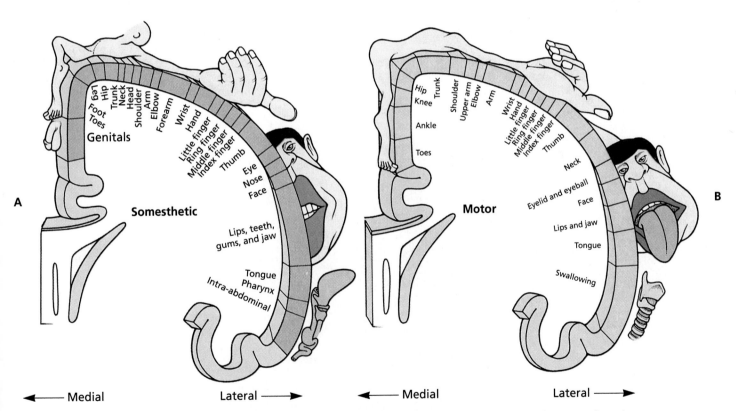

Fig. 22-6 Topography of the somesthetic and motor cortex. Cerebral cortex seen in coronal section on the left side of the brain. The figure of the body (homunculus) depicts the relative nerve distributions; the size indicates relative innervation. Each cortex occurs on both sides of the brain but appears on only one side in this illustration. The inset shows the motor and somesthetic regions of the left hemisphere. **A,** Somesthetic cortex. **B,** Motor cortex. *(From Seeley, Stephens, Tate, 1995.)*

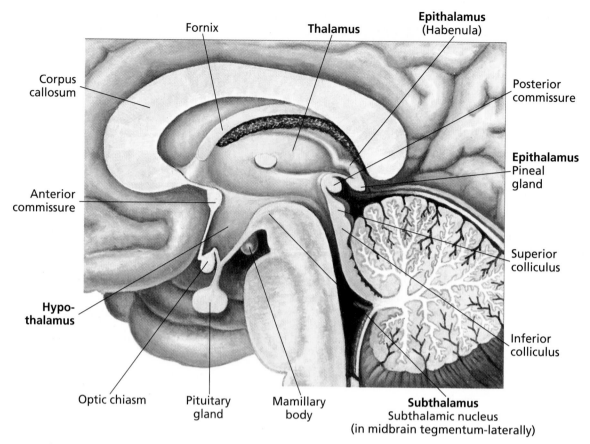

Fig. 22-7   Diencephalon. Lateral view of the brain.   *(From Chipps, Clanin, Campbell, 1992.)*

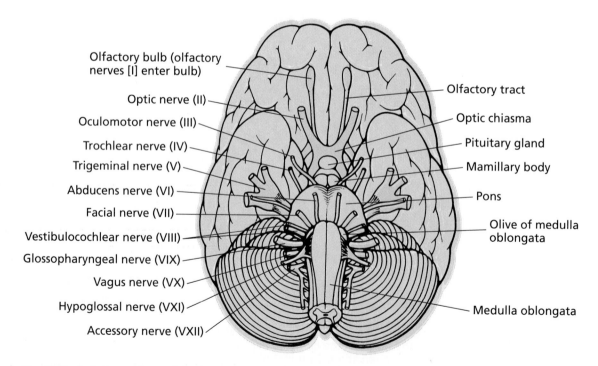

Fig. 22-8   Inferior surface of the brain showing the origin of the cranial nerves.   *(From Seeley, Stephens, Tate, 1995.)*

The occipital lobe contains the primary visual cortex and is responsible for receiving and interpreting visual information.

Diencephalon. The diencephalon lies on top of the brainstem and contains the thalamus, hypothalamus, epithalamus, and subthalamus (Fig. 22-7). The thalamus is a relay and inte- gration station from the spinal cord to the cerebral cortex and other parts of the brain. The hypothalamus has a variety of func- tions and plays an important role in maintaining homeostasis. Some of these functions include regulation of body tempera- ture, hunger, and thirst; formation of autonomic nervous system responses; and storage and secretion of hormones from the pituitary gland. The epithalamus contains the pineal gland, which is believed to have a role in physical growth and sexual development. The subthalamus is part of the extrapyramidal system of the autonomic nervous system and the basal ganglia.

Basal ganglia. Between the cerebral cortex and midbrain and adjacent to the diencephalon lies the basal ganglia structures. The basal ganglia's function is the refinement of voluntary motor activity via a balanced production of the neurotransmitters acetylcholine and dopamine.

Brainstem. The brainstem consists of the midbrain, pons, and medulla oblongata. The major function of the midbrain is to relay stimuli concerning muscle movement to other brain structures. It contains part of the motor tract pathways that control reflex motor movements in response to visual and auditory stimuli. The oculomotor nerve (cranial nerve III) and trochlear nerve (cranial nerve IV) originate in the midbrain. The pons relays impulses to the brain centers and lower spinal nerves. The cranial nerves (CN) that originate in the pons are trigeminal (CN V), abducens (CN VI), facial (CN VII), and acoustic (CN VIII). The medulla oblongata contains reflex centers for controlling involuntary functions such as breathing, sneezing, swallowing, coughing, vomiting, and vasoconstriction. The cranial nerves that originate in the medulla are glossopharyngeal (CN IX), vagus (CN X), spinal accessory (CN XI), and hypoglossal (CN XII) (Fig. 22-8).

Limbic system. The limbic system is on the medial surface of each cerebral hemisphere. It is involved in short-term memory, as well as the mediation of the visceral and behavioral responses to emotions such as fear, affection, and aggression.

Cerebellum. The cerebellum is separated from the cerebral cortex by the tentorium cerebelli (see Fig. 22-1). Functions of the cerebellum include coordinating movement, equilibrium, muscle tone, and proprioception. Each of the cerebellar hemispheres controls movement for the same (ipsilateral) side of the body.

Spinal cord. The spinal cord is a continuation of the medulla oblongata, which begins at the foramen magnum and ends at the first and second lumbar (L1 and L2) vertebrae. At L1 and L2 the spinal cord branches into lumbar and sacral nerve roots called the cauda equina. The spinal cord consists of 31 segments, each giving rise to a pairs of spinal nerves (Fig. 22-9). Nerve fibers, grouped into tracts, run through the spinal cord transmitting sensory, motor, and autonomic impulses between the higher centers in the brain and the body. The myelinated white matter of the spinal cord contains ascending and descending tracts of nerve fibers. The ascending or sensory tracts carry sensory information from the body to the parietal lobe. The posterior (dorsal) column spinal tract carries fibers for the sensations of touch, deep pressure, vibration, position of joints, stereognosis, and two-point discrimination. The spinothalamic tract carry fibers for sensations of light touch, pressure, temperature, and pain. The descending or motor tracts carry impulses from the frontal lobe and communicate impulses to muscle groups.

They also play a role in muscle tone and posture. The pyramidal tract is the great motor pathway that conveys impulses for voluntary movement. The gray matter, which contains the nerve cell bodies, is arranged in a butterfly shape with anterior and posterior horns (see Fig. 22-11).

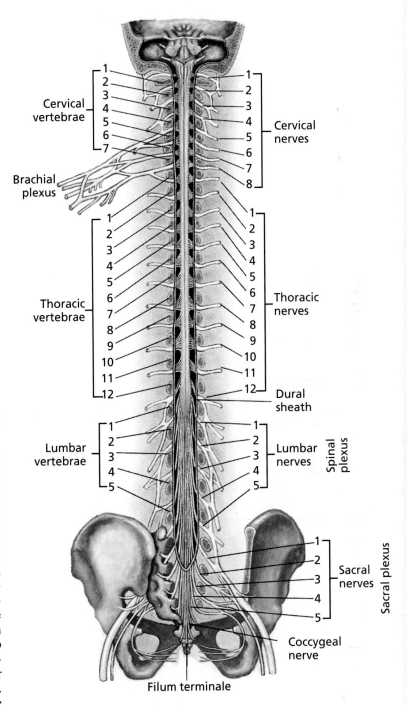

Fig. 22-9 View of the spinal column showing vertebrae, spinal cord, and spinal nerves exiting. *(From Chipps, Clanin, Campbell, 1992.)*

Upper motor neurons originate and terminate within the central nervous system and comprise the descending pathways from the frontal lobe to the spinal cord. Lower motor neurons originate in the anterior horn of the spinal cord and terminate in muscle fibers.

PERIPHERAL NERVOUS SYSTEM

Cranial nerves.   Of the twelve pairs of cranial nerves some nerves have only motor fibers (five pairs) or sensory fibers (three pairs), while others have both (four pairs). Table 22-1 lists the 12 cranial nerves and their functions.

Spinal nerves.   The 31 pairs of spinal nerves emerge from different segments of the spinal cord. There are 8 pairs of cervical nerves, 12 pairs of thoracic nerves, 5 pairs of lumbar nerves, and 1 pair of coccygeal nerves. The first 7 cervical nerves exit above their corresponding vertebrae. The remaining spinal nerves exit below the corresponding vertebrae (see Fig. 22-9).

Each pair of spinal nerves is formed by the union of an efferent or motor (ventral) root and an afferent or sensory (dorsal) root attached to the spinal cord. The motor fibers carry impulses from the brain through the spinal cord to muscles and glands, while sensory fibers carry impulses from the sensory receptors of the body through the spinal cord to the brain. Each pair of spinal nerves and its corresponding part of the spinal cord make up a spinal segment and innervates specific body segments. The dorsal root of each spinal nerve supplies the sensory innervation to a segment of the skin known as a *dermatome*. Knowledge of the distribution of dermatomes is useful for assessment of sensory perception (Fig. 22-10).

Reflex arc.   Some sensory impulses may initiate a reflex response when synapsing immediately with a motor fiber after a stimulus, such as a tap on a stretched tendon. Structures needed for a reflex arc are a receptor, an afferent (sensory) nerve, an efferent (motor) nerve, and an effector muscle or gland (Fig. 22-11). Deep tendon reflexes are segmental responses to stimulation of a tendon, stretching the neuromuscular spindles of a muscle group. Table 22-2 (see p. 647) shows the deep tendon reflexes and superficial reflexes and the segments of the spinal cord that innervates each reflex.

AUTONOMIC NERVOUS SYSTEM

The autonomic nervous system (ANS) is considered part of the peripheral nervous system (Fig. 22-12). It regulates the body's internal environment in conjunction with the endocrine system. The ANS has two components: the sympathetic nervous system and the parasympathetic nervous system. The sympathetic nervous system arises from the thoracolumbar segments of the spinal cord and is activated during stress (the fight-or-flight response). Sympathetic responses include increased blood pressure and heart rate, vasoconstriction of peripheral blood vessels, inhibition of gastrointestinal peristalsis, and bronchodilation. By contrast, the parasympathetic nervous system arises from craniosacral segments of the spinal cord and controls vegetative functions. It is involved in functions associated with conserving energy. These functions include decreasing heart rate and force of myocardial contraction, decreasing blood pressure and respirations, and stimulating gastrointestinal peristalsis.

TABLE 22-1	The Cranial Nerves and Their Functions

CRANIAL NERVES	FUNCTION
Olfactory (1)	Sensory: smell reception and interpretation
Optic (II)	Sensory: visual acuity and visual fields
Oculomotor (III)	Motor: raise eyelids, most extraocular movements
	Parasympathetic: pupillary constriction, change lens shape
Trochlear (IV)	Motor: downward, inward eye movement
Trigeminal (V)	Motor: jaw opening and clenching, chewing and mastication
	Sensory: sensation to cornea, iris, lacrimal glands, conjunctiva eyelids, forehead, nose, nasal and mouth mucosa, teeth, tongue, ear, facial skin
Abducens (VI)	Motor: lateral eye movement
Facial (VII)	Motor: movement of facial expression muscles except jaw, close eyes, labial speech sounds (b, m, w, and rounded vowels)
	Sensory: taste—anterior two thirds of tongue, sensation to pharynx
	Parasympathetic: secretion of saliva and tears
Acoustic (VIII)	Sensory: hearing and equilibrium
Glossopharyngeal (IX)	Motor: voluntary muscles for swallowing and phonation
	Sensory: sensation of nasopharynx, gag reflex, taste—posterior one third of tongue
	Parasympathetic: secretion of salivary glands, carotid reflex
Vagus (X)	Motor: voluntary muscles of phonation (guttural speech sounds) and swallowing
	Sensory: sensation behind ear and part of external ear canal
	Parasympathetic: secretion of digestive enzymes; peristalsis; carotid reflex; involuntary action of heart, lungs, and digestive tract
Spinal accessory (XI)	Motor: turn head, shrug shoulders, some actions for phonation
Hypoglossal (XII)	Motor: tongue movement for speech sound articulation (l, t, n) and swallowing

From Seidel et al: Mosby's guide to physical examination, *ed 3, St Louis, 1995, Mosby.*

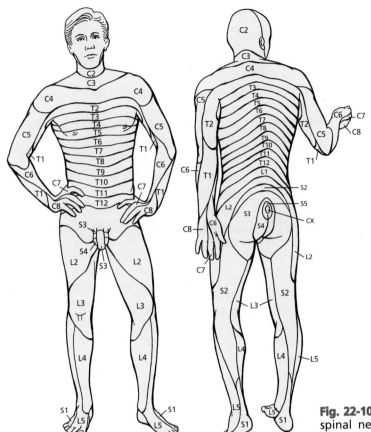

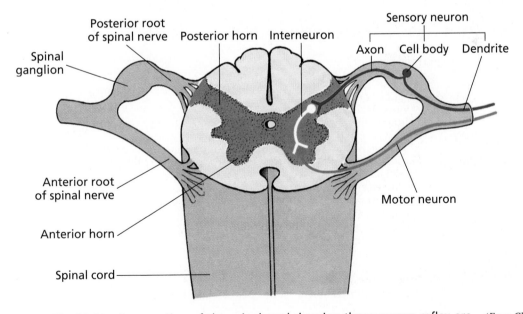

Fig. 22-10 Dermatomal map. Letters and numbers indicate the spinal nerves innervating a given region of skin. *(From Seeley, Stephens, Tate, 1995.)*

Fig. 22-11 Cross-section of the spinal cord showing three-neuron reflex arc. *(From Chipps, Clanin, Campbell, 1992.)*

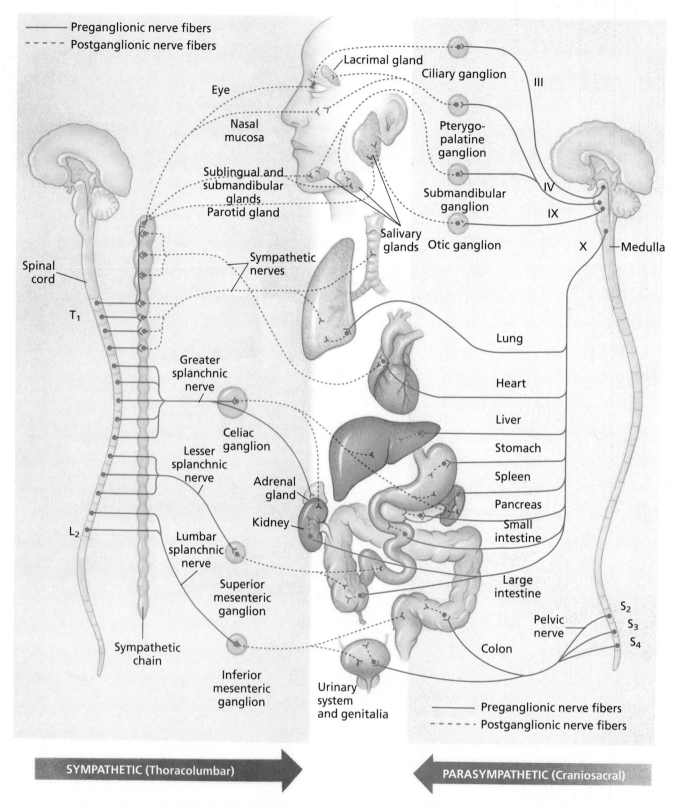

Fig. 22-12 Innervation of organs by the autonomic nervous system. Preganglionic fibers are indicated by solid lines, and postganglionic fibers are indicated by broken lines. *(From Seeley, Stephens, Tate, 1995.)*

TABLE 22-2	Superficial and Deep Tendon Reflexes

REFLEX	SPINAL LEVEL
Superficial	
Upper abdominal	T7, T8, and T9
Lower abdominal	T10 and T11
Cremasteric	T12, L1, and L2
Plantar	L4, L5, S1, and S2
Deep	
Biceps	C5 and C6
Brachioradial	C5 and C6
Triceps	C6, C7, and C8
Patellar	L2, L3, and L4
Achilles	S1 and S2

From Seidel et al: Mosby's guide to physical examination, *ed 3, St Louis, 1995, Mosby.*

DEVELOPMENTAL CONSIDERATIONS

INFANTS AND CHILDREN

In infants during the first year of life, major brain growth and myelinization of the brain and nervous system occur. Initial reflexes that should be evident in the newborn include the following: yawning, sneezing, hiccupping, blinking at both bright lights and loud noises, constricting pupils in response to light, and withdrawing from painful stimuli.

Later, as the brain develops, advanced cortical functions and voluntary control will take over, diminishing or inhibiting some of the more primitive reflexes.

Motor control develops in a cephalocaudaul direction, from head and neck to trunk and extremities. Functions generally develop in an orderly sequence but may vary considerably in timing from one child to the next, sometimes occurring simultaneously.

PREGNANT WOMEN

Neurologic changes occur in response to hypothalamic-pituitary neurohormonal changes, but specific neurologic alterations in pregnancy are not easily identified. There may be some loss of balance from changes in the center of gravity, lightheadedness, or fainting (as a response to vasodilation, hypoglycemia, and hypotension). Some of the more common physiologic alterations include headaches due to contraction or tension factors and acroesthesia, a numbness and tingling in the hands. Also, the woman may have a waddling, broad-based stride from softened pelvic joints.

OLDER ADULTS

Starting as early as age 30, the velocity of the conduction of nerve impulses—and thus responses—diminishes by about 10% over the next 60 years or so. Touch and pain sensation may also diminish. From about age 50, the number of brain cells may decrease by about 1% per year, but the vast number of reserve cells are usually sufficient to protect the individual from any real functional damage as a result.

Only a systemic or neurologic disorder will cause a distinct decline in an older adult's general intelligence; vocabulary and information inventory (stored knowledge) should not change significantly. In addition, any sign of the more commonly noted declines in problem-solving skills will most likely be due to mere disuse. In some individuals, remote memory may be more efficient than recent memory; this change, too, is usually a reflection of that individual's overall health.

HEALTH HISTORY   Neurologic System and Mental Status

The disorders involving neurologic system impairment are headache, dizziness or vertigo, seizures, changes in consciousness, altered mobility (tremors, weakness, or incoordination), altered sensation (numbness or tingling) dysphagia, dysphasia, pain, and altered mental status. Medications that a client is taking should be noted, since they may alter behavior.

QUESTIONS	RATIONALE
HEADACHE	
■ Have you had any unusually frequent or severe headaches? When did these headaches begin? Where are they located? Is there any specific event or triggering circumstance associated with these headaches? What relieves the headache?	◀ *For a more complete headache history outline, see Chapter 10, "Head and Neck."*
DIZZINESS OR VERTIGO	
■ Do you feel dizzy or lightheaded, as if you cannot keep your balance and may fall? Do you feel as if you may faint? When do you feel this way? How often? Is it associated with a change in position or with activity? What relieves the dizziness?	◀ *It is important to distinguish between dizziness and vertigo when questioning the client about this symptom. Fainting is a loss of consciousness caused by a lack of cerebral blood flow.*
■ Have you ever experienced vertigo? Does the room seem to spin or do you feel that you are spinning? Does this happen suddenly or gradually? What relieves the vertigo?	◀ *Vertigo may be caused by a neurologic dysfunction (usually with a gradual onset), or a problem with the vestibular apparatus such as an inner ear infection (labyrinthitis) or Meniere's disease (usually with a sudden onset).*
SEIZURES	
■ Have you ever had seizures or convulsions? When? What were they like? How often did they occur?	◀ *Seizure may be caused by idiopathic epilepsy or result from a pathologic process, endogenous or exogenous poison, metabolic disturbances, or fever (see the Common Problems section at end of chapter for further description).*
■ Do you have any warning signs before the seizure starts? Describe what happens.	◀ *An aura may precede a seizure; it can involve auditory, gustatory, olfactory, visual, or motor sensations. The area in the brain that corresponds to the aura provides information about seizure origin.*
■ Describe how the seizure proceeds through your body. Where does it begin? Does it travel? Where? Do your muscles feel limp or tense? Have you noted any other signs, such as a change in color of the face or lips, loss of consciousness (note how long), automatisms (lip smacking or eyelid fluttering, for example), or incontinence?	◀ *Responses to these questions help identify the areas of the brain involved in the seizure activity.*

QUESTIONS

- After the seizure, are you confused? Have a headache or aching muscles? Feel weak? Do you spend time sleeping?
- Are there any factors that seem to start these seizures, such as stress, fatigue, activity, or discontinuing medication? Are you taking any medication for the seizure? What is the drug and how often are you taking it? Do you take any actions to prevent hurting yourself during seizures?
- How have the seizures affected your life? Your occupation?

CHANGES IN CONSCIOUSNESS

- Have you ever lost consciousness? Had a blackout? Fainted? Felt you were not aware of your surroundings? Did the change occur suddenly? Can you describe what happened to you just before you lost consciousness? Were there other symptoms associated with the change of consciousness? Have you ever had a stroke? Did you have any aftereffects from the stroke? Have you ever had an injury to your head? Have you had a psychiatric illness? Do you have diabetes mellitus, liver failure, or kidney failure?

ALTERED MOBILITY

- Have you noticed any tremors or shaking of the hands or face? When did they start? Do they seem worse when you are anxious or at rest? When you focus on doing something (intention)? What relieves the tremors—rest, activity, or alcohol? Do they affect your performance of daily activities? Do you have thyroid disease?
- Have you noted any twitches or sudden jerks? Where? When did these begin? Does anything seem to make the twitches worse? What relieves twitching?
- Have you felt any sense of weakness in or difficulty moving parts of your body? Is this confined to one area or generalized? Is it associated with anything in particular (activity, etc.)? Do you do anything to prevent the weakness? To relieve the weakness?

- Do you have problems with coordination? Do you have difficulty keeping your balance when you walk? Do you lean to one side or fall? Which direction? Do you feel clumsy? Do your legs suddenly give way?

ALTERED SENSATION

- Have you noted any numbness or tingling? Where? How does it feel? Like pins and needles? Is it associated with any activity in particular?

DYSPHAGIA

- Have you noted any problems swallowing? Do these problems involve liquids or solids? Both? Do you have excessive saliva or drooling?

RATIONALE

◄ *Answers to these questions help determine the extent and location of seizures.*
◄ *Answers to these questions help plan prevention strategies for seizures or any injury experienced during the seizure.*

◄ *Loss of consciousness may be due to cardiovascular disorders, which tend to cause symptoms more rapidly, or neurologic disorders. Changes in consciousness are also associated with drugs, psychiatric illness, or metabolic diseases such as liver or kidney failure or diabetes mellitus.*

◄ *Parkinson's disease causes tremor at rest but no tremor with intentional movement. Hyperthyroidism can cause tremors.*

◄ *These symptoms are related to a variety of neurologic disorders such as tics.*

◄ *Decreased circulation to the brain can cause these symptoms. Some types of transient ischemic attack (TIA) or cerebrovascular accident (CVA) may have occurred.*
◄ *A CVA may be considered, but dysfunction of the cerebellum or inner ear should also be considered when balance is impaired. Parkinson's disease may also be considered.*

◄ *These questions relate to some types of central nervous system disorder (e.g., multiple sclerosis or CVA [stroke]) or peripheral nerve disorder (e.g., diabetics may develop peripheral neuropathy).*

◄ *These may be due to cranial nerve dysfunction or muscle weakness, e.g., from a stroke. Parkinsonism and myasthenia gravis may cause excessive salivation.*

QUESTIONS	**RATIONALE**

DYSPHASIA

- Have you had any problems speaking? With forming words or finding the right words? Have you had difficulty understanding things that are said to you? Has your handwriting changed? When did this begin? How long did it last?

Dysphasia may be associated with dysfunction in the temporal lobe by tumor or stroke. Parkinson's disease may cause some of these symptoms too.

PAIN

- Describe the location and quality of the pain you have had. Describe the pain intensity (on a scale of 1 to 10, with 10 being the most severe pain ever experienced). Is the pain constant or intermittent? Does it radiate? What relieves the pain? Medications? Position? What makes the pain worse? Light? Position? Stress?

Pain may be a symptom of a variety of disorders in other body systems, or it may indicate pressure on a sensory nerve from a variety of causes.

USE OF MEDICATIONS AND DRUGS

- What medications are you taking currently? How much alcohol do you drink per day? Per week? Do you use or have you ever used substances such as marijuana, cocaine, barbiturates, tranquilizers, or any other mood-altering drugs?

Note especially any anticonvulsant medications, antitremor drugs, antivertigo agents, or pain medications that could alter a client's mental status and neurologic examination.

INFANTS

Neuromuscular assessment is a vital part of evaluation of newborns and infants. The prenatal history may affect the infant's development and should be outlined carefully.

- Did you (the mother) have any health difficulties while you were pregnant? Any infections or illnesses? Toxemia? Hypertension (high blood pressure)? Did you take any medications? Use alcohol or drugs? Do you have diabetes?

These factors may have affected the fetal development of the neurologic system.

- Describe the baby's birth. Was the infant born at term or prematurely? What was the baby's birth weight? Were there any problems with the birth? Trauma? Did the baby breathe right away? Do you remember the newborn's Apgar scores? Were any congenital defects found?
- Describe the infant's behavior. Does the baby seem to have coordinated sucking and swallowing reflexes? When you touch his or her cheek, does the baby turn toward the touch? Does the baby startle when there is a loud noise or when the crib is shaken? Does the baby hold onto your finger when you place it in his or her palm?

These behaviors result from expected infantile reflexes (Table 22-3).

- Has the infant had any seizures? Was this associated with a high fever? Describe the seizure. How long did it last? Did the infant lose consciousness? How many seizures did the infant have with this illness (if the seizures were associated with a high fever)?
- Is there any family history of seizures, cerebral palsy, muscular dystrophy, or other neuromuscular diseases?

Seizures can occur in infants and children with high fevers or can be evidence of a neurologic disorder.

CHILDREN

In addition to the questions asked concerning infants, ask the parent or guardian the following.

- Does the child appear to have problems with balance? Does he or she seem to fall unexpectedly, be clumsy or unsteady in gait, have progressive muscular weakness, have problems going up and down stairs, or getting up from a lying position?

QUESTIONS

RATIONALE

■ Did the child achieve motor and developmental milestones at approximately the right times? Does he or she seem to be growing and maturing normally? Is the child's development comparable to that of siblings or others of the same age?

◀ *Failure to achieve developmental milestones may indicate a neurologic disorder.*

🌐 Racial Variation

African-American children tend to develop motor skills more rapidly than children of other ethnic groups. This developmental difference persists until the child is 3 to 4 years of age.

■ Has the child been exposed to environmental lead?

◀ *Long-term exposure to lead may produce developmental delay or loss of skills; it is possible that no clinical signs of abnormality may be present.*

■ Have you been notified of any problems the child may be having in school, such as short attention span, lack of concentration, or hyperactivity?

◀ *Parental report of hyperactivity is usually the first sign of an attention deficit hyperactivity disorder (AD/HD).*

OLDER ADULTS

■ Do you feel dizzy when you first sit down, stand up, move your head, get up in the morning, or walk after eating?
■ Do you ever have to get up at night to urinate and feel faint as you stand?
■ Has the dizziness affected your performance of daily activities? Can you drive safely and maneuver within your house without incident? What safety modifications have you made?
■ Have you noticed any difficulty remembering or other changes in mental functions? Do you feel confused? Does this occur suddenly or gradually?
■ Do your muscles feel weak? Where? In one area or all over? Is this associated with any particular activity?

◀ *Problems with dizziness may result from diminished cerebral blood flow, vestibular response, or orthostatic hypotension. The resultant staggering with position change increases the risk of falling.*

◀ *Altered memory may be caused by a variety of disorders such as malnutrition, Alzheimer's disease, depression, organic brain syndrome, or CVA.*

■ Have you experienced any tremors in your hands or face? Anywhere else? Does this seem worse when you are anxious, at rest, or busy? What relieves this tremor? Rest? Activity? Alcohol? Does the tremor interfere with your performance of daily activities?

◀ *Senile tremor can be relieved with alcohol, although this is not recommended treatment. If the client reports using alcohol to relieve tremor, review the pattern of use for possible abuse.*

■ Do you have any problems with vision? Feel that you have fleeting blindness? When this occurs, is it associated with weakness? Have you lost consciousness?

◀ *These symptoms may indicate stroke.*

CLIENTS WITH SPECIAL NEEDS

Clients with expressive dysphasia are able to receive information, but may have difficulty answering questions about their history. This type of dysphasia can accompany a stroke or head injury involving Wernicke's area in the temporal lobe. When answering questions, these clients may require more time to respond. Patience is needed on the part of the examiner to determine how this person communicates best.

Clients taking medications, for example, anticonvulsants, may be slow to answer questions due to the medications they take to reduce seizures. These clients may include those diagnosed with epilepsy, as well as those who have had craniotomy or head injury. One of the side effects of slowing neuronal responses to reduce seizures may be a slowed thought process, requiring additional time and patience from the examiner.

EXAMINATION Procedure and Findings

Guidelines The major areas to be examined are mental and speech patterns, the cranial nerves, proprioception and cerebellar function, the motor system, the sensory system, and reflexes.

EQUIPMENT

Penlight to test pupillary reaction (CN III)
Tongue blade to test uvula (CN IX and X)
Bent paper clip or broken tongue blade to test sharp and dull sensation
Cotton ball to test light touch (sensation)
Cotton-tipped applicator to test two-point discrimination;
    test corneal reflex (CN V)
Tuning fork (128 Hz) to test vibratory sensation;
    test air and bone conduction (CN VIII)
Percussion hammer to test deep tendon reflexes
Aromatic materials to test sense of smell (CN I)

TECHNIQUES and NORMAL FINDINGS

ABNORMAL FINDINGS

ASSESS speech for Articulation, Comprehension, Coherence, and Voice Quality. Voice should have inflections and sufficient volume with clear speech.

- ■ Note errors in the choice of words or syllables; difficulty in articulation, which could involve thought processes, tongue, or lips; slurred speech (tone sounds slurred); poorly coordinated or irregular speech; monotone or weak voice; nasal tone, rasping, or hoarseness; whispering voice; and stuttering.

ASSESS nose for Smell. Evaluate olfactory cranial nerve (CN I). Have client close eyes and properly identify common aromatic substance held under the nose; test one nostril at a time. Examples include coffee, toothpaste, orange, or oil of cloves (Fig. 22-13).

- ■ Note if the client cannot smell anything or incorrectly identifies the odor. Allergic rhinitis or excessive tobacco smoking may interfere with ability to distinguish odors. Loss of smell may be caused by trauma to the cribriform plate or by an olfactory tract lesion.

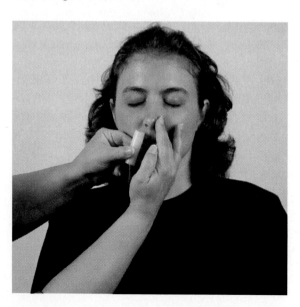

Fig. 22-13 Examination of the olfactory cranial nerve (CN I). *(From Chipps, Clanin, Campbell, 1992.)*

ASSESS eyes for Visual Acuity and Peripheral Vision. Test the optic nerve (CN II) for *visual acuity* using the Snellen eye chart (see Chapter 13) and *peripheral vision* by the confrontation test. The latter test is done by facing the client, standing or sitting 2 to 3 feet (60 to 90 cm) apart. Have the client cover one eye with an opaque card as you cover your own eye directly opposite the client's covered eye. (*Note:* An alternate technique involves not covering the eyes but instead testing them simultaneously in each of the four directions.) Stare directly at one another. Hold a pencil or use your finger midway between you and the client. Ask the client to report when he or she first sees the object; you should see the object at the same time. Slowly move the object in from the periphery in four directions: anteriorly (from above the head down into field of vision); inferiorly (from upper chest up toward field of vision), temporally (move laterally into field of vision), and nasally (move medially into the field of vision). If the client cannot see the pencil or finger at the same time as the examiner, peripheral field loss is suggested. Refer the client for more precise testing. Estimate the angle between the anteroposterior axis of the eye and the peripheral axis when the pencil or finger is first seen. Normal values are 50° upward, 90° temporal peripheral, 70° downward, and 60° degrees toward the nose. (*Note:* This test assumes that the examiner has normal peripheral visual fields.)

■ Lesions in the central nervous system (e.g., tumors) may cause peripheral visual defects such as loss of vision in one half or one quarter of the visual field, either medially or laterally. (See Fig. 13-33 in Chapter 13, *Eyes and Visual System.*)

ASSESS eyes for Extraocular Movement. The oculomotor (CN III), trochlear (CN IV), and abducens (CN VI) nerves are tested together since they control muscles that provide eye movement.

Test the movement of the eyes in the six cardinal fields of gaze as follows (see Fig. 13-9):

1. Have client look directly ahead at you.
2. Ask client to move his or her eyes only to follow your finger or an object in your hand.
3. Move an object from center position to upper outer extreme, hold there, move back to center, to lower inner extreme, and hold there.
4. Move an object to temporal-nasal extremes, holding there momentarily.
5. Move an object to opposite upper outer extreme and back to opposite lower inner extreme.

Normally there will be parallel tracking of the object with both eyes. Mild nystagmus at extreme lateral gaze is also normal.

(*Note:* An alternative method to steps 3 to 5 above is to move your finger in a clockwise circle to each of the six directions. Stop in each position so that the client can hold the gaze briefly before moving to the next position.)

■ Eye movement that is not parallel indicates an extraocular muscle weakness or a dysfunction of cranial nerve III, IV, or VI. Note any nystagmus other than that noted as normal. Note any ptosis (eyelid droop) that may occur with ocular myasthenia gravis.

ASSESS eyes for Pupillary Constriction and Accommodation. Further test the CN III for pupillary reaction and accommodation. Shine a light into the eye to note whether the iris constricts, making the pupil smaller (referred to as pupillary constriction). Accommodation is tested by observing pupillary constriction when the client changes gaze from a distant object to a near object (pencil or examiner's finger at 10 cm [4 inches] from bridge of the nose).

■ Increased intracranial pressure on or trauma to the midbrain may cause pressure on CN III, resulting in diminished to absent pupillary constriction, ptosis of the eye, and altered superior and inferior movement of the eyeball.

■ Clients with diabetes or syphilis may lose pupillary constriction to light, but retain accommodation.

ASSESS face for Movement and Sensation. Evaluate the trigeminal nerve (CN V) for facial movement and sensation. Test motor function by having the client clench his or her teeth, then palpate the temporal and masseter muscles. There should be bilaterally strong muscle contractions (Fig. 22-14, *A*).

■ Note any inequalities in muscle contractions, pain, twitching, or asymmetry. Any disorders of the pons, (e.g., a tumor) may cause altered function of CN V, VI, VII, or VIII.

TECHNIQUES and NORMAL FINDINGS

To test light sensation, have the client close his or her eyes, then wipe a cotton wisp lightly over the anterior scalp, paranasal sinuses, and jaw. A tickle sensation should be present equally over the palpated areas.

To test deep sensation, use alternating blunt and sharp ends of a paper clip over the client's forehead and paranasal sinuses. He or she should be able to feel pressure and pain equally throughout these areas and should be able to differentiate between sharp and dull (Fig. 22-14, *B*).

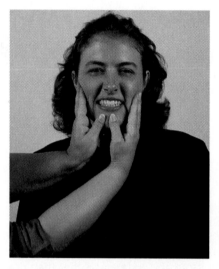 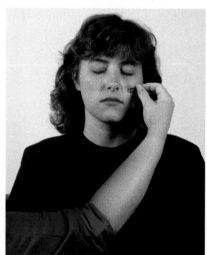

A   B

Fig. 22-14   Examination of the trigeminal nerve (CN V) for motor function, **A,** and sensory function, **B.**   *(From Chipps, Clanin, Campbell, 1992.)*

To test the sensation of a branch of CN V and motor function of CN VII by the corneal reflex, have the client look up and approach him or her from the side. Lightly touch the cornea with a wisp of cotton. There should be a bilateral blink to corneal touch.

Evaluate the facial nerve (CN VII) for facial movement. Inspect the face both at rest and during conversation. Have the client raise the eyebrows, frown, close the eyes tightly, show the teeth, smile, and puff out the cheeks. He or she should be able to correctly follow each command and the results should be symmetric (Fig. 22-15, *A-F*).

ABNORMAL FINDINGS

■ Note any decreased or unequal sensation.

■ Note any decreased or unequal sensation. Trigeminal neuralgia is characterized by stablike pain radiating along the trigeminal nerve, caused by degeneration of or pressure on the nerve.

■ Record if no blink occurs. Be sure to check that this abnormal response is not caused by the presence of contact lenses.

■ Note asymmetry, unequal movements, facial weakness, drooping of one side of the face or mouth, or inability to maintain position until instructed to relax.

TECHNIQUES and NORMAL FINDINGS

ABNORMAL FINDINGS

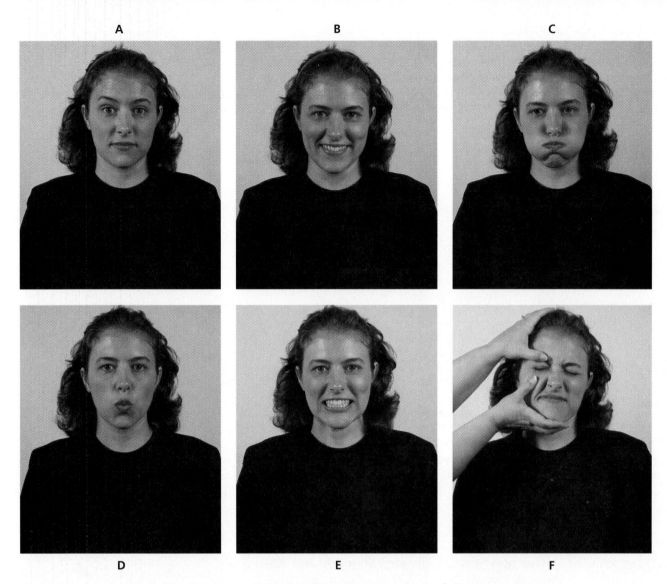

Fig. 22-15 Examination of the facial nerve (CN VII). Ask the client to make the following movements: **A,** Raise eyebrows and wrinkle forehead. **B,** Smile. **C,** Puff out cheeks. **D,** Purse lips and blow out. **E,** Show teeth. **F,** Squeeze eyes shut while you try to open them. *(From Chipps, Clanin, Campbell, 1992.)*

ASSESS ears for Hearing. Evaluate acoustic nerve (CN VIII) for hearing and balance. Hearing initially can be screened while taking the history. The following tests are also discussed in Chapter 12.

Whisper voice: Stand 1 to 2 feet (30 to 60 cm) slightly behind client, occlude the client's opposite ear, then whisper in one- and two-syllable words in a low voice. Client should hear 50% of time.

Rinne test uses a tuning fork to compare air and bone conduction. Strike tuning fork and place on client's mastoid process, noting the starting time in seconds; when client can no longer hear tone, note time, then move tuning fork in front of the ear; note time when client can no longer hear tone. Air-conducted sound should be heard twice as long as bone-conducted sound (AC > BC). This is a positive (expected) result.

Weber test assesses bone conduction by testing lateralization of sound. Strike tuning fork and place on midline of forehead. Client should perceive the sound equally.

■ Bone-conducted sound heard as long as or longer than air-conducted sound (BC>AC) is called a negative test; it is a sign of conductive hearing loss. Sensorineural hearing loss may be present when AC>BC in affected ear; but less than 2:1 ratio.

■ If client has conductive loss, sound lateralizes to affected ear. If client has sensorineural loss, sound lateralizes to unaffected ear.

ASSESS mouth for Taste. Evaluate taste over the anterior half of the tongue (CN VII). Instruct the client to stick out the tongue and leave it out during the testing process. Use a cotton applicator to place quantities of salt, sugar, and lemon on the client's tongue. He or she should be able to correctly identify each taste (Fig. 22-16).

Test glossopharyngeal nerve for taste of the posterior portion of the tongue or pharynx (CN IX). The client should be able to taste sweet, salty, and sour.

■ Note if the client cannot identify any of the tastes or consistently identifies a substance incorrectly.

■ Note if the client is unable to differentiate tastes.

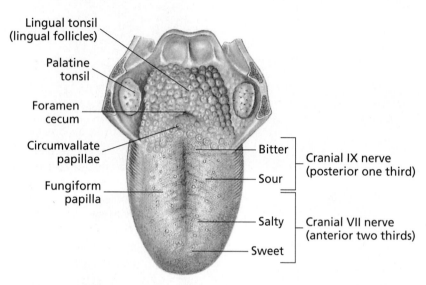

Fig. 22-16   Location of the taste bud regions tested for the sensory function of the facial and glossopharyngeal cranial nerves.   *(From Seidel et al, 1995.)*

ASSESS mouth for Gag Reflex and Movement of Soft Palate. Evaluate glossopharyngeal nerve (CN IX) and vagus nerve (CN X) together for movement and gag reflex. Instruct the client to say "Ah"; there should be bilaterally equal upward movement of the soft palate and uvula; gagging will occur; and speech should be smooth.

■ Note any asymmetry of the soft palate or tonsillar pillar movement, any lateral deviation of the uvula, or absence of the gag reflex. Disorders of the medulla oblongata, for example, tumors, may cause pressure on CN IX, X, XI, and XII.

ASSESS mouth for Tongue Movement, Symmetry, Strength, and Absence of Tumors. Evaluate hypoglossal nerve (CN XII) for symmetry and movement. Client protrudes tongue. Note symmetry, atrophy, and absence of tumors. Then ask client to move tongue toward nose, chin, and side to side. Strength of tongue can be tested by pressing it against your gloved index finger (Fig. 22-17).

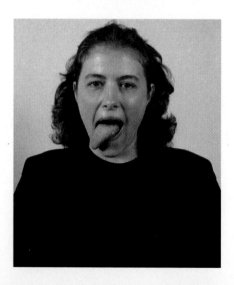

Fig. 22-17   Examination of the hypoglossal nerve (CN XII). *(From Chipps, Clanin, Campbell, 1992.)*

TECHNIQUES and NORMAL FINDINGS	ABNORMAL FINDINGS

ASSESS shoulder and neck muscles for Strength and Movement. Evaluate spinal accessory nerve (CN XI) for movement. First, have the client shrug his or her shoulders upward against your hands. Note strength and symmetry of contraction of the trapezius muscles.

Have the client turn his or her head to the side against your hand; repeat with the other side. Observe the contraction of the opposite sternocleidomastoid muscle and note the force of movement against your hand.

ASSESS cerebellar function for Balance and Coordination. To test proprioception (awareness of position and movement) and cerebellar function for an asymptomatic client, use at least two techniques for each area assessed. Choose these techniques based on the client's age and overall physical ability. For example, not every client should have to perform deep knee bends.

General: Observe gait by having the client walk across the room, turn, and walk back. He or she should be able to maintain upright posture, walk unaided, maintain balance, and use opposing arm swing.

Balance: Perform the Romberg test. Have the client stand with feet together, arms resting at sides, eyes open, then eyes closed. The examiner stands close to the client with arms ready to "catch" client if he or she begins to fall off balance. There will be slight swaying, but the upright posture and foot position should be maintained.

Have the client close his or her eyes and stand on one foot, then the other. He or she should be able to maintain position for at least 5 seconds.

Have the client walk in tandem, placing the heel of one foot directly against the toes of the other foot. The client should be able to maintain this heel-toe walking pattern along a straight line (Fig. 22-18).

■ Note any muscle weakness, whether unilateral or bilateral, and any pain or discomfort.

■ Note any inability to maintain the contracted muscle position, asymmetry, or difficulty of movement.

■ Unexpected findings may be due to a variety of causes, such as cerebellar tumors, stroke, Parkinson's disease, or inner ear problems.

■ Note poor posturing, ataxia, unsteady gait, rigid or absent arm movements, wide-based gait, trunk and head held tight, legs bent from hips only, lurching or reeling, scissors gait, or parkinsonian gait (stooped posture, flexion at hips, elbows, and knees).

■ If client sways with eyes closed but not open, the problem is probably proprioceptive. If client sways with eyes open and closed, the problem is probably cerebellar.

■ Note if the client cannot maintain single-foot balance for 5 seconds.

■ Note if the client is unable to maintain the heel-toe walking pattern or steps to a wider-based gait to maintain the upright posture.

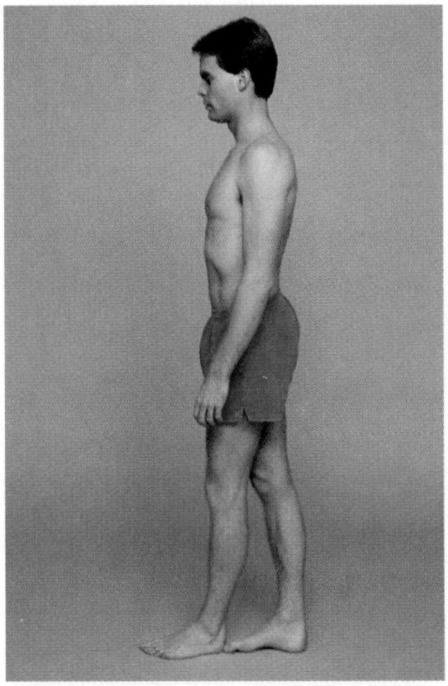

Fig. 22-18 Evaluation of balance with heel-toe walking on a straight line. *(From Seidel et al, 1995.)*

TECHNIQUES and NORMAL FINDINGS

ABNORMAL FINDINGS

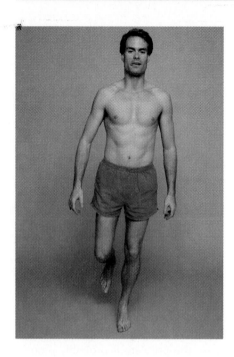

Fig. 22-19 Evaluation of balance with the client hopping in place on one foot. *(From Seidel et al, 1995.)*

Have the client hop first on one foot and then on the other. The client should be able to follow directions successfully and have enough muscle strength to follow through (Fig. 22-19).

Have the client hold a hand outward and perform several shallow or deep knee bends. He or she should be able to follow directions successfully, with muscle strength adequate to follow through.

Have client walk on toes, then heels. The client should be able to follow directions, walking several steps on the toes and then on the heels. He or she may need to use the hands to maintain balance.

Coordination: *Upper extremity:* Have the client alternately tap thighs with hands using rapid pronation and supination movements. Timing should be equal bilaterally and movement purposeful; the client should have no problem maintaining a rapid pace (Fig. 22-20, *A* and *B*).

Have the client stretch arms outward and use index fingers to alternately touch the nose rapidly; eyes are closed. The client should be able to repeatedly touch the nose in a rhythmic pattern.

- ▪ Note if the client is unable to hop or maintain single-leg balance.

- ▪ Note if the client is unable to perform activity because of difficulty with balance or lack of muscle strength.
- ▪ Note inability to retain balance, poor muscle strength, or inability to complete the activity.
- ▪ Any inability to maintain rapid pace is abnormal.

- ▪ Note missing the nose several times, or arms unable to maintain the testing position, tending to drift downward.

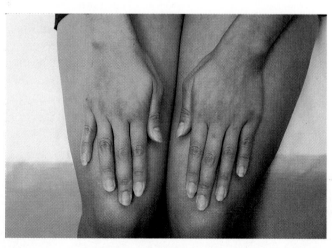 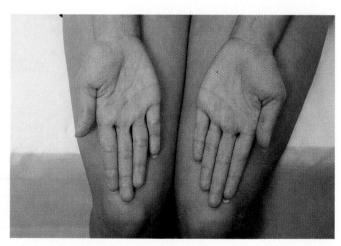

A   **B**

Fig. 22-20 Examination of coordination with rapid alternating movements. Ask client to tap top of thighs with both hands, alternately with **A,** palms down, and **B,** palms up.

TECHNIQUES and NORMAL FINDINGS

Evaluate the client's ability to perform rapid, rhythmic, alternating movement of fingers by having the client touch each finger to the thumb in rapid sequence. Test each hand separately. The client should have no problem rapidly and purposefully touching each finger to thumb (Fig. 22-21).

Have the client rapidly move his or her index finger back and forth between his or her nose and your finger 18 inches (46 cm) apart. Test one hand at a time. The client should be able to maintain the activity with a conscious coordinated effort (Fig. 22-22).

ABNORMAL FINDINGS

■ An inability to coordinate fine, discrete, rapid movement is abnormal.

■ Note if the client is unable to maintain continuous touch with both his or her own nose and your finger; if he or she is unable to maintain the rapid movement; or if there is obvious difficulty coordinating these movements.

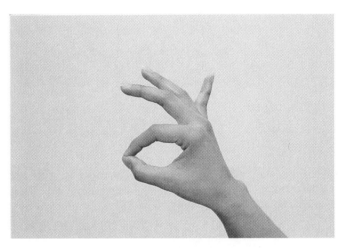

Fig. 22-21 Examination of finger coordination. Ask client to touch each finger to thumb in rapid sequence.

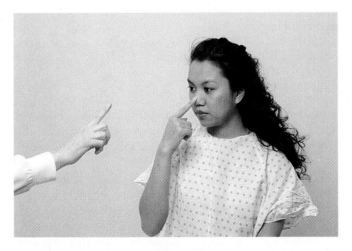

Fig. 22-22 Examination of fine motor function. Ask client to alternately touch own nose and the examiner's index finger with the index finger of one hand.

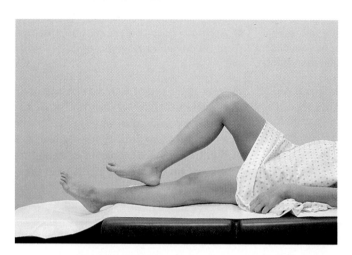

Fig. 22-23 Examination of fine motor function. Ask client to run heel of one foot down shin of other leg. Repeat with opposite leg.

Lower extremity: With the client seated, ask him or her to place the heel of one foot just below the opposite knee on the tibia (Fig. 22-23). Then ask the client to run the heel down the shin to the toe; repeat with the other foot. The client should be able to run the heel down the opposite shin purposefully, with bilaterally equal coordination.

ASSESS extremities for Muscle Strength, Sensation, and Deep Tendon Reflexes. *Muscle function:* Test muscle function according to the procedures outlined in Chapter 21.

Sensory function: Test the peripheral extremities in several areas for sensation. If intact, no further evaluation is needed; if impaired, move up extremities, testing periodically until a level or area of sensation is identified. Also evaluate the forehead, cheeks, and abdomen if necessary. If a deviation is identified, try to map out the area involved. Compare bilateral responses in each sensory testing area. Refer to dermatome chart (see Fig. 22-10) to identify the spinal nerve providing sensation to that area of the body.

Test light touch sensation by using a cotton wisp to lightly touch each designated area (client's eyes are closed) (Fig. 22-24, *A*). The client should perceive light sensation and be able to correctly point to or name the spot touched.

Test sharp and dull sensation by using the pointed tip of a paper clip to lightly prick each designated area (client's eyes are closed) (Fig. 22-24, *B*). Alternate sharp and dull sensations to more accurately evaluate the client's response. The client should perceive sensation and be able to identify the area touched.

Place a vibrating tuning fork on a bony area of the wrist, ankle, and sternum and ask the client to describe the sensation (Fig. 22-24, *C*). He or she should feel a sense of vibration. Repeat the procedure. Ask client when he or she no longer feels vibration, then stop vibration with tuning fork still touching bony prominence.

Test kinesthetic sensation by grasping the client's finger or toe and moving its position 0.4 inch (1 cm) up or down (client's eyes are closed) (Fig. 22-24, *D*). The client should be able to describe how the position has changed.

■ Note if the client cannot coordinate this activity, if the heel keeps moving off the shin, if the responses are unequal side to side, or if there are tremors or awkwardness.

■ Note specific areas of the body where sensation is impaired and whether there is absence of sensation or abnormal sensation.

■ Note if the client is unable to perceive the touch, incorrectly identifies the touched area, or exhibits an asymmetric response.
■ Note whether the client cannot perceive the sensation, incorrectly identifies touch location, or exhibits an asymmetric response.
■ Note unequal or decreased vibratory sensation. This may be found in clients with diabetes, as well as those who have had a stroke or spinal cord injury.
■ Note if the client cannot distinguish the change in position.

TECHNIQUES and NORMAL FINDINGS   **ABNORMAL FINDINGS**

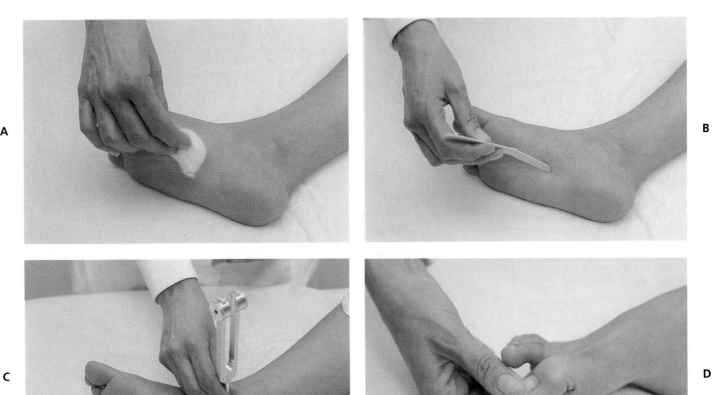

Fig. 22-24 Evaluation of peripheral nerve sensory function. **A,** Superficial tactile sensation. **B,** Superficial pain sensation. **C,** Vibratory sensation. **D,** Position sense of joints.

Test stereognosis by placing a small familiar object in the client's hand and asking the client to identify it (eyes closed) (Fig. 22-25, *A*). It should be properly identified.

Test two-point discrimination by touching selected parts of the body simultaneously while the client remains with eyes closed (Fig. 22-25, *B*). Use two sharp objects and ask the client to tell if one or two objects are used. The client should be able to distinguish two-point discrimination to the following distances: fingertips, 2.8 mm; palms, 8 to 12 mm; chest/forearm, 40 mm; back, 40 to 70 mm; and upper arm/thigh, 75 mm.

Evaluate graphesthesia using a blunt instrument to draw a number or letter on the client's hand, back, or other area (client has eyes closed) (Fig. 22-25, *C*). He or she should be able to recognize the number or letter drawn.

■ Note if the client cannot identify the object properly. Altered stereognosis may indicate a parietal lobe dysfunction.
■ Note if client cannot distinguish two-point discrimination.

■ If client cannot distinguish the number or letter, it may indicate a parietal lobe lesion.

A

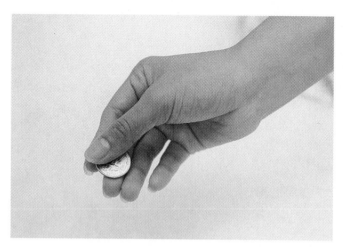

B

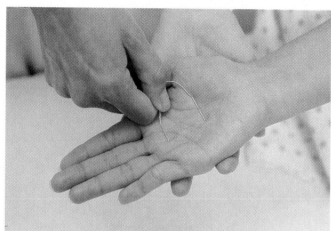

C

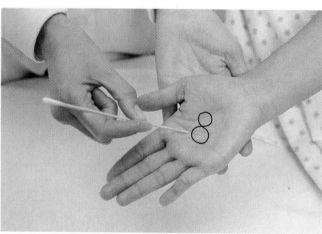

Fig. 22-25 Evaluation of cortical sensory function. **A,** Stereognosis: identification of a familiar object by touch. **B,** Two-point discrimination. **C,** Graphesthesia: draw letter or number on palm and ask client to identify by touch.

Reflexes: Test deep tendon reflexes for muscle contraction in response to direct or indirect percussion of a tendon. See the box below for scoring system. Hold reflex hammer between your thumb and index finger, and briskly tap the tendon with a flick of the wrist.

◼ Note if there is a hyperactive or diminished response or if the responses are unequal bilaterally for each of the reflexes. Unexpected findings indicate alteration of peripheral nerves or an area of the spinal cord from infection, compression, or trauma. See Table 22-2 for the spinal level of each reflex.

Scoring Deep Tendon Reflexes

Test the five deep tendon reflexes (triceps, biceps, brachioradial, patellar and achilles) using a reflex hammer. Compare the reflexes bilaterally. Reflexes are graded on a scale of 0 to 4+, with 2+ being the expected findings. Findings are recorded as follows:

0 = no response
1+ = sluggish or diminished
2+ = active or expected response
3+ = slightly hyperactive, more brisk than normal; not necessarily pathologic
4+ = brisk, hyperactive with intermittent clonus associated with disease

The client must be relaxed and sitting or lying down. To elicit the *triceps reflex,* ask client to let a relaxed arm fall onto your arm. Hold his or her arm, with elbow flexed at a 90° angle, in one hand. Palpate and strike the triceps tendon just above the elbow with either end of the reflex hammer (Fig. 22-26, *A*). (Some examiners prefer the flat end due to the wider striking surface.) The expected response is the contraction of the triceps muscle that causes visible or palpable extension of the elbow. An alternate arm position is to grasp the upper arm and allow the lower arm to bend at the elbow and hang freely, and then to strike the triceps tendon.

The *biceps reflex* is elicited by asking the client to let his or her relaxed arm fall onto your arm. Hold the arm with elbow flexed at a 90° angle, and place your thumb over the biceps tendon in the antecubital fossa and your fingers over the biceps muscle. Using the pointed end of the reflex hammer, strike your thumb instead of striking the tendon directly (Fig. 22-26, *B*). The expected response is the contraction of the biceps muscle that causes visible or palpable flexion of the elbow.

The *brachioradial reflex* is elicited by asking the client to let his or her relaxed arm fall into your hand. Hold the arm with the hand slightly pronated. Using either end of the reflex hammer, strike the brachioradialis tendon directly about 1 to 2 inches (2.5 to 5 cm) above the wrist (Fig. 22-26, *C*). The expected response is pronation of the forearm and flexion of the elbow.

The *patellar reflex* is tested by flexing the client's knee at a 90° angle, with the lower leg hanging freely. Strike the patellar tendon just below the patella (Fig. 22-26, *D*). The expected response is the contraction of the quadriceps muscle, causing extension of the lower leg. When no response is found, divert the client's attention to another muscular activity by asking him or her to pull the fingers of each hand against the other. While the client is pulling, strike the patellar tendon.

The *Achilles tendon* is assessed by flexing the client's knee and dorsiflexing the ankle 90°. Hold your hand against the bottom of the client's foot while you strike the Achilles tendon at the level of the ankle malleolus with the flat end of the reflex hammer (Fig. 22-26, *E*). The expected response is the contraction of the gastrocnemius muscle, causing plantar flexion of the foot.

Check for the plantar (Babinski) reflex. Using a moderately sharp object, stroke the lateral aspect of the sole of the foot from heel to ball, curving medially across the ball of the foot (Fig. 22-26, *F*). There should be flexion of the great toe, with fanning of the other toes.

Test for ankle clonus if reflexes are hyperactive. Support the client's knee in partly flexed position. With the other hand, sharply dorsiflex the foot and maintain it in flexion (Fig. 22-26, *G*). There should be no movement of the foot.

■ Note if extension of the great toe, with fanning of the other toes, occurs; this indicates pyramidal tract disease.

■ Note if there are rhythmic oscillations between dorsiflexion and plantar flexion.

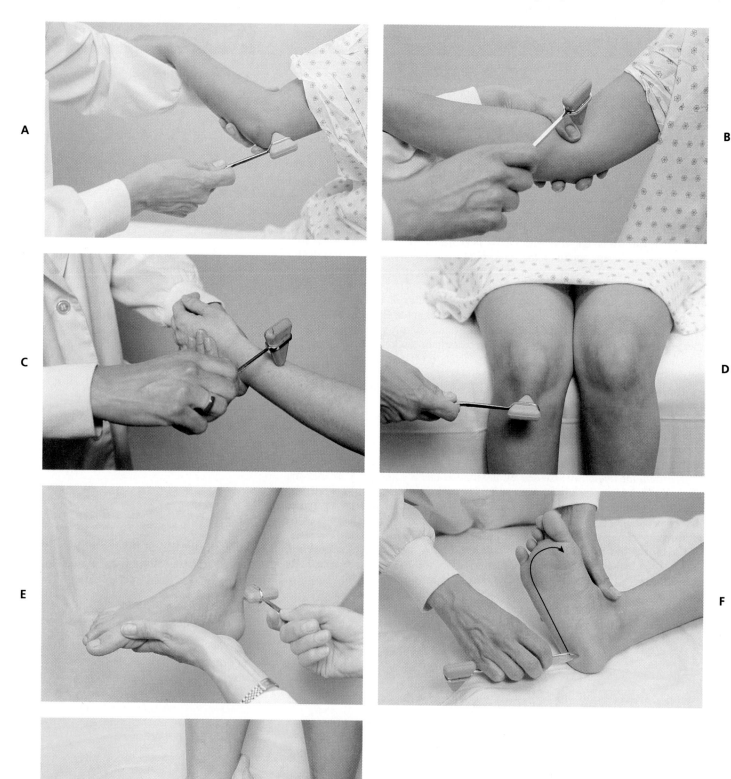

Fig. 22-26 Location of tendons for evaluation of deep tendon reflexes. **A,** Triceps reflex. **B,** Biceps reflex. **C,** Brachioradialis reflex. **D,** Patellar reflex. **E,** Achilles reflex. **F,** Babinski reflex. **G,** Ankle tonus.

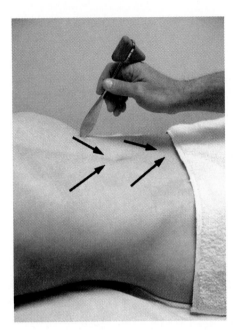

Fig. 22-27 Examination of the superficial abdominal reflexes. One of several approaches is illustrated. *(From Seidel et al, 1991.)*

ASSESS abdomen for Superficial Reflexes. Test abdominal reflexes for reaction. With the client lying down, use a sharp instrument to lightly stroke both above and below the umbilicus diagonally (Fig. 22-27). The abdominal muscles contract slightly, and the umbilicus moves slightly toward the area of stimulation. The response should be equal bilaterally. See Table 22-2 for spinal level of these reflexes.

(For male clients:) Check the cremasteric reflex. Lightly stroke the inner aspect of the thigh with the reflex hammer or tongue blade. The ipsilateral testicle should rise slightly.

ASSESS Mental Status. Most information needed for the assessment of the "normal" client's mental status is obtained from the psychosocial history. The "minimental state" test is a standardized screening tool of mental status (Fig. 22-28).

Appearance and Grooming. Observe whether appearance is appropriate for the season.

■ Lack of concern for appearance or inappropriate dress for the season in a previously well-groomed person may indicate an emotional problem, psychiatric disturbance, or organic brain syndrome.

■ Positive responses may indicate anxiety or depressive states.

Behavior. Ask the following questions: Do you have difficulty falling asleep, staying asleep, or being wakeful early in the morning? Describe your mood in the morning. Have you noticed any marked changes in appetite or eating habits? Have you recently gained or lost weight? Do you have periods of depression or nervousness to the extent that you feel unable to cope? If so, how do you treat yourself? Is the treatment effective? Do you have crying spells? Have you noticed a change in the amount of energy you have to accomplish daily functions? Do you have difficulty making decisions? Have you noticed an increase in irritability? Restlessness? Listlessness? Do you ever feel as though you do not care about anything? Do you spend much time alone? (Estimate the number of waking hours per day, per week.) Do you have friends whom you can trust and who are available when you need them? Have you ever thought about hurting yourself or ending your life? (If so, describe past methods and any specific plans for the future.)

Patient.................................
Examiner..............................
Date ....

"MINI-MENTAL STATE"

Maximum
Score   Score

ORIENTATION

5   ( )   What is the (year) (season) (date) (day) (month)?
5   ( )   Where are we: (state) (county) (town) (hospital) (floor).

REGISTRATION

3   ( )   Name 3 objects: 1 second to say each. Then ask the patient all 3 after you have said them.
              Give 1 point for each correct answer. Then repeat them until he learns all
              3. Count trials and record.
                            Trials

ATTENTION AND CALCULATION

5   ( )   Serial 7's. 1 point for each correct. Stop after 5 answers. Alternatively spell "world"
              backwards.

RECALL

3   ( )   Ask for the 3 objects repeated above. Give 1 point for each correct.

LANGUAGE

9   ( )   Name a pencil, and watch (2 points)
              Repeat the following "No ifs, ands or buts." (1 point)
              Follow a 3-stage command:
                      "Take a paper in your right hand, fold it in half, and put in on the floor"
                      (3 points)
              Read and obey the following:
                      CLOSE YOUR EYES (1 point)
              Write a sentence (1 point)
              Copy design (1 point)
_____   Total score

ASSESS level of consciousness along a continuum _____
                                      Alert   Drowsy   Stupor   Coma

INSTRUCTIONS FOR ADMINISTRATION OF MINI-MENTAL STATE EXAMINATION

ORIENTATION

(1) Ask for the date. Then ask specifically for parts omitted, e.g., "Can you also tell me what season it is?" One point for each correct.

(2) Ask in turn "Can you tell me the name of this hospital?" (town, county, etc.). One point for each correct.

REGISTRATION

Ask the patient if you may test his memory. Then say the name of 3 unrelated objects, clearly and slowly, about one second for each. After you have said 3, ask him to repeat them. The first repetition determines his score (0-3) but keep saying them until he can repeat all 3, up to 6 trials. If he does not eventually learn all 3, recall cannot be meaningfully tested.

ATTENTION AND CALCULATION

Ask the patient to begin with 100 and count backwards by 7. Stop after 5 subtractions (93,86,79,72,65). Score the total number of correct answers.

If the patient cannot or will not perform this task, ask him to spell the word "world" backwards. The score is the number of letters in correct order. E.g. dlrow = 5, dlorw = 3.

RECALL

Ask the patient if he can recall the 3 words you previously asked him to remember. Score 0-3.

LANGUAGE

Naming: Show the patient a wrist watch and ask him what it is. Repeat for pencil. Score 0-2.

Repetition: Ask the patient to repeat the sentence after you. Allow only one trial. Score 0 or 1.

3-Stage command: Give the patient a piece of plain blank paper and repeat the command. Score 1 point for each part correctly executed.

Reading: On a blank piece of paper print the sentence "Close your eyes", in letters large enough for the patient to see clearly. Ask him to read it and do what it says. Score 1 point only if he actually closes his eyes.

Writing: Give the patient a blank piece of paper and ask him to write a sentence for you. Do not dictate a sentence, it is to be written spontaneously. It must contain a subject and verb to be sensible. Correct grammer and puncuation are not necessary.

Copying: On a clean piece of paper, draw intersecting pentagons, each side about 1 in., and ask him to copy it exactly as it is. All 10 angles must be present and 2 must intersect to score 1 point. Tremor and rotation are ignored.

Estimate the patient's level of sensorium along a continuum, from alert on the left to coma on the right.

Fig. 22-28   "Mini-mental state" test, a standardized screening tool of mental status. The maximum score is 30. Depressed clients without dementia usually score between 24 and 30. A score of 20 or less is found in clients with dementia, delirium, schizophrenia, or an affective disorder.   *(From Folstein et al, 1985.)*

TECHNIQUES and NORMAL FINDINGS

ABNORMAL FINDINGS

Cognitive Abilities. Assess client's orientation to time, place, and person.

Some people have difficulty keeping up with dates and places; do you know what today's date is? Do you know where you are? What is your name and address?

- *Time* disorientation is associated with anxiety, depression, and organic brain syndrome. *Place* disorientation may occur with psychiatric disorders and organic brain syndrome. *Person* disorientation may result from cerebral trauma, seizures, or amnesia.

Assess client's memory.

Recent: What did you have for breakfast this morning? What time did you arrive at the agency today? What time was your appointment?

Remote: (Ask questions about medical history, first job, when married.)

Assess ability to make judgments:

What would you do if you saw a man picking someone's pocket right in front of you? What would you do if you needed to use a vending machine and had no change?

Assess abstract reasoning:

Ask the client to explain the meaning of the following proverbs.

- A bird in the hand is worth two in the bush.
- Not to decide is to decide.
- Every cloud has a silver lining.

- Impaired memory occurs in various neurologic and psychiatric disorders.

- Inability to give an adequate explanation may indicate organic brain syndrome, brain damage, or lack of intelligence.

Emotional Stability. Assess emotional status alteration:

(Inquire about stressors such as money, intimate relationships, death or illness of a family member or friend, employment problems.) How are you feeling right now? Do you consider your present feeling to be a problem in your daily life? If so, do you feel the problem is temporary or curable?

Assess thought content disruptions. Do you have certain thoughts or feelings that consistently return or disrupt your thinking? Are you able to control them? Do you ever lose control of your thoughts? Do you have any dreadful or uncontrollable fears that keep returning? Do you have the feeling that something dreadful is going to happen? Do you feel you have enemies or that someone is trying to hurt, discredit, or control you? Do you feel guilty about your behavior or your feelings? Do you ever have the feeling you are losing touch with what is happening around you? Perception distortion: Do you ever hear voices or strange noises? Do you see visions, lights, or people that others cannot see? Do you ever experience strange odors or tastes? Have you ever experienced strange sensations (warmth, pressure, cold) on your skin?

- Thought content disruptions may occur in various neurologic or psychiatric disorders.

Additional Assessment Techniques for Special Cases. Meningeal signs are assessed when meningitis is suspected. These include tests for Kernig's sign and Brudzinski's sign. Kernig's sign is tested by flexing one of the client's legs at the hip and knee, then extending the knee (Fig. 22-29, *A*). No pain reported is a negative Kernig's sign. The second test is performed with the client supine. The examiner flexes the client's neck (Fig. 22-29, *B*). The client should report no pain or resistance to neck flexion.

The Glasgow Coma Scale assesses level of consciousness using a 15-point scale (Fig. 22-30). Clients are assessed for the best response to eye opening, motor response, and verbal response. For example, when a client who is paralyzed on one side due to a stroke is assessed, the best motor response is assessed on the client's unaffected side.

- If a client has inflammation of the meninges, he or she will report pain along the vertebral column when the leg is extended; a positive Kernig's sign indicating irritation of the meninges.
- A positive Brudzinski's sign occurs when client passively flexes hip and knee in response to head flexion and reports pain along vertebral column.

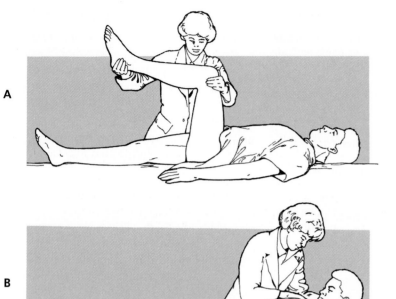

A

B

Fig. 22-29   Kernig's sign and Brudzinski's sign are tests of meningeal irritation. **A,** Kernig's sign. Flex one of the client's legs at the hip and knee. Note resistance or pain. **B,** Brudzinski's sign. With the client recumbent, place your hands behind the client's head and flex the neck forward. Note resistance or pain. Watch also for flexion of the client's hips and knees in reaction to your maneuver.   *(From Chipps, Clanin, Campbell, 1992.)*

Glasgow Coma Scale

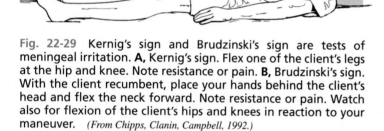

Best eye-opening response	Spontaneously	4
	To verbal command	3
	To pain	2
	No response	1
Best verbal response	Oriented, converses	5
	Disoriented, converses	4
	Inappropriate words	3
	Incomprehensible sounds	2
	No response	1
Best motor response		
To verbal command	Obeys	6
To painful stimulus	Localizes pain	5
	Flexion-withdrawal	4
	Flexion-decorticate	3
	Extension-decerebrate	2
	No response	1
	TOTAL	(3-15)

Decorticate   Rigid flexion; upper arms held tightly to the sides of body; elbows, wrists, and fingers flexed; feet are plantar flexed, legs extended and internally rotated; may have fine tremors or intense stiffness

Decerebrate   Rigid extension; arms fully extended; forearms pronated; wrists and fingers flexed; jaws clenched, neck extended, back may be arched; feet plantar flexed; may occur spontaneously, intermittently, or in response to a stimulus

Fig. 22-30   Glasgow coma scale.   *(Modified from Chipps, Clanin, Campbell, 1992.)*

NEWBORNS/INFANTS

■ APPROACH

There is more neurologic maturation during the first year of life than in any other period. The examiner must closely evaluate this development month by month. If the infant is quiet before the exam, his or her slumber will be disturbed, because the neurologic examination requires moving the infant in many positions.

■ FINDINGS

Newborns

Note the responses of the newborn or ask parents about them. Newborns should respond to touch, pressure, and temperature. They yawn, blink, sneeze, and hiccup. Reflexes to evaluate posture and movement and feeding responses are described in Table 22-3. As the newborn's neurologic system matures, these reflexes disappear. *Abnormal findings* would include abnormal or absent response to reflexes or asymmetric or weak movement.

Infants

Assess the infant for achievement of expected developmental milestones for fine- and gross-motor, social/adaptive, and language skills described in Chapter 2. Observe the infant's waking activity, responses to environmental stimuli, and social interactions with parents and others. Observe spontaneous motor activity; it should be smooth and symmetric. Assess resting posture for muscle tone. Cranial nerves are assessed by observing eye movements, wrinkling of forehead, turning head toward a sound, swallowing, and sucking. Flex the infant's knees onto the abdomen and quickly release them. They should unfold gradually. Flex the infant's head forward; the baby should comply. With the baby supine, pull to a sitting position holding the wrists; observe head control. Some head flexion (head lag) is normally present. Three-month-old babies raise the head and arch the back; this reflex persists until 18 months of age. Note muscle strength as reflected in sucking and spontaneous motor activity. There should be no tremors or constant overshooting when reaching for something.

Abnormal findings include lethargy, hyporeactivity, hyperirritability, and a report by the parent(s) of any significant change in behavior. Motor activity delays may indicate brain damage, mental retardation, peripheral neuromuscular damage, illness, or neglect. Abnormal postures include frog position (hips abducted, almost flat on table, externally rotated) and opisthotonos (stiff neck, head arched backward, arms and legs extended). Any continued asymmetry of posture is also abnormal. Note any spasticity, which may be an early sign of cerebral palsy. If present, the legs quickly extend and adduct, possibly even in a scissoring pattern. The baby will resist head movement and push back against the examiner's hand. Note any head lag, which could indicate brain damage.

TABLE 22-3	Infantile Reflexes			

REFLEX	TECHNIQUE FOR EVALUATION	APPEARANCE AGE	DISAPPEARANCE AGE	NORMAL RESPONSE
Reflexes to evaluate position and movement				
Moro	Startle infant by making loud noise, jarring examination surface, or slightly raising infant off examination surface and letting him fall quickly back onto examining table	Birth	1 to 4 months	Infant abducts and extends arms and legs; index finger and thumb assume C position; then infant pulls both arms and legs up against trunk as if trying to protect self
Tonic neck	Infant supine; rotate head to side so that chin is over shoulder	Birth to 6 weeks	4 to 6 months	Arm and leg on side to which head turns extend; opposite arm and leg flex; infant assumes fencing position (some normal infants may never show this reflex)
Plantar grasp	Touch object to sole of infant's foot	Birth	8 to 10 months	Toes will flex tightly downward in attempt to grasp
Palmar grasp	Touch object against ulnar side of infant's hand; then place finger in palm of hand	Birth	3 to 4 months	Infant will grasp finger; grasp should be tight, and examiner may be able to pull infant into sitting position by infant's grasp

TABLE 22-3	Infantile Reflexes—cont'd			
REFLEX	**TECHNIQUE FOR EVALUATION**	**APPEARANCE AGE**	**DISAPPEARANCE AGE**	**NORMAL RESPONSE**
Reflexes to evaluate position and movement—cont'd				
Babinski	Stroke lateral surface of infant's sole, using inverted J-curve from sole to great toe	Birth	18 months	Infant response: positive response showing fanning of toes
		Starting 18 months		Adult response: occurs after child has been walking for some time; flexion of great toe with slight fanning of other toes
Step in place	Infant in upright position, feet flat on surface	Birth	3 months	Will pace forward using alternating steps
Clonus	Dorsiflex foot; pinch sole of foot just under toes	Birth	4 months	May get clonus movement of foot (not always present)
Feeding reflexes				
Rooting response (awake)	Brush infant's cheek near corner of mouth	Birth	3 to 4 months	Infant will turn head in direction of stimulus and will open mouth slightly
Sucking	Touch infant's lips	Birth	10 to 12 months	Sucking motion follows with lips and tongue

CHILDREN

Follow the same sequence of evaluation as for adults when dealing with children, making the following alterations.

■ APPROACH

The examiner may need to make careful observations of the child during spontaneous activity, since the child may not be able to cooperate with requests as an adult would. Making the examination a game helps in data collection.

■ FINDINGS

Assess the child for achievement of expected developmental milestones for fine- and gross-motor, social/adaptive, and language skills described in Chapter 2. Evaluate the child's general behavior while he or she is at play, interacting with parents, and cooperating with parents and with the examiner. Usually the sense of smell is not tested; if it is, use a scent familiar to the child, such as orange or peanut butter. In testing visual fields and gaze (CN II, III, IV, and VI), gently immobilize the head so that the child cannot follow objects with the whole head but only with the eyes. For testing CN VII, approach it like a game, asking the child to make "funny faces" as the examiner models them. Evaluate motor skills as the child performs the activities of dressing, undressing, and manipulating buttons. This provides information concerning fine motor skills, muscle strength, symmetry, and range of motion of the various joints.

Observe the child's gait while running as well as walking. Toddlers normally have a wide-based gait, and preschoolers walk in a knock-kneed fashion. Normally children can balance on one foot for 5 seconds by age 4 and 8 to 10 seconds at age 5. They hop at 4 years of age.

Observe the child as he or she rises from a supine position on the floor to a sitting and then a standing position. Note in particular the muscles of the neck, abdomen, and extremities. Note weakness of the pelvic muscles (Gower's sign). Use the finger-to-nose test to evaluate fine-motor coordination. Use the Denver II to assess fine-motor coordination in children under 6 years of age. For children older than 6 years, use the finger-to-nose test, with the examiner's finger held 1 to 2 inches (2.5 to 5 cm) away from the child's nose

Sensory function is not normally tested before age 5. Carefully explain what is being done when children are tested, and use descriptions that the child can understand, such as "this will feel like a tickle or a mosquito bite." Use simple numbers for graphesthesia testing (such as 0, 7, 5, 3, or 1) and X and O for younger children. The responses should be the same as those listed for adults. It is not necessary to test reflexes if the child shows all other healthy neurologic signs.

The screening assessment for neurologic "soft" signs in school-age children is controversial (Table 22-4). It is used to describe vague and minimal dysfunctions signs, such as clumsiness, language disturbances, motor overload, mirroring movement of extremities, or perceptual development difficulties. These signs may be considered normal in the young child, but as the child matures, the signs should disappear. Their continued presence represents a developmental delay or lag in the sensory or motor system. The identification of soft signs indicates failure of the child to perform age-specific activities. If the examiner finds responses indicating difficulty in performing tasks, the responses should be clustered as described in Table 22-4 and the child referred.

Abnormal findings include muscle hypertrophy, atrophy, weakness, or incoordination. Note any persistence of broad-based gait beyond the toddler stage, scissor gait, or failure to hop after 5 years of age.

TABLE 22-4	Screening Assessment of Neurologic "Soft" Signs	
INSTRUCTIONAL TECHNIQUE	**IMPORTANT OBSERVATIONS**	**VARIABLES AND CONSIDERATIONS**
1. Evaluation of fine motor coordination: observe child during:		
a. Undressing, unbuttoning	Note child's general coordination	
b. Tying shoe		
c. Rapidly touching alternate fingers with thumb	Note if similar movement on opposite side	For items c to e and b and i, movement of other side noted as associated motor movements, adventitious overflow movements, or synkinesis
d. Rattling imaginary doorknob	Note if similar movement on other side	
e. Unscrewing imaginary light bulb	Note if similar movement on other side	
f. Grasping pencil and writing	Note excessive pressure on pen point; fingers placed directly over point, or placed greater than 1 inch (2.5 cm) up shaft	May indicate difficulty with fine-motor coordination
g. Moving tongue rapidly		
h. Demonstrating hand grip	Note if similar movement on opposite side	
i. Inverting feet	Note if similar movement on opposite side	
j. Repeating several times "pa, ta, ka" or "kitty, kitty, kitty"	Accurate reproduction of these sounds indicates auditory coordination	
2. Evaluation of special sensory skills		
a. Dual simultaneous sensory tests (face-hand testing): first demonstrate technique, then instruct child to close eyes; examiner performs simultaneously:		
(1) Touch both cheeks	Failure to perceive hand stimulus when face simultaneously touched referred to as *rostral dominance*	About 80% of normal children able to perform this test by age 8 years without rostral dominance
(2) Touch both hands		
(3) Touch right cheek and right hand		
(4) Touch left cheek and right hand		
(5) Touch left cheek and left hand		
(6) Touch right cheek and left hand		
b. Finger localization test (finger agnosia test): touch two spots on one finger or two fingers simultaneously; child has eyes closed; ask, "How many fingers am I touching, one or two?"	Evaluate number of correct responses with four trials for each hand Six out of eight possible correct responses passes	About 50% of all children pass test by age 6 years About 90% of all children pass by age 9 years This test reflects child's orientation in space, concept of body image, sensation of touch, and position sense
3. Evaluation of child's laterality and orientation in space		
a. Imitation of gestures: instruct child to use same hand as examiner and to imitate the following movements ("Do as I do"): (1) Extend little finger (2) Extend little and index fingers	Note difficulty with fine finger movements, manipulation, or reproduction of correct gesture Note any marked right-left confusion regarding examiner's right and left hands	This test helps to evaluate child's finger discrimination and awareness of body image, right, left, front, back, and up and down orientation Especially important after age 8 years if there continues to be marked right-left confusion

Data from McMillan J. Nieburg P. Oski F: The whole pediatrician catalog, *Philadelphia, 1977, WB Saunders.*

Continued

TABLE 22-4	Screening Assessment of Neurologic "Soft" Signs—*cont'd*

INSTRUCTIONAL TECHNIQUE	IMPORTANT OBSERVATIONS	VARIABLES AND CONSIDERATIONS
(3) Extend index and middle fingers (4) Touch two thumbs and two index fingers together simultaneously (5) Form two interlocking rings—thumb and index finger of one hand, with thumb and index finger of other hand (6) Point index finger of one hand down toward cupped finger of opposite hand held below		
b. Following directions: ask child to: (1) Show me your left hand (2) Show me your right eye (3) Show me your left elbow (4) Touch your left knee with your left hand (5) Touch your right ear with your left hand (6) Touch your left elbow with your right hand (7) Touch your right cheek with your right hand	Note any incorrect response Note any difficulty with following sequence of directions	Items *1* through *7* mastered by approximately age 6 years
(8) Point to my left ear (9) Point to my right eye (10) Point to my right hand (11) Point to my left knee		Items *8* through *11* mastered by age 8 years

OLDER ADULTS

■ APPROACH

The neurologic examination for older adults is the same as for younger adults.

■ FINDINGS

The examiner should be aware that some older adults have slowed responses, move more slowly, or show a decline in function (for example, the sense of taste). Other normal changes with aging include decline in muscle bulk, especially in the hands; occasionally senile tremors or dyskinesias (defects in voluntary movements) deviation of gait from midline; difficulty with rapidly alternating movements; and some loss of reflexes and sensations (for example, the knee jerk or ankle jerk reflexes and light touch and pain sensations). Older adults may have difficulty relaxing their limbs and may require reinforcement when you are eliciting deep tendon reflexes. Often a normal flexor response is indistinct, and the plantar reflex may be missing or hard to interpret. An extensor response is abnormal, however. Superficial abdominal reflexes may be missing.

CLIENTS WITH SITUATIONAL VARIATIONS

PREGNANT WOMEN

■ FINDINGS

Although the examination proceeds as for other adults, pregnancy alters gait and balance and produces vascular symptoms. The pregnant woman normally has a side-waddling gait with broad-based support as a result of softening of the pelvic joints and instability. She may appear clumsy and tend to lose balance because of the shift in her center of gravity. In addition, she may experience light-headedness or fainting from vasodilation, hypoglycemia, or hypotension.

Abnormal findings are seizures, increased seizures from a preexisting condition, signs of multiple dystrophy or myasthenia gravis, carpal tunnel syndrome (burning, pain, tingling in hand, wrist, or elbow), or hand numbness as a result of brachial plexus traction. Conditions return to prepregnant state after delivery.

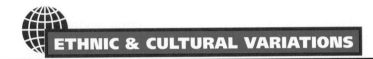

ETHNIC & CULTURAL VARIATIONS

■ FINDINGS

The structure and function of the neurologic system is consistent across racial lines. Some differences have been noted in early motor development. Young African-American children tend to develop more rapidly than other children.

Stroke is the third leading cause of death in the United States and cultural differences are noted among various ethnic groups in morbidity and mortality from this disease. African-American men are at particular risk. Depression and resultant suicide is seen at a much higher rate among young American Indian/Alaskan Native men than any other group in the United States.

E X A M I N A T I O N   S U M M A R Y

Neurologic System and Mental Status

- Assess speech *(p. 652)* for:
  Articulation
  Comprehension
  Coherence
  Voice quality
- Assess nose *(p. 652)* for:
  Smell (olfactory nerve CN I)
- Assess eyes *(p. 654)* for:
  Visual acuity and peripheral vision (optic nerve CN II)
  Extraocular movement (oculomotor nerve CN III, trochlear nerve CN IV, and abducens nerve CN VI)
  Pupillary constriction and accommodation (oculomotor nerve CN III)
- Assess face *(pp. 653-654)* for:
  Movement (trigeminal nerve CN V and facial nerve CN VII)
  Sensation (trigeminal nerve CN V)
- Assess ears *(p. 655)* for:
  Hearing (acoustic nerve CN VIII)
- Assess mouth *(p. 656)* for:
  Taste (anterior tongue: facial nerve CN VIII;

posterior tongue: glossopharyngeal nerve CN IX)
  Gag reflex and movement of soft palate (glossopharyngeal CN IX and vagus nerve CN X)
  Tongue movement, symmetry, strength, and absence of tumors (hypoglossal nerve CN XII)
- Assess shoulder and neck muscles *(p. 657)* for:
  Strength (spinal accessory CN XI)
  Movement
- Assess cerebellar function *(p. 657-660)* for:
  Balance and coordination (also tests CN VIII)
- Assess extremities *(p. 660-664)* for:
  Muscle strength
  Sensation
  Deep tendon reflexes
- Assess abdomen *(p. 665)* for:
  Superficial reflexes
- Assess mental status *(p. 665-668)* for:
  Physical appearance
  Behavior
  Cognitive abilities
  Emotional stability

COMMON PROBLEMS / CONDITIONS
associated with the Nervous System and Mental Status

DISORDERS OF ALTERED MENTAL STATUS

■ **Depression:** An abnormal emotional state characterized by exaggerated feelings of sadness, melancholy, dejection, worthlessness, emptiness, and hopelessness that are inappropriate and out of proportion to reality. The overt manifestations, which are extremely variable, range from a slight lack of motivation and inability to concentrate to severe physiologic alterations of body function and may represent symptoms of a variety of mental and physical conditions, a syndrome related to symptoms associated with a particular disease, or a specific mental illness.

 Cultural Note

> The suicide rates among American Indian and Alaskan Native men aged 15 to 24 is 2½ times that of the general population.

■ **Delirium:** An acute confusional state that can be completely reversed. A cluster of cognitive impairments include a clouded awareness involving sensory misperceptions and disordered thought. Disordered thought processes include disturbed attention, memory thinking, and orientation. There also may be disturbances in activity patterns and the wake-sleep cycle. Generally there is a rapid onset with a brief course of illness. Signs may include restlessness; frightened facial expression; garbled, incoherent speech; agitation; and disorientation to time and place.

■ **Dementia:** A progressive, organic mental disorder characterized by chronic personality disintegration, confusion, disorientation, stupor, deterioration of intellectual capacity and function, and impairment of memory, judgment, and impulses. Dementia may be improved when the cause is related to drug intoxication, pernicious anemia, paresis, subdural hematoma, benign brain tumor, hydrocephalus, or insulin shock. Dementia usually is not amenable to treatment when caused by Alzheimer's disease, Pick's disease, Huntington's chorea, and traumatic brain injury.

■ **AIDS dementia complex (HIV encephalopathy):** A progressive dementia related to HIV infection of the brain. It is a neurologic effect of encephalitis or brain inflammation experienced by nearly one-third of all AIDS clients. There is an insidious onset with headaches, loss of memory and concentration, and inability to follow complex instructions. Motor findings include hyperreflexia, inability to perform rapid rhythmic movements, clumsiness and weakness of arms and legs, and gait ataxia. Incontinence of stool and urine may also occur.

■ **Alzheimer's disease:** A type of dementia characterized initially by memory loss and disintegration of personality. Later symptoms include disorientation, restlessness, speech disturbances, and inability to carry out purposeful movements. There is severe progressive deterioration in mental functions with subtle, insidious onset.

DISORDERS OF THE CENTRAL NERVOUS SYSTEM

■ **Multiple sclerosis:** A progressive disease characterized by disseminated demyelination of nerve fibers of the brain and spinal cord. It is thought to be caused by an autoimmune disorder initiated by a virus that attacks the myelin at various areas of the central nervous system. Since the sites of demyelination are varied, the symptoms of the disease are varied. It begins slowly in young adulthood and continues throughout life with period of exacerbations and remissions. The first signs may be paresthesia of extremities or of one side of the face. Other early signs include muscle weakness, vertigo, and visual disturbance such as nystagmus, diplopia, and partial blindness. Later in the disease there may be emotional lability, ataxia, or paralysis.

■ **Seizure disorder:** A hyperexcitation of neurons in the brain leading to a sudden violent involuntary series of muscle contractions that may be paroxysmal and episodic, as in a seizure disorder, or transient and acute, as after a concussion. A seizure may be partial, such as localized seizures, or generalized, such as tonic-clonic.

■ **Meningitis:** An inflammation of the meninges that surround the brain and spinal cord. It may result from invasion of bacteria, viruses, fungi, parasites, or other toxins. Bacterial meningitis is most common and can result in death if not treated promptly. By contrast, viral meningitis is a self-limiting infection with full recovery. Symptoms of meningitis include severe headache, fever, and generalized malaise. Signs of meningeal irritation are common; these include stiff neck and positive Brudzinski's and Kernig's signs. Level of consciousness may decrease with drowsiness and reduced attention span, which may progress to stupor and coma. Confusion, agitation, and irritability may occur.

■ **Encephalitis:** An inflammation of the brain tissue and meninges. It is caused by bacteria, viruses, fungi, and parasites, with viral encephalitis being most common. Symptoms of encephalitis are variable, depending on the invading organism and the part of the brain involved. The onset may be gradual or sudden with symptoms of fever, headache, nuchal rigidity, irritability, lethargy, nausea, and vomiting. Over several days the client may develop reduced consciousness, motor weakness, tremors, seizures, aphasia, and Babinski's sign.

■ **Spinal cord injury:** Any traumatic disruption of the spinal cord, often associated with extensive musculoskeletal involvement. Common spinal cord injuries are vertebral fractures and dislocations, such as those suffered by individuals involved in car accidents, sports injuries, and other violent impacts. Injury to the cervical spinal cord may result in quadriplegia, while injury to the thoracic and lumbar spinal cord may result in paraplegia. Signs and symptoms include paresthesia or anesthesia and paralysis below the level of injury with loss of bowel and bladder control.

■ *Head injury:* Called craniocerebral injury. These injuries can result from primary or secondary injury to the head. Primary injury occurs when the head is subjected to traumatic forces. Head injuries may be open or closed. Open head injuries result from fractures or penetrating wounds; closed head injuries result from blunt head injury producing cerebral concussion, contusion, or laceration. Manifestations of head injury are variable depending on the severity of the trauma and the areas of the brain involved.

■ *Parkinson's disease:* A chronic, slowly progressive degeneration of the brain's dopamine-producing neurons in the substantia nigra, part of the basal ganglia. Parkinson's disease is characterized by the clinical symptoms of masklike facies, trunk-forward flexion, muscle weakness and rigidity, shuffling gait, resting tremor, finger pill-rolling, and bradykinesia (Figs. 22-31 and 22-32).

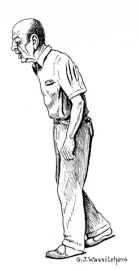

Fig. 22-32 Posture and shuffling gait associated with Parkinson's disease. *(From Rudy, 1984.)*

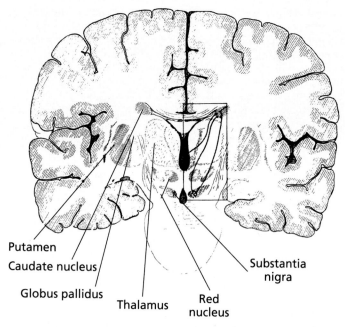

Putamen
Caudate nucleus
Globus pallidus
Thalamus
Red nucleus
Substantia nigra

Fig. 22-31 Coronal section of the brain shows the basal ganglia. Pathways controlling normal and abnormal motor function are depicted in portion of basal ganglia named in the drawing. *(From Cutler, 1983.)*

■ *Cerebrovascular accident (stroke):* Occurs when a cerebral blood vessel is occluded by a thrombus or embolus, or when cerebrovascular hemorrhage occurs. Both mechanisms result in ischemia of the brain tissue. Manifestations depend on which areas of the brain are involved and the extent of ischemic area. For example, ischemia to the frontal lobe on the left side of the brain may result in paralysis of the right arm or leg.

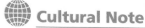 **Cultural Note**

The morbidity and mortality from cerebral vascular disease and stroke is greatly increased for African Americans, particularly African-American men. There are nearly twice as many deaths (60 to 76 per 100,000) among African Americans as there are among the general population (35 to 42 per 100,000). Hispanics and whites have the next highest rates, which are comparable to general population rates. Asian Americans, Pacific Islanders, and American Indians and Alaskan Natives all have rates considerably lower (25 to 34 per 100,000) than the general population.

DISORDERS OF THE PERIPHERAL NERVOUS SYSTEM

■ *Myasthenia gravis:* A neuromuscular disease characterized by abnormal weakness of voluntary muscles that improves with rest and administration of anticholinesterase drugs. The receptor sites for acetylcholine at the myoneuronal junctions are destroyed by autoantibodies against them, resulting in the muscle weakness. Symptoms vary from ocular myasthenia (ptosis and diplopia) to weakness of face, limbs, and muscles of breathing.

■ *Guillain-Barré syndrome:* An acute syndrome characterized by widespread demyelination of nerves of the peripheral nervous system due to a cell-mediated autoimmune response. Clients usually have a viral infection weeks before onset of symptoms. Symptoms often begin with weakness and paresthesia in the lower extremities and ascend the body to the upper extremities and face. A functional recovery occurs in 85% of clients.

DISORDERS FOUND IN CHILDREN

■ *Cerebral palsy:* A motor function disorder caused by a permanent, nonprogressive brain defect or lesion present at birth or shortly thereafter. It is usually associated with premature or abnormal birth and intrapartum asphyxia, causing damage to the central nervous system. The neurologic deficit may result in spasticity, paralysis, seizures, varying degrees of mental retardation and impaired vision, speech, and hearing.

■ *Attention-deficit/hyperactivity disorder (AD/HD):* A combination of behavior problems that interfere with a child's ability to learn. This disorder is characterized by impulsivity, inattention, and motor restlessness. Because these signs are typically seen in preschoolers, a diagnosis usually cannot be made until at least 5 years of age. Indications of inattention include frequent forgetfulness, distractability, poor attention to detail, and difficulty in maintaining attention. Indications of hyperactivity include excessive talking, motor restlessness, difficulty remaining seated, interrupting others, and impatience. These manifestations may continue into adulthood.

&Nursing Diagnosis

CASE 1   25-year-old Japanese man with depression

Subjective

25-year-old Japanese man presents with fatigue and difficulty sleeping. States he was laid off at work 6 weeks ago and has been unsuccessful in finding another job. Has been married 1 year, lives in an apartment. Wife working, supportive of his efforts to find a job. Feels he has let his wife down; he should be supporting her. Reports feeling sad, hopeless, worthless, and a failure. Trouble concentrating. Awakens during night, can't go back to sleep, gets about 4 to 5 hours sleep per night. Decreased appetite. Reports no thoughts of suicide or of hurting himself. No history of psychiatric illness or suicide.

Objective

Mental status   Cooperative man. Dress and behavior appropriate. Responds to questions appropriately. Looks at floor, rare eye contact. Oriented to person, place, and time. Recent and remote memory intact. Speech articulate, understandable.

Neurologic status   CN II-XII intact. Cerebellum: Rapid alternating movement and heel down shin slow, but coordinated bilaterally. Negative Romberg. Able to balance on one foot, walk in tandem. Sensation intact for light touch, sharp and dull sensation, and vibration. Stereognosis: Identified comb. Deep tendon reflexes 2+ bilaterally.

● ●

Nursing Diagnosis #1

Hopelessness related to loss of job.

Defining characteristics   Fatigue, report of worthlessness, feeling sad, decreased sleep.

Nursing Diagnosis #2

Self-esteem disturbance; situational related to loss of job.

Defining characteristics   Lack of eye contact, feeling of inadequacy.

Nursing Diagnosis #3

Fatigue related to depression.

Defining characteristics   Fatigue reported, inability to concentrate, inadequate sleep.

&Nursing Diagnosis

Sample Documentation

CASE 2 60-year-old African-American woman with cerebrovascular accident

Subjective

60-year-old African-American woman who had a cerebrovascular accident 18 months ago with left side paralysis. Dropped hammer on left foot yesterday helping husband with repairs to their one-story home. Applied ice and elevated foot. Able to walk with cane and leg brace, but wheelchair is faster. History of accidents while trying to be independent. History of hypertension; family history of strokes.

Objective

BP 138/88.

Pulse 88.

Rate 14.

Temperature 98.8° F (37.1° C).

Cooperative, alert woman in wheelchair accompanied by husband. Communicates and dresses appropriately. CN I-XII intact. Upper extremity (UE): Voluntary, symmetric, coordinated movement with full range of motion, sensation to vibration, cotton, pin prick bilaterally. Lower extremity (LE): Right, voluntary, symmetric, coordinated movement with full range of motion, sensation to vibration, cotton, pin prick. Left, paralysis and anesthesia; foot edematous, red, no sensation. Cerebellum: Alternating movement both arms; right heel down left leg; deep tendon reflexes 2+ bilaterally.

••

Nursing Diagnosis #1

Impaired physical mobility related to altered sensory and neuromuscular status.

Defining characteristics Paralysis and anesthesia of left leg from stroke, uses wheelchair.

Nursing Diagnosis #2

High risk for injury, trauma related to desire to be as independent as possible.

Defining characteristics Injured self helping husband, history of injuries from trying to be independent.

HEALTH PROMOTION

■ **Risk Factors for Cerebrovascular Disease** Cerebrovascular disease is the third leading cause of death in the United States, accounting for nearly 150,300 deaths annually, 60% of whom are women. It has been estimated that 500,000 strokes occur each year and that almost 3 million living Americans have had a stroke (American Heart Association, 1991). Hypertension is the major risk factor that predisposes individuals to a stroke. Nonmodifiable risk factors include family history of stroke, as well as a diagnosis of diabetes mellitus or cardiac disease. Modifiable risk factors, however, are high serum lipids, obesity, cigarette smoking, sedentary life style, and stress. Periodic screening of serum blood cholesterol and triglycerides is recommended. Regular screening of blood pressure in all persons over the age of 3 is also recommended (Report of the U.S. Preventive Services Task Force, 1989). Counselling clients to stop smoking, engage in regular exercise, and reduce dietary intake of fat have been shown to be effective interventions.

■ **Safe Travel** The number of nervous system injuries from motor vehicle accidents (MVA) can be reduced by wearing seat belts and using a designated driver program to prevent those under the influence of alcohol or drugs to drive. Approximately 15,000 to 20,000 people sustain spinal cord injuries each year in the United States. Vehicular accidents account for 48% of these injuries. An estimated 7000 people die annually from traumatic brain injury, and 50,000 to 60,000 survive but have injuries with varying levels of permanent deficits.

■ **Safe Recreation** The number of nervous system injuries from recreational activities can be reduced in a variety of ways. Helmets are recommended for skateboarding and riding bicycles, motorbikes, and motorcycles. Sports injuries also account for 14% of the spinal cord injuries, with diving injuries accounting for 66% of those injuries. The highest incidence occurs in men between the ages of 16 and 32. Diving accidents can be reduced by using the strategy of "Feet first, first time" to encourage divers to get into water feet-first to determine the water depth before diving in. Near-drowning accidents can be reduced when all occupants of a boat wear life jackets, swimmers swim with a buddy, and young children are closely supervised around swimming pools.

   Many unintentional injuries from firearms in the home and while hunting involve children, adolescents, and young adult men. Strategies to prevent firearm injuries include keeping guns stored unloaded and in a locked compartment. When hunting, preventive strategies are supervising children and adolescents and wearing fluorescent orange clothing to increase visibility (Report of the U.S. Preventive Services Task Force).

??????? STUDY QUESTIONS ???????

1. What is the function of the nervous system? Identify and describe the two structural categories of the nervous system.
2. Identify and describe the three meningeal layers that cover the brain.
3. What is the purpose of the cerebrospinal fluid? What is its composition?
4. Identify and describe the major structures of the brain. Describe the anatomy of the spinal cord.
5. Distinguish between the spinal nerves and the cranial nerves.
6. What comprises a reflex arc? What is the purpose of a reflex arc?
7. Identify and describe the two components of the autonomic nervous system.
8. An individual presents with a chief complaint of headaches and dizziness. What additional information about this complaint do you need to collect during history-taking?
9. An individual is brought to the emergency department after an apparent seizure. What information do you need to collect from the individual? What information do you need from the friend who witnessed the "seizure event"?
10. An older woman reports a recent jerking and twitching in her hands. What areas do you need to explore while taking the history?
11. What additional areas need explored when obtaining a neurologic history on an infant? A young child? An older adult?
12. What areas do you want to focus on in the physical exam? What equipment is needed?
13. Match the cranial nerve with the appropriate exam procedure:

   CN II   Cardinal gaze fields
   CN IV   Rinne test
   CN VII   Confrontation test
   CN VIII   Corneal reflex test

14. What cranial nerves control taste? What nerve controls tongue movement? What nerves affect movement of the palate and gag reflex?
15. When performing a gait assessment, what is important to observe? Describe how to perform a Romberg test. What are normal results in a Romberg test?
16. Describe what is involved in performing an upper extremity exam. What findings would be considered abnormal in this exam?
17. Describe what procedures you should perform if sensation is impaired in the left leg.
18. Describe how to test for a) pain sense, b) vibratory sense, c) stereognosis, and d) two-point discrimination.
19. Identify the five deep tendon reflexes. How are reflexes graded? What is the expected grade if reflexes are normal? What does a 4+ mean?
20. Describe the procedure involved in testing reflexes in the knee, the ankle, and the elbow.

21. Describe how to test abdominal reflexes. How do you test the cremasteric reflex? What is the expected response when testing these reflexes?

22. What is the "mini-mental state" exam used for? What five major areas are assessed in this exam? What is the maximum score?

23. What mental history information do you need to collect to assist in deciding whether an individual is depressed?

24. How would you assess an individual for a) recent memory, b) remote memory, c) judgment ability, and d) abstract reasoning ability?

25. What areas would you explore when assessing for an alteration in emotional status? Alteration in thought processes?

26. What is the purpose of testing for a positive Kernig's sign? A positive Brudzinski's sign?

27. What is the Glasgow coma scale used for? Identify the three categories being assessed. What would a score of 14 indicate? What would a score of 3 indicate?

28. What reflex responses are normal in the neonate but abnormal in a 2-year-old?

29. List at least three alterations you would make when doing a neurologic exam on a child. What normal changes would you expect in neurologic findings when examining an older individual?

30. Distinguish between delirium and dementia. Distinguish between AIDS dementia complex and dementia related to Alzheimer's disease.

31. What is the difference between meningitis and encephalitis? What are their similarities?

32. Distinguish between myasthenia gravis and Guillain-Barré syndrome.

33. List the risk factors for stroke. Which of those factors can be modified by the individual? Who is at the greatest risk of dying from a stroke?

34. What single health promotion activity, if adhered to, would do the most to reduce the incidence of head injury and spinal cord injury?

CHAPTER 23

Head-To-Toe Examination and Documentation

Now that you have studied and practiced assessing all of the body systems separately, it is time to put everything together. This is tricky, because you start with your knowledge and techniques for each single system, but the client presents to you as a whole person. You must then organize your approach and techniques to collectively examine the person, literally from "head to toe." This means that when you start at the top with the head, you should examine the facial characteristics, skin, hair, eyes, ears, mouth, throat, and range of motion of the neck in a systematic and collective fashion. When you have done this, you have assessed the neurologic, integumentary, musculoskeletal, visual, and auditory systems, and the head, neck, nose, and mouth regions. Then you must move on to the next area of the body and do the same. After all body regions are examined, you must then take the information apart again so that it may be systematically analyzed and accurately recorded on the client's record.

How each examiner actually "puts together" the approach of performing a head-to-toe examination is usually unique. No two examiners do things exactly the same, nor are any two clients exactly the same. Therefore it is important that, as a student, you take time to determine what total examination method works best for you. It is of utmost importance to try to learn a systematic method so that you do not leave things out.

SPECIAL CONSIDERATIONS

Even after you spend hours, days, weeks, and months learning how to do a complete physical examination in a systematic and thorough manner, the unexpected always occurs:

- The baby is crying so hard that there is no way you can listen to the infant's heart or lungs during the examination of the chest.
- Every time the client tries to lie down for the abdominal examination, she becomes short of breath.
- The client is paralyzed and confined to a wheelchair, but she needs her annual examination and pap smear.

- The client arrived in the United States 2 weeks ago from Puerto Rico and does not speak a word of English.

In each of these cases, an examination must be performed. Each case described means that you must individualize your approach and perhaps the order of the actual assessment procedures. Think about each situation just described and plan your approach.

THE MODEL INTEGRATED PHYSICAL ASSESSMENT

In the model situation, the assessment should begin as you first meet the client. During this introductory period, watch the client enter the room, noting gait, posture, and ease of movement. Shake hands with the client and note eye contact and firmness of the hand grip. Introduce yourself to the client and conduct introductory conversation. Note language spoken, as well as cursory hearing and speech capability. Additionally, observe such things as obvious vision difficulties or blindness; difficulty standing, sitting, or rising from sitting; obvious musculoskeletal difficulties; general affect; appearance of interest and involvement; dress and posture; general mental alertness, orientation, and integration of thought processes; difficulty hearing; obvious shortness of breath or posture that would facilitate breathing; and obesity, emaciation, or malnourishment.

After the introductions, assessment of vital signs, vision examination, and cursory evaluation, prepare the client for the examination. Instruct the client to first empty the bladder (collect specimen if necessary) and then remove all clothing (including shoes, socks, bra, and underwear), put on a gown, and sit on the examination table in the examination room. You are now ready to conduct the model examination as follows or use the components of the model examination to conduct a customized examination that accommodates the client's special circumstances.

Use the following information only as a guide. It was developed to show how each body system, as thoroughly described in the preceding chapters, must now be taken apart and integrated with other body systems to permit comprehensive regional examination of the client. Note in the following example that all relevant body systems are assessed when the examiner is examining a certain area of the client's body. For example, when the nurse is examining the client's anterior chest, he or she must think about all of the individual body systems that must be assessed at that time and incorporate them into an individual but integrated examination. Body systems that should be assessed during the anterior chest examination include skin; thorax and lungs; lymphatic; cardiovascular; musculoskeletal; and breast. Collectively these individual assessments make up the anterior chest assessment.

Exactly how the examination and the documentation will be formatted depends greatly on the purpose of the assessment and the individual ability and needs of the client. It is anticipated that, as you actually examine the client, the sample format described below will need to be modified, expanded, or simplified to meet the client's situational needs.

The purpose of providing this guide is to make the point that every time you examine a client, you should regiment your mind and your methods so that you think about each individual and all of what needs to be assessed in a single, systematic, head-to-toe evaluation. Nothing is worse for a client than having a disorganized examiner who jumps around the client's body assessing areas that were previously forgotten.

Most important are the following points:

- Be organized.
- Develop a routine. This will help with consistency.

- Before you ever begin the actual examination, have a clear picture in your mind of what you plan to do in what order.
- Practice, practice, practice so that you will learn to become systematic and inclusive.
- Imagine yourself as the client and prepare as you would want an examiner to be prepared if he or she were to examine you.

Equipment for Physical Examination

Eye examination charts, such as Snellen and Jaeger charts	Patient examination gown
Ophthalmoscope	Vaginal speculum (for female clients)
Otoscope with pneumatic bulb	Pap smear materials (for female clients)
Stethoscope with bell and diaphragm	Percussion hammer
Tongue blades	Tuning fork
Penlight	Aromatic material
4 × 4-inch gauze pads	Cotton balls
Examination gloves	Sharp and dull testing instruments
Cotton-tipped applicators	Ruler and tape measure
Lubricant	Goniometer
Drape sheet	Marking pen
Gooseneck light	Cup for water
Examination table with stirrups	Objects for stereognosis
Writing surface for examiner	

Clinical Guidelines for Adult Head-To-Toe Examination

PROCEDURE	BODY PART OR SYSTEMS INVOLVED	CLINICAL STRATEGIES (ADULT AND ELDERLY)
Begin examination with client fully dressed (client may remove shoes for height measurement).		
1. **Assess vital functions and other baseline measurements before asking client to get undressed.** Temperature Blood pressure (both arms) Radial pulse Respirations Height Weight Vision testing Snellen chart		If deviation from normal discovered, reevaluate when associated system assessed
Instruct client to undress, put on a gown, and sit on the end of the examination table.		
2. **Examine client's hands** Skin surface characteristics Temperature and moisture of hands Characteristics of nails Clubbing	Skin, hair, and nails Heart and peripheral vascular Lungs and respiratory	Both examiner and client will be at ease if examiner starts with client's hands

Clinical Guidelines for Adult Head-To-Toe Examination—*cont'd*

PROCEDURE	BODY PART OR SYSTEMS INVOLVED	CLINICAL STRATEGIES (ADULT AND ELDERLY)
Examine client's hands—cont'd		
Skeletal characteristics and/or deformities of fingers and hands	Musculoskeletal	Fine motor neurologic assessment may be included at this point; others find it more convenient to perform neurologic assessment as a clustered procedure toward end of evaluation period
Range of motion and motor strength of fingers and hands		
Muscle wasting		
Asymmetry		
3. Examine client's arms from wrists to shoulders		
Skin surface characteristics	Skin, hair, and nails	Examine each arm separately
Muscle wasting	Musculoskeletal	
Asymmetry		
Radial pulses: compare one arm to other	Heart and peripheral vascular	May have already been done during vital signs evaluation
Range of motion and motor strength of wrists, elbows, forearms, upper arms, shoulders	Musculoskeletal Neurologic	Note that, again, neurologic assessment has been delayed Use make/break techniques
Palpation of epitrochlear lymph nodes	Lymphatic	
4. Examine client's head and neck		
Facial characteristics and symmetry	Head and neck Neurologic	Observe head and neck, gathering as much information as possible
Skin surface characteristics	Skin and hair	Do not touch until after thorough observation
Symmetry and external characteristics of eyes and ears		
Hair characteristics: texture, distribution, quantity		
Palpate hair and scalp		Palpate thoroughly; do not be intimidated by hair spray or dirty hair (may need to wash hands before progressing)
Palpate facial bones	Musculoskeletal	
Client opens and closes mouth for evaluation of temporomandibular joint		
Clench teeth	Neurologic—CN V (trigeminal nerve)	
Palpate sinus regions	Paranasal sinuses	
Clench eyes tight, wrinkle forehead, smile, stick out tongue, and puff out cheeks	Neurologic—CN VII, XII (facial, hypoglossal nerves)	Be straightforward; provide client with step-by-step instructions
Eye and near-vision assessment	Eyes and visual	
External eye examination: eyebrows, eyelids, eyelashes, surface characteristics, lacrimal apparatus, corneal surface, anterior chamber, iris		
Near-vision screening and eye function: pupillary response, accommodation, cover-uncover test	Neurologic—CN II, III (optic, oculomotor nerves)	
Extraocular eye movements; vision field testing	Neurologic—CN III, IV, VI, (oculomotor, trochlear, abducens nerves)	Hold chin if head movement occurs
Internal eye examination: red reflex, disc, cup margins, vessels, retinal surface, vitreous	Eyes and visual	Room must be darkened; should have small amount of secondary light Instruct client to focus on single object at distance

Continued

Clinical Guidelines for Adult Head-To-Toe Examination—*cont'd*

PROCEDURE	BODY PART OR SYSTEMS INVOLVED	CLINICAL STRATEGIES (ADULT AND ELDERLY)
Examine client's head and neck—cont'd		
Ear and hearing assessment External ear examination: alignment, surface characteristics, external canal	Ears and auditory	
Use whisper test to evaluate hearing	Neurologic—CN VIII (acoustic nerve)	Room must be quiet
Otoscopic examination: characteristics of external canal, cerumen, eardrum (landmarks, deformities, inflammation)		Use largest speculum that will fit into canal; if necessary, review technique guidelines for using otoscope
Rinne and Weber tests	Ears and auditory; neurologic—CN VIII (acoustic nerve)	
Nasal examination: note structure, septum position; use nasal speculum or otoscope to evaluate patency, turbinates, meatuses	Nose, paranasal sinuses, mouth, and oropharynx	Even though uncomfortable, should be part of every thorough assessment
Evaluate sense of smell	Neurologic—CN I (olfactory nerve)	
Mouth examination: inspect gingivobuccal fornices, buccal mucosa, and gums	Nose, paranasal sinuses, mouth, and oropharynx	
Inspect teeth: number, color, surface characteristics		If client has dentures, they should be removed
Inspect and palpate tongue: symmetry, movement, color, surface characteristics		
Inspect floor of mouth: color, surface characteristics		
Inspect hard and soft palates: color, surface characteristics		
Inspect oropharynx: note mouth odor, anterior and posterior pillars, uvula, tonsils, posterior pharynx		
Palpate tongue and gums		
Evaluate gag reflex	Neurologic—CN IX, X (glossopharyngeal, vagus nerves)	
Evaluate range of motion of head and neck: instruct client to shrug shoulders against resistance; head movement positions, neck flexion and extension, ear-to-shoulder flexion, chin-to-shoulder rotation	Musculoskeletal Neurologic—CN XI (accessory nerve)	
Observe symmetry and smoothness of neck and thyroid region	Head and neck	Client's gown should be lowered slightly so that examiner may fully inspect neck
Palpate carotid pulses	Heart and peripheral vascular	
Observe for jugular venous distention		
Palpate trachea, thyroid (isthmus and lobes), lymph nodes (preauricular, postauricular, occipital, tonsillar, submaxillary, submental, superficial cervical chain, posterior cervical, deep cervical chain, and supraclavicular)	Head and neck; lymphatic	Client may need drink of water to facilitate swallowing during thyroid evaluation

Clinical Guidelines for Adult Head-To-Toe Examination—*cont'd*

PROCEDURE	BODY PART OR SYSTEMS INVOLVED	CLINICAL STRATEGIES (ADULT AND ELDERLY)
Examine client's head and neck—cont'd		
Auscultate thyroid and carotid for bruits	Head and neck; heart and peripheral vascular	
Complete assessment of cranial nerves: use cotton swab to evaluate sensitivity of forehead to light touch, cheeks, chin (trigeminal nerve sensory tract)	Neurologic—CN V (trigeminal nerve)	Client should be instructed to close eyes and identify where and when light touch felt
5. Assess posterior chest: examiner moves behind client; client seated; gown to waist for men; gown removed but pulled up to cover breasts for women		
Observe posterior chest: symmetry of shoulders, muscular development, scapular placement, spine straightness, posture	Musculoskeletal	
Observe skin: intactness, color, lesions	Skin	
Observe respiratory movement: excursion, quality, depth, and rhythm of respirations	Lungs and respiratory	
Palpate posterior chest: evaluate muscles and bone structure, palpate excursion of chest expansion; palpate down vertebral column; note straightness	Musculoskeletal Lungs and respiratory	
Palpate posterior chest for fremitus		Palpate with pads of fingers while client says "one-two-three"
Percuss posterior chest for resonance, respiratory excursion	Lungs and respiratory	During excursion evaluation, demonstrate to client how to take deep breath and hold it Measure amount of excursion with ruler
Percuss with fist along costovertebral angle for kidney tenderness	Kidney	
Inspect, bilaterally palpate, and percuss along lateral axillary chest walls	Lungs and respiratory	
Auscultate posterior and lateral chest walls for breath sounds; note quality of sounds heard and presence of adventitious sounds	Lungs and respiratory	Instruct client to breathe deeply by mouth
Assess for bronchophony, egophony, and whispered pectoriloquy if adventitious sounds are present		
6. Assess anterior chest: move to front of client; client should lower gown to waist		
Inspect skin color, intactness, presence of lesions, muscular symmetry, bilaterally similar bone structure	Skin Musculoskeletal	

Continued

PROCEDURE	BODY PART OR SYSTEMS INVOLVED	CLINICAL STRATEGIES (ADULT AND ELDERLY)
Assess anterior chest—cont'd		
Observe chest wall for pulsations or heaving	Heart and peripheral vascular	
Observe movement during respirations	Lungs and respiratory	
Observe client's ease with respirations, posture, pursing lips		
Female breasts: Note size, symmetry, contour, moles or nevi, breast or nipple deviation, dimpling, or lesions; evaluate range of motion of shoulders and regularity of breast tissue during various movements: a. Client's arms extended over head b. Client's arms behind head c. Client's hands behind small of back d. Client's hands pushed tightly against each other at shoulder level e. Client leaning forward slightly so that breasts hang away from chest wall; note symmetry and pull on suspensory ligaments	Musculoskeletal Breasts and axillae	It is helpful to explain to client basically what she will be expected to do and why before actual examination; may help to alleviate client anxiety as well facilitate active participation During examination, it may be helpful to discuss what is being observed; breast self-examination instruction should follow at some point to reiterate these and other aspects of breast examination
Male breasts: Note size, symmetry, breast enlargement, nipple discharge, or lesions		
All clients: Palpate anterior chest wall for stability, crepitations, muscular or skeletal tenderness	Musculoskeletal	
Palpate precordium for thrills, heaves, pulsations	Heart and peripheral vascular	Evaluate chest while client is sitting upright and then leaning forward
Palpate left chest wall to locate point of maximum impulse (PMI)	Heart	
Palpate chest wall for fremitus, as with posterior chest	Lungs and respiratory	If examiner has difficulty percussing woman's anterior chest because of large breasts, percuss downward until breast tissue reached; then postpone further percussion until client lies down
Percuss anterior chest for resonance		
For female clients: Palpate breasts, including all four quadrants, tail of Spence, and areolar area; note firmness, tissue qualities, lumps, areas of thickness, or tenderness	Breasts and axillae	Client should be comfortably seated with arms resting at side As before, discuss what is being done so that client can incorporate similar techniques into breast self-examination
Palpate nipples; note elasticity, tissue characteristics, discharge	Breasts and axillae	

Clinical Guidelines for Adult Head-To-Toe Examination—*cont'd*

PROCEDURE	BODY PART OR SYSTEMS INVOLVED	CLINICAL STRATEGIES (ADULT AND ELDERLY)
Assess anterior chest—cont'd		
All clients: Palpate lymph nodes associated with lymphatic drainage of breasts; including supraclavicular and infraclavicular, central, lateral, axillary, pectoral, subscapular, scapular, brachial, intermediate, and internal mammary areas	Lymphatic	
For male clients: Palpate breasts; note swelling or presence of excessive tissue or lumps, nipple discharge, or lesions		
All clients: Auscultate breath sounds of anterior chest from apex to base; note quality, rate, type, presence of adventitious sounds	Lungs and respiratory	Instruct client to breathe deeply through mouth
Auscultate heart: aortic area, pulmonic area, Erb's point, tricuspid area, apical area; note rate, rhythm, location, intensity, frequency, timing, and splitting of S_1, S_2, S_3, S_4 murmurs	Heart and peripheral vascular	Examiner must decide whether to start at apical area and work upward or start at aortic area and work downward; examiner should develop routine method of procedure If examining large-breasted woman, part of auscultatory evaluation may be deferred until client lying down
Assist client to lying or low Fowler position		
7. Assess anterior chest in recumbent position		
Inspect and measure jugular venous pressure for height seen above sternal angle	Heart and peripheral vascular	Extend footrest for client's legs
Female breast inspection: Note symmetry, contour, venous pattern, skin color, areolar area (note size, shape, surface characteristics), nipples (note direction, size, shape, color, surface characteristics, possible crusting)	Breasts and axillae	Provide drape for legs and abdomen Place towel under shoulder of the breast to be evaluated Instruct client to abduct arm overhead Explain procedures to client as performed
Female breast palpation: Note firmness, tissue qualities, lumps, areas of thickness, or tenderness; areolar and nipple area (note elasticity, tissue characteristics, discharge)		After breast palpation, may teach client to palpate own breasts
All clients: Palpate anterior chest wall for cardiac movements or thrills, heaves, pulsations	Heart and peripheral vascular	

Continued

Clinical Guidelines for Adult Head-To-Toe Examination—*cont'd*

PROCEDURE	BODY PART OR SYSTEMS INVOLVED	CLINICAL STRATEGIES (ADULT AND ELDERLY)
Assess anterior chest—cont'd		
Auscultation of heart: aortic area, pulmonary area, Erb's point, tricuspid area, apical area; note S_1, S_2, S_3, S_4 murmurs (location, rate, rhythm, intensity, frequency, timing, splitting); turn client slightly to left side; repeat assessment of these areas	Heart and peripheral vascular	
Provide chest drape for females; expose abdomen from pubis to epigastric region		
8. **Assess abdomen**		
Observe skin characteristics from pubis to midchest region; note scars, lesions, vascularity, bulges, navel	Skin and hair	Client should be comfortably positioned with pillow under head and knees slightly flexed to relax abdominal muscles
Observe abdominal contour	Abdomen and gastrointestinal	
Observe movement of abdomen, peristalsis, pulsations	Heart and peripheral vascular Abdomen and gastrointestinal	
Auscultate abdomen (all quadrants); note bowel sounds, bruits, venous hums	Heart and peripheral vascular	
Percuss abdomen (all quadrants) and epigastric region for tone	Abdomen and gastrointestinal	
Percuss upper and lower liver borders and estimation of liver span		Liver percussion should occur at midclavicular line
Percuss left midaxillary line for splenic dullness		
Lightly palpate all four quadrants; note tenderness, guarding, masses		Allow client to become accustomed to examiner's hands
Deeply palpate all four quadrants; note tenderness, guarding, masses		Gently but firmly move palpation deeper and deeper until examiner convinced that abdomen sufficiently assessed
Deeply palpate right costal margin for liver border		Examiner must decide whether to use one-hand or two-hand approach
Deeply palpate left costal margin for splenic border		
Deeply palpate abdomen for right and left kidneys		
Deeply palpate midline epigastric area for aortic pulsation	Heart and peripheral vascular	Tenderness in epigastric area normal
Test abdominal reflexes with pointed instrument	Neurologic	
Client raises head to evaluate flexion and strength of abdominal muscles	Musculoskeletal	Note use of arms or hand to assist; older client may have difficulty with this technique
Lightly palpate inguinal region for lymph nodes, femoral pulses, and bulges that may be associated with hernia	Lymphatic Heart and peripheral vascular Abdomen and gastrointestinal	

Clinical Guidelines for Adult Head-To-Toe Examination—*cont'd*

PROCEDURE	BODY PART OR SYSTEMS INVOLVED	CLINICAL STRATEGIES (ADULT AND ELDERLY)
Client remains lying; abdomen and chest should be draped		
9. Assess lower limbs and hips		
Inspect client's feet and legs for skin characteristics, vascular sufficiency, pulses; note deformities of toes, feet, nails, ankles, legs	Skin, hair, and nails Heart and peripheral vascular Musculoskeletal	
Palpate feet and lower legs; note temperature, pulses, tenderness, deformities	Heart and peripheral vascular Musculoskeletal	
Range of motion and motor strength of toes, feet, ankles, and knees	Musculoskeletal Neurologic	Motor strength testing may be postponed until patient seated
Range of motion and motor strength of hips		
Palpate hips for stability	Musculoskeletal	
Client is lying and adequately draped		This may be performed last
10. Assess genitalia, pelvic region, and rectum		
For males: Inspect and palpate external genitalia, including pubic hair, penis and scrotum, testes, epididymides, and vas deferens	Genitalia Anus, rectum, and prostate Genitalia and reproductive	If mass in scrotal sac suspected, transilluminate
Inspect sacrococcygeal and perianal areas and anus for surface characteristics		Position client lying on left side with right hip and knee flexed
Palpation of anus, rectum, and prostate gland with gloved finger		Lubricate gloved finger and slowly insert; wait for sphincter to relax before advancing finger
Note characteristics of stool when gloved finger removed	Anus, rectum, and prostate	
For females (client should be lying in lithotomy position): inspect and palpate external genitalia, including pubic hair, labia, clitoris, urethral and vaginal orifices, perineal and perianal area and anus for surface characteristics	Genitalia and reproductive Urinary	
Insert vaginal speculum and inspect surface characteristics of vagina and cervix		
Collect Pap smear and culture specimen		
Perform bimanual palpation to assess form, size, and characteristics of vagina, cervix, uterus, adnexa		Lubricate first two fingers of gloved hand to be inserted internally; other hand should be positioned on abdomen directly above internal hand
Perform vaginal-rectal examination to assess rectovaginal septum and pouch, surface characteristics, broad ligament tenderness		When examination completed, client should be offered tissue for drying of genital area

Continued

Clinical Guidelines for Adult Head-To-Toe Examination—*cont'd*

PROCEDURE	BODY PART OR SYSTEMS INVOLVED	CLINICAL STRATEGIES (ADULT AND ELDERLY)
Assess genitalia—cont'd		
Perform rectal examination to assess anal sphincter tone, surface characteristics (anal culture may be obtained)	Anus and rectum	
Note characteristics of stool when gloved finger removed		

Client resumes seated position; client should have gown on and be draped across lap

11. Assess neurologic system

PROCEDURE	BODY PART OR SYSTEMS INVOLVED	CLINICAL STRATEGIES (ADULT AND ELDERLY)
Observe client moving from lying to sitting position; note use of muscles, ease of movement, and coordination	Neurologic Musculoskeletal	
Test sensory function by using light and deep (dull and sharp) sensation on forehead, paranasal sinus area, hands, lower arms, feet, lower legs	Neurologic (sensory function)	Client's eyes should be closed; instruct client to either point to or verbally report area that has been touched
Bilaterally test and compare vibratory sensations of ankle, wrist, sternum		Alternate light, dull, and pin-prick sensations Test bilaterally
Test two-point discrimination of palms, thighs, back	Neurologic	Evaluate cortical, discriminatory, and sensory functions
Test stereognosis or graphesthesia		
Test fine-motor functioning and coordination of upper extremities by instructing client to perform at least two of following:	Neurologic	Perform technique bilaterally and compare responses; evaluates the proprioception and cerebellar function
a. Alternating pronation and supination of forearm		
b. Touching nose with alternating index fingers		
c. Rapidly alternating finger movements to thumb		
d. Rapidly moving index finger between nose and examiner's finger		
Test and bilaterally compare fine-motor functioning and coordination of lower extremities by instructing client to run heel down tibia of opposite leg		
Alternately cross legs over knee	Musculoskeletal	
Test proprioception by moving the toe up and down	Neurologic	If client shows any neurologic problems, evaluate by Babinski and ankle clonus tests. Evaluates the client's reflex status.
Test and bilaterally compare deep tendon reflexes, including:		
a. Biceps tendon		
b. Triceps tendon		
c. Brachioradialis tendon		
d. Patellar tendon		
e. Achilles tendon		

Clinical Guidelines for Adult Head-To-Toe Examination—*cont'd*

PROCEDURE	BODY PART OR SYSTEMS INVOLVED	CLINICAL STRATEGIES (ADULT AND ELDERLY)
Instruct client to stand		
12. **Palpate scrotum and inguinal region (male)**	Genitalia	
Palpate scrotum and inguinal region for characteristics and hernias	Genitalia	Instruct client to bear down or cough during hernia evaluation
13. **Assess neurologic and musculoskeletal system**		
Assessment of client's gait: observe and palpate straightness of client's spine as client stands and bends forward to touch toes	Musculoskeletal Neurologic	Elderly clients may not be able to do this Client's age and general ability may help define which technique to use
With client's waist stabilized, evaluate hyperextension, lateral bending, rotation of upper trunk	Musculoskeletal	
Assess proprioception and cerebellar and motor functions by using at least two of the following: a. Romberg test (eyes closed) b. Walking straight heel-to-toe formation c. Standing on one foot and then other (eyes closed) d. Hopping in place on one foot and then other e. Knee bends	Neurologic	Protect client from falling by remaining close and ready to catch him or her if necessary Elderly clients may not be able to do this

INTEGRATION OF THE INFANT AND PEDIATRIC EXAMINATION

The procedure for integrating the pediatric examination depends entirely on the age and cooperation of the child. By the time the child reaches school age, he or she should be able to participate fully in a cooperative manner. It is the younger child who will present the challenge. The following sample format changes should facilitate a thorough assessment.

Clinical Guidelines for Neonatal and Pediatric Examination

AGE AND PREPARATION	ASSESSMENT PROCEDURES	BODY PART OR SYSTEM INVOLVED
Newborn to 6 months: infant undressed, lying on examination table	Obtain history, highlighting developmental or problem areas	
	Check vital signs: temperature, pulse, respiration	
	Record weight, length, chest and head circumference	
	Observe child lying on examination table; note color, general health, body symmetry, gross motor movement, alertness, gross and fine motor development, language development, social adaptive development, skin characteristics, and response to sound and vision stimulation	Heart and peripheral vascular, neurologic, musculoskeletal, skin, eyes and visual, ears and auditory
	Examine and manipulate hands, arms, shoulders, feet, legs; note range of motion and tone	Musculoskeletal, neurologic
	Examine skin over extremities, chest, abdomen, and back	Skin and hair
	Auscultate thorax, lungs, heart, abdomen	Lungs and respiratory, heart and peripheral vascular, abdomen and gastrointestinal
	Palpate and examine external characteristics of head, neck, face, axillary region	Lymphatic, head and neck, eyes and visual, ears and auditory, nose, mouth, and oropharynx
	Palpate thorax, abdomen, and umbilical area	Lungs and respiratory, abdomen and gastrointestinal
	Observe and palpate external genitalia, inguinal area, and hip stability	Genitalia, musculoskeletal
	Examine eyes with ophthalmoscope	Eyes and visual
	Examine mouth, teeth (development), tongue, posterior pharynx, nose	Nose, mouth, and oropharynx
	Examine ears with otoscope	Ears and auditory
Six months to 2 years: child in diaper, sitting on parent's lap; examiner's chair should be in front of parent's chair, and examiner's knees should touch parent's; during supine examination, child may lie on parent's and examiner's lap	Obtain history highlighting developmental or problem areas	
	Perform developmental, social, vision, speech, hearing, and fine and gross motor assessment during play and initial "get acquainted" period	Neurologic, eyes and visual, speech, ears and auditory, musculoskeletal
	Record weight, length, and chest and head circumferences (until 18 months)	
	Check vital signs, including blood pressure in children over 18 months of age (may be postponed until later if child becomes agitated)	
	Auscultate lungs and heart	Lungs and respiratory, heart and peripheral vascular
	Examine skin over extremities, chest, abdomen, and back	Skin and hair
	Examine and manipulate hands, arms, shoulders, feet, legs; note range of motion and tone	Neurologic, musculoskeletal
	Palpate and examine external characteristics of head, neck, face, axillary region	Lymphatic, head and neck, eyes and visual, ears and auditory, nose, mouth, and oropharynx
	Auscultate abdomen with child in supine position on parent's and examiner's lap	Abdomen and gastrointestinal

Clinical Guidelines for Neonatal and Pediatric Examination—*cont'd*

AGE AND PREPARATION	ASSESSMENT PROCEDURES	BODY PART OR SYSTEM INVOLVED
Six months to 2 years—cont'd	Palpate thorax, abdomen, and umbilical area	Lungs and respiratory, abdomen
	Observe and palpate external genitalia, inguinal area, and hip stability	Genitalia, musculoskeletal
	Examine eyes with ophthalmoscope	Eyes and visual
	Examine mouth, teeth (development), tongue, posterior pharynx, nose	Nose, mouth, and nasopharynx, head and neck
	Examine ears with otoscope	Ears, auditory
Two to 4 years: Child undressed to underpants; may be examined either on parent's lap or examination table; much of assessment may be informal as examiner observes and plays with child	Same assessment procedures as for child age 6 months to 2 years.	
Four to 6 years: child undressed to underpants, sitting on examination table; assessment should move toward adult format; child's developmental immaturity may necessitate that examiner alter various examination techniques to facilitate child's participation and correct response	Same assessment procedures as for child age 6 months to 2 years	
Over 6 years old: child in gown on examination table	Same assessment procedures and approach as for adult client	

Comparison of Documentation Forms

PLAIN PAPER	PREDEVELOPED FORM
Advantages	**Advantages**
Documentation space is not a problem.	Departmental continuity is maintained.
Specific data for individual client may be emphasized as necessary.	Data will be easy to locate by other examiners.
	Preprinted forms serve as reminder for completeness.
Disadvantages	**Disadvantages**
The examiner must be organized; if not, rambling and insignificant data may be a problem.	Individual situations may be difficult to emphasize.
All examiners in the agency may not use the same format.	Examiner may not have adequate space for documentation.
	If form was developed without examiner's input, it may not include all data the examiner wants to collect.
	Separate forms necessary for different types of clients (e.g., children, older adults).

PHYSICAL EXAMINATION WRITE-UP

The database and the information collected during the physical assessment must be organized and documented. The components of the documentation are (1) subjective data (history), (2) objective data (physical assessment), (3) risk profile, and (4) problem list/nursing diagnoses. Before the actual documentation, the examiner must decide whether to record the data on plain paper or on a predesigned form. Each has advantages and disadvantages. See the box at left for a comparison.

Once the style of documentation to be used is determined, the examiner must decide how to synthesize the client's history and physical data and then record the information. The examiner is urged to record *what* is observed, heard, percussed, or palpated and to avoid using vague and nondescriptive terms such as *normal, negative, good,* or *poor.* Always be specific and precise.

Following is a documentation model that should be viewed as a guide to the comprehensiveness of the types of information that are recorded. The information presented here is not intended to be an exhaustive list of all content areas included in the text. For complete and detailed descriptions of the information that may be recorded, refer to the individual body system chapters.

DOCUMENTATION FORMAT

Subjective Database (History)
- Biographic data
- Reason for visit
- Present health status
- Current health data
  Immunizations
  Allergies
  Last examination
- Past health status
  Childhood illnesses
  Serious or chronic illnesses
  Serious accidents or injuries
  Hospitalizations
  Surgeries
  Emotional health
  Obstetric health
- Family history
- Review of physiologic systems
  General
  Nutritional
  Integumentary
  Head and neck
  Eyes
  Ears, nose and mouth
  Breasts
  Cardiovascular
  Respiratory
  Hematolymphatic
  Gastrointestinal
  Urinary
  Genital
  Musculoskeletal
  Central nervous system
  Endocrine
  Allergic and immunologic responses
- Psychosocial history
  General status
  Response to illness
  Significant others
  Occupational history
  Educational level
  Activities of daily living
  Habits
  Financial status

- Health maintenance efforts
  Maintenance of self-health
  Health care patterns
- Environmental health
  General assessment
  Employment
  Home
  Neighborhood
  Community

Objective Database (Physical Examination)
- Vital statistics
  Age
  Race
  Nutritional status
  Height
  Weight
  Temperature
  Pulse
  Blood pressure (both arms, lying and sitting)
  Communication skills
- General statement of appearance
- Integumentary system (skin, hair, and nails)
  Color
  Integrity
  Texture
  Presence or absence of lesions, edema, unusual odors
  Distribution and texture of hair
- Head and neck
  Size, symmetry, and contour of head and face
  Edema or puffiness
  Palpation of lymph nodes
  Palpation of thyroid
  Palpation of sinuses
- Nose
  Position, including septum
  Nasal patency
  Presence of polyp(s)
  Appearance of turbinates
- Mouth and pharynx
  Condition and alignment of teeth
  Color and characteristics of tongue, mucosa, pharynx, gums
  Position and appearance of tonsils and palate
  Symmetry and movement of tongue and uvula
  Taste and gag reflex
- Ears and auditory system
  Position and alignment of auricles
  Surface characteristics of external ear and canal
  Characteristics of temporomandibular joint
  Rinne and Weber tests
- Eyes and visual system
  Visual acuity and visual fields
  Surface characteristics of eyes
  Extraocular movements
  Corneal light reflex
  Characteristics of cornea
  Consensual response to light
  Findings from ophthalmoscopic examination
- Lungs and respiratory system
  Chest wall configuration and anteroposterior diameter

Respiratory rate and depth

Palpation to evaluate symmetry and tactile fremitus

Percussion to evaluate tones and diaphragm excursion

Auscultation to identify breath sound characteristics and adventitious sounds

Auscultation of other sounds

■ Heart and peripheral vascular system

Location and characteristics of the apical impulse

Auscultation of S_1 and S_2 to note location, pitch, intensity, timing, splitting, systole, and diastole

Presence and characteristics of extra sounds, such as murmurs, clicks, snaps, S_3 and S_4

Jugular vein distention

Peripheral pulses: quality of pulses, bilaterally equal

Allen's test

■ Breasts and axillae

Size and surface characteristics

Symmetry

Presence of masses, tenderness, discharge, dimpling

Presence of scars

Lymphatic assessment

■ Abdomen and gastrointestinal system

Contour, visible aortic pulsations

Auscultation of all four quadrants to identify bowel sounds

Palpation of all four quadrants to identify organs, tenderness, masses

Costovertebral angle tenderness

Hernia

■ Female genitalia and reproductive system

Characteristics of external genitalia

Speculum examination: note discharge, pain, surface characteristics of vagina, cervix, adnexa

Bimanual examination: note tenderness, masses, size of uterus and ovaries

Rectal examination

■ Male genitalia

Characteristics of external genitalia

Palpation of penis and scrotum to note tenderness, discharge, lesions

Investigation of inguinal hernia to note swelling or tenderness

■ Anus, rectum, and prostate

Prostate evaluation

Rectal examination

■ Musculoskeletal system

Gait

Alignment of extremities and spine, symmetry of body

Joint evaluation

Muscle development, symmetry, and strength

Range of motion

Drawer test

McMurray's test

■ Neurologic system

Mental status, thought processes, cognitive assessment

Cranial nerve assessment

Fine and gross motor function

Sensory evaluation

Reflexes

Risk Profile.   The risk profile should include those items from the client's history and physical assessment that might indicate risk to the overall health state. They are potential problems. After you have determined any risk factors that the client may have, you should discuss with the client how some or all of these may be modified. (Remember that not all risk factors are modifiable.) During the history and physical assessment is an excellent opportunity to discuss health promotion with the client (see Health Promotion boxes in Chapters 8-22).

Problem List/Nursing Diagnosis.   The problem list should be a synthesis of those items that are currently identified as stressors for the client. The stressors may be physiologic, sociologic, psychologic, or a combination. The problems are those items that reduce the client's overall level of health. Once the problems or nursing diagnoses are listed and assigned a priority, it can be decided which are within the examiner's scope of practice to handle and which must be referred to other health care providers.

It is important for the examiner to cluster subjective and objective data to describe problems. The following unrelated examples demonstrate a holistic approach to problem identification. From this problem list, the nurse can formulate appropriate nursing diagnoses and then determine expected client outcomes and appropriate nursing interventions (see boxes on Sample Documentation & Nursing Diagnosis in each body system chapter for examples of documentation and formulation of nursing diagnoses).

■ Weight gain: 18 pounds in past year; exercise limited to game of tennis twice a month; expresses desire to diet but needs direction

■ Shortness of breath when walking up more than one flight of stairs; moderate edema below midcalf bilaterally; fine rales in lower bases bilaterally

■ Limited range of motion in right shoulder, which interferes with activities of daily living, for example, dressing, preparing meals

■ Cataracts bilaterally, which interfere with reading and driving at night

■ BP 180/120 (right arm) lying, 172/112 (right arm) sitting, retinal A-V ratio appears to be 2/4; arteriolar narrowing

■ Periodic urinary incontinence since birth of child 3 years ago; cystocele noted during vaginal examination

■ Complaints of LLQ discomfort for 6 months; cyclic with menses; increased discomfort at ovulation time and just before menses; thickening in left adnexa area; increased tenderness with palpation of left adnexa area; menses regular; pinpoint tenderness on deep palpation in LLQ

■ Smokes one pack of cigarettes a day for past 15 years; deep, nonproductive cough for past 5 years, becoming worse; increased breathing difficulty when climbing more than one flight of stairs; decreased breath sounds on right; bilateral rales or rhonchi in base of lungs; slight clearing with cough

■ Death of spouse 2 months ago; since then increased periods of depression, 10-pound weight loss, decreased desire to maintain own health state

Always remember to properly and completely document subjective and objective findings. Your record will become the basis for subsequent care and health promotion delivered to the client.

??????? STUDY QUESTIONS ???????

1. You are doing a head-to-toe examination. What equipment do you need to have on hand before you start the examination?

2. Describe how you would prepare an individual for an assessment.

3. What things are important to assess early in the examination in order to avert problems later in the examination?

4. During your practice assessment sessions, which elements have been the easiest for you? Which elements have presented the most challenge?

5. Have you attempted to do a complete assessment yet? If so, describe what the experience felt like. How long did it take? Did anything unexpected happen? Did all of your equipment work? What elements, if any, did you forget? Did you feel overwhelmed? What would you do differently next time?

6. Compare and contrast the advantages and disadvantages of using plain paper versus a predeveloped form for documentation.

7. Select at least one body system and perform a history and physical exam. Document your results. Evaluate your documentation. Is it complete? Are the results clearly and concisely presented? Is your terminology specific, clear, and descriptive?

8. What is the purpose of conducting a risk profile? How might a risk profile assist you in teaching the client about health promotion?

9. What is a problem list? Where do you get data to formulate a problem list? What is the problem list used for?

10. Select two of the example problems cited in the chapter and formulate appropriate nursing diagnoses. Prioritize your diagnoses.

Sample Documentation

ADULT CLIENT

Date: **1-8-96**

BIOGRAPHIC DATA

Name:	Sara Jane Borden 1001 S. Gloucester St. Richland, TX 76092-2415
Telephone:	(214) 650-7650
Date of Birth:	7-5-17
Gender:	Female
Race:	Caucasian
Religion:	Protestant
Marital Status:	Widow
Soc. Security No.:	459-67-9980
Occupation:	Retired
Birth Place:	Topeka, Kansas
Source of Referral:	Daughter: Karan Marsh
Usual Source of Health Care:	Dr. Murphy, who retired
Source and Reliability of Information:	Self; reliable
Advanced Directive:	Yes, copy in file.
Insurance:	Medicare and private insurance
REASON FOR SEEKING HEALTH CARE:	Pain in right leg and knee when walking for last 2 months.
PRESENT ILLNESS	Pain is burning and radiates from right hip to knee, worse when getting up in the morning; has to hobble to bathroom; after she is up for a few hours, pain is better, but never completely relieved; tried water exercise and ibuprofen to relieve pain; pain sometimes prevents her from grocery shopping, because pain is worse the longer she stands; pain relieved somewhat by sitting; unable to take daily walks since pain occurred.

PAST MEDICAL HISTORY

Allergies:	Morphine and codeine "make me deathly ill" Sulfa drugs "break me out in a rash"
Current meds at home:	Dyazide 1 tab daily Lanoxin 0.25 mg daily Captopril 50 mg bid Premarin 0.625 mg daily Vitamin E 400 units daily Calcium supplement daily
Immunizations:	Tetanus—doesn't remember date Annual flu and pneumonia immunization

Last Exams:	Eyes—3 months ago
	Ears—wears hearing aide R ear since 1970, nerve deafness
	Dental—8 months ago
	Physician—for annual physical
	ECG—today
	Mammogram—one year ago

Surgeries:	Tonsillectomy as a child
	Cholecystectomy 1993
	Carpal tunnel 1991
	C-section 1935, 1937, 1940
	Appendectomy 1940
	Total hysterectomy with anterior/posterior (A & P) repair 1954

Chronic Diseases:	Hypertension for 30 years
	Type II diabetes mellitus controlled with diet for 25 years
	Fibrocystic breast disease for 7 years

| **Obstetric History:** | Gravida 4 para 3 (1 miscarriage) |

Family History:	Father died age 82—prostate cancer
	Mother died age 87—myocardial infarction
	Brother, alive and well—diabetes mellitus

Genogram

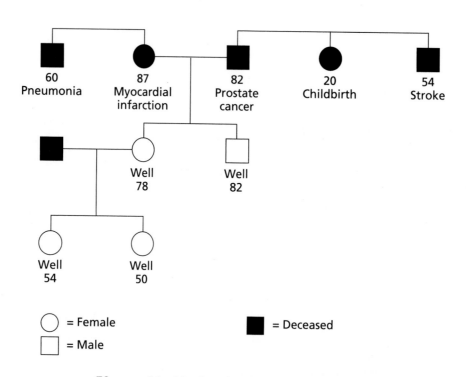

Social History: 78-year-old white female who lives alone in a 3-bedroom, 2-bath, one-story home with a cat. She is a retired school teacher with three adult children who live in surrounding towns and provide social and emotional support for her. Plays bridge twice a week at churches in her community; drives herself. Makes clothes for her four grandchildren.

Current Health Habits: Smokes ½ pack cigarettes, walks with a friend 1½ miles around track at local high school 4 to 5 times/week. Eats diet consistent with food pyramid. Stopped drinking coffee and eating chocolate because of fibrocystic breast disease. Drinks one bourbon with water nightly while fixing dinner.

REVIEW OF SYSTEMS In good health until 2 months ago

Skin, hair, nails: Skin itches on feet due to diabetes neuropathy; skin thin, bleeds easily when she bumps her arm or her cat scratches her while playing; bathes daily, applies body lotions; has hair fixed weekly, keeps nails manicured and polished.

Head:	Reports no headaches unless her blood pressure is elevated
Eyes:	Wears bifocals, has black floaters, photophobia; able to see to read, watches television, drives; reports no blurred vision, itching, drainage
Ears:	Wears bilateral hearing aides due to nerve deafness; reports no tinnitus, pain, drainage
Nose and sinuses:	Reports no congestion, drainage, sinus pain
Throat and mouth:	Reports no sore throat, hoarseness, dysphagia, bleeding gums, or difficulty in chewing; no dental appliances, brushes and flosses teeth twice daily, no slipping or crepitation of temporomandibular joint
Neck:	Reports no stiffness or tenderness
Breasts:	Reports no tenderness or nipple drainage; performs breast self-exam when she remembers, about every 3 months; has annual mammogram; has fibrocystic disease that has improved since she started taking vitamin E and decreased coffee and chocolate
Cardiovascular:	Last blood pressure was normal, chest pain 1993, hospitalized, palpitation 2 years ago, feet swell; no report of shortness of breath, dyspnea, or chest pain; extremities warm and with no discoloration
Respiratory:	Had pneumonia last year, treated at home with antibiotics; no reports of wheeze, cough, dyspnea, SOB, or hemoptysis
Endocrine:	No report of changes in thyroid function, skin or hair. Has polyuria when she goes off her diet; occurs several times per year, usually during holidays
Hematologic:	No report of excess bruising; bleeds easily when bumps arm or cat scratches her "due to thinner skin since I'm getting old"
Gastrointestinal:	No report of diarrhea, constipation, rectal bleeding, nausea, or emesis; has bowel movement each morning after breakfast, formed brown stool; no report of laxative use, eats fresh vegetables instead
Genitourinary:	Voids about 5 times each day, clear light yellow; reports no nocturia, dysuria, itching, or discharge; had hysterectomy in 1954, takes estrogen replacement
Musculoskeletal:	No report of weakness, spasms, or pain until 2 months ago when hip and leg pain began
Neurologic:	No report of difficulty performing activities of daily living until pain in hip and leg began; has tingling in her feet periodically from diabetic neuropathy, rubbing her feet helps; reports no changes in cognition

PHYSICAL EXAMINATION

Vital signs:	BP 140/88; P 88; R 16; T 98.8° F (37.1° C); Wt 130 lb (59 kg); Ht 5'4" (163 cm) = 50th percentile weight for height for medium women
General:	Cooperative, oriented, alert woman, maintains eye contact, appropriately groomed
Skin, hair, nails:	Smooth, pink, moist, thin with elastic turgor; ecchymosis on forearms bilaterally from previous trauma, no tenderness to palpation, no drainage noted; hair, gray with female distribution, soft texture
Head:	Scalp intact, no lesions of tenderness; symmetric
Eyes:	Snellen 20/20 each eye with glasses, near vision, able to read newspaper at 14" with glasses; brows, lids, and lashes intact with no crusting; no tearing; conjunctiva pink without discharge, sclera white; corneal light reflex symmetric; pupils equal, round, and react to light and accommodation; extraocular movement intact, peripheral bilaterally, discs with well-defined borders bilaterally, vessels present in all quadrants without crossing defects, no hemorrhages or exudates; retina pink, macula present; cornea, lens, and vitreous clear
Ears:	Auricles aligned with eyes without lesions, masses or tenderness; tympanic membranes gray, translucent with light reflex and bony landmarks present; no perforations. Weber lateralizes to right ear, negative Rinne (BC>AC) right ear; positive

Rinne (AC>BC) left ear; repeats whispered words at ½ feet bilaterally (with hearing aid)

Noses and sinuses: Septum midline, patent bilaterally, mucous membranes moist and pink without exudate, no pain or palpation of sinuses; correctly identified coffee and orange odors bilaterally

Mouth and throat: Mucosa and gingiva pink and moist without lesions, 28 teeth in good repair, tongue midline without lesions or tremor, uvula midline with elevation of soft palate, gag reflex intact, pharynx pink, moist without exudate, no hoarseness

Neck: Trachea midline and movable, thyroid not palpable or tender, no lymph nodes palpable, full range of motion with strong movement, no tenderness or masses; carotid arteries full, round, rate = 88, jugular veins flat at 45°

Chest and lungs: AP diameter < lateral, muscle and respiratory effort symmetric, equal excursion, tactile fremitus equal, resonant percussion throughout, diaphragmatic excursion 4 cm bilaterally, vesicular breath sounds throughout with no adventitious sounds; even, quiet breathing

Breasts: Symmetric, moderate size, nodular, granular consistency bilaterally; nipples soft without discharge, areolas equal in size, no dimpling, masses, tenderness or lesions; no lymphadenopathy

Heart: Apical pulse full and round fifth ICS left MCL; no lifts, heaves, thrills, or abnormal pulsations; S_1 and S_2 normal with regular rate and rhythm without murmurs

Abdomen: Rounded, striae noted; skin smooth with no lesions, aorta midline, no visible pulsations; bowel sounds in all quadrants, no bruits; tympanic percussion tones over most of abdomen; liver span 6 cm at right midclavicular line; abdomen soft, liver, spleen and kidney not palpable, no tenderness, no CVA tenderness, no inguinal lymphadenopathy; superficial abdominal reflexes intact

Peripheral vascular: Extremities pink, no edema, clubbing; pulses strong, round, warm, no tenderness

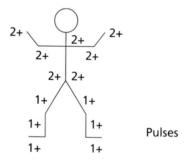

Pulses

Musculoskeletal: Vertebral column symmetric, no tenderness or curvature; full extension, lateral bending and rotation; arms and left leg symmetric, range of motion without pain or crepitation; right leg pain with hip and knee flexion and straight leg raises; muscle strength 4/5

Neurologic: Oriented to time, place, and person; appearance, behavior, speech and clothing appropriate; thought coherent, remote and recent memory intact; cranial nerves I-XII intact; upper extremity (UE) sensation intact to pinprick, vibration, and light touch bilaterally; lower extremity (LE) sensation decreased to pinprick and vibration and absent to light touch; deep tendon reflexes 2+ UE and 1+ LE; babinski negative bilaterally, no clonus; negative Romberg, cerebellum finger to nose intact, unable to walk on toes of right foot

Genitalia: Female hair distribution, sparse amount of hair; external genitalia pink, dry, no lesions or discharge; vaginal walls nontender; anus, no hemorrhoids, fissures, or lesions; rectal wall no tenderness, no masses, strong sphincter tone, stool soft brown, guaiac negative

Sample Documentation

CHILD CLIENT

Date: **1-5-96**

BIOGRAPHIC DATA

Name:	Roberto Aquera
Address:	912 West Rochelle, Apt. 101 Fort Worth, TX 76129
Telephone:	(817) 921-7659
Date of Birth:	12-1-95
Birth Place:	Medical Center Hospital Fort Worth, Texas
Race:	Hispanic
Culture:	Mexican-American
Religion:	Catholic
Marital Status:	Single
Family in Home:	Lives with parents and older brother
Soc. Security No.:	Not applicable
Occupation:	Not applicable Parents employed full time: mother as teacher aide, father as plumber
Contact Person:	Arturo and Esther Aquero
Advanced Directive:	Not applicable
Dual Power of Attorney:	Not applicable
Usual Source of Health Care:	Private
Health Insurance:	Yes—health maintenance organization
Description of Home:	Two-bedroom apartment, ground floor
Source of Data:	Parents, reliable sources
REASON FOR SEEKING CARE	"Cough and runny nose for 3 days"
PRESENT HEALTH STATUS	He was well until 3 days ago. Nasal drainage is slightly thick and yellow, cough is nonproductive. No fever, sneezing, or rash reported. He coughs more when lying down, nose runs more when he is sitting up. No medications have been given due to his age.

PAST MEDICAL HISTORY

Health of mother:

Prenatal care:	In 2nd and 3rd trimesters
Complications during pregnancy:	None
Planned pregnancy:	Yes
Mother's attitude:	Pleased with healthy baby, wanted a girl
Father's attitude:	Pleased with healthy baby

| **Hospitalizations:** | Vaginal delivery with epidural anesthesia 4 weeks ago, breech presentation, 38 weeks gestation, no complications during labor or delivery |

Health of Neonate:

| **Birthweight:** | 7 lb 13 oz; length: 22½ inches |

Previous health care:

Immunizations:	1st hepatitis B at birth
Allergies:	None
Family History:	Father, alive and well, age 26
	Mother, alive and well, age 23
	Brother, alive and well, age 5

Genogram

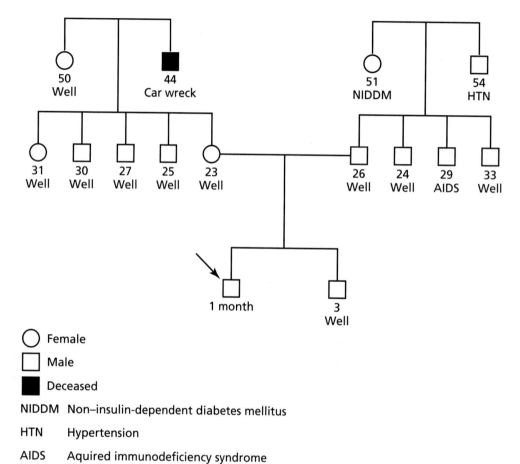

REVIEW OF SYSTEMS

Nutrition:	Bottle feeding, Similac formula 4 to 5 ounces per feeding, 7 to 8 feedings per day
Sleep:	6 to 7 hours at night, several naps during the day; sleeps on side or back
Skin, hair, nails:	Reports no changes in skin, hair, or nails; has darker area over buttocks
Eyes:	Opens eyes to sounds, follows movement
Ears:	Turns head to noises, no discharges reported
Nose:	Has had moderately thick yellow discharge, previously able to breath without difficulty
Throat:	No difficulty reported, swallows formula without difficulty, strong suck

Neck:	No swollen areas reported, turns head to noises
Respiratory:	Cough for 3 days, no sneezing, wheezing. Stops frequently to take breaths during feeding
Cardiovascular:	No difficulty reported
Gastrointestinal:	See nutrition above; has 1 to 2 soft stools each day, no abdominal distention reported
Genitourinary:	Urinates 7 to 8 times a day
Musculoskeletal:	Moves all extremities symmetrically
Central nervous system:	Cry is normal, parents able to console him; likes to be held

PSYCHOSOCIAL STATUS

Sibling rivalry:	Older child is adjusting to new brother; was jealous at first, now helps with care of younger brother
Return to work:	Mother returns to work in 2 weeks; baby's aunt will keep him while parents work

ENVIRONMENTAL HEALTH

Safety:	Using infant car seat and seat belts, parents supported baby's head appropriately, neither parent smokes

PHYSICAL EXAMINATION

General:	Alert, active infant—age 1 month, 4 days
Vital signs:	T 98.2° F (36.8° C); P 130 bpm; R 40 rpm Height (length): 22½" (56 cm) (90th percentile) Weight: 11 lb 12 oz (5.3 kg) (90th percentile) Head circumference: 14¾" (37 cm) (90th percentile) Chest circumference: 13½" (33 cm)
Skin:	Light brown, smooth, soft; turgor elastic; mongolian spot over buttocks
Head:	Anterior fontanel soft, diamond-shaped 1¼" (3.5 cm); posterior fontanel soft, triangular-shaped ½" (1.25 cm); skull symmetric, hair evenly distributed
Eyes:	Symmetric, sclera white, conjunctiva moist, pink, no tears; red reflex bilaterally; pupils equal, round, and react to light, symmetric corneal light reflex, able to follow to midline
Ears:	Lateral edge of eye aligned with top of pinna, pinna flexible, cartilage present; startle reflex elicited by loud noise; tympanic membrane pearly gray bilaterally
Nose:	Symmetric, patent, small amount yellow exudate
Mouth and throat:	Mucous membranes moist, uvula midline, sucking, rooting, and gag reflexes present
Neck:	Short thick neck
Chest and lungs:	Anteroposterior and lateral diameters equal, no retraction noted; abdominal respirations, bilateral bronchial breath sounds
Heart:	Apex fourth ICS, MCL, S_2 slightly sharper and higher in pitch than S_1
Abdomen:	Round; bowel sounds in all quadrants; liver, spleen, kidneys not palpable; equal bilateral femoral pulses
Genitalia:	Urethral opening at tip of glans penis, circumcised; testes palpable in scrotum
Musculoskeletal:	Hands closed, full range of motion, nail beds pink; spine intact, vertebral column straight patent; hips stable
Neurologic:	Extension of extremity followed by some degree of flexion, head lag while sitting, able to turn head side to side when prone, grasp reflex strong, tonic neck reflex present

Appendix B

American Nurses Association (ANA) Screening Guidelines

CHILD PREVENTIVE CARE TIME LINE

Checkup visits are important for a child's health. Some authorities recommend these visits at the following ages: 2 to 4 weeks; 2, 4, 6, 9, 12, 15, and 18 months; and 2, 3, 4, 5, 6, 8, 10, 12, 14, 16, and 18 years. A child's physician or other health care provider will discuss the individual needs of the child. At checkup visits, a child may receive a physical examination and the types of preventive care shown at right.

Please note:
Children with special risk factors may need more frequent and additional types of preventive care. Some examples:

Risk factor	Preventive service(s) needed
Exposure to TB	TB test
Sexually active	Pap test (females); syphilis, gonorrhea, chlamydia tests
High-risk sexual behavior	AIDS test, hepatitis immunization
Drug abuse	AIDS, TB test, hepatitis immunization

Key:

▮ Recommended by all major authorities.

▮ Recommended by some major authorities.

708

YEARS OF AGE

TESTS

Newborn screening

Head Size

Height and weight

Blood pressure

Anemia

Lead

Urinalysis

Tuberculosis

Hearing

Vision

EXAMS

Eye

Dental

IMMUNIZATIONS

Hepatitis B (HBV)

Polio (OPV)

Haemophilus influenzae (Hib)

Diphtheria, tetanus, pertussis (DTP, Td)

Measles, mumps, rubella (MMR)

Chickenpox (VZV)

HEALTH GUIDANCE

Development, nutrition, oral health, physical activity, injuries and poisons, sun exposure, smoking, alcohol and drugs, AIDS, sexual behavior, family planning

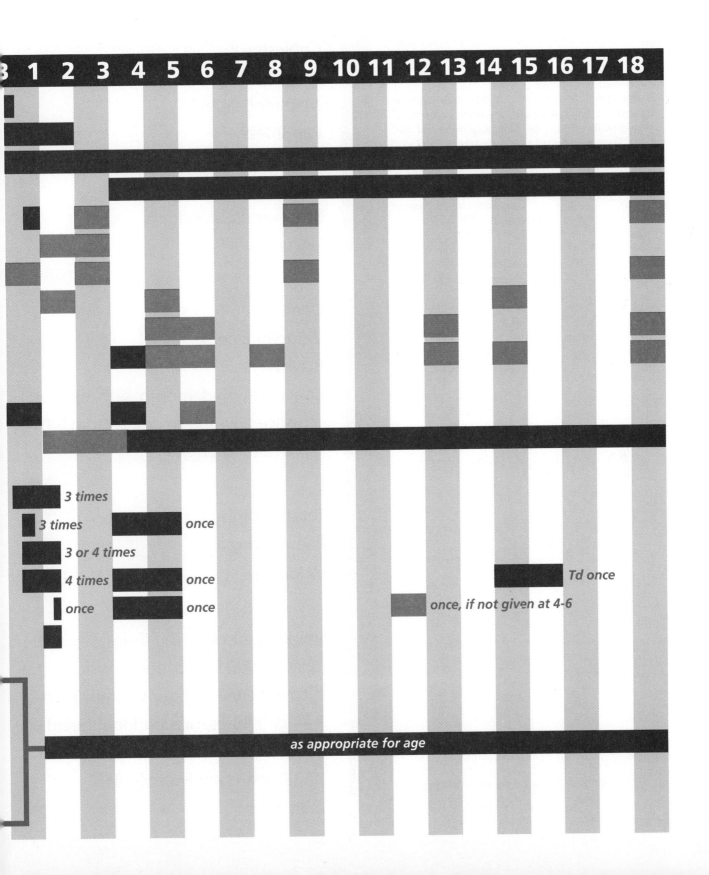

ADULT PREVENTIVE CARE TIME LINE

Checkup visits with a physician or other health care provider are important for good health. Most authorities recommend these visits every 1 to 3 years until age 65 and yearly thereafter. Each individual should speak with a physician or other health care provider about the proper schedule of checkup visits. This chart shows the different types of preventive care that is needed at each age.

Please note:
Recommended intervals for each type of preventive care may vary among authorities. Individuals with special risk factors may need more frequent and additional types of preventive care. Some examples:

Risk factor	**Preventive service(s) needed**
Diabetes	Eye, foot examinations, urine test
Drug abuse	AIDS, TB tests, hepatitis immunization
Alcoholism	Influenza, pneumococcal immunizations, TB test
Overweight	Blood sugar test
Homeless, recent refugee or immigrant	TB test
High-risk sexual behavior	AIDS, syphilis, gonorrhea, chlamydia tests

Key:

▮ Recommended by all major authorities.

▮ Recommended by some major authorities.

YEARS OF AGE

TESTS

Blood pressure
Height and weight
Cholesterol
Hearing
Mammography
Pap smear
Prostate-specific antigen
Sigmoidoscopy
Stool occult blood
Urinalysis

EXAMS

Dental
Vision/glaucoma
Breast
Cancer (thyroid, mouth, skin, ovaries, testicles, lymph nodes, rectum (40+), prostate (men 50+)

IMMUNIZATIONS

Tetanus-diphtheria
Pneumococcal
Influenza

HEALTH GUIDANCE

Smoking, alcohol and drugs, sexual behavior, AIDS, nutrition, physical activity, violence and guns, family planning, injuries, occupational health, folate (women 12-45), aspirin (men 40+), estrogen (women 45+)

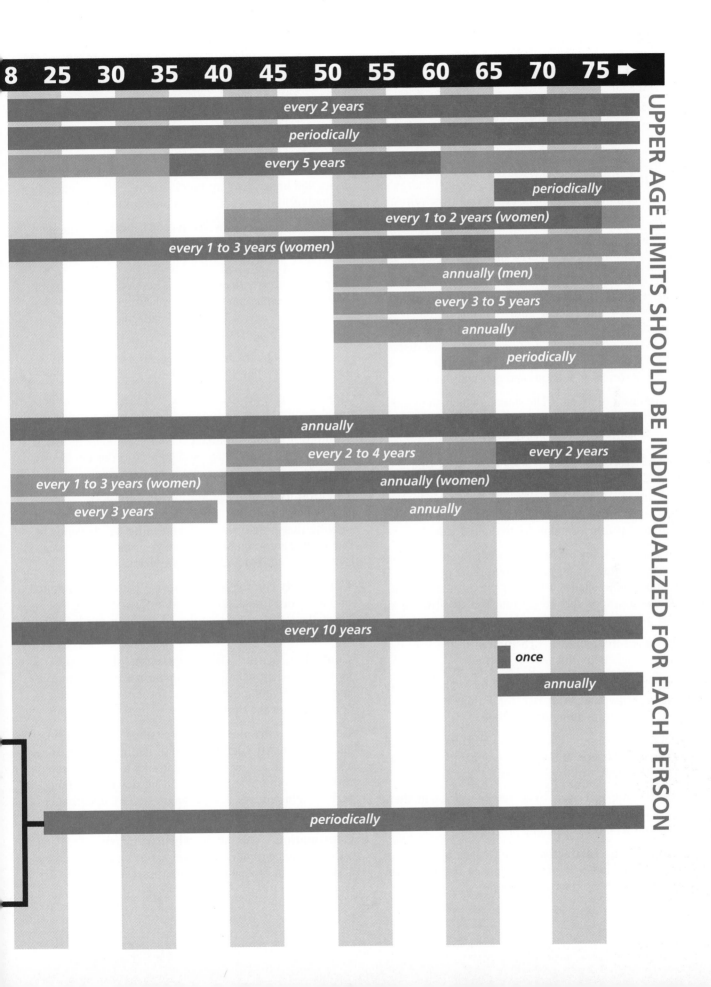

Alphabetical List of North American Nursing Diagnosis Association (NANDA) Diagnoses

Activity intolerance The state in which an individual has insufficient physiological or psychological energy to endure or complete required or desired daily activities.

Activity intolerance, risk for The state in which an individual is at risk of experiencing insufficient physiological or psychological energy to endure or complete required or desired daily activities.

Adaptive capacity, decreased intracranial A clinical state in which intracranial fluid dynamic mechanisms that normally compensate for increases in intracranial volumes are compromised, resulting in repeated disproportionate increases in intracranial pressure (ICP) in response to a variety of noxious and non-noxious stimuli.

Adjustment, impaired The state in which an individual is unable to modify his/her lifestyle behavior in a manner consistent with a change in health status.

Airway clearance, ineffective The state in which an individual is unable to clear secretions or obstructions from the respiratory tract to maintain airway patency.

Anxiety A vague, uneasy feeling, the source of which is often nonspecific or unknown to the individual.

Aspiration, risk for The state in which an individual is at risk for entry of gastric secretions, oropharyngeal secretions, or exogenous food or fluids into tracheobronchial passages due to dysfunction or absence of normal protective mechanisms.

Body image disturbance Disruption in the way one perceives one's body image.

Body temperature, altered, risk for The state in which an individual is at risk for failure to maintain body temperature within normal range.

Bowel incontinence The state in which an individual experiences a change in normal bowel habits characterized by involuntary passage of stool.

Breast-feeding, effective The state in which a mother-infant dyad/family exhibits adequate proficiency and satisfaction with breast-feeding process.

Breast-feeding, ineffective The state in which a mother, infant, and/or family experiences dissatisfaction or difficulty with the breast-feeding process.

Breast-feeding, interrupted A break in the continuity of the breast-feeding process as a result of inability or inadvisability to put baby to breast for feeding.

Breathing pattern, ineffective The state in which an individual's inhalation and/or exhalation pattern does not enable adequate ventilation.

Cardiac output, decreased The state in which the blood pumped by an individual's heart is sufficiently reduced to the extent that it is inadequate to meet the needs of the body's tissues.

Caregiver role strain A caregiver's felt difficulty in performing the family caregiver role.

Caregiver role strain, risk for Vulnerability for feeling difficulty in performing the family caregiver role.

Communication, impaired verbal The state in which an individual experiences a decreased or absent ability to use or understand language in human interaction.

Community coping, potential for enhanced A pattern of community activities for adaptation and problem solving that is satisfactory for meeting the demands or needs of the community but can be improved for management of current and future problems/stressors.

Community coping, ineffective A pattern of community activities for adaptation and problem solving that is unsatisfactory for meeting the demands or needs of the community.

Confusion, acute The abrupt onset of a cluster of global, transient changes and disturbances in attention, cognition, psychomotor activity, level of consciousness, and/or sleep/wake cycle.

Confusion, chronic An irreversible, long-standing, and/or progressive deterioration of intellect and personality characterized by decreased ability to interpret environmental stimuli and decreased capacity for intellectual thought processes. It is manifested by disturbances of memory, orientation, and behavior.

Constipation The state in which an individual experiences a change in normal bowel habits characterized by a decrease in frequency and/or passage of hard, dry stools.

Constipation, colonic The state in which an individual's pattern of elimination is characterized by hard, dry stool that results from a delay in passage of food residue.

Constipation, perceived The state in which an individual makes a self-diagnosis of constipation and ensures a daily bowel movement through use of laxatives, enemas, and suppositories.

Coping, defensive The state in which an individual experiences falsely positive self-evaluation based on a self-protective pattern that defends against underlying perceived threats to positive self-regard.

Coping, family: potential for growth Effective managing of adaptive tasks by family member involved with the patient's health challenge, who now is exhibiting desire and readiness for enhanced health and growth in regard to self and in relation to the patient.

Coping, ineffective family: compromised Insufficient, ineffective, or compromised support, comfort, assistance, or encouragement—usually by a supportive primary person (family member or close friend); patient may need it to manage or master adaptive tasks related to his/her health challenge.

Coping, ineffective family: disabling Behavior of significant person (family member or other primary person) that disables his/her own capacities and the patient's capacities to effectively address tasks essential to either person's adaptation to the health challenge.

Coping, ineffective individual Impairment of adaptive behaviors and problem-solving abilities of a person in meeting life's demands and roles.

Decisional conflict (specify) A state of uncertainty about the course of action to be taken when choice among competing actions involves risk, loss, or challenge to personal life values. (Specify focus of conflict; e.g., choices regarding health, family relationships, career, finances, or other life events.)

Denial, ineffective A conscious or unconscious attempt to disavow the knowledge or meaning of an event to reduce anxiety/fear to the detriment of health.

Diarrhea The state in which an individual experiences a change in normal bowel habits characterized by the frequent passage of loose, fluid, unformed stools.

Disuse syndrome, risk for The state in which an individual is at risk for deterioration of body systems as the result of prescribed or unavoidable inactivity.

Diversional activity deficit The state in which an individual experiences a decreased stimulation from or interest or engagement in recreational or leisure activities.

Dysreflexia The state in which an individual with spinal cord injury at T7 or above experiences or is at risk of experiencing life-threatening uninhibited sympathetic response of the nervous system attributable to a noxious stimulus.

Energy field disturbance A disruption of the flow of energy surrounding a person's being, which results in a disharmony of the body, mind, or spirit.

Environmental interpretation syndrome, impaired Consistent lack of orientation to person, place, time, or circumstances over more than 3 to 6 months, necessitating a protective environment.

Family processes, altered: alcoholism The state in which the psychosocial, spiritual, and physiological functions of the family unit are chronically disorganized, leading to conflict, denial of problems, resistance to change, ineffective problem-solving, and a series of self-perpetuating crises.

Family processes, altered The state in which a family that normally functions effectively experiences a dysfunction.

Fatigue An overwhelming sense of exhaustion and decreased capacity for physical and mental work regardless of adequate sleep.

Fear Feeling of dread related to an identifiable source that the person validates.

Fluid volume deficit The state in which an individual experiences vascular, cellular, or intracellular dehydration related to failure of regulatory mechanisms.

Fluid volume deficit (2) The state in which an individual experiences vascular, cellular, or intracellular dehydration related to active loss.

Fluid volume deficit, risk for The state in which an individual is at risk for experiencing vascular, cellular, or intracellular dehydration.

Fluid volume excess The state in which an individual experiences increased fluid retention and edema.

Gas exchange, impaired The state in which an individual experiences an imbalance between oxygen uptake and carbon dioxide elimination at the alveolar–capillary membrane gas exchange area.

Grieving, anticipatory Intellectual and emotional responses and behaviors by which individuals work through the process of modifying self-concept based on the perception of potential loss.

Grieving, dysfunctional Extended, unsuccessful use of intellectual and emotional responses by which individuals attempt to work through the process of modifying self-concept based on the perception of loss.

Growth and development, altered The state in which an individual demonstrates deviations in norms from his/her age-group.

Health maintenance, altered Inability to identify, manage, and/or seek help to maintain health.

Health-seeking behaviors (specify) The state in which a patient in stable health is actively seeking ways to alter personal health habits and/or the environment in order to move toward optimal health. (*Stable health status* is defined as age-appropriate illness prevention measures achieved; the patient reports good or excellent health, and signs and symptoms of disease, if present, are controlled.)

Home maintenance management, impaired Inability to independently maintain a safe growth-promoting immediate environment.

Hopelessness The subjective state in which an individual sees limited or no alternatives or personal choices available and is unable to mobilize energy on own behalf.

Hyperthermia The state in which an individual's body temperature is elevated above his/her normal range.

Hypothermia The state in which an individual's body temperature is reduced below his/her normal range but not below 35.6° C (rectal)/ 36.4° C (rectal, newborn).

Incontinence, functional The state in which an individual experiences an involuntary, unpredictable passage of urine.

Incontinence, reflex The state in which an individual experiences an involuntary loss of urine occurring at somewhat predictable intervals when a specific bladder volume is reached.

Incontinence, stress The state in which an individual experiences a loss of urine of less than 50 ml occurring with increased abdominal pressure.

Incontinence, total The state in which an individual experiences a continuous and unpredictable loss of urine.

Incontinence, urge The state in which an individual experiences involuntary passage of urine occurring soon after a strong sense of urgency to void.

Infant behavior, disorganized Alteration in integration and modulation of the physiological and behavioral systems of functioning (i.e., autonomic, motor, state, organizational, self-regulatory, and attentional-interactional systems).

Infant behavior, disorganized: risk for Risk for alteration in integration and modulation of the physiological and behavioral systems of functioning (i.e., auto-

nomic, motor, state, organizational, self-regulatory, and attentional-interactional systems).

Infant behavior, organized: potential for enhanced A pattern of modulation of the physiologic and behavioral systems of functioning of an infant (i.e., autonomic, motor, state, organizational, self-regulatory, and attentional-interactional systems) that is satisfactory but that can be improved, resulting in higher levels of integration in response to environmental stimuli.

Infant feeding pattern, ineffective A state in which an infant demonstrates an impaired ability to suck or coordinate the suck-swallow response.

Infection, risk for The state in which an individual is at increased risk for being invaded by pathogenic organisms.

Injury, perioperative positioning: risk for A state in which the client is at risk for injury as a result of the environmental conditions found in the perioperative setting.

Injury, risk for The state in which an individual is at risk of injury as a result of environmental conditions interacting with the individual's adaptive and defensive resources. See also Poisoning, risk for; Suffocation, risk for; Trauma, risk for.

Knowledge deficit (specify) Absence or deficiency of cognitive information related to specific topic.

Loneliness, risk for A subjective state in which an individual is at risk of experiencing vague dysphoria.

Management of therapeutic regimen, community: ineffective A pattern of regulating and integrating into community processes programs for treatment of illness and the sequelae of illness that are unsatisfactory for meeting health-related goals.

Management of therapeutic regimen, families: ineffective A pattern of regulating and integrating into family processes a program for treatment of illness and the sequelae of illness that is unsatisfactory for meeting specific health goals.

Management of therapeutic regimen, individuals: effective A pattern of regulating and integrating into daily living a program for treatment of illness and its sequelae that is satisfactory for meeting specific health goals.

Management of therapeutic regimen, individuals: ineffective A pattern of regulating and integrating into daily living a program for treatment of illness and the sequelae of illness that is unsatisfactory for meeting specific health goals.

Memory, impaired The state in which an individual experiences the inability to remember or recall bits of information or behavioral skills. Impaired memory may be attributed to pathophysiological or situational causes that are either temporary or permanent.

Mobility, impaired physical The state in which an individual experiences a limitation of ability for independent physical movement.

Noncompliance (specify) A person's informed decision not to adhere to a therapeutic recommendation.

Nutrition, altered: less than body requirements The state in which an individual experiences an intake of nutrients insufficient to meet metabolic needs.

Nutrition, altered: more than body requirements The state in which an individual is experiencing an intake of nutrients that exceeds metabolic needs.

Nutrition, altered: risk for more than body requirements The state in which an individual is at risk of experiencing an intake of nutrients that exceeds metabolic needs.

Oral mucous membrane, altered The state in which an individual experiences disruptions in the tissue layers of the oral cavity.

Pain The state in which an individual experiences and reports the presence of severe discomfort or an uncomfortable sensation.

Pain, chronic The state in which an individual experiences pain that continues for more than 6 months.

Parent/infant/child attachment, altered, risk for Disruption of the interactive process between parent or significant other and infant that fosters the development of a protective and nurturing reciprocal relationship.

Parental role conflict The state in which a parent experiences role confusion and conflict in response to a crisis.

Parenting, altered

Parenting, altered, risk for The state in which the ability of nurturing figure(s) to create an environment that promotes the optimal growth and development of another human being is altered or at risk.

Peripheral neurovascular dysfunction, risk for A state in which an individual is at risk of experiencing a disruption in circulation, sensation, or motion of an extremity.

Personal identity disturbance Inability to distinguish between self and nonself.

Poisoning, risk for Accentuated risk of accidental exposure to or ingestion of drugs or dangerous products in doses sufficient to cause poisoning.

Post-trauma syndrome The state in which an individual experiences a sustained painful response to (an) overwhelming traumatic event(s).

Rape-trauma syndrome Forced, violent sexual penetration against the victim's will and consent. The trauma syndrome that develops from this attack or attempted attack includes an acute phase or disorganization of the victim's lifestyle and a long-term process of reorganization of lifestyle.

Rape-trauma syndrome: compound reaction An acute stress reaction to a rape or attempted rape, experienced along with other major stressors, that can include reactivation of symptoms of a previous condition.

Rape-trauma syndrome: silent reaction A complex stress reaction to a rape in which an individual is unable to describe or discuss the rape.

Relocation stress syndrome Physiological and/or psychosocial disturbances as a result of transfer from one environment to another.

Role performance, altered Disruption in the way one perceives one's role performance.

Self-care deficit, bathing/hygiene The state in which one experiences an impaired ability to perform or complete bathing/hygiene activities for oneself.

Self-care deficit, dressing/grooming The state in which one experiences an impaired ability to perform or complete dressing and grooming activities for oneself.

Self-care deficit, feeding The state in which one experiences an impaired ability to perform or complete feeding activities for oneself.

Self-care deficit, toileting The state in which one experiences an impaired ability to perform or complete toileting activities for oneself.

Self-esteem disturbance Negative self-evaluation/feelings about self or self-capabilities, which may be directly or indirectly expressed.

Self-esteem, chronic low Long-standing negative self-evaluation/feelings about self or self-capabilities.

Self-esteem, situational low Negative self-evaluation/feelings about self that develop in response to a loss or change in an individual who previously had a positive self-evaluation.

Self-mutilation, risk for A state in which an individual is at high risk to perform an act on the self to injure, not kill, that produces tissue damage and tension relief.

Sensory/perceptual alterations (specify) (visual, auditory, kinesthetic, gustatory, tactile, olfactory) The state in which an individual experiences a change in the amount or patterning of incoming stimuli accompanied by a diminished, exaggerated, distorted, or impaired response to such stimuli.

Sexual dysfunction   The state in which an individual experiences a change in sexual function that is viewed as unsatisfying, unrewarding, or inadequate.

Sexuality patterns, altered   The state in which an individual expresses concern regarding his/her sexuality.

Skin integrity, impaired   The state in which an individual's skin is adversely altered.

Skin integrity, impaired, risk for   The state in which an individual's skin is at risk of being adversely altered.

Sleep pattern disturbance   Disruption of sleep time that causes discomfort or interferes with desired lifestyle.

Social interaction, impaired   The state in which an individual participates in an insufficient or excessive quantity or ineffective quality of social exchange.

Social isolation   Aloneness experienced by an individual and perceived as imposed by others and as a negative or threatened state.

Spiritual distress (distress of the human spirit)   Disruption in the life principle that pervades a person's entire being and that integrates and transcends one's biological and psychosocial nature.

Spiritual well-being, potential for enhanced   The process of an individual's developing or unfolding of mystery through harmonious interconnectedness that springs from inner strengths.

Suffocation, risk for   Accentuated risk of accidental suffocation (inadequate air available for inhalation).

Swallowing, impaired   The state in which an individual has decreased ability to voluntarily pass fluids and/or solids from the mouth to the stomach.

Thermoregulation, ineffective   The state in which an individual's temperature fluctuates between hypothermia and hyperthermia.

Thought processes, altered   The state in which an individual experiences a disruption in cognitive operations and activities.

Tissue integrity, impaired   The state in which an individual experiences damage to mucous membrane or corneal, integumentary, or subcutaneous tissue. See also Oral mucous membrane, altered.

Tissue perfusion, altered (specify type) (renal, cerebral, cardiopulmonary, gastrointestinal, peripheral)   The state in which an individual experiences a decrease in nutrition and oxygenation at the cellular level due to a deficit in capillary blood supply.

Trauma, risk for   Accentuated risk of accidental tissue injury (e.g., wound, burn, fracture).

Unilateral neglect   The state in which an individual is perceptually unaware of and inattentive to one side of the body.

Urinary elimination, altered   The state in which an individual experiences a disturbance in urine elimination. See also Incontinence (functional, reflex, stress, total, urge).

Urinary retention   The state in which an individual experiences incomplete emptying of the bladder.

Ventilation, inability to sustain spontaneous   A state in which the response pattern of decreased energy reserves results in an individual's inability to maintain breathing adequate to support life.

Ventilatory weaning process, dysfunctional   A state in which an individual cannot adjust to lowered levels of mechanical ventilator support, which interrupts and prolongs the weaning process.

Violence, risk for: self-directed or directed at others   The state in which an individual experiences behaviors that can be physically harmful either to the self or to others.

From NANDA: Proceedings of the Eleventh National Conference of the North American Nursing Diagnosis Association, *1994.*

Appendix D

Conversion Tables

TABLE D-1	Length		
IN	**CM**	**CM**	**IN**
1	2.54	1	0.4
2	5.08	2	0.8
4	10.16	3	1.2
6	15.24	4	1.6
8	20.32	5	2.0
10	25.40	6	2.4
20	50.80	8	3.1
30	76.20	10	3.9
40	101.60	20	7.9
50	127.00	30	11.8
60	152.40	40	15.7
70	177.80	50	19.7
80	203.20	60	23.6
90	228.60	70	27.6
100	254.00	80	31.5
150	381.00	90	35.4
200	508.00	100	39.4

1 in = 2.54 cm
1 cm = 0.3937 inch

TABLE D-2	Weight		
LB	**KG**	**KG**	**LB**
1	0.5	1	2.2
2	0.9	2	4.4
4	1.8	3	6.6
6	2.7	4	8.8
8	3.6	5	11.0
10	4.5	6	13.2
20	9.1	8	17.6
30	13.6	10	22
40	18.2	20	44
50	22.7	30	66
60	27.3	40	88
70	31.8	50	110
80	36.4	60	132
90	40.9	70	154
100	45.4	80	176
150	66.2	90	198
200	90.8	100	220

1 lb = 0.454 kg
1 kg = 2.204 lb

TABLE D-3	Temperature

To *convert Centigrade or Celsius degrees to Fahrenheit degrees:* multiply the number of Centigrade degrees by ⅝ and add 32 to the result. To *convert Fahrenheit degrees to Centigrade degrees:* Subtract 32 from the number of Fahrenheit degrees and multiply the difference by ⅝.

Fahrenheit and Celsius equivalents: body temperature range

F°	C°	F°	C°	F°	C°	F°	C°	F°	C°
94.0	34.44	97.0	36.11	100.0	37.78	103.0	39.44	106.0	41.11
94.2	34.56	97.2	36.22	100.2	37.89	103.2	39.56	106.2	41.22
94.4	34.67	97.4	36.33	100.4	38.00	103.4	39.67	106.4	41.33
94.6	34.78	97.6	36.44	100.6	38.11	103.6	39.78	106.6	41.44
94.8	34.89	97.8	36.56	100.8	38.22	103.8	39.89	106.8	41.56
95.0	35.00	98.0	36.67	101.0	38.33	104.0	40.00	107.0	41.67
95.2	35.11	98.2	36.78	101.2	38.44	104.2	40.11	107.2	41.78
95.4	35.22	98.4	36.89	101.4	38.56	104.4	40.22	107.4	41.89
95.6	35.33	98.6	37.00	101.6	38.67	104.6	40.33	107.6	42.00
95.8	35.44	98.8	37.11	101.8	38.78	104.8	40.44	107.8	42.11
96.0	35.56	99.0	37.22	102.0	38.89	105.0	40.56	108.0	42.22
96.2	35.67	99.2	37.33	102.2	39.00	105.2	40.67		
96.4	35.78	99.4	37.44	102.4	39.11	105.4	40.78		
96.6	35.89	99.6	37.56	102.6	39.22	105.6	40.89		
96.8	36.00	99.8	37.67	102.8	39.33	105.8	41.00		

Appendix E

Conversion Factors to International System of Units (SI Units)

TABLE E-1	Conversion Factors (SI Units)

COMPONENT	NORMAL RANGE IN UNITS AS CUSTOMARILY REPORTED	CONVERSION FACTOR	NORMAL RANGE IN SI UNITS, MOLECULAR UNITS, INTERNATIONAL UNITS, OR DECIMAL FRACTIONS
Biochemical Components of Blood*			
Acetoacetic acid (S)	0.2-1.0 mg/dL	98	19.6-98.0 µmol/L
Acetone (S)	0.3-2.0 mg/dL	172	51.6-344.0 µmol/L
Albumin (S)	3.2-4.5 g/dL	10	32-45 g/L
Ammonia (P)	20-120 µg/dL	0.588	11.7-70.5 µmol/L
Amylase (S)	60-160 Somogyi units/dL	1.85	111-296 U/L
Base, total (S)	145-160 mEq/L	1	145-160 mmol/L
Bicarbonate (P)	21-28 mEq/L	1	21-28 mmol/L
Bile acids (S)	0.3-3.0 mg/dL	10	3-30 mg/L
		2.547	0.8-7.6 µmol/L
Bilirubin, direct (S)	Up to 0.3 mg/dL	17.1	Up to 5.1 µmol/L
Bilirubin, indirect (S)	0.1-1.0 mg/dL	17.1	1.7-17.1 µmol/L
Blood gases (B)			
PCO_2 arterial	35-40 mm Hg	0.133	4.66-5.32 kPa
PO_2 arterial	95-100 mm Hg	0.133	12.64-13.30 kPa
Calcium (S)	8.5-10.5 mg/dL	0.25	2.1-2.6 mmol/L
Chloride (S)	95-103 mEq/L	1	95-103 mmol/L
Creatine (S)	0.1-0.4 mg/dL	76.3	7.6-30.5 µmol/L
Creatinine (S)	0.6-1.2 mg/dL	88.4	53-106 µmol/L
Creatinine clearance (P)	107-139 mL/min	0.0167	1.78-2.32 mL/s
Fatty acids (total) (S)	8-20 mg/dL	0.01	0.08-2.00 mg/L
Fibrinogen (P)	200-400 mg/dL	0.01	2.00-4.00 g/L
Gamma globulin (S)	0.5-1.6 g/dL	10	5-16 g/L
Globulins (total) (S)	2.3-3.5 g/dL	10	23-35 g/L
Glucose (fasting) (S)	70-110 mg/dL	0.055	3.85-6.05 mmol/L
Insulin (radioimmunoassay) (P)	4-24 µlU/ml	0.0417	0.17-1.00 µg/L
	0.20-0.84 µg/L	172.2	35-145 pmol/L
Iodine, BEI (S)	3.5-6.5 µg/dL	0.079	0.28-0.51 µmol/L
Iodine, PBI (S)	4.0-8.0 µg/dL	0.079	0.32-0.63 µmol/L
Iron, total (S)	60-150 µg/dL	0.179	11-27 µmol/L
Iron-binding capacity (S)	300-360 µg/dL	0.179	54-64 µmol/L
17-Ketosteroids (P)	25-125 µg/dL	0.01	0.25-1.25 mg/L
Lactic dehydrogenase (S)	80-120 units at 30°C	0.48	38-62 U/L at 30°C
	Lactate → pyruvate 100-190 U/L at 37°C	1	100-190 U/L at 37°C
Lipase (S)	0-1.5 U/ml (Cherry-Crandall)	278	0-417 U/L

From Tilkian SM, Conover MB, Tilkian AG: Clinical implications of laboratory tests, *ed. 3, St. Louis, 1983, Mosby*

* This is a selected (not a complete) list of biochemical components. The ranges listed may differ from those accepted in some laboratories and are shown to illustrate the conversion factor and the method of expression in SI molecular units. For a more complete listing, see Henry JB, editor: Todd-Sanford-Davidsohn clinical diagnosis and management by laboratory methods, *ed. 16, Philadelphia, W.B. Saunders Co.*

TABLE E-1 Conversion Factors (SI Units)—*cont'd*

Component	Normal Range in Units as Customarily Reported	Conversion Factor	Normal Range in SI Units, Molecular Units, International Units, or Decimal Fractions
Biochemical Components of Blood—cont'd			
Lipids (total) (S)	400-800 mg/dL	0.01	4.00-8.00 g/L
Cholesterol	150-250 mg/dL	0.026	3.9-6.5 mmol/L
Triglycerides	75-165 mg/dL	0.0114	0.85-1.89 mmol/L
Phospholipids	150-380 mg/dL	0.01	1.50-380 g/L
Free fatty acids	9.0-15.0 mM/L	1	9.0-15.0 mmol/L
Nonprotein nitrogen (S)	20-35 mg/dL	0.714	14.3-25.0 mmol/L
Phosphatase (P)			
Acid (units/dL)	Cherry-Crandall	2.77	0-5.5 U/L
	King-Armstrong	1.77	0-5.5 U/L
	Bodansky	5.37	0-5.5 U/L
Alkaline (units/dL)	King-Armstrong	1.77	30-120 U/L
	Bodansky	5.37	30-120 U/L
	Bessey-Lowry-Brock	16.67	30-120 U/L
Phosphorus, inorganic (S)	3.0-4.5 mg/dL	0.323	0.97-1.45 mmol/L
Potassium (P)	3.8-5.0 mEq/L	1	3.8-5.0 mmol/L
Proteins, total (S)	6.0-7.8 g/dL	10	60-78 g/L
Albumin	3.2-4.5 g/dL	10	32-45 g/L
Globulin	2.3-3.5 g/dL	10	23-35 g/L
Sodium (P)	136-142 mEq/L	1	136-142 mmol/L
Testosterone: Male (S)	300-1,200 ng/dL	0.035	10.5-42.0 nmol/L
Female	30-95 ng/dL	0.035	1.0-3.3 nmol/L
Thyroid tests (S)			
Thyroxine (T_4)	4-11 μg/dL	12.87	51-142 nmol/L
T_4 expressed as iodine	3.2-7.2 μg/dL	79.0	253-569 nmol/L
T_3 resin uptake	25%-38% relative uptake	0.01	0.25%-0.38% relative uptake
TSH (S)	10 μU/mL	1	$<10^{-3}$ IU/L
Urea nitrogen (S)	8-23 mg/dL	0.357	2.9-8.2 mmol/L
Uric acid (S)	2-6 mg/dL	59.5	0.120-0.360 mmol/L
Vitamin B_{12} (S)	160-950 pg/mL	0.74	118-703 pmol/L
Hematology Values*			
Red cell volume (male)	25-35 mL/kg body weight	0.001	0.025-0.035 L/kg body weight
Hematocrit	40%-50%	0.01	0.40-0.50
Hemoglobin	13.5-18.0 g/dL	10	135-180 g/L
Hemoglobin	13.5-18.0 g/dL	0.155	2.09-2.79 mmol/L
RBC count	$4.5\text{-}6 \times 10^6/\mu L$	1	$4.6\text{-}6 \times 10^{12}/L$
WBC count	$4.5\text{-}10 \times 10^3/\mu L$	1	$4.5\text{-}10 \times 10^9/L$
Mean corpuscular volume	80-96 μm^3	1	80-96 fL

The International Committee for Standardization in Hematology recommends that the numbers remain the same but that the units change, so that hemoglobin is expressed as grams per deciliter (g/dL) even though other measurements are expressed as units per liter (U/L).

Abbreviations

A & P	Anterior and posterior; auscultation and percussion
A & W	Alive and well
abd	Abdomen; abdominal
a̅c	Before meals
ADL	Activities of daily living
AJ	Ankle jerk
AK	Above knee
ANS	Autonomic nervous system
AP	Anteroposterior
bid	Twice a day
BK	Below knee
BP	Blood pressure
BPH	Benign prostatic hypertrophy
BS	Bowel sounds; breath sounds
c̅	With
CC	Chief complaint
CHD	Childhood disease; congenital heart disease; coronary heart disease
CHF	Congestive heart failure
CNS	Central nervous system
c/o	Complains of
COPD	Chronic obstructive pulmonary disease
CV	Cardiovascular
CVA	Costovertebral angle; cerebrovascular accident
CVP	Central venous pressure
Cx	Cervix
D & C	Dilation and curettage
D/C	Discontinued
DM	Diabetes mellitus
DOB	Date of birth
DOE	Dyspnea on exertion
DTRs	Deep tendon reflexes
DUB	Dysfunctional uterine bleeding
Dx	Diagnosis
ECG, EKG	Electrocardiogram; electrocardiograph
EENT	Eye, ear, nose, and throat
ENT	Ear, nose, and throat
EOM	Extraocular movement
FB	Foreign body
FH	Family history
FROM	Full range of motion
FTT	Failure to thrive
Fx	Fracture
GB	Gallbladder
GE	Gastroesophageal
GI	Gastrointestinal
GU	Genitourinary
GYN	Gynecologic
HA	Headache
HCG	Human chorionic gonadotropin
HEENT	Head, eyes, ears, nose, and throat
HOPI	History of present illness
HPI	History of present illness
Hx	History
ICS	Intercostal space
IOP	Intraocular pressure
IUD	Intrauterine device
IV	Intravenous
JVP	Jugular venous pressure
KJ	Knee jerk
KUB	Kidneys, ureters, and bladder
lat	Lateral
LCM	Left costal margin
LE	Lower extremities
LLL	Left lower lobe (lung)
LLQ	Left lower quadrant (abdomen)
LMD	Local medical doctor
LMP	Last menstrual period
LOC	Loss of consciousness; level of consciousness
LS	Lumbosacral; lumbar spine
LSB	Left sternal border
LUL	Left upper lobe (lung)
LUQ	Left upper quadrant (abdomen)
M	Murmur
MAL	Midaxillary line
MCL	Midclavicular line
MGF	Maternal grandfather
MGM	Maternal grandmother
MSL	Midsternal line
MVA	Motor vehicle accident
N & T	Nose and throat
N & V	Nausea and vomiting
NA	No answer; not applicable
NKA	No known allergies
NPO	Nothing by mouth
NSR	Normal sinus rhythm

OD	Oculus dexter; right eye	**RCM**	Right costal margin
OM	Otitis media	**REM**	Rapid eye movement
OS	Oculus sinister; left eye	**RLL**	Right lower lobe (lung)
OTC	Over the counter	**RLQ**	Right lower quadrant (abdomen)
OU	Oculus uterque; each eye	**RML**	Right middle lobe (lung)
		ROM	Range of motion
p̄	After	**ROS**	Review of systems
P & A	Percussion and auscultation	**RSB**	Right sternal border
p̄c	After meals	**RUL**	Right upper lobe (lung)
PE	Physical examination	**RUQ**	Right upper quadrant (abdomen)
PERRLA	Pupils equal, round, react to light and accommodation		
		s̄	Without
PGF	Paternal grandfather	**SCM**	Sternocleidomastoid
PGM	Paternal grandmother	**SQ**	Subcutaneous
PI	Present illness	**Sx**	Symptoms
PID	Pelvic inflammatory disease		
PMH	Past medical history	**T & A**	Tonsillectomy and adenoidectomy
PMI	Point of maximum impulse; point of maximum intensity	**TM**	Tympanic membrane
		TPR	Temperature, pulse, and respiration
PMS	Premenstrual syndrome		
prn	As necessary	**UE**	Upper extremities
Pt	Patient	**URI**	Upper respiratory infection
PVC	Premature ventricular contraction	**UTI**	Urinary tract infection
q	Every	**WD**	Well developed
qd	Every day	**WN**	Well nourished
qh	Every hour		
qod	Every other day	**x**	Times; by (size)

A

abduction Movement of the limbs or the trunk and head away from the median plane of the body.

accommodation Process of visual focusing from far to near; accomplished by contraction of the ciliary muscle, which thickens and increases the convexity of the crystalline lens.

active listening State of selective attention and alertness that encompasses the skill of observation so that verbal and nonverbal cues are registered and clarified in an interaction; involves data absorption, retention, and exchange for clarification of meaning.

adduction Movement of the limbs or the trunk and head toward the median plane of the body.

adnexa General term meaning adjacent or related structures.
> EXAMPLE: The ovaries and fallopian tubes are adnexa of the uterus.

adventitious sounds Sounds that are not normal within the lungs.

affect Observable behaviors indicating an individual's feelings or emotions.

ageusia Absence or impairment of the sense of taste.

alopecia Absence or loss of hair.

alveolar ridge Bony prominences of the maxilla and mandible that support the teeth; in edentulous clients these structures support dentures.

amblyopia Reduced vision that occurs after deprivation of visual stimulation during visual maturation (birth to 2 years); eye appears normal during examination; also called *suppression amblyopia*.

amenorrhea The absence of menstruation.

ametropia General term denoting a condition involving a refractive error.
> EXAMPLES: Myopia, hyperopia.

anesthesia Partial or complete loss of sensation.

angina pectoris Paroxysmal pain in chest, often associated with myocardial ischemia; pain patterns and severity vary among individuals; pain sometimes radiates to neck, jaw, or left arm; may be accompanied by choking or smothering sensations.

angle of Louis Point of tracheal bifurcation.

ankylosis Fixation of a joint, often in an abnormal position, usually resulting from destruction of articular cartilage, as in rheumatoid arthritis.

anular Describes a lesion that forms a ring around a clear center of normal skin.

anosmia Absence or impairment of the sense of smell.

anterior triangle (of neck) Landmark area for palpating the submaxillary, submental, and anterior cervical lymph nodes; sectioned by the anterior surface of the sternocleidomastoid muscle, the mandible, and an imagined line running from the chin to the sternal notch.

anulus Dense fibrous ring surrounding the tympanic membrane.

anuria Absence of urine production or the inability to produce more than 250 ml of urine per day.

apathy Lack of emotional expression; indifference to stimuli or surroundings.

aphakia Absence of the crystalline lens of the eye.

aphasia Absence or impairment of the ability to communicate through speech.

aphthous ulcer (canker sore) A painful ulcer on the mucous membrane of the mouth.

apocrine sweat glands Secretory dermal structures located in the axillae, nipples, areolae, scalp, face, and genital area; develop at puberty and respond to emotional stimulation.

arcus senilis Gray ring composed of lipids deposited in the peripheral cornea; commonly seen in older adults; also called *arcus cornealis*.

areola A circular, darkly pigmented area around the nipple of the breast.

arteriosclerosis General term denoting hardening and thickening of the arterial walls; *atherosclerosis* is one type of arteriosclerosis.

ascites Accumulation of serous fluid in the perintoneal cavity.

assessment Process of gathering and analyzing subjective and objective client data for summarization of a client's status.

asthenopia General eye discomfort or fatigue resulting from use of the eyes.

asthma Paroxysmal dyspnea that is accompanied by wheezing and caused by spasm of the bronchial tubes or by swelling of their mucous membranes.

astigmatism Visual distortion resulting from an irregular corneal curvature that prevents light rays from being focused clearly on the retina.

ataxia Inability to coordinate muscular movement.

atherosclerosis The formation of plaques within arterial walls resulting in thickening of the walls and narrowing of the lumen; end organs supplied by these vessels receive diminished circulation.

athetosis Condition in which there are slow, irregular, involuntary movements in the upper extremities, especially the hands and fingers.

atrial fibrillation Rapid, involuntary, random atrial contractions that cause rapid, irregular ventricular contractions and diminished cardiac output; this arrhythmia results from chaotic electrical impulses within the atrial myocardium.

atrial flutter Rapid atrial rhythm (approximately 300 per minute) that may or may not cause ventricular tachycardia, depending on the degree of A-V (atrioventricular) blocking.

atrophy Diminution of size or wasting; can also refer to loss of elastic tissue resulting in a slightly sunken epidermis that wrinkles easily when pulled to the side.

attrition of teeth Wearing away of the occlusal surfaces of the teeth from many years of chewing or excessive grinding.

auricle Flap of the external ear; also called the *pinna*.

auscultatory gap A phenomenon sometimes noted by an examiner listening for blood pressure sounds; temporary silent interval between systolic and diastolic sounds that may cover a range of 40 mm Hg.; commonly occurs with hypertensive clients with a wide pulse pressure.

B

balano- Combining form denoting the glans penis.
EXAMPLE: *Balanitis* means inflammation of the glans penis.

ballottement Technique of palpating a floating structure by bouncing it gently and feeling it rebound.

Bartholin glands Two mucus-secreting glands located within the posterolateral vaginal vestibule.

bigeminal pulse Abnormal pulse characterized by a strong beat and a weaker one in close succession, followed by a pause when no beat is felt; pulse is irregular in rhythm; associated with premature contractions, digitalis toxicity, or a partial heart block.

Biot breathing Breathing characterized by several short breaths followed by long, irregular periods of apnea.

bisferiens pulse Abnormal pulse characterized by two main peaks; occurs with aortic stenosis and/or regurgitation.

blepharitis Inflammation of the eyelid.

blocking Interruption in a train of thought, loss of an idea, or repression of a feeling or idea from conscious awareness; can be a normal behavior or, in extreme form, indicative of abnormality.

borborygmi Abdominal sounds produced by hyperactive intestinal peristalsis, audible at a distance.

bradycardia An abnormally slowed heart rate, usually under 50 beats per minute. *Note:* Conditioned athletes often manifest a normally slowed rate of 50 beats, or slightly less, per minute.

bradypnea Breathing that is abnormally slow.

bronchitis Inflammation of the bronchi.

bronchophony Increased vocal resonance detected over a bronchus that is surrounded by consolidated lung tissue.

bronchovesicular breathing Refers to breath sounds at a pitch intermediate between bronchial or tracheal sounds and alveolar sounds.

bruit Audible murmur (a blowing sound) heard in auscultating over a peripheral vessel or an organ.

bruxism Grinding of the teeth; usually an unconscious act occurring during sleep.

buccal Pertaining to the inside of the cheek.

bulbar conjunctiva Thin, transparent mucous membrane that covers the sclera and adjoins the palpebral conjunctiva, which lines the inner eyelid.

bulla Elevated, circumscribed, fluid-filled lesion greater than 1 cm in diameter.

bunion Abnormal prominence on the inner aspect of the first metatarsal head, with bursal formation; results in lateral or valgus displacement of the great toe.

bursa Fibrous, fluid-filled sac found between certain tendons and the bones beneath them.

bursitis Inflammation of a bursa.

C

callus Hyperkeratotic area caused by pressure or friction; usually not painful.

canthus Outer or inner angle between the upper and lower eyelids.

carpal tunnel syndrome Painful disorder of the wrist and hand induced by compression of the median nerve between the inelastic carpal ligament and other structures within the carpal tunnel.

cataract Opacity of the crystalline lens of the eyes.

cerebellar system Receives sensory and motor input and coordinates muscular activity; also helps to maintain posture and equilibrium.

cerumen Waxy secretion of the glands of the external acoustic meatus; earwax.

chalazion Small, localized swelling of the eyelid caused by obstruction and dilation of a meibomian gland.

chordee Ventral curvature of the penis; congenital anomaly caused by a restrictive band of tissue between the meatus and the glans; usually associated with hypospadias.

circinate Circular.

circumduction Circular movement of a limb.

circumscribed Well defined, limited, and encircled.

clonus Abnormal pattern of neuromuscular functioning characterized by rapidly alternating involuntary contraction and relaxation of skeletal muscles.

clonus Spasmodic alternation of muscular contraction and relaxation.

coarctation Stricture or narrowing of the wall of a vessel.

cochlea Conical bony structure of the inner ear; perforated by numerous appertures for passage of the cochlear division of the acoustic nerve.

cognitive functioning Appraisal of an individual's perception of his intellectual awareness, his potential for growth, and his recognition by others for his mental skills and contributions.

cogwheel rigidity Abnormal motion in the muscle tissues characterized by jerky movements when the muscle is passively stretched.

coherency Conversation and behavior that convey thoughts, feelings, ideas, and perceptions in a logical and relevant manner.

compulsive behavior A repetitive act that usually originates from an obsession; extreme anxiety emerges if the act is not completed.

condyloma acuminatum (wart) Soft, warty, papillomatous projection that appears on the labia and within the vaginal vestibule; viral in origin and sexually transmitted.

condyloma latum Slightly raised, moist, flattened papules that appear on the labia or within the vaginal vestibule; a sign of secondary syphilis; sexually transmitted.

confabulation The fabrication of events or sequential experiences often recounted to cover up memory gaps.

confluent Describes lesions that run together.

consolidation Increasing density of lung tissue caused by pathologic engorgement.

contusion (bruise) Swelling, discoloration, and pain without a break in the skin; caused by a blow to the area.

Cooper ligaments Suspensory ligaments of the breast.

corn Hyperkeratotic, slightly raised, circumscribed lesion caused by pressure over a bony prominence; usually on the fourth or fifth toe; painful if pressure or friction is persistent.

costal angle Costal margin angle formed on the anterior chest wall at the base of the xiphoid process, where the ribs separate.

crackles Abnormal respiratory sound heard during auscultation characterized by discontinuous bubbling sounds; heard over distal bronchioles and alveoli that contain serous secretions; formerly called *rales.*

crepitus Dry, crackling sound or sensation heard or felt as a joint is moved through its range of motion.

cricoid cartilage Lowermost cartilage of the larynx.

crust Dried serum, blood, or purulent exudate on the skin surface.

cryptorchism (undescended testis) Failure of one or both of the testicles to descend into the scrotum.

cyanosis Bluish-gray discoloration of the skin resulting from the presence of or abnormal amounts of reduced hemoglobin in the blood.

cycloplegia Paralysis of the ciliary muscle resulting in a loss of accommodation and a dilated pupil; usually induced with medication to allow for examination or surgery of the eye.

cystocele Bulging of the anterior vaginal wall caused by protrusion of the urinary bladder through relaxed or weakened musculature.

D

darwinian tubercle Blunt point projecting up from the upper part of the helix of the ear.

database Collection or store of information.
    subjective Portion of the client data that is supplied by the client; the client's perceptions of himself.
    objective Portion of the client data that is perceived by the examiner through physical examination or obtained from other external sources (such as laboratory studies).

delusion Persistent belief or perception that is illogical or improbable.

dementia A broad term that indicates impairment of intellectual functioning, memory, and judgment.

depersonalization Sense of being out of touch with one's environment; loss of a sense of reality and association with personal events.

desquamation Sloughing process of the cornified layer of the epidermis; when accelerated, the process can cause peeling, scaling, and loss of the deeper layers of skin.

diaphragmatic excursion The extent of movement of the diaphragm.

diastasis recti Lateral separation of the two halves of the rectus abdominis muscle.

diastole Period of time within the cardiac cycle in which ventricles are relaxed and filling with blood.

diffuse Spread out, widely dispersed, copious.

diplopia Double vision; usually caused by an extraocular muscle malfunction or a muscle innervation disorder.

dizziness Sensation of faintness.

dorsiflexion Backward bending or flexion of a joint.

dura mater Tough, fibrous connective tissue that lies directly beneath the periosteum of the cranium.

dysarthria Speech disorder involving difficulty with articulation and pronunciation of specific sounds; results from loss of control over muscles of speech.

dysesthesia Sensation of something crawling on the skin or of pricks of pins and needles.

dyslexia Impairment of the ability to read (with no impairment of mental or intellectual function); letters or words may appear reversed, or the reader may have difficulty distinguishing right from left.

dysmenorrhea Abnormal pain associated with the menstrual cycle. Mild, self-limiting premenstrual pain is considered normal. Pain becomes abnormal when it is severe, disabling, or accompanied by other severe symptoms, such as nausea, vomiting, fainting, or intestinal cramping.

dysmetria Inability to fix the range of movement in a muscular activity.

dyspareunia Pain associated with sexual intercourse. The term is most often applied to female conditions, including vaginal spasms, lack of lubrication, or genital lesions.

dysphasia Speech disorder involving difficulty with use of language and words to convey meaning to others; often associated with cerebral vascular accidents.

dysphonia Difficulty in controlling laryngeal speech sounds; can be a normal event, such as male vocal changes occurring at puberty.

dyspnea Breathing that is labored or difficult.

dyssynergia Failure of muscular coordination; also known as *ataxia*.

dysuria Difficulty, pain, or burning sensation with urination.

ecchymosis Discoloration of skin or a mucous membrane caused by leakage of blood into the subcutaneous tissue; can also be a bruise.

eccrine sweat glands Secretory dermal structures distributed over the body that secrete water and electrolytes and regulate body temperature; heat, emotional reactions, and physical exercise are the primary stimulants for secretion.

ectopic Describes an event that occurs away from its usual location; in reference to the heart, it could pertain to an extra beat or contraction.

ectropion Abnormal outward turning of the margin of the eyelid.

eczematous A superficial inflammation characterized by scaling, thickening, crusting, weeping, and redness.

egophony An abnormality in vocal resonance; when lungs are auscultated the client says "e-e-e," but nurse hears sound of "a-a-a"; suggests pleural effusion.

embolus A foreign object (composed of air, fat, or clustered cellular elements) that circulates through the blood and usually lodges in a vessel, causing some degree of occlusion.

emotional functioning Appraisal of an individual's access to his own feelings, his satisfaction with his feelings, his ability to express his feeling effectively, and his capacity to resolve or deal with stressors.

empathic response State of mind that enables one to view another as that person views himself; coupled with interviewing skills that enable an examiner to verbally or nonverbally respond to a client statement without coloring or altering the client's intended meaning.

silence A deliberate examiner response (sometimes very difficult for the examiner) to a client statement; allows time for client reflection.

facilitative behaviors Examiner behaviors (verbal or nonverbal) that encourage the client to continue.
EXAMPLES: Leaning forward, nodding head, maintaining eye contact, or saying, "Um-hum," "Yes," "Please go on," etc.

reflection Repetition of key words from the client's last statement to encourage elaboration.
EXAMPLE: The client says, "I feel as though I'm going to explode." The examiner responds, "Explode?"

interpretive reflection Rearrangement or rewording of the client's statement.

EXAMPLE: The client says, "When you have that much pain, you just want to give up." The examiner responds, "You feel frustrated and helpless."

emphysema A chronic pulmonary disease characterized by overdistended lung tissue.

enophthalmos Abnormal backward placement of the eyeball.

entropion Abnormal inward turning of the margin of the eyelid.

enuresis Any involuntary urination, especially during sleep.

environment Composition of physical facilities, resources, and people that affect an individual's capacity to exist to his or her satisfaction.

epicondyle Round protuberance above the condyle (at the end of a bone).

epididymitis Inflammation of the epididymis (tightly coiled, comma-shaped structure overlying posterolateral surface of testis); infection can be acute or chronic; area is extremely tender, usually involving the scrotal wall and occasionally extending along the spermatic cord.

epiphysis End of a long bone that is cartilaginous during early childhood and becomes ossified during late childhood.

epispadias Congenital defect in which the urinary meatus opens on the dorsum of the penis; opening may be located on the glans or anywhere along the penile shaft, or extend into the pubic symphysis.

epistaxis Bleeding from the nose.

epulis Any growth on the gum.

erosion Wearing away or destruction of the mucosal or epidermal surface; often develops into an ulcer.

erythematous Redness (of the skin).

escutcheon General term meaning a surface that is shield-shaped. In female anatomy it denotes the visible surface of the lower abdomen, the mons pubis, and the inverted-triangle–shaped patch of hair covering the area.

euphoria Sense of elation or well-being; can be a normal feeling or exaggerated to the extent of distorting reality.

eustachian tube Tube, lined with mucous membrane, that joins the nasopharynx and the tympanic cavity, allowing equalization of air pressure with atmospheric pressure.

exacerbation Increase in intensity of signs or symptoms.

excoriation Scratch or abrasion on the skin surface.

exophthalmos Abnormal forward placement of the eyeball.

extension Movement that brings a joint into a straight position.

external rotation Outward turning of a limb.

extrapyramidal system Motor pathways lying outside the pyramidal tract that help to maintain muscle tone and to control body movements such as walking; includes nerve pathways between the cerebral cortex, basal ganglia, brain stem, and spinal cord.

F

fasciculation Localized, uncoordinated, uncontrollable twitching of a single muscle group innervated by a single motor nerve fiber.

fissure Linear crack in the skin.

flank Part of the body between the bottom of the ribs and the upper border of the ilium.

flatulence Presence of excessive amounts of gases in the stomach or intestines.

flexion Movement that brings a joint into a bent position.

fontanel Unossified space or soft spot lying between the cranial bones of an infant.

Fordyce spots Small, yellow spots on the buccal membrane that are visible sebaceous glands; a normal phenomenon seen in many adults, but sometimes mistaken for abnormal lesions; also called *Fordyce granules.*

fornix (plural: fornices) General term designating a fold or an archlike structure. The vaginal fornix is the ringed recess (pocket) that forms around the cervix as it projects into the vaginal vault; although continuous, this fornix is anatomically divided into the anterior, posterior, and lateral fornices.

fourchette Small fold of membrane connecting the labia minora in the posterior part of the vulva.

frenulum (lingual) Band of tissue that attaches the ventral surface of the tongue to the floor of the mouth.

friction rub Sound produced by the rubbing of the pleura around the lung or pericardium around the heart.

frontal bone Forehead bone.

functional assessment Appraisal of an individual's perception of his capacity to maneuver within a defined environment.

G

gallop rhythm Audible extra heart sound produced by an abnormal third or fourth heart sound.

general well-being assessment Appraisal of an individual's view of his worth and his capability for maintaining and/or enhancing his quality of life.

gingiva Pertaining to the gum.

glaucoma Eye disease characterized by abnormally increased intraocular pressure caused by obstruction of the outflow of aqueous humor.

glossitis An inflammation of the tongue.

goiter Hypertrophy of the thyroid gland, usually evident as a pronounced swelling in the neck.

gout Metabolic disease associated with abnormal uric acid metabolism that is a form of acute arthritis; marked by inflammation of the joints.

graphesthesia Ability to recognize symbols, numbers, or letters traced on the skin.

gravida Denotes number of pregnancies.
EXAMPLE: *Multigravida* designates more than one pregnancy.

guarding Protective withdrawal or positioning of a body part during pain or injury.

gynecomastia Abnormally large mammary glands in the male.

H

hallucination Sensory perception that does not arise from an external stimulus; can be auditory, visual, tactile, gustatory, or olfactory.

heave Palpable, diffuse, sustained lift of the chest wall or a portion of the wall.

helix Margin of the external ear.

hematuria Presence of blood in the urine.

hemoptysis The expectoration of blood from the lungs or bronchial tubes.

hepatojugular reflux A phenomenon indicating right heart failure, in which venous pressure rises when the upper abdomen is compressed for 30 to 45 seconds; upon upper right quadrant compression, increased prominence of the jugular vein is noted.

hernia Abnormal opening in a muscle wall or cavity that permits protrusion of its contents.
direct inguinal hernia Protrusion of abdominal contents through external ring of inguinal canal, usually in region superior to the canal.
indirect inguinal hernia Protrusion of abdominal contents into internal ring of inguinal canal; contents may remain in the canal, emerge through external ring, or extend downward into scrotal sac; occurs more commonly than direct inguinal herniation.
femoral hernia Protrusion of abdominal contents through femoral canal (below inguinal ligament); occurs more often with women than men and is less common than inguinal hernias.

herpetiform Describes a cluster of vesicles resembling herpes lesions.

hirsutism Excessive body hair, usually in a masculine distribution, owing to heredity, hormonal dysfunction, porphyria, or medication.

holosystolic (pansystolic) Pertaining to the entire systolic interval; usually refers to an audible murmur.

Homans sign Calf pain associated with rapid dorsiflexion of the foot, often indicative of thrombophlebitis.

hordeolum (stye) Infection of a sebaceous gland at the margin of the eyelid.

hydrocele Nontender, serous fluid mass located within the tunica vaginalis (layered, hollow membrane adjacent to testis).

hymenal caruncles Small, irregular, fleshy projections that are remnants of a ruptured hymen; they are a normal phenomenon and may or may not be present at the vaginal introitus in varied sizes and shapes.

hyoid Single bone suspended from the styloid process of the temporal bone.

hyperesthesia Abnormally increased sensitivity to sensory stimuli, such as touch or pain.

hyperkinesis Hyperactivity or excessive muscular activity.

hyperkinetic Hyperactive.

hyperopia (farsightedness) Refractive error in which light rays focus behind the retina.

hyperpnea Respiration that is deeper and more rapid than that usually experienced during normal activity.

hyperresonance Sound elicited by percussion; its pitch lies between that of resonance and tympany.

hypoesthesia Decreased or dulled sensitivity to stimulation.

hyposmia Decreased sense of smell.

hypospadias Congenital defect in which the urinary meatus opens on the ventral aspect of the penis; opening may be located in the glans, penile shaft, scrotum, or perineum.

hypothesis Formation of an idea that relates available information to a probable cause. (*Note:* In the context of research, *hypothesis* has a broader meaning.)

hypovolemic Pertaining to decreased blood volume; usually refers to a state of shock resulting from massive blood loss and inadequate tissue perfusion.

I

illusion Perceptual distortion of an external stimulus.
EXAMPLE: Mirage in a desert.

"inching" Recommended method for moving the stethoscope over the precordium while listening for heart sounds; small, sliding movements (versus lifting and lowering stethoscope from side to side) may enable the listener to hear more sounds.

incidence The number of times an event occurs.

incus One of three ossicles in the middle ear; resembling an anvil, it communicates sound vibrations from the maleus to the stapes.

induration Hardening of the skin, usually caused by edema or infiltration by a neoplasm.

infarct Localized area of tissue necrosis caused by prolonged anoxia.

injection Redness or congestion of a part of the body caused by dilation of blood vessels secondary to an inflammatory or infectious process.

intermittent claudication Condition characterized by symptoms of pain, aching, cramping, and localized fatigue of the legs that occur while walking but can be quickly relieved by rest (2 to 5 minutes); discomfort occurs most often in the calf but may arise in the foot, thigh, hip, or buttock; caused by prolonged ischemia.

internal rotation Inward turning of a limb.

introitus General term denoting an opening or the orifice of a cavity or hollow structure.
    EXAMPLE: Vaginal introitus.

inverted nipple Nipple that is turned inward.

ischemia Diminished supply of blood to a body organ or surface; characterized by pallor, coolness, and pain.

isthmus (glandulae thyroideae) Narrow portion of the thyroid gland connecting the left and right lobes.

K

keloid Hypertrophic scar tissue; prevalent in non-white races.

keratosis Overgrowth and thickening of the cornified epithelium.

kinesthetic sensation Ability to detect the position of a body part when it is moved through space.

Korotkoff sounds Sounds heard during the taking of blood pressure; an inflated cuff encircles a limb and obstructs normal blood flow through the arteries; as the cuff is released, turbulent blood flow creates a series of sounds that enable the listener to determine systolic and diastolic pressures.

Kussmaul respiration Deep, gasping type of respiration, often associated with diabetic acidosis.

kyphosis Abnormal convexity of the posterior curve of the spine.

L

labile emotions Unpredictable, rapid shifting of expression of feelings.

labyrinth Complex structure of the inner ear that communicates directly with the acoustic nerve, transmitting sound vibrations from the middle ear through the fluid-filled network of three semicircular canals that join at a vestibule connected to the cochlea.

leukoplakia Thickened, white, well-circumscribed patch that can appear on any mucous membrane; sometimes precancerous; often a response to chronic irritation, such as pipe smoking.

leukorrhea White, vaginal discharge; can be a normal phenomenon that occurs (or increases) with pregnancy, the use of birth control medication, or as a postmenstrual phase; can also be an abnormal sign indicating malignancy or infection.

lichenification Thickening of the skin characterized by accentuated skin markings; often the result of chronic scratching.

light reflex Triangular landmark area on the tympanic membrane that most brightly reflects the examiner's light source.

linea alba White line of connective tissue in the abdomen extending from sternum to pubis.

lordosis Abnormal anterior concavity of the spine.

lower motor neurons Nerve cells that originate in the anterior horn cells of the spinal column and travel to innervate the skeletal muscle fibers. Injury or disease of this area will result in decreased muscle tone, reflexes, or strength.

lymphadenitis Inflammation of the lymph nodes.

lymphoma General term for growth of new tissue in the lymphatic area; ordinarily a malignant growth.

M

macule Flat, circumscribed lesion of the skin or mucous membrane; 1 cm or less in diameter.

malleus Innermost ossicle of the middle ear; resembling a hammer, it is connected to the tympanic membrane and transmits sound vibrations to the incus, which communicates with the stapes.

manubrium Upper segment of the sternum that articulates with the clavicle and the first pair of costal cartilages.

mastitis An inflammation of the breast.

mastoid process Conical projection of the temporal bone extending downward and forward behind the external auditory meatus.

McBurney point Point of specialized tenderness in acute appendicitis, situated on a line between the umbilicus and the right anterosuperior iliac spine, about 1 or 2 inches above the latter.

menarche Onset of menstruation in adolescence or young adulthood.

menorrhagia Abnormally heavy or extended menstrual periods.

metrorrhagia Any uterine bleeding that is not related to menstruation.
> EXAMPLE: A bleeding lesion within the vagina, cervix, or uterus.

miosis Condition in which the pupil is constricted; usually drug-induced (agent is called a *miotic*).

Montgomery tubercles Small sebaceous glands located on the areola of the breast.

Murphy's sign Sign of gallbladder disease consisting of pain on taking a deep breath when the examiner's fingers are pressing on the approximate location of the gallbladder.

myalgia Tenderness or pain in the muscle.

mydriasis Dilation of the pupil; usually drug-induced (agent is called a *mydriatic*).

myoclonus Twitching or clonic spasm of a muscle group.

myopia (nearsightedness) Refractive error in which light rays focus in front of the retina.

N

nabothian cyst (retention cyst) Small, white or purple, firm nodule that commonly appears on the cervix; forms within the mucus-secreting nabothian glands, which are present in large numbers on the uterine cervix.

nares (singular: naris) Nostrils; the anterior openings of the nose.

necrosis Localized death of tissue.

neurosis Ineffective or troubled coping mechanism stemming from anxiety or emotional conflict.

nevus Congenital, pigmented area on the skin.
> EXAMPLES: Mole, birthmark.

nicking Abnormal condition showing compression of a vein at an arteriovenous crossing; visible through an ophthalmoscope during a retinal examination.

nodule Solid skin elevation that extends into the dermal layer; 1 to 2 cm in diameter.

NSR (normal sinus rhythm) The heart rate that originates within sinoatrial (S-A) node in right atrium.

nystagmus Involuntary rhythmical movement of the eyes; oscillations may be horizontal, vertical, rotary, or mixed.

O

obsession Persistent thought or idea that preoccupies the mind; not always realistic and may result in compulsive behavior.

occipital bone Bone in the lower back part of the skull between the parietal and temporal bones.

O.D. (oculus dexter) Right eye.

O.S. (oculus sinister) Left eye.

O.U. (oculus uterque) Each eye.

oligomenorrhea Abnormally light or infrequent menstruation.

oliguria Inadequate production or secretion of urine (usually less than 400 ml in a 24-hour period).

orchi- Combining form denoting the testes.
> EXAMPLE: *Orchitis* means inflammation of one or both of the testes.

orthopnea Difficulty in breathing in any position other than an upright one.

osteoarthritis Form of arthritis in which one or many of the joints undergo degenerative changes.

otalgia Pain in the ear.

otitis Inflammation or infection of the ear.

otitis externa Inflammation on infection of the external canal or auricle of the external ear.

otitis media Inflammation or infection of the middle ear.

P

Paget's disease of the nipple Condition characterized by an excoriating or scaling lesion of the nipple, extending from an intraductal carcinoma of the breast.

palpebral conjunctiva Thin, transparent mucous membrane that lines the inner eyelid and adjoins the bulbar conjunctiva, which covers the sclera.

palpebral fissure Opening between the upper and lower eyelids.

palpitation Sensation of pounding, fluttering, or racing of the heart; can be a normal phenomenon or caused by a disorder of the heart.

papilla General term for a small projection; dorsal surface of the tongue is composed of a variety of forms of papillae that contain openings to the taste buds.

papule Solid, elevated, circumscribed, superficial lesion; 1 cm or less in diameter.

paradoxical pulse Diminished pulse amplitude on inspiration and increased amplitude on expiration; an exaggeration of a normal response to respiration; often associated with obstructive lung disease.

paranoia Sense of being persecuted or victimized; suspicion of others.

paraphimosis Condition characterized by the inability to pull the foreskin forward from a retracted position; glans is usually swollen and inflamed.

paresthesia Abnormal sensation, such as numbness or a tingling feeling.

parietal bone One of the pair of bones that form the sides of the cranium.

parity Denotes the number of viable births.
　EXAMPLES: *Nulliparous* means having experienced no viable births (also indicated as *para 0*); *multiparous* designates more than one viable birth.

paronychia Inflammation of the skinfold that adjoins the nail bed; characterized by redness, swelling, and pain; may be pustular.

paroxysmal nocturnal dyspnea (PND) Periodic acute attacks of shortness of breath while recumbent; relieved by sitting or standing.

pars flaccida Small portion of the tympanic membrane between the mallear folds.

pars tensa Larger portion of the tympanic membrane.

patch Flat, circumscribed lesion of the skin or mucous membrane; more than 1 cm in diameter.

peau d'orange Dimpling of the skin that resembles the skin of an orange.

pectoralis major muscle One of the four muscles of the anterior upper portion of the chest.

pectus carinatum Abnormal prominence of the sternum.

pectus excavatum Abnormal depression of the sternum.

periodontitis (pyorrhea) Inflammation and deterioration of the gums and supporting alveolar bone; occurs in varying degrees of severity; if neglected, this condition will result in loss of teeth.

perlèche (cheilosis, cheilitis) Fissures at the corners of the mouth that become inflamed; causes are overclosure of the mouth in an edentulous client, marked loss of alveolar ridge, or riboflavin deficiency; saliva irritates the area, and moniliasis is a common complication.

PERRLA Stands for "pupils equal, round, react to light, and accommodation."

petechiae Tiny, flat, purple or red spots on the surface of the skin resulting from minute hemorrhages within the dermal or submucosal layers.

phimosis Tightness of the foreskin that results in an inability to retract it; usually caused by adhesions of the prepuce to the underlying glans.

phobia Uncontrollable, often unreasonable, and intense fear of a specific object or event.

photophobia Ocular discomfort caused by exposure of the eyes to bright light.

physical functioning Appraisal of an individual's perception of his ability to control and manipulate his physical environment, as well as his judgment of the ability of his inner resources to control and use his body effectively.

pilonidal fistula (or sinus) Abnormal channel containing a tuft of hair, situated most frequently over or close to the tip of the coccyx but also occurring in other regions of the body.

pinna Auricle or projected part of the external ear.

plantar flexion Extension of the foot so that the forepart is depressed with respect to the position of the ankle.

plaque Solid, elevated, circumscribed, superficial lesion; more than 1 cm in diameter.

plaque, dental Film that accumulates on the surface of teeth; made up of mucin and colloidal material from saliva, plaque is subject to bacterial invasion.

pleximeter Finger placed on the skin surface to receive the taps from the percussion hammer or plexor; used in percussion.

PMI (point of maximum impulse) Specific area of the chest where the heartbeat is palpated most clearly; usually the apical impulse, a brief systolic beat in the fourth or fifth intercostal space, midclavicular line.

posterior triangle (of neck) Landmark area for palpating the posterior cervical chain, the supraclavicular chain, and the occipital lymph chain; sectioned along the anterior border by the sternocleidomastoid muscle, the posterior border by the trapezius muscle, and the bottom by the clavicle.

Poupart's ligament Inguinal ligament.

precipitating factor Event or entity that hastens the onset of another event.
　EXAMPLE: Chronic overeating is a precipitating factor for obesity.

precordium Area of the chest that overlies the heart and adjacent great vessels.

predisposing factor (risk factor) Event or entity that contributes to the cause of another event.
　EXAMPLE: A family history of obesity increases the risk for obesity.

presbycusis Impairment of hearing in old age.

presbyopia Loss of accommodation (ability to focus on near objects) associated with aging.

problem list Compilation of findings that appear at the end of the database; may be diagnoses (medical or nursing), clusters of interrelated findings, or isolated findings that the examiner wishes to pursue but cannot label or attach to other findings.

EXAMPLE: *diagnoses*—herpes simplex, knowledge deficit; *clusters*—polydipsia, polyuria, polyphagia; *finding*—lower back pain.

pronate To turn the forearm so that the palm faces downward, or to rotate the leg or foot inward.

proprioception Awareness of posture, movement, and changes in equilibrium.

pruritus Itching.

psychosis Any major mental disorder characterized by greatly distorted perceptions and severe disorganization of personality.

psychosocial functioning Appraisal of an individual's capacity to attain and maintain satisfactory intimate and social relationships with others.

ptosis Drooping of the upper eyelid; can be unilateral or bilateral; usually results from innervation or lid muscle disorder.

ptyalism Excessive salivation.

pudendum Collective term denoting the external genitalia; for the female it includes the mons pubis, labia majora, labia minora, vaginal vestibule, and vestibular glands; for the male it includes the penis, scrotum, and testes.

pulse deficit A discrepancy between the ventricular rate auscultated over the heart and the arterial rate palpated over the radial artery; caused by a ventricle that contracts with a partially filled chamber and is unable to produce a palpable pulse with each beat.

pulse pressure The difference between systolic and diastolic pressures, usually within the range of 30 to 40 mm Hg; tends to increase as systolic pressure rises with arteriosclerosis of the large vessels (specifically the aorta); can be altered with vigorous exercise, fever, or other disease states.

pulsus alternans Alternating pulse; abnormal pulse characterized by a regular rhythm in which a strong beat alternates with a weaker one; sometimes differences in amplitude are subtle and more easily distinguished during taking of blood pressure; associated with severe hypertension, coronary artery disease, and left ventricular failure.

purpura Hemorrhage into the tissue, usually circumscribed; lesions may be described as petechiae, ecchymoses, or hematomas, according to size.

pustule Vesicle or bulla that contains pus.

pyramidal tract Bundle of upper motor neurons that coordinate voluntary movements originating in the motor cortex of the brain; nerve fibers travel through the brain stem and the spinal cord, where they synapse with anterior horn cells, responsible for the coordinated response of voluntary movements.

pyrosis Burning sensation in the epigastric and sternal region with the raising of acid liquid from the stomach; also called *heartburn.*

pyuria Presence of white cells (pus) in the urine.

Q

questions

closed Question posed in such a way that the respondent is directed toward a brief answer or a "yes" or "no"; does not encourage the respondent to elaborate.

EXAMPLE: "Has your back pain improved since the last visit?"

open A broadly stated question that encourages a free-flowing, open response.

EXAMPLE: "How has your back been feeling since your last visit?"

directive A question or series of questions that leads the client in the questioner's channel of thinking. (*Note:* Most of the questions in the review of systems are directive.)

EXAMPLES: "What problems have you had with your vision?"

probing Form of directive questioning that enables the examiner to pursue a line of thinking to prove or disprove a hypothesis.

leading A question worded in such a way that it suggests the answer to the respondent.

EXAMPLE: "Do you find that your chest pain radiates to your left arm or shoulder?" versus "Does your chest pain ever move around or locate in another area?"

R

rebound tenderness Sign of inflammation in the peritoneum in which pain is elicited by sudden withdrawal of a hand pressing on the abdomen; often found in appendicitis.

rectocele Bulging of the rectum and posterior vaginal wall through relaxed or weakened musculature of the vagina.

refraction Deviation of light rays as they pass from one transparent medium into another of different density.

remission Disappearance or diminishment of signs or symptoms.

reticular Describes a netlike pattern or structure of veins on a tissue surface.

retraction Shortening or drawing backward of the skin.

rheumatoid arthritis Chronic, destructive collagen disease characterized by inflammation, thickening, and swelling of the joints.

rhino- Combining form pertaining to the nose.

EXAMPLE: *Rhinitis* is an inflammation of the mucous membrane of the nose.

rhonchus Loud, low-pitched, coarse sound like a snore heard on auscultation of an airway obstructed by thick secretions, muscular spasm, neoplasm, or external pressure; also called *sonorous wheeze.*

Riedel lobe Tongue-shaped mass of tissue projecting from the right lobe of the liver.

Romberg test Evaluates an individual's ability to maintain a given position when standing erect with feet together and eyes closed.

S

scale Small, thin flakes of epithelial cells.

schizoid Exhibiting behaviors or having characteristics that resemble schizophrenia.

schizophrenia Any one of a large group of psychotic disorders characterized by marked distortion of reality and disorganization of personality characteristics.

scoliosis Lateral curvature of the spine.

scotoma Defined area of blindness within the visual field; can involve one or both eyes.

sebaceous glands Secretory dermal structures that produce sebum, an oily substance; puberty stimulates production, and the primary areas for secretion are in the face, chest, and upper part of back.

seborrhea Group of skin conditions characterized by non-inflammatory, excessively dry scales or by excessive oiliness.

sensorium Status of level of consciousness and orientation to surroundings.

shifting dullness Change in the dull sounds heard with palpation; at first the dull sound is heard in one location, then in a different location.

shotty node Small lymph node that feels hard and nodular; generally movable and nontender; may show evidence of having been infected many times in the past.

sign Objective finding; one perceived by the examiner.

significant negative Absence of a finding that is often significant in clarifying the client's status.
EXAMPLE: A client with diagnosed congestive heart failure shows no sign of ankle edema. (This is significant and should be reported as negative, or not present, because it clarifies the client's physical status for the reader.)

singultus Hiccup.

Skene glands (periurethral) Mucus-secreting glands that lie just inside the urethral orifice of women; not visible during examination.

smegma A secretion of sebaceous glands, especially the cheesy, foul-smelling secretion sometimes found under the foreskin of the penis and at the base of the labia minora near the glans clitoris.

spasticity Increased tone or contractions of muscles causing stiff and awkward movements; seen with upper motor neuron lesions.

spermatocele (epididymal cyst) Painless, fluid-filled epididymal mass that contains spermatozoa.

spiritual state An individual's version of his effectiveness in developing and sustaining a belief and value system that assists him in self-acceptance and in his relationship to others and to a Higher Being.

spondylitis Inflammation of one or more of the spinal vertebrae, usually characterized by stiffness and pain.

sprain Traumatic injury to the tendons, muscles, or ligaments around a joint; characteristics are pain, swelling, and discoloration of the skin over the joint.

stapes One of the ossicles in the middle ear; it resembles a tiny stirrup and transmits sound vibrations from the incus to the internal ear.

stereognosis Ability to recognize objects by the sense of touch.

sternocleidomastoid muscle Major muscle that rotates and flexes the head; originates by two heads from the sternum and clavicle and inserts on the mastoid process and the occipital bone.

stoma General term that means opening or mouth.
EXAMPLE: *Stomatitis* refers to a general inflammation of the oral cavity.

strabismus Condition in which the eyes are not directed at the same object or point.

strain Temporary damage to the muscles, usually caused by excessive physical effort.

striae Streaks of linear scars that often result from rapidly developing tension in the skin; also called *stretch marks.*

stridor Shrill, harsh sound heard during inspiration and caused by laryngeal obstruction.

subluxation Partial or incomplete dislocation.

supernumerary nipple Extra nipple.

supinate To turn the forearm so that the palm faces upward, or to rotate the foot and leg outward.

suspended judgment State of mind that permits the examiner to pose questions without allowing the answers to convey a meaning that would alter the completion or direction of the ensuing questions; suspended meaning allows both the examiner and the client to maintain an open state of inquiry versus pursuing a narrowed line of questioning to support the meaning of a given answer.

symptom Subjective indicator or sensation perceived by the client.

systole Period of time within the cardiac cycle in which the ventricles are contracted and ejecting blood into the aorta and pulmonary arteries.

tachycardia Rapid heart rate (more than 100 beats per minute); normally occurs with exercise, excitement, anxiety, or fever, but can also indicate abnormal states, such as anemia, heart failure, or shock.

tactile fremitus Vibratory sensations of the spoken voice felt through the chest wall on palpation.

tail of Spence Upper outer tail of the breast that extends into the axillary region.

telangiectasia Dilation of a superficial capillary or network of small capillaries that produces fine, irregular red lines on the skin surface.

tendinitis Inflammation of a tendon.

tenesmus Spasmodic contraction of the anal or vesical sphincter with pain and a persistent desire to empty the bowel or bladder; involves involuntary, ineffective straining efforts.

thrill Palpable murmur described as feeling like the throat of a purring cat.

thrombophlebitis An inflammation of a vein often associated with clot formation; can be induced by trauma, prolonged immobility, postoperative venous stasis, infection, or blood hypercoagulation disorder.

thrombus Blood clot attached to the inner wall of a vessel; usually causes some degree of occlusion.

tic Spasmodic muscular contraction most commonly involving the face, head, neck, or shoulder muscles.

tinnitus Tinkling or ringing sound heard in one or both ears.

tophus Calculus, containing sodium urate deposits, that develops in periauricular fibrous tissue; associated with gout.

torsion (of spermatic cord) Twisting of the spermatic cord resulting in an infarction of the testis; severe pain, redness, and swelling are present; loss of the testis can be prevented if the condition is diagnosed and treated quickly.

torus palatinus Exostosis, or benign outgrowth of bone, located on the midline of the hard palate; a fairly common finding that appears in a variety of shapes and sizes.

tragus Cartilaginous projection in front of the exterior meatus of the ear.

trapezius muscle Major muscle that rotates and extends the head; originates along the superior curved line of the oc-ciput and the spinous processes of the seventh cervical and all thoracic vertebrae and inserts at the clavicle, acromion, and base of the scapula.

tremor Continuous involuntary trembling movement of a part or parts of the body.

tumor Solid skin elevation extending into the dermal layer; more than 1 cm in diameter.

turbinates Extensions of the ethmoid bone located along the lateral wall of the nose; these fingerlike projections are covered with erectile mucosal membranes that become swollen or inflamed in response to allergy or viral invasion.

turgor Normal resiliency of the skin.

two-point discrimination Ability to identify being touched by two sharp objects simultaneously.

tympany Low-pitched note heard on percussion of a hollow organ such as the stomach.

ulcer Circumscribed crater on the surface of the skin or mucous membrane that leaves an uncovered wound.

umbo Central depressed portion of the concavity on lateral surface of the tympanic membrane; marks the spot where the malleus is attached to the inner surface

upper motor neurons Nerve cells that originate in the cerebral cortex and project downward; make up the corticobulbar and pyramidal tracts and end in the anterior horn of the spinal cord; responsible for the fine and discrete conscious movements.

urticaria (hives) Pruritic wheals, often transient and allergic in origin.

vaginitis Inflammation of the vaginal vault; has various causes.

   atrophic Associated with aging and diminished vaginal lubrication; itching, redness, a thin, yellow discharge, and superficial erosions may be present; leukoplakia or petechiae may appear.

   monilial Related to a common yeastlike organism (*Candida albicans*), normally present in mucous membranes, that may cause a superficial infection; presenting symptoms are itching, redness, swelling, a white, cheesy discharge, and white patches that bleed when scraped off.

   trichomoniasis Caused by a protozoan parasite that is sexually transmitted; itching, burning, and a malodorous, frothy, yellow-green discharge are commonly seen.

valgus Bending outward.

varicocele Abnormal tortuosity and dilation of spermatic veins; spermatic cord is described as feeling like a bag of worms; condition is not painful but involves a pulling or dragging sensation.

varus Turning inward.

verge (anal) External ring opening of the anus.

vermilion border Demarcation point between the mucosal membrane of the lips and the skin of the face; common site for recurrent infections, such as herpes infections, and carcinoma; blurring of this border may be an early sign of lesion development.

vertigo Sensation of moving around in space (whirling motion) (subjective vertigo) or of objects moving about oneself (objective vertigo); results in disturbance of the individual's equilibrium.

vesicle Fluid-filled, elevated, superficial lesion; 1 cm or less in diameter.

vesicular breathing The normal breath sounds heard over most of the lungs.

vestibule Middle part of the inner ear, located behind the cochlea and in front of the semicircular canals.

vocal fremitus The sensation of vibrations heard during auscultation when the client speaks.

wheal Elevated, solid, transient lesion; often irregularly shaped but well demarcated; an edematous response.

wheeze High-pitched, musical noise sounding like a squeak heard on auscultation of a narrowed airway.

whispered pectoriloquy Transmission of whispered words through the chest wall, heard during auscultation; indicates solidification of the lungs.

xerostomia Dryness of the mouth.

Al-Azzawi F: *Color atlas of childbirth and obstetric techniques,* St. Louis, 1990, Mosby.

Baden HP: *Diseases of the hair and nails,* Chicago, 1987, Year Book.

Baran R, Dawber RR, Levene GM: *Color atlas of the hair, scalp, and nails,* St. Louis, 1991, Mosby.

Barkauskas VH et al: *Health and physical assessment,* St. Louis, 1994, Mosby.

Beaven DW, Brooks SE: *Color atlas of the nail in clinical diagnosis,* ed 2, London, 1994, Times Mirror International.

Bedford MA: *Color atlas of ophthalmological diagnosis,* London, 1986, Wolfe.

Belcher AE: *Cancer nursing,* St. Louis, 1994, Mosby.

Bingham BJG, Hawke M, Kwok P: *Atlas of clinical otolarynology,* St. Louis, 1992, Mosby.

Bobak IM, Jensen MD: *Maternity and gynecologic care: the nurse and the family,* ed 5, St. Louis, 1993, Mosby.

Bowers AC, Thompson JM: *Clinical manual of health assessment,* ed 4, St. Louis, 1992, Mosby.

Canobbio MM: *Cardiovascular disorders,* St. Louis, 1990, Mosby.

Centers for Disease Control: Recommended childhood immunization schedule—United States, 1995, *MMWR 43*(51 & 52): 959-960, 1995.

Chipps EM: Clanin NJ, Campbell VG: *Neurologic disorders,* St. Louis, 1992, Mosby.

Cohen BA: *Pediatric dermatology,* London, 1993, Wolfe.

Crichlow RW et al: *Ann Surg* 175:490, 1972.

Cummings CW, ed: *Otolaryngology—head and neck surgery,* vol 4, St. Louis, 1993, Mosby.

Cutler WP: *Degenerative and hereditary diseases,* ed 7, Washington, DC, 1983, Scientific American Medicine.

Dickason EJ, Silverman, BL, Schult MO: *Maternal-infant nursing care,* ed 2, St. Louis, 1994, Mosby.

Doughty DB, Jackson DB: *Gastrointestinal disorders,* St. Louis, 1993, Mosby.

Droegemueller W et al: *Comprehensive gynecology,* St. Louis, 1987, Mosby.

Dyken PR, Miller MD: *Facial features of neurologic syndrome,* St. Louis, 1990, Mosby.

Edge V, Miller M: *Women's health care,* St. Louis, 1994, Mosby.

Farrar WE, Martin JW, Innes JA, Tubbs H: *Infectious diseases,* ed 2, London, 1992, Gower.

Finkbeiner BL, Johnson CS: *Mosby's comprehensive dental assisting,* St. Louis, 1995, Mosby.

Fitzpatrick RE: *Laser surgery of the cutaneous vascular lesions, Am J Cosmetic Surg* 9:107, 1992.

Folstein M et al: *The meaning of cognitive impairment in the elderly, J Am Geriatr Soc* 33(4):228, 1985.

400 more self-assessment picture tests in clinical medicine, London, 1988, Wolfe Medical Publications Ltd.

400 self-assessment picture tests in clinical medicine, London, 1984, Wolfe.

Gallager HS et al: *The breast,* St. Louis, 1978, Mosby.

Goldman MP, Fitzpatrick RE: *Cutaneous laser surgery: the art and science of selective photo thermolysis,* St. Louis, 1994, Mosby.

Goodman RM, Gorlin RJ: *Atlas of the face in genetic disorders,* ed 2, St. Louis, 1977, Mosby.

Grimes DE, Grimes RM: *AIDS and HIV infection,* St. Louis, 1994, Mosby.

Grimes DE, Grimes RM, Hamelink M: *Infectious diseases,* St. Louis, 1991, Mosby.

Habif TP: *Clinical dermatology: a color guide to diagnosis and therapy,* ed 2, St. Louis, 1990, Mosby.

Hart CA, Broadhead RL: *Color atlas of pediatric infectious diseases,* St. Louis, 1992, Mosby.

Helveston EM: *Surgical management of strabismus: an atlas of strabismus surgery,* ed 4, St. Louis, 1993, Mosby.

Hill MJ: *Skin disorders,* St. Louis, 1994, Mosby.

Institutes of Medicine: *Nutrition during pregnancy and lactation: an implementation guide,* Washington, D.C., 1993, National Academy Press.

Issacs JH: *Textbook of breast disease,* St. Louis, 1992, Mosby.

Kaufman RH et al: *Benign diseases of the vulva and vagina,* ed 4, St. Louis, 1994, Mosby.

Lawrence RA: *Breast-feeding: a guide for the medical profession,* ed 2, St. Louis, 1994, Mosby.

Lloyd-Davies RW et al: *Color atlas of urology,* ed 2, London, 1994, Wolfe.

Marshall WA, Tanner JM: *Arch Dis Child* 44:291, 1969.

Meheus A, Ursi JP: *Sexually transmitted diseases,* 1982, Kalamazoo, Michigan: The Upjohn Company.

Mourad LA: *Orthopedic disorders,* St. Louis, 1991, Mosby.

Newell FW: *Ophthalmology,* ed 7, St. Louis, 1992, Mosby.

Oklahoma Dietetic Association: *Oklahoma diet manual,* ed. 9, Oklahoma City, Oklahoma, 1993, The Association.

Potter PA, Perry AG: *Basic nursing: theory and practice,* ed 3, St. Louis, 1995, Mosby.

Rimoin DL: *N Engl J Med* 272:923, 1965.

Rocca RCD, Nesi FA, Lisman RD, eds.: *Ophthalmic plastic and reconstructive surgery,* vol 1, St. Louis, 1992, Mosby.

Rowland M: *A monogram for computing body mass index,* vol. 1, City (?) 1989, Dietetic Currents.

Rudy E: *Advanced neurological and neurosurgical nursing,* St. Louis, 1984, Mosby.

Scully C, Welbury R: *Color atlas of oral diseases in children and adolescents,* London, 1994, Wolfe.

Seeley RR, Stephens TD, Tate P: *Anatomy and physiology,* St. Louis, 1995, Mosby.

Seidel HM et al: *Mosby's guide to physical examination,* ed 3, St. Louis, 1995, Mosby.

Sigler BA, Schuring LT: *Ear, nose, and throat disorders,* St. Louis, 1993, Mosby.

Stark DD, Bradley WG Jr: *Magnetic resonance imaging,* ed 2, vol 2, St. Louis, 1992, Mosby.

Swartz MJ: *Textbook of physical diagnosis,* ed 2, Philadelphia, 1994, Saunders.

Tanner JM: *Growth at adolescence,* ed 2, Oxford, England, 1962, Blackwell Scientific Publications.

Tennant F: *Is your patient abusing drugs? Postgrad Med* 84:108-114, 1988.

Thibodeau GA, Patton K: *Anatomy and physiology,* ed 2, St. Louis, 1993, Mosby.

Thibodeau GA, Patton KT: *The human body in health and disease,* St. Louis, 1992, Mosby.

Thompson et al: *Mosby's clinical nursing,* ed 4, St. Louis,1993, Mosby.

Tyldesley WR: *Color atlas of oral medicine,* London, 1994, Wolfe.

Van Wieringen JC: *Growth diagrams 1965 Netherlands, second national survey on 0-24-year-olds,* Groningen, Netherlands, 1971, Wolters-Noordhoff.

Von Noorden GK: *Binocular vision and ocular motility: theory and management of strabismus,* ed 4, St. Louis, 1990, Mosby.

Wilson SF, Thompson JM: *Respiratory disorders,* St. Louis, 1990, Mosby.

Wong DL: *Nursing care of infants and children,* ed. 5, St. Louis, 1995, Mosby.

Zitelli BJ, Davis HW: *Atlas of pediatric physical diagnosis,* ed 2, London, 1992, Gower.

References

Alexander J, Scheller K: The Harlaxton experience: transcultural nursing education in the United Kingdom, *Nurse Educator* 15:20-25, 1990.

Allen D, Sanders L: (Letters) The excess mortality of Black adults in the United States, *JAMA* 264:571, 1990.

American Heart Association: *1990 Stroke facts,* Dallas, TX, 1991, American Heart Association.

American Nurses Association: *Standards of clinical nursing practice,* Kansas City, 1991, the Association.

American Nurses Association: *Standards of clinical nursing practice,* Washington, D.C., 1991, the Association.

American Psychiatric Association: *Diagnostic and statistical manual of mental disorders,* ed 3, Washington, D.C., 1987, the Association.

A support group for those with sarcoidosis, *Urban Health* 15:9, 1994.

Baden A, Karkeck J, Chernoff R: *Geriatrics.* In Gottschlich MM, Matarese LE, Shronts EP, eds: *Nutrition support dietetics core curriculum,* ed 2, Gaithersburg, MD, 1993, Aspen Press.

Barkauskas VH, Stolenberg-Allen K, Bauman LC, Darling-Fisher C: *Health and physical assessment,* St. Louis, 1994, Mosby.

Basset A, Liautaud B, Bassirou N (translated by Andrew Pembroke): *Dermatology of black skin,* New York, 1986, Oxford University.

Bayley N: *Bayley scales of infant development,* New York, 1993, Psychological Corporation.

Bennett MA, Stucko J, Ross E, et al: *Task force on the implications for darkly pigmented intact skin in the prediction and prevention of pressure ulcers,* Brooklyn, NY, 1994, Woodhull Medical and Mental Health Center.

Bess FH, Lichtenstein MJ, Logan SA et al: Hearing impairment as a determinant of function in the elderly, *J Am Geriatr Soc* 37:123-8, 1989.

Bess FH, Paradise JL: Universal screening for infant impairment: not simple, not risk free, not necessarily beneficial, and not presently justified, *Pediatrics* 92:330-334, 1994.

Black-White disparities in health care. Council on Ethical and Judicial Affairs, *JAMA* 263:2344-2346, 1990.

Blackburn GL, Bestrian BR, Maini BS et al: *Nutritional and metabolic assessment of the hospitalized patient,* JPEN 1:15, 1977.

Block B: Nursing care of Black patients. In Orque MS, Block B, Monrroy LSA: *Ethnic nursing care: a multicultural approach,* St. Louis, Mosby.

Block B: Nursing intervention in Black patient care. In Luckraft D, ed: *Black awareness: implications for Black patient care,* New York, 1976, American Journal of Nursing

Bluma SM, Shearer MS, Frohman AH, Hilliard J: *Portage guide to early education,* 1976, Cooperative Educational Service Agency No. 12, Box 564, Portage, Wisconsin, 53901.

Bobak IM, Jensen MD: *Essentials of maternity nursing,* ed 3, St. Louis, 1991, Mosby.

Bowers AC, Thompson JM: *Clinical manual of health assessment,* ed 4, St. Louis, 1992, Mosby.

Bowman JE, Murray RF: *Genetic variation and disorders in peoples of African origin,* Baltimore, MD, 1990, Johns Hopkins University.

Brazelton TB: *Neonatal behavioral assessment scale,* Clinics in Developmental Medicine, No. 50, Spastics International Medical Publications, Philadelphia, 1973, Lippincott.

Brazelton TB: *Neonatal behavioral scale,* ed 2, Clinics in Developmental Medicine, No. 88. Spastics International Medical Publications, Philadelphia, 1983, Lippincott.

Brazelton TB: Saving the bathwater, *Child Development* 61:1661-1671, 1990.

Brazelton TB, Nugent JK, Lester BM: Neonatal behavioral assessment scale, 1987. In Osofsky J, ed: *The handbook of infant development,* New York, Wiley, pp. 780-817.

Breastfeeding Task Force, St. Louis Model Standards. Missouri Department of Health, 1991.

Brown M: *Readings in gerontology,* St. Louis, 1978, Mosby.

Cancer facts & figures, Atlanta, 1995, National American Cancer Society.

Canobbio MM: *Cardiovascular disorders,* St. Louis, 1990, Mosby.

Carlson SJ: *Neonatology.* In Gottschlich MM, Matarese LE, Shronts EP, eds: *Nutrition support dietetics core curriculum,* ed 2, Gaithersburg, MD, 1993, Aspen Press.

Centers for Disease Control: Recommendations for prevention of HIV transmission in health-care settings, *MMWR* 41(2S):3-17, 1987.

Centers for Disease Control: Revised classification system for HIV infection and expanded surveillance case definition for AIDS among adolescents and adults, *MMWR* 41(RR-17):1, 1993.

Cerrato P: Improving the odds of a healthy birth, *RN* 71-73, Sept. 1992

Chew AL: *The Lollipop Test: a diagnostic screening test of school readiness,* Atlanta, 1981, Humanics Limited.

Chew AL: *Developmental and interpretive manual for the Lollipop Test: a diagnostic screening test of school readiness,* Atlanta, 1989, Humanics Limited.

Chew AL: *The Lollipop Test: a diagnostic screening test of school readiness,* Atlanta, 1992, Humanics Limited.

Chew AL, Morris JD: Validation of the Lollipop Test: a diagnostic screening test of school readiness, *Educational and Psychological Measurement,* 1984. 44, 987-991.

Chew AL, Morris JD: Investigation of the Lollipop Test as a prekindergarten screening instrument, *Educational and Psychological Measurement,* 1987. 47, 467-471.

Chipps E, Clanin N, Campbell V: *Neurologic disorders,* St. Louis, 1992, Mosby.

Chumlea WC: Growth and development. In Queen P, Lang C, eds: *Handbook of pediatrics nutrition,* Gaithersburg, MD, 1993, Aspen Publishers, pp. 3-23.

Clinical Preventive Services, Baltimore, 1994, Williams & Wilkins.

Coddington RD: The significance of life events as etiologic factors in diseases of children. Part I: A survey of professional workers, *J Psychosomatic Res* 16:7-18, 1972.

Coddington RD: The significance of life events as etiologic factors in diseases of children. Part II: A study of a normal population, *J Psychosomatic Res* 16:205-213, 1972.

Cornblath M, Schwartz R: Hypoglycemia in the neonate, *J Pediatr Endrincol* 6:113-129, 1993.

Crocker R: *Childhood obesity.* In Queen P, Lang C, eds: *Handbook of pediatric nutrition,* Gaithersburg, MD, Aspen Publishers.

Cropley C, Lester P, Pennington S: Assessment tool for measuring maternal attachment behavior. In McNall LK, Galeener JT, eds: *Current practice in obstetrics and gynecologic nursing,* vol. 1, St. Louis, 1976, Mosby.

Davis MA, Murphy SP, Neuhaus JM, Lein D: Living arrangements and dietary quality of older U.S. adults, *J Am Diet Assoc* 90:1667-1672, 1990.

Denver Developmental Materials Catalog of Screening and Training Materials, Denver, 1994, DDM, Inc.

Detsky AS, McLaughlin JR, Baker JP et al: What is Subjective Global Assessment of Nutritional Status? *J Parenteral Enteral Nutr* 11:8-13, 1987.

Dewey KG, Heinig MJ, Nommsen LA: Maternal weight-loss patterns during prolonged lactation, *Am J Clin Nutr* 58:162-166, 1993.

Doan MA, Wollenburg K, Wilson E: *Portage guide to early education,* 2nd revision, 1994, Portage Project, Cooperative Educational Service Agency 5, Box 564, Portage, WI 53901.

Duvall EM: *Marriage and family development,* ed 5, New York, 1977, Harper & Row.

Duvall EM, Miller BC: *Marriage and family development,* ed. 6, 1985, New York: Harper & Row.

Edelman CL, Mandle CL: *Health promotion through the lifespan,* St. Louis, 1994, Mosby.

Erikson EH: *Childhood and society,* New York, 1993, Norton.

Erikson EH: Generativity and ego-integrity. In Neugarten B, ed: *Middle age and aging,* Chicago, 1968, University of Chicago Press.

Erikson EH: *Identity and the life cycle,* New York/London, 1980, Norton.

Erikson E, Erikson J, Kivnick H: *Vital involvement in old age,* New York, 1986, Norton.

Family Stress, Coping & Health Project. Madison, WI, 1995, University of Wisconsin-Madison.

Finkbeiner BL, Johnson CS: *Mosby's comprehensive dental assisting,* St. Louis, 1995, Mosby.

Fitzpatrick TB, Eisen AZ, Wolff K et al, eds: *Dermatology of general medicine,* ed 4, New York, 1993, McGraw-Hill.

Flavell JH: *The developmental psychology of Jean Piaget,* New York, 1963, D. Van Nostrand Company.

Ford E, Cooper R, Castaneo A, et al: Coronary arteriography and coronary by-pass surgery among whites and other racial groups relative to hospital based incidence rate for coronary artery disease: findings from NHDS, *Am J Public Health,* 79:437-440, 1989.

Frankenburg WK, Dodds J, Archer et al: The Denver II: a major revision and restandardization of the Denver Developmental Screening Test, *Pediatrics* 89:91-97, 1992.

Frongilli EA, Rauschenbach BS, Roe DA, Williamson DR: Characteristics related to elderly persons not eating for 1 or more days: implications for meal programs, *Am J Public Health* 82:600-602, 1992.

Garfinkel L: The epidemiology of cancer in Black Americans, *Stat Bull* 72:11-17, 1991.

Garry PJ, Hunt WC, Bandrofchak JL et al: Vitamin A intake and plasma retinol levels in healthy elderly men and women, *Am J Clin Nutr* 46:898-894, 1987.

Gaskin FC: *Teaching ethnic and racial variations: erythema in the person with the dark skin,* Presentation at the First National Eldercare Institute on Older Women National Council of Negro Women, Washington, DC. 1993.

Gaskin FC: Detection of cyanosis in the person with dark skin, *J Nat Black Nurses Assoc* 1:52-60, 1986.

Geissler EM: *Pocket guide to cultural assessment,* St. Louis, 1994, Mosby.

Georgieff MK, Sasanow SR: Nutritional assessment of the neonate, *Clin Perinatol* 13:73-89, 1986.

Gibes RM: Clinical uses of the Brazelton Neonatal Behavioral Assessment Scale in nursing practice, *Pediatr Nurs* 7:23, 1981.

Giger JN, Davidhizar RE: *Transcultural nursing: assessment and intervention,* ed 2, St. Louis, 1995, Mosby.

Giotta MP: Nutrition during pregnancy: reducing obstetric risk, *J Perinatol Neonatal Nurs* 6:1-12, 1993.

Glenn MB, Carfi J, Belle SE et al: Serum albumin as a predictor of course and outcome on a rehabilitation service, *Arch Phys Med Rehabil* 66:294-296, 1985.

Goldenring JM, Cohen E: Getting into adolescent heads, *Contemporary Pediatrics* 75-90, July 1988.

Goldstein G, Hersen M: *Handbook of psychological assessment,* New York, 1984, Pergamon Press.

Goodenough FL: *Measurement of intelligence by drawings,* New York, 1926, World Book.

Grant A, DeHoog S: *Anthropometrics.* In Grant A, DeHoog S, eds: *Nutritional assessment and support,* ed 3, Seattle, WA, 1985, Anne Grant and Susan DeHoog.

Gray M, Dobkin K: *Genitourinary system.* In Thompson J, McFarland G, Hirsch J and Tucker S: *Clinical nursing,* ed 3, St. Louis, ed 3, Mosby.

Grimes DE, Grimes RM: *AIDS and HIV infection,* St. Louis, 1994, Mosby.

Grimes DE: *Infectious diseases,* St. Louis, 1991, Mosby.

Groh-Wargo SL, Antonelli K: *Normal nutrition during infancy.* In Queen PM, Lang CE, eds: *Handbook of pediatric nutrition,* Gaithersburg, MD. 1993, Aspen Publishers.

Grundy SM, Bilheimer D, Chait A et al: Summary of the Second Report of the National Cholesterol Education Program Expert Panel on Detection, Evaluation, and Treatment of High Blood Cholesterol in Adults, *JAMA* 269:3015-3023, 1993.

Guide to Clinical Preventive Services: *An assessment of the effectiveness of 169 interventions,* Report of the U.S. Preventative Series Task Force, Baltimore, MD, 1989, Williams and Wilkins.

Harris DB: *Children's drawing as measures of intellectual maturity,* San Diego, CA, 1963, Harcourt Brace Jovanovich.

Herbst KRG: Psychosocial consequences of disorders of hearing in the elderly. In Hinchcliffe R, ed: *Hearing and balance in the elderly,* Edinburgh, 1983, Churchill Livingstone.

Hill MJ: *Skin disorders,* St. Louis, 1994, Mosby.

Himes JH, Dietz WH: Guidelines for overweight in adolescent preventive services: recommendations from an expert committee, *Am J Clin Nutr* 54:307-316, 1994.

Holmes TH, Rahe RH: The social readjustment rating scale, *Psychosom Res* 11:213-218, 1967.

Hopkins B: *Assessment of nutritional status.* In Gottschlich MM, Matarese LE, Shronts EP, eds: *Nutrition support dietetics core curriculum,* ed 2, Gaithersburg, MD, 1993, Aspen Publishers.

Institutes of Medicine: *Nutrition during lactation,* Washington, DC, 1991, National Academy Press.

Institutes of Medicine: *Nutrition during pregnancy, part I: Weight gain; part II: Nutrient supplements,* Washington, DC, 1991, National Academy Press.

Institutes of Medicine: *Nutrition during pregnancy and lactation: an implementation guide,* Washington, DC, 1993, National Academy Press.

Isselbacher KJ, Braunwald E, Wilson JD et al, eds: *Harrison's principles of internal medicine,* ed 13, New York, 1994, McGraw-Hill.

Jacobs AH, Walton RG: Incidence of birthmarks in the neonate, *Pediatrics* 58:218-222, 1976.

James SA, Strongatz DS, Wing SB, Ramsey DL: Socioeconomic status, John Henryism, and hypertension in Black and Whites, *Am J Epidemiol* 126:664-673, 1987.

Johansson CB, Johansson JC: *Manual supplement for the career assessment inventory,* Minneapolis, 1978, National Computer Systems.

Kane R, Kane RL: *Assessing the elderly,* Lexington, MA, 1984, Lexington Books.

Kaufman M, McMurrian TT: *Humanics national child assessment form,* 1992, Humanics Limited, P O Box 7447, Atlanta, GA 30309.

Kemper DW, Giuffre J, Drabinski G: *Pathways,* Idaho, 1986, Healthwise, Inc.

Kenney Jr JA: Skin problems of Blacks, *J Nat Med Assoc* 236:301-303, 1976.

Kerfoot KM: Managing cultural diversity: turning demographic factors into a competitive advantage. Nursing management considerations, *Nurs Econ* 8:352, 360, 362, 1994.

Kicklighter RH, Richmond BO: *Children's adaptive behavior scale revised and expanded manual,* Atlanta, 1983, Humanics Limited.

Krause MV, Mahan LK: *The assessment of nutritional status.* In Krause MV, Mahan LK, eds: *Food, nutrition, and diet therapy: a textbook of nutritional care,* ed 7, Philadelphia, 1984, Saunders.

Kreiger N, Rowley DL, Herman AA et al: Racism, sexism and social class: implications for studies of health, disease, and well being, *Racial Differences in Preterm Delivery,* 14, 82-122, 1992.

Krug-Wispe S: *Nutritional assessment.* In Queen PM, Lang CE, eds: *Handbook of pediatric nutrition,* Gaithersburg, MD, 1993, Aspen Publishers.

Krumholz H, Seeman T, Merrill SS et al: Lack of association between cholesterol and coronary heart disease mortality and morbidity and all-cause mortality in persons older than 70 years, *JAMA* 272:1335-1340, 1994.

Lawrence PB: Breast milk: best source of nutrition for term and preterm infants, *Pediatr Clin North Am* 41:925-941, 1994.

Lawrence R: *Breastfeeding: a guide for the medical professional,* ed 4, St. Louis, 1994, Mosby.

Leininger MM: The transcultural nurse, specialist: imperative in today's world. *Nurs Health Care* 10:251-256, 1989.

Leininger MM: Leininger's theory of nursing: cultural care diversity and universality, *Nurs Sci Q* 1:152-160, 1988.

Libertino JA, ed: *International perspectives in urology,* vol. 5, Baltimore, MD, 1982, Williams and Wilkins.

Lipschultz LI, Howards SS, eds: *Infertility in the male,* ed 2, St. Louis, 1991, Mosby.

Lucas B: *Normal nutrition from infancy through adolescence.* In Queen PM, Lang CE, eds: *Handbook of pediatric nutrition,* Gaithersburg, MD, 1993, Aspen Publishers.

Lueckenotte, AG: *Pocket guide to gerontologic assessment,* St. Louis, 1994, Mosby.

Lunneborg PW: *Vocational interest inventory manual,* Los Angeles, 1981, Western Psychological Services.

MacBurney M: *Pregnancy.* In Gottschlich MM, Matarese LE, Shronts EP, eds: *Nutrition support dietetics core curriculum,* ed 2, Gaithersburg, MD, 1993, Aspen Publishers.

Matteson MA, McConnell ES: *Gerontological nursing concepts and practices,* Philadelphia, 1988, Saunders.

McCubbin HI, Thompson AI, eds: *Family assessment inventories for research and practice,* Madison, WI, 1987, The University of Wisconsin-Madison.

Metcoff J: Clinical assessment of nutritional status at birth, *Pediatr Clin North Am* 41:875, 1994.

Moos RH, Moos BS: A typology of family social environments, *Fam Process* 15:357-371, 1976.

Mosby's patient teaching guides, St. Louis, 1995, Mosby.

Mourad LA: *Orthopedic disorders,* St. Louis, 1991, Mosby.

Murphy C: Assessment of fathering behaviors. In Johnson SH: *High-risk parenting: nursing assessment and strategies for the family at risk,* Philadelphia, PA, 1979, Lippincott.

Myers I, Briggs-Myers PB: *Gifts differing,* Palo Alto, CA, 1980, Consulting Psychologists Press.

NANDA: Proceedings of the Eleventh National Conference of the North American Nursing Diagnosis Association, 1994.

National Institutes of Health: *NIH consensus statement: early identification of hearing impairment in infants and young children,* vol. 11, no. 1, Washington, DC, 1993, NIH.

National Research Council: *Recommended dietary allowances,* ed 10, Washington DC, 1989, National Academy Press.

Neinstein LS: *Adolescent health care: a practical guide,* ed 2, Baltimore, 1991, Williams & Wilkins.

Nichols BL: Failure to thrive in the infant, *Pediatric Rounds* 1:3-8, 1992.

Olefsky JM. Diabetes mellitus. In Wyngaarden JB, Smith LH, Bennett JC, eds: *Cecil textbook of medicine,* Philadelphia, 1992, Saunders.

Olson DH: Circumplex model VII: validation studies and FACES III, *Family Process 25:337-351, 1986.*

Overton T: *Biological variations in health and illness: race, age and sex differences,* Reading, MA, 1985, Addison-Wesley.

Pennington JAT: *Bowe's and Church's food values of portions commonly used,* ed 16, Philadelphia, 1994, Lippincott.

Peterson KE: *Failure to thrive.* In Queen PM, Lane CE, eds: *Handbook of pediatric nutrition,* Gaithersburg, MD, 1993, Aspen Publishers.

Piaget J, Inhelder B (translated by Helen Weaver): *The psychology of the child,* New York, 1969, Basic Books.

Pipes PL, Trahms CM: *Nutrition in infancy and childhood,* ed 5, St. Louis, 1993, Mosby.

Pi-Sunyer F: Obesity. In Wyngaarden JB, Smith LH, Bennett JC, eds: *Cecil textbook of medicine,* Philadelphia, 1992, Saunders.

Polednak AP: *Racial and ethnic differences in disease,* New York, 1989, Oxford University.

Portage Project, 1994, Portage, WI: CESA 5.

Porter LW: A study of perceived need satisfactions in bottom and middle management jobs, *Personnel Journal* 59:907-912, 1961.

Potter AF, Perry PA: *Clinical nursing skills and techniques,* ed 3, St. Louis, 1994, Mosby.

Prager DA, Stone DA, Rose DN: Hearing loss screening in the neonatal intensive care unit: auditory brain stem response versus crib-o-gram, a cost-effective analysis, *Ear Hear* 213-278, 1987.

Psychological Corporation: *Tests and other products for psychological assessment,* San Antonio, TX, 1995, Harcourt Brace.

Ray LU, Yuwiler J: *Child and adolescent fatal injury data book,* San Diego, CA, 1994, Children's Safety Network: Injury Data Technical Assistance Center, Center for Childhood Injury Prevention, San Diego State University.

Redel C, Shulman RJ: Controversies in the composition of infant formulas, *Pediatr Clin North Am* 4:909-924, 1994.

Reidy M, Thibaudeau MF: Evaluation of family functioning: development and validation of a scale which measures family competence in measures of health, *Nursing Papers* 16:42-56, 1984.

Report of the Second Task Force on blood pressure on children, *Pediatr* 79:1-25, 1987.

Report of the U.S. Preventive Services Task Force: *Guide to clinical preventive services: an assessment of the effectiveness of 169 interventions,* Baltimore, MD, 1989, Williams & Wilkins.

Riko K, Hyde ML, Alberti PW: Hearing loss in early infancy; incidence, detection and assessment, *Laryngoscope* 95:137-45, 1985.

Roach L: *Color changes in dark skins,* Nursing 72:48-51, 1977.

Roberts A: *Biological perspectives on human pigmentation,* New York, 1991, Cambridge.

Roberts RJ: Drug therapy in infants. In *Pharmacologic principles and clinical experience,* 1984, Philadelphia, PA.

Robinson RA: The diagnosis and prognosis of dementia. In W.F. Anders, ed: *Current achievements in geriatrics,* London, 1964, Cassell.

Roland DA: Nutrition in adulthood and the later years. In *Food, nutrition, and diet therapy,* Philadelphia, 1984, Saunders.

Rolfes SR, DeBruyne LK: *Life span nutrition: conception through life,* New York, 1990, West Publishing Company.

Rosen T, Martin S: *Atlas of black dermatology,* Boston, MA, 1981, Little, Brown.

Rush D: Periconceptional folate and neural tube defect, *Am J Clin Nutr* 59(suppl):511S-6S, 1994.

Satter E: *How to get your kid to eat. . .but not too much,* Palo Alto, CA, 1987, Bull Publishing.

Schaefer MT, Olson DH: Assessing intimacy: the pair inventory. *J Marital Family Therapy* 7:47-60, 1981.

Scully C, Welbury R: *Color atlas of oral diseases in children and adolescents,* London, 1994, Wolfe.

Seeley RR, Stephens TD, Tate P: *Anatomy and physiology,* ed 3, St. Louis, 1995, Mosby.

Seidel HM, Ball JW, Dains JE, Benedict JW: *Mosby's guide to physical examination,* ed 3, St. Louis, 1995, Mosby.

Shader RI, Harmatz JS, Salzman C: A new scale for clinical assessment in geriatric populations: Sandoz Clinical Assessment Geriatric (SCAG). *J Am Geriatr Soc* 22:107-113, 1974.

Sigler BA, Schuring LT: *Ear, nose, and throat disorders,* St. Louis, 1993, Mosby.

Smith AD: Causes and classifications of impotence, *Urology Clin North Am* 8:79, 1981.

Smith PC, Kendall LM, Hulin CL: *The measurement of satisfaction in work and retirement,* Chicago, 1969, Rand-McNally.

Spark A: Children's diet and health requirements: preschool age through adolescence, *Compr Ther* 18:9-20, 1992.

Spector RE: *Cultural diversity in health and illness,* ed 3, Norwalk, CT, 1991, Appleton & Lange.

Sperhac AM, Salzer JL: A new developmental screening test: The Denver II. *J Am Acad Nurse Practitioners* 3:152-157, 1991.

Stewart, Sundeen: *Principles of psychiatric nursing,* ed 5, St. Louis, 1995, Mosby.

Stokes S, Gordon S: Development of a tool to measure stress in the older individual, New York, 1986, Stewart Research Conference, Nursing in the 21st Century, Perspectives and Possibilities.

Swanson CA, Mansourian R, Dirren H, Rapin CH: Zinc status of healthy elderly adults: response to supplementation, *Am J Clin Nutr* 48:343-349, 1988.

Swartz MH: *Textbook of physical diagnosis: history and examination,* ed 2, Philadelphia, 1994, Saunders.

Tennant F: The rapid eye test to detect drug abuse, *Postgrad Med* 84(1), 1988.

Thompson JM, McFarland GK, Hirsh JE, Tucker SM: *Mosby's clinical nursing,* ed 3, St. Louis, 1993, Mosby.

Tyldesley WR: *Color atlas of oral medicine,* London, 1994, Mosby-Wolfe.

Unti SM: The critical first year of life: history, physical examination, and general developmental assessment, *Pediatr Clin North Am* 41:849-873, 1994.

U.S. Department of Health and Human Services: *Clinician's handbook for preventative services,* Washington, DC, 1994, U.S. Government Printing Office.

U.S. Department of Health and Human Services: *Healthy people 2000: national health promotion and disease prevention objectives,* 1992, Fall Report with commentary, DHHS Publication No. (PHS) 91-40212.

U.S. Department of Health and Human Services: *National cholesterol education program: report of the expert panel on blood cholesterol levels in children and adolescents,* 1991, NIH Publication.

Valassi K, Clark HM: Nutrition and digestive function. In Burke MM, Walsh MB, eds: *Gerontologic nursing,* St. Louis, 1992, Mosby.

Visher ED, Visher JS: *Step-families: a guide to working with stepparents and stepchildren,* Secaucus, NJ, 1979, The Citadel Press.

Walker O, Beauchene RE: The relationship of loneliness, social isolation, and physical health to dietary adequacy of independently living elderly, *J Am Diet Assoc* 91:300-34, 1991.

Weinberg A, Pals JK, Campbell SM: Preventing dehydration in the elderly: the challenge of assessment and treatment, *Dietetic Currents* 21:9-10, 1994.

Whaley LF, Wong DL: *Essentials of pediatric nursing,* ed 3, St. Louis, 1989, Mosby.

Whaley LF, Wong DL: *Whaley and Wong's nursing care of infants and children,* ed 5, St. Louis, 1995, Mosby.

Whitney EN, Rolfes SR: *Life cycle nutrition: childhood, adolescence and aging.* In Whitney EN, Rolfes SR, eds: *Understanding nutrition,* ed 6, St. Paul, MN, 1993, West Publishing.

Wilson S, Thompson J: *Respiratory disorders,* St. Louis, 1990, Mosby.

Wong DL: *Whaley and Wong's essentials of pediatric nursing,* ed 4, St. Louis, 1993, Mosby.

Zeman FJ: *Nutritional assessment.* In *Clinical nutrition and dietetics,* ed 2, New York: Macmillian Publishing Co.

Zeman FJ: Ney DM: *Evaluating nutritional status.* In *Applications of clinical nutrition,* Englewood Cliffs, NJ, 1988, Prentice Hall.

Index

A

Abdomen; *see also* Gastrointestinal system
  connective tissue of, 437-438
  distention of, 444, 450
    4 "Fs" and, 450
  dullness of, 452, 454, 462
  examination of, 450-452, 454-458, 461-465, 471
    deep palpation in, 456
    in integrated assessment, 692
  floating mass in, 465, 471
  fluid in, 462-463, 471
  landmarks of, 449
  musculature of, 437-438
  pain in; *see* Abdominal pain
  percussion of, 74, 75
  quadrants of, 448
  reflexes of, 461
    superficial, neurologic examination of, 647, 665
  regions of, 449
  rigidity of, 454
  vasculature of, 440
Abdominal aneurysm, 442
Abdominal floating mass, 465, 471
Abdominal fluid, 462-463, 471
Abdominal pain, 441
  differentiation of, 456-457
  examination of, 463-464, 471
  lower, 489
Abdominal reflexes
  examination of, 461
  superficial, neurologic examination of, 647, 665
Abducens nerve, 642, 643, 644, 653
  eye movement and, 277, 286
Abduction, 585
Abrasions, corneal, 306
  Wood's lamp for detecting, 70
Abscess, 153
  pelvic, 464
  perianal, 567
Abuse
  child, 493-494
  drug
    documentation of, 58
    eye signs of, 299-300
    in pregnancy, 103
  sexual, 540
Accessory nerve, 642, 643, 644
  head turning and, 197
  tests for, 657
Accidents, history of, 44
Accommodation, 653
  inspection of, 292
  loss of, 280, 284
Acetylsalicylic acid, ototoxicity of, 250
Achilles tendon reflex, 662-664
Acne, 128, 139
  in acne vulgaris, 139, 140

Acoustic nerve, 642, 643
  ear anatomy and, 247, 248
  testing of, 259, 261, 655
Acoustic stethoscope, 61, 62
Acquired immunodeficiency syndrome, 179
  health history and, 492
  oral Kaposi's sarcoma in, 243
  safe sex and, 528
Acrochordons, 41, 140
Acrocyanosis, 382
Acromegaly, 196, 204
Acromioclavicular joint, 605
Active listening, 41
Activities of daily living
  limitations of self-care behaviors in, 593-594
  of older adult, 54
Acute pain as nursing diagnosis
  in earache, 273
  in epigastric pain, 478
Acute renal failure, 476
Adduction, 585
Adenoids, 170
AD/HD; *see* Attention deficit/hyperactivity disorder
Adie's pupil, 310
ADL; *see* Activities of daily living
Adnexa, uterine, 509, 510
Adolescent, 17-18
  assessment of, 17-18
    external genitalia in, 511
    nutrition in, 110-111
  development of, 17-18
  health history of, 52, 53
  heart rates of, 78
  pregnancy in, 32-33
  pregnancy of
    ethnic and cultural influences on, 32-33
    high-risk nutritional conditions during, 104
  respiratory rates of, 79
  weight and height of, 87
Adolescent-Family Inventory of Life Events and Changes, 24
Adrenarche, 486
Adult
  anthropometrics in, 93-95
  assessment of; *see also* Assessment
    developmental, 18-19
    nutrition in, 93-97; *see also* Nutrition
  heart rates of, 78
  intelligence in, 8
  older; *see* Older adult
  respiratory rates of, 79
Adventitious breath sounds, 340, 341
Afferent fibers of spinal nerves, 644
A-FILE; *see* Adolescent-Family Inventory of Life Events and Changes
African-American culture, 30-36
AGA; *see* Appropriate for gestational age

Age
  blood pressure and, 81
  health history variations and, 48-55
  physical assessment variations and, 83-87, 88-91, 111
Agenesis of third molar, 215
Aglossia, 234
AIDS; *see* Acquired immunodeficiency syndrome
AIDS dementia complex, 677
Air
  in body cavities, transilluminator for differentiation of, 70
  obstruction of nasal flow of, 219
  trapping of, 333
Alaskan natives, 31-37
Albumin, serum
  in neonate and infant, 107
  nutrition and, 95
  in older adult, 112
  in pregnancy, 100-101
Alcohol
  documentation of use of, 58
  excess consumption of, 478
    ethnic and cultural influences on, 33
  eye signs and, 300
  food pyramid and, 102
  in pregnancy, 103
  sexual function and, 541
Alimentary tract, 438-440; *see also* Gastrointestinal system
  common problems or conditions of, 472-473
Allen test, 297
Allergies, 219, 220, 324
  eye problems and, 282
  in health history, 43
  skin and, 146
Alopecia, 132
  in alopecia areata, 156
  in child, 139
Altered breathing pattern in cough, 355
Altered growth and development
  high risk for, in child with ear disorders, 273
  potential for, in male genitalia problems, 555
Altered health maintenance as nursing diagnosis
  in breast lumps, 433
  in epigastric pain, 478
  in hypertension, 396
  in skin lesions, 160
Altered mobility, health history and, 649
Altered nutrition
  less than body requirements, in temporomandibular joint dysfunction, 244
  more than body requirements
    in child, 477
    in male breast enlargement, 434
    in older adult, 314

Altered patterns of elimination in urinary difficulties, 579
Altered peripheral tissue perfusion in arterial insufficiency, 397
Altered sensation
  in eye disorders, 314, 315
  health history and, 649
Altered skin integrity in arterial insufficiency, 397
Alternative folk remedies, 27, 34-35
Alternative health care providers, 27, 34-35
Alveolar-capillary membranes, 361
Alveoli
  in older adult, 322
  transfer of gases in, 317, 319
Alzheimer's disease, 677
  in older adult, 651
American Indian/Alaskan native culture, 31-37
American Nurses Association, Standards of Practice of, 39
Amulets, 34
ANA; see American Nurses Association
Anal sphincter tone, 509
Androgens, 538
Anemia
  in adolescent, 110
  in pregnancy, 100
  in toddler, 108
Aneroid sphygmomanometer, 63
Anesthesia, stocking, 374
Aneurysm
  abdominal, pain in, 442
  aortic, 378
  arterial, 395
Anger in interview, 42-43
Angina, 363-364, 390
Angiomas, 125, 137
Angle
  costal, 320
  of Louis, 320
Angular stomatitis, 98
Anisocoria, 291, 309
Ankle
  assessment of, 616-617, 627
    ankle clonus in, 662-664
  range of motion of, 617
  supporting structures of, 590
Anorectal fissure, 563, 575
Anorexia nervosa, 446
  in pregnancy, 104
Antacids, food interaction with, 113
Anteflexed uterus, 508
Anterior chamber of eye, 277
Anteverted uterus, 507
Anthropometrics
  in adolescent, 110
  in adult, 93-95
  defined, 93
  in neonate and infant, 106-107
  in older adult, 111-112
  in postpartum and lactating women, 105
  in pregnancy, 100
  in preschooler and school-age child, 109
  in toddler, 108
Antibodies, 165
Anticonvulsants, 650
Antihelix, 247

Antihypertensives, 369
  galactorrhea and, 431
  sexual function and, 538, 541
Antiinflammatory drugs, food interaction with, 113
Antitremor medications, 650
Antivertigo medications, 650
Anus, 559-581
  of adolescent, 572
  age-related variations in, 572
  anatomy and physiology of, 559, 560
  of child, 561, 565, 572
  common problems or conditions of, 575-576
    nursing diagnoses for, 578-579
    sample documentation of, 578-579
  developmental considerations for, 561
  ethnic and cultural variations in, 574
  examination of, 567-569, 570
  fissures of, 563, 575
  health history and, 562-566
  health promotion and, 580
  imperforate, 564
  of infant, 561, 564-565, 572
  inspection of, 499
  in male, health history and, 566
  of older adult, 561, 566, 572
  in pregnancy, 573
    developmental considerations for, 561
    health history and, 565-566
  situational variations in, 573-574
Anxiety
  as nursing diagnosis
    in blurred vision, 314
    in ear disorders, 272
    in infant check-ups, 210
  skin lesions and, 160
Aorta, 359, 361
  bruits and, 451
  coarctation of, 393
    in infant, 382
  palpation of, 457
Aortic aneurysm, 378
Aortic valves, 359
  heart sounds and, 379, 380
    abnormal, 388
  regurgitation or stenosis of, 378, 388-389
Aperture setting for ophthalmoscope, 66
Aphthous ulcer, 241
Apical pulse, 371, 377
  in infant, 382
Apley test, 621
Apnea in newborn, 327
Apocrine sweat glands, 116
  in adolescent, 117
Appearance, mental status and, 665
Appendages, 116
Appendicitis
  iliopsoas muscle test in, 464
  obturator muscle test in, 464
  pain in, 442, 456-457
  rebound tenderness in, 463
Appendicular skeleton, 589-590
Appendix, rupture of, 464
Appetite, decrease in, 444
Appropriate for gestational age, 106
Aqueous humor, 278
ARC; see Auditory response cradle

Areola, variations in, 412-413
Areolar lymphatic drainage, 401
Argyll Robertson pupil, 309
Arm
  assessment of, 608-609, 626
    in integrated examination, 687
  lymph nodes in, 168, 169
    examination of, 175
  muscles of, 586
  racial variation of, 590
  supporting structures of, 589
Arterial aneurysm, 395
Arterial insufficiency, nursing diagnoses and documentation for, 397
Arterial oxygen saturation, 64
Arterial peripheral vessels, examination of, 368-374
Arterial pulses, 78; see also Pulse
Arteries, 361, 362
Arteriosclerosis obliterans, 394
Arthritis
  assessment in, 597
  rheumatoid, 592, 629
Ascites, 454
ASD; see Atrial septal defect
Asian/Pacific Islander culture, 31-37
Aspen guidelines for serum albumin in older adult, 112
Aspirin
  food interaction with, 113
  as ototoxic drug, 250
Assessment
  of activities of daily living, 54
  health; see Health assessment
  in nursing process, 1, 2
  nutritional, 93-114; see also Nutrition
  physical; see Physical assessment
Assessment alert
  for adolescent, 111
  for adult nutrition, 97
  for preschool and school-age child, 110
Assessment Tool for Measuring Maternal Attachment, 21
Asthma, 324, 348
  documentation and nursing diagnosis in, 354
Ataxic respirations, 80, 333
Atelectasis, 348
Atherosclerosis, peripheral, 394
Athlete's foot, 151
Atresia, biliary, 476
Atrial kick, 360
Atrial septal defect, 392
Atrioventricular nodes, 359, 360
Atrioventricular valves, 359-360
Atrophy, 131
  of muscle mass, 595
Attention deficit/hyperactivity disorder, 651, 679
Audiometer, 68
Auditory canal
  common problems or conditions of, 268-269
  examination of, 255-259
    in infant, 262
  external, 247
    common problems or conditions in, 267-268
    infection of, 249, 250, 256
    otoscope for, 67

Auditory response cradle, 262
Auditory system, 247-276
  of adolescent, 264
  age-related variations in, 262-264
  anatomy and physiology of, 247-248
  of child, 263
    developmental considerations for, 248
    health history and, 252-253
  common problems or conditions in, 267-271
    auditory canal in, 268-269
    documentation for, 272-273
    external ear in, 267-268
    hearing loss in, 271
    middle ear in, 270-271
    nursing diagnoses for, 272-273
    tympanic membrane in, 270-271
    vestibular function in, 271
  developmental considerations for, 248
  ethnic and cultural considerations of, 251, 258, 265
  examination of, 254-266
    auditory canal and, 255-259
    ear, 254-255
    hearing and, 259-261
    screening, 67, 68, 259-261
    tympanic membrane and, 255-259
  health history and, 249-253
  health promotion for, 274-275
  of infant, 262-263
    developmental considerations for, 248
    health history and, 252
  of older adult, 264
    developmental considerations for, 248
    health history and, 253
  in pregnancy, 264
    developmental considerations for, 248
  racial variations in, 257
  screening examination for, 269-261
    audiometer for, 68
    tuning fork for, 67
  situational variations in, 264-265
Aura, 648
Auricle, 247
Auscultation
  brachial artery, 368
  characteristics of sounds heard by, 76
  of chest, 338-340, 341
  of heart, 379-381
  in physical assessment, 74-76
Authoritarian data collection interview, 42
Autonomic nervous system, 644, 646
A-V nicking, 293
AV nodes; see Atrioventricular nodes
Axial skeleton, 589
Axilla, 401-436
  anatomy and physiology of, 401, 402
  breast and; see Breast
  characteristics of, 405
  developmental considerations for, 402-403
  examination of, 416-417
    lymph nodes in, 169, 174
  hair development and, 486
  health history and, 404-409
  lymph nodes in, 166, 168, 169
    examination of, 169, 174
  temperature measurement and, 76
Axillary lines, 320-322

B

B lymphocytes, 165
B vitamins, deficiency of, 98, 99
Babinski reflex, 671
  testing for, 662-664
Back pain, 614
  in kidney infection, 444
  in lumbar disk Injury, 622
Bacterial infection
  endocarditis in, 391
  otitis media in, 270
  of skin, hair, and nails, 151-153
Bag of worms, 554
Balance, 251
  examination of, 657-658
Balanitis, 544
Ballottement, 465, 619
Barlow-Ortolani maneuver, 623, 624
Barrel chest, 322, 331
Barrier protection, 71
Bartholin glands, 482
  inflamed, 520
  inspection of, 499-500
Basal cell carcinoma, 154
  prevention of, 161
Basal ganglia, 643
  Parkinson's disease and, 678
Basilar arteries, 637, 640
Bayley Infant Neurodevelopmental Screener, 21
Bayley Scale of Infant Development, 21
Beans in food pyramid, 102
Behavior, mental status and, 665
Behavioral development
  of infant, 9, 10-11
  of preschooler, 12, 16
  of school-age child, 13
  of toddler, 12
Beliefs about health and illness, 28, 34-35
Bell of stethoscope, 62
Bell's palsy, 193
Benign breast disease, 404, 405, 429
Benign prostatic hypertrophy, 576
Beriberi, 99
Biceps reflex, testing for, 662-664
Bigeminal pulse, 370
Biischial diameter of pelvis, 515
Bilateral hemianopia, 307
Bile, 439
Bile ducts
  in biliary atresia, 476
  common problems or conditions of, 458, 474-475
  obstruction of, 458
Bilingualism, 36-37
Bilirubin, 439
Bimanual examination for female internal genitalia, 506-509
BINS; see Bayley Infant Neurodevelopmental Screener
Biochemical tests
  in adolescent, 110
  defined, 93
  in neonate and infant, 107
  in nutritional assessment, 95-96
  in older adult, 112
  in pregnancy, 100-101

Biochemical tests—cont'd
  in preschooler and school-age child, 109
  in toddler, 108
Biographic data in health history, 43
  documentation of, 56
  of infant and child, 50
  of newborn, 48
  of pregnant woman, 55
Biot respiration, 80, 333
Birth control, 490
Birth history, hearing loss and, 252
Birthmarks, 123, 136
Bitot's spots, 98
Blackheads, 139
Bladder, urinary, 440
  in infant and child, 466
Bleeding
  postmenopausal, 495
  rectal, 563
    nursing diagnosis and documentation in, 578
Blepharitis, 304
Blind spot, 281
Blindness, legal, 284
Blood
  circulation of, 361, 362; see also Peripheral vessels
    personal habits and, 363
  coughing up, 364
  universal precautions for, 71
Blood chemistry; see Biochemical tests
Blood flow, 361, 362; see also Peripheral vessels
Blood glucose
  in neonate and infant, 107
  nutritional status and, 96
  in pregnancy, 101
Blood pressure, 79-81, 82, 368-369
  in child, 87
  diurnal variation in, 81
  examiner error in, 81
  measurement of
    equipment for, 63-64, 79
    mechanisms of, 80-81, 82
    procedure for, 79, 81, 368-369
  normal, 80
  in older adult, 383
  in pregnancy, 87, 362, 384
  racial variations in, 369, 385, 394
Blood pressure cuffs, 64, 368
Blood urea nitrogen in neonate and infant, 107
BMI; see Body mass index
BNBAS; see Brazelton Neonatal Assessment Scale
Body cavities, transilluminator and, 70
Body fluids
  transilluminator for differentiation of, 70
  universal precautions for, 71
Body hair, 133
  increased growth of, 157
Body image disturbance as nursing diagnosis
  in female reproductive system disorders, 525, 526
  in male breast enlargement, 434
  in skin lesions, 159
  in thyroid dysfunction, 211
Body mass index, 94, 95, 96
Body temperature, 76
Bones
  of head and neck, 185
    in infant, 188

Bones—*cont'd*
    inspection of, 595
    of nasal cavity, 213
    pain in, 592
    of pelvis, 585
    percussion of, 75
    racial variation of, 590
    of trunk, 585
Bony pelvis, female, 483, 486
Bony prominences vulnerable to pressure, 143, 144
Borborygmi, 451
Bouchard's nodes, 610, 611
Bounding pulsations, 378
Boutonniere deformity, 610
Bowel function, changes in, 456-457, 562
Bowel sounds, 451
Bowleg, 614
BPH; *see* Benign prostatic hypertrophy
Brachial artery auscultation, 368
Brachial pulse, 78, 372
Brachioradial reflex, testing for, 662-664
Bradycardia, 369
Bradypnea, 80, 332, 333
Brain, 637, 640
    arteries of, 637, 640
Brainstem, 643
Brazelton Neonatal Assessment Scale, 21
Breads in food pyramid, 102
Breast, 401-436
    of adolescent, 424
        developmental considerations for, 402, 403
        health history and, 407-408
    age-related variations in, 423-424
    anatomy and physiology of, 401, 402
    cancer of, 429, 430
        ethnic and cultural variations in, 427
        history of, 405
        in men, 406, 422, 432
        prevention and screening for, 435
        risk factors for, 406
    of child, 423-424
        developmental considerations for, 402
        health history and, 406-407
    common problems or conditions of, 429-432
        documentation in, 433-434
        in female, 429-431
        in male, 432
        nursing diagnoses in, 433-434
    cystic disease of, 404, 405, 429
    development of, 402-403, 486
    engorgement of, 409, 425, 426
    ethnic and cultural variations in, 427
    examination of, 410-428
        female, 410-421, 428
        inspection in, 410-416
        in integrated assessment, 690-692
        male, 422, 428
        mass characteristics in, 418
        nipple discharge cytology in, 414
        palpation in, 417-421
        self-, 421, 435
    female
        anatomy and physiology of, 401, 402
        common problems or conditions of, 429-431
        examination of, 410-421, 428

Breast—*cont'd*
    female—*cont'd*
        in lactation, 403, 409, 425-426
        in pregnancy, 101, 402, 408, 425
    fibroadenoma of, 429
    health history and, 404-409
    health promotion and, 435
    hyperpigmentation and erythema of, 411
    of infant, 423
        developmental considerations for, 402
        health history and, 406
    intraductal papilloma of, 430
    lumps or thickening of, 404, 405, 429
    lymph nodes in, 166-169, 401
        examination of, 169, 174
    male
        common problems or conditions of, 403, 406, 432, 522
        developmental considerations for, 403
        examination of, 422, 428
        health history and, 406, 408
    masses in
        characteristics of, 418
        differentiation of, 431
        palpation of, 417
        subareolar, in adolescent male, 424
    of older adult, 424
        developmental considerations for, 403
        health history and, 408
    Paget's disease of, 405, 414, 430
    pain or tenderness in, 404
    racial variations in, 415, 417
    in review of systems, 46
        documentation of, 57
        of infant and child, 51
        in pregnant woman, 55
    screening recommendation for, 435
    self-examination of, 421, 435
    situational variations in, 425-427
    skin characteristics of, 405
Breast-feeding, 488
    health promotion and, 435; *see also* Lactation
    stools and, 565
Breath
    odor of, 227
    shortness of, 364
Breath sounds, 337, 338-340, 341
    in infant, 343
Breathing; *see also* Respirations
    abnormal, 332-333
    altered pattern of, as nursing diagnosis in cough, 355
    chest pain with, 325
    ineffective pattern of, as nursing diagnosis in asthma, 354
Breathing distance, 344
Breathing problems, 323-325
Bronchi, 317, 319
Bronchial breath sounds, 338-340
Bronchiectasis, 349
Bronchitis, 324, 349
Bronchophony, 340-342
Bronchovesicular breath sounds, 339-340
Brudzinski's sign, 667, 668
Bruising, 119, 124
    in child, 138-139

Bruising—*cont'd*
    inspection of, 125
    in newborn, 136
    in older adults, 594
Bruits, 199, 371
    in abdominal examination, 451
    stethoscope and, 62
BSID-II; *see* Bayley Scale of Infant Development
Buccal mucosa, 230
    common problems or conditions of, 241-243
Bulbar conjunctiva
    in infant, 296
    in older adult, 298
Bulge sign, 619
Bulimia, 446
    in adolescent, 110
    in pregnancy, 104
Bulla, 128
BUN; *see* Blood urea nitrogen
Bundle of His, 360
Burning, rectal, 563-564
Bursae, 587, 590
Bursitis, 629

C

CABS; *see* Children's Adaptive Behavior Scale Revised
Café au lait spots, 136
Caffeine
    documentation of intake of, 58
    in pregnancy, 103
CAI; *see* Career Assessment Inventory
Calcaneovarus, 631
Calcium
    in older adult, 112
    in pregnancy, 103
    recommended dietary allowances of, 101
Calculi
    gallbladder, 475
    renal, 476
Calgary Family Assessment, 24
Caliente, 34
Callus, 122, 155
    of feet, 616
Calories, deficiency of, 98, 99
Canal of Schlemm, 278
Cancer; *see* Carcinoma; specific organ
Candida albicans, 505; *see also* Candidiasis
Candidiasis
    oral, 241
    on skin, 152
    venereal, 505, 522
Canker sore, 241
Caput succedaneum, 193
Carbon dioxide transfer in respiratory system, 317
Carcinoma; *see also* specific organ
    basal cell, 154
        prevention of, 161
    squamous cell, of skin, 154
Cardiac glycosides, food interaction with, 113
Cardiac output, fatigue and, 365
Cardiac sphincter, 438
Cardiovascular system; *see also* Heart; Peripheral vessels
    in nutritional assessment, 99
    in review of systems, 46

Cardiovascular system—*cont'd*
 documentation of, 57
 of infant and child, 51
 in pregnant woman, 55
Career Assessment Inventory, 22
Career choice, 18
Caretakers of infant and child, psychosocial status
 of, 51
Carotid arteries, 637, 640
Carotid pulse, 371
Carpal tunnel syndrome, 628
 tests for, 618
Cartilage, 587, 590
Cartilaginous joints, 583-584
Cataracts, 292, 308
 nursing diagnoses and documentation in, 314
Cauliflower ear, 267
Cavernous hemangioma, 137
Cavities
 air in
  paranasal sinuses and, 213
  transilluminator for differentiation of, 70
 lung; *see* Lung
 nasal
  bones of, 213
  inspection of, 223-224, 225
CC; *see* Chief complaint
CDC; *see* Centers for Disease Control and Prevention
Cellulitis, 151
Centers for Disease Control and Prevention
 on personal protective equipment, 71
 pregnancy recommendations of, 104
Centigrade temperature conversion, 76
Central nervous system
 anatomy and physiology of, 637-644, 645
 basal ganglia in, 643
 brain in, 637, 640
 brainstem in, 643
 cerebellum in, 643
 cerebrospinal fluid and, 637, 639
 cerebrum in, 637-642
 diencephalon in, 642-643
 disorders of, 677-678
 limbic system in, 643
 protective structures of, 637, 638
 in review of systems, 47
  documentation of, 57
  of infant and child, 51
  of newborn, 49
 spinal cord in, 643-644, 645
 ventricular system of, 637, 639
Central neurogenic hyperventilation, 80
Cephalhematoma, 193, 200
Cereals in food pyramid, 102
Cerebellar function, 657-660
Cerebellum, 643
Cerebral cortex topography, 641
Cerebral palsy, 679
Cerebrospinal fluid, 637, 639
Cerebrovascular accident, 678
 health history and, 649
 health promotion and, 682
 nursing diagnoses and sample documentation
  of, 681
 in older adult, 651

Cerebrum, 637-642
Cerumen
 cleaning of ears for, 275
 dry, 248
 ear examination and, 256
 excessive, 268
 impacted, 249, 268
Cervical lymph nodes, 166, 167, 168
 examination of, 173
Cervical vertebrae, 185
 assessment of, 601, 626
Cervix, 482
 bimanual examination for, 507
 cancer of, 518
  risk for, 491, 504-505
 collection of smears from, 504-505
 common problems and conditions of, 518
 dilation of, for infant delivery, 515
 discharge from, 504
 inspection of, 503-504
  vaginal speculum for, 70
 during pregnancy, 486, 488
Chalazion, 304
Change in Life Events Scale for Children, 22
Cheese in food pyramid, 102
Cheilosis, 98
Chemistry, blood; *see* Biochemical tests
Cherry angioma, 125
Chest
 barrel, 322, 331
 circumference of
  in child, 86, 87
  in newborn and infant, 83-84, 86, 87,
   106-107
 examination of, 333-342
  in integrated examination, 689-692
 expansion of, 334
 funnel, 331, 332
 pain in, 325, 363-364
 percussion of, 74, 75
 pigeon, 331
 thoracic cage and, 317-320
 wall of
  configuration of, 330-332
  expansion of, 334
  retractions of, 377
Cheyne-Stokes respirations, 80, 333
Chicken pox, 149
Chief complaint, 43
Child; *see also* Preschooler; School-age child;
 Toddler
 developmental assessment of, 12-17
 external genitalia examination for, 510-511
 health history of, 49-52
 school-age, 13-17
 vital signs of, 86-87
 weight and height of, 86, 87-91
Child abuse, history of, 493-494
Childhood illnesses in health history, 43
Children's Adaptive Behavior Scale Revised, 22
Chinese health practices, 35, 37
Chlamydial infection, 522
 collection of cultures for, 505
 health history and, 492
 signs and symptoms of, 524
Chloasma melasma, 142

Choking in infant and child, 327
Cholecystitis, 458
 with cholelithiasis, 475
 pain in, 456-457
Cholelithiasis, 475
Cholesterol
 cardiovascular system and, 363, 398
 in health eating guidelines, 97
 in older adult, 112
 total, nutritional status and, 96
Choroid, 277
Chronic disability, 594
Chronic illness in health history, 44
Chronic obstructive pulmonary disease, 345, 349
Chronic renal failure, 476
Cigarette smoking; *see* Smoking
Ciliary body, 277-278
Cimetidine, breast milk and, 409
Circle of Willis, 637, 640
Circulatory system, 361, 362; *see also* Peripheral
 vessels
 personal habits and, 363
Circumcision, 539, 543
 examination of infant and, 548
Circumduction, 585
Cirrhosis, 452, 474
Clarification in data collection interview, 41
Clavicles, 320
Clavus, 155
Claw toes, 616
Cleft lip, 240
Clicking of joints, 593
Client
 communication with, in interview, 40-43
 interruption of, 42
 personal beliefs about health and illness of, 28
 positioning of
  for female reproductive system assessment,
   497-498
  for physical assessment, 76, 77
Clinical evaluation
 in adolescent, 110
 in nutritional assessment, 93
  of adult, 96-97, 98-99
  of neonate and infant, 107-108
 in pregnancy, 101-104
 in older adult, 112
 in preschooler and school-age child, 109
 in toddler, 108
Clitoris, 481, 482
 inspection of, 499
Clonus reflex, 671
Closed-ended questions, 41
Clubbing of nails, 134, 374
Clubfoot, 624, 631
Cluster headache, 189, 203
Cluster respirations, 80
CMV infection; *see* Cytomegalovirus infection
Coarctation of aorta, 393
 in infant, 382
Cocaine
 cardiovascular system and, 363
 eye signs and, 300
Coccygeal area, 568
Coccyx, 483, 486
COG; *see* Crib-o-gram

Cognitive abilities
  development of, 8
  mental status and, 667
Coining, 119
Colchicine, food interaction with, 113
Cold extremities, 374
Cold sores, 148, 239
Colds, 219
Colicky pain, 442
Colitis, 562
  ulcerative, 473, 563
Coloboma, 310
Colon, 438; see also Gastrointestinal system
Color vision testing in child, 297
Colorectal cancer, 575
  health promotion in, 580
  risk factors for, 562
Colostomy, 573-574
Colostrum, 402, 403
Columns of Morgagni, 559
Coma, Glasgow Coma Scale for, 667, 668
Comedones, 139
Communication
  ethnic and cultural influences on, 29, 36-37
  in interview for health history, 40-43
  primary method of, 29
Community access of older adult, 54
Comprehensive health assessment, 39-40
Condoms, female, 528
Conductive hearing loss, 248, 260, 271, 655
Condyloid joints, 584-585
Condylomata
  in female, 522
  in male, 552
Cones, 279
Confrontation in data collection interview, 41
Confrontation test, 285
Confusion, nutritional assessment and, 99
Congenital dislocation of hip, 630
  tests for, 623, 627
Congenital heart defects, 382, 391-393
  health history and, 366, 367
Congenital hypothyroidism, 212
Congenital lymphedema, 179
Congenital rubella, 366
Congestion, sinus, 219
Congestive heart failure, 364, 365, 390
  in infant, 367
Conjunctiva, 277
  in infant, 296
  inspection of, 289-290
  in nutritional assessment, 98
  in older adult, 298
Conjunctivitis, 289, 306
Connective tissue of abdomen, 437-438
Consciousness
  changes in, 649
  loss of, in head injury, 191
Constipation, 563
  health promotion and, 580
  as nursing diagnosis
    in rectal bleeding, 578
    in thyroid dysfunction, 211
  in pregnancy, 103, 561, 566
Contact dermatitis, 146

Contraceptives, 528
  fluid retention and, 365
  use of, 490
  vaginal discharge and, 490
Contracture of hip, flexion, 621
Convergence, drug intoxication and, 300
Cooper's ligaments, 401
Coordination, examination of, 658-660
COPD; see Chronic obstructive pulmonary disease
Coping
  ineffective, as nursing diagnosis in asthma, 354
  psychosocial status of child and, 52
Copper, deficiency of, 98, 99
Cor pulmonale, 390
Corn, 155
Cornea, 277, 278
  abrasion or ulcer of, 306
    Wood's lamp for detecting, 70
  inspection of, 291
  nutrition and, 98
  in older adult, 298
Corneal arcus, 291
Corneal reflex, 286-287
  drug intoxication and, 300
  in older adult, 280
Corona, 531
Coronary arteries, 359
Corpora cavernosa, 531
  thrombosis of, 536
Corpus spongiosum, 531
Costal angle, 320
Costovertebral angle, 74
  tenderness at, 461-462
Cough, 323-324
  cardiovascular system and, 364
  nursing diagnoses and documentation in, 355
Cover-uncover test, 287
Crackles, 74, 341
Cradle cap, 138, 146
Cramps, leg, 366
Cranial bones of infant, 591
Cranial nerves, 642, 643, 644; see also Peripheral nervous system
  I, 223, 642, 644, 652
  II, 642, 643, 644
    destruction of, 309
    in eye anatomy and physiology, 277, 279, 280
    pupils of eye and, 292
  III, 642, 643, 644, 654
    damage to, 310
    destruction of, 309
    eye anatomy and, 277-278, 279, 280
    eye movement and, 286
    in pupil size and shape, 292
  IV, 642, 643, 644, 653
    eye movement and, 277, 286
  V, 600, 642, 643, 644
    edema of brainstem and, 291
    eye and, 277
    in neck, 185
    tests for, 653-654, 655
  VI, 642, 643, 644, 653
    eye movement and, 277, 286
  VII, 642, 643, 644
    edema of brainstem and, 291

Cranial nerves—cont'd
  VII—cont'd
    eye movement and, 277
    in neck, 185
    teeth alignment and, 228
    tests for, 654, 655
  VIII, 642, 643
    ear anatomy and, 247, 248
    testing of, 259, 261, 655
  IX, 642, 643, 644
    tests for, 656
  X, 642, 643, 644
    tests for, 656
  XI, 642, 643, 644
    in neck, 197
    tests for, 657
  XII, 642, 643, 644
    tests for, 656
    tongue movement and, 231
  brainstem and, 643
  in child, 672
Craniotabes, 98
Cremasteric reflex, 665
Crepitus, 334, 595, 596, 600
Crib-o-gram, 262
CRICHT; see Crichton Geriatric Rating Scale
Crichton Geriatric Rating Scale, 23
Crohn's disease, 472
Croup, 350
Cruciate ligament tears, 620
Crying, interview and, 42
Cryptorchidism, 548
Crystallized intelligence, 8
Cuerandera, 27
Cuffs, blood pressure, 64, 368
Cultural diversity, 27; see also Ethnic and cultural considerations
  in interview, 42
Cultural groups, 30-37
Cultural sensitivity, 27
Cupping, 119
Cushing syndrome, 206
Cutaneous tags, 41, 140
Cutaneous tenderness of abdomen, 454, 455
CVA; see Costovertebral angle
Cyanosis, 119, 122, 124, 332
  in infant or child, 367, 382
  peripheral, 375, 376
Cycles per second of sound wave, 68
Cyst, 128
  gingival, in infant, 234
  Meibomian, 288
  Nabothian, 518
  pilonidal, 567, 575
  sebaceous, 128, 268
Cystic disease of breast, 404, 405, 429
Cystic fibrosis, 346, 350
Cystitis, acute, 537
Cystocele, 501, 521
Cytology of nipple discharge, 414
Cytomegalovirus infection, 311

D

Dacryocystitis, 289, 306
Darwinian tubercle, 254, 267

Data
  collection of, for health history
    extent of, 39-40
    scope of, 43-48
  recording of, 3
  types of, 2
Death rate, ethnic and cultural influences on, 33
Decibels, 68
Deciduous teeth, 217
Decongestants, hypertension and, 363
Deep tendon reflexes, 644, 647
  percussion hammer for, 68
  testing for, 662-664
Deformities
  muscular, 593
  of toes, 616
Dehydration
  in child, 139
  in older adult, 112
Delirium, 677
Delivery, trauma during, 594
Dementia, 677
Demographic trends, 30-31
Dental care
  cultural considerations in, 229
  health history and, 221
  in health promotion, 246
  in older adult, 236
Dentition of permanent teeth, 216
Dentures, health history and, 221
Denver II assessment test, 14-15, 22
Dependent leg edema, 365
Depression, 677
  nursing diagnoses and sample documentation
    of, 680
  in older adult, 651
Dermatitis, 146-147
  stasis, 129, 147
Dermatologic problems, 146-148
Dermatomes, 644, 645
Dermis, 115-116
Development, theories of, 7-8
Developmental assessment, 7-25
  of adolescent, 17-18
  of adult, 18-19
    in early adulthood, 18, 19
    in middle adulthood, 18, 19
    in older adulthood, 19
  of child, 12-17
  of family, 20
  of infant, 9-11
  instruments for, 21-24
  theories of development and, 7-8
Developmental dysplasia, 630
Developmental tasks
  of family, 20
  of infant and toddler, 9, 10-11
  of middle adults, 19
  of older adult, 19
  of preschooler, 16
  of school-age child, 17
  of toddler, 9, 24
  of young adult, 19
Deviation
  of nasal septum, 224

Deviation—cont'd
  tracheal, 330, 333
Dextrocardia, 379, 382
Diabetes mellitus
  blood glucose in, 96
  cardiovascular disease in, 384
Diabetic retinopathy, 311
Diagnoses
  NANDA, 4-5
  in nursing process, 1, 2
Diagonal conjugate, 513, 514
Diameters of pelvis, 513-515
Diaper rash, 138, 493, 539
Diaphragm, 317
  of stethoscope, 61-62
Diaphragmatic excursion, 336-338
Diarthrotic joints, 584, 586, 589
Diastasis recti
  in child, 466
  in pregnancy, 440, 467
Diastole
  blood pressure and, 79, 368-369
  heart and, 359-360, 361
Diastolic murmurs, 388-389
Diencephalon, 642-643
Diet
  adequacy of, 97, 100-101, 102
  of child, 445
  documentation of, 56
  ethnic and cultural influences on, 29
  fiber in, 563
  iodine in, 212
  stool characteristics and, 565, 566
Dietary assessment, 93
  in adolescent, 110-111
  in adult, 97, 100-101, 102
  in neonate and infant, 108
  in older adult, 112-113
  in postpartum and lactating women, 106
  in pregnancy, 104-105
  in preschooler and school-age child, 109-110
  in toddler, 108-109
Diffusion, 79, 317
Digitalis, food interaction with, 113
Dilation of cervix for infant delivery, 515
Diphtheria, tetanus, and pertussis immunization,
    162-163
Diphtheria and tetanus toxoids and acellular per-
    tussis vaccine, 162-163
Diplopia, 282, 310
Direct inguinal hernia, 550
Directive questions, 41
Disability, chronic, 594
Dislocations, 629
  congenital hip, 630
    test for, 623, 627
Disorientation, 667
Disposable, single-use thermometer strips, 61, 62
Distention, abdominal, 444, 450
Diuretics
  food interaction with, 113
  sexual function and, 538
Diverticular disease, 473
  pain in, 456-457
Diverticulitis, 473

Diverticulosis, 473
Diverticulum, Meckel, 476
Dizziness, 190
  auditory system and, 251
  in health history, 648
  in older adult, 194
Documentation
  forms for, 697
  of health assessment data, 3, 697-699
    format for, 698-699
  of health history, 56, 699
Doppler ultrasonic stethoscope, 64, 87
Dorsal recumbent position, 77
Dorsal roots of spinal nerves, 644
Dorsalis pedis pulse, 373
Dowager hump, 632
Down syndrome, 205
Drawer test, 620
Drugs
  abuse of
    documentation of, 58
    eye signs of, 299-300
    in pregnancy, 103
  bowel habits and, 563
  breast milk and, 409
  food interactions with, in older adult, 112, 113
  in health history, 43
    documentation and, 56, 58
    of older adult, 54
  intoxication from, eye in, 299-300
  nausea and vomiting from, 443
  neurologic health history and, 650
  ototoxic, 250
  sexual function and, 541
Dry cerumen, 248
Dry eyes in older adult, 280
Dry skin, 131
  history of, 118
Dry smear, vaginal or cervical, 505
DTaP; see Diphtheria and tetanus toxoids and acel-
    lular pertussis vaccine
DTP; see Diphtheria, tetanus, and pertussis immu-
    nization
Ductus arteriosus, patent, 391
Dull chest tones, 336
Dullness, 74
  abdominal, 452, 454, 462
Duodenum, 438
Dura mater, 637, 638
Duration of sound, 76
Dysphagia, 220, 444
  health history and, 649
Dysphasia
  expressive, 651
  health history and, 650
Dysplasia, developmental, 630
Dyspnea, 364
  paroxysmal nocturnal, 324
Dystrophy, muscular, 631

E

"E" chart, 65, 284
  for child, 297
Ear; see also Auditory system
  anatomy and physiology of, 247-248

Ear—*cont'd*
  cauliflower, 267
  of child, 51, 253
  cleaning of, 275
  color of, 255
  discharge from, 249, 255, 257
  examination of, 254-255
  external, 247; *see also* Auditory canal, external
    common problems or conditions in, 267-268
    infection of, 247
    otoscope for, 67
  foreign body in, 269, 275
  in health history, 249-250
  of infant, 51, 262-263
    alignment of, 263
  infection of, in child, 253
  injury to, 249
  inner, 247
  itching of, 250
  low-set, 254
  middle, 247, 248
    common problems or conditions of, 270-271
  otoscope for, 67
  pain in
    in child, 253
    health history and, 249-250
  in review of systems, 46
    documentation of
    of infant and child, 51
    of newborn, 49
    in pregnant woman, 55
  ringing in, 250
Ear canal, external; *see* Auditory canal, external
Ear pieces of stethoscope, 61, 62
Earache
  in child, 253
  health history and, 249-250
  nursing diagnosis in, 273
Early adulthood, developmental assessment in, 18, 19
Eating; *see also* Nutrition
  in adolescent, 110, 446
  assessment of, 54
  difficulty in, 444
    in older adult, 112
  guidelines for healthy, 97
  in preschool and school-age child, 110
Eating disorders
  in adolescent, 446
  in pregnancy, 104
Ecchymosis, 98, 119, 124
  inspection of, 125
Eccrine sweat glands, 116
ECG; *see* Electrocardiogram
Ectopic pregnancy, 456-457
Ectropion, 303
Eczema, 146
Edema
  in nutritional assessment, 99
  peripheral, 375, 376
    dependent leg, 365
    popliteal, 616
  in pregnancy, 362
  in tumor or inflammation, 595
Education, ethnic and cultural influences on, 30-31
Efferent fibers of spinal nerves, 644

Effusion
  pericardial, 379
  pleural, 352
Eggs in food pyramid, 102
Egophony, 342
Ejaculation, 531
  difficulty with, 537-538
Elbow
  assessment of, 608-609, 626
  range of motion of, 609
  supporting structures of, 590
Electric conduction of heart, 360, 361
Electrocardiogram, 360
Electronic sphygmomanometer, 63
Electronic thermometer, 61, 62, 76
Elimination, altered
  in bowel function changes, 562
  in fecal incontinence, 564
  in irritable bowel disease, 456-457, 562
  urinary, 579
Ellipsoidal joints, 584-585
Embryonic ridge, milk line from, 415
Emotions
  blood pressure and, 81
  displays of, in interview, 42-43
  mental status and, 667
Emphysema, 350
Employment, ethnic and cultural influences on, 30-31
Encephalitis, 677
Encephalopathy, HIV, 677
Endocarditis, bacterial, 391
Endocrine system in review of systems, 47
  documentation of, 57
  of infant and child, 51
Endometriosis, 518
Endometrium, 483
  cancer of, 520
Enemas, 563
Energy intake per centimeter of height, 109
Engorgement, 425, 426
Enophthalmos, 288, 303
Environmental health
  of adolescent, 52
  documentation of, 58
  exposure to respiratory irritants and, 325-326
  in health history, 48, 49
  of infant and child, 52
  of newborn, 49
  of older adult, 55
  of pregnant woman, 56
Ephelides, 122, 123
Epicondylitis, 609
Epidermis, 115
Epididymides
  anatomy and physiology of, 531
  examination of, 546
  inflammation of, 554
Epididymitis, 554
Epigastric pain, nursing diagnoses and documentation in, 478
Epilepsy, 648
Epiphora, 282, 289
Epispadias, 544
Epistaxis, 220
Epithelial tissue, nutrition and, 98

Epstein-Barr mononucleosis, 180
Epstein's pearls, 234
Equilibrium, 251
Equipment, 61-72, 686
  audiometer in, 68
  for blood pressure measurement, 63-64, 79
  Doppler, 64
  goniometer in, 69
  nasal speculum in, 67
  near vision chart in, 66
  ophthalmoscope in, 66-67
  otoscope in, 67
  penlight in, 69
  percussion or reflex hammer in, 68
  personal protective, 71
  pulse oximetry in, 64
  ruler in, 69
  skin calipers in, 69, 82, 83-85, 94
  Snellen visual acuity chart in, 65
  stethoscope in, 61-62, 74-75
    Doppler ultrasonic, 87
  tape measure in, 69
  thermometers in, 61, 62, 76
  transilluminator in, 70
  tuning fork in, 67
  vaginal speculum in, 70
  Wood's lamp in, 70
Erb's palsy, 624
Erb's point, 379, 380
Erection, difficulty with, 537-538
Erikson's theory of personality development, 7, 8
Erosion, 130
Erythema, 124
  of breast, 411
Erythema toxicum, 138
Esophageal motility in older adult, 441
Esotropia, 286, 308
  nursing diagnoses and documentation in, 313
Essential fatty acids, deficiency of, 98
Estrogens, 483
  fluid retention and, 365
  galactorrhea and, 431
  gynecomastia and, 432
  lactation and, 403
  during pregnancy, 486
  in replacement therapy, 491
    breast cancer and, 408
Ethacrynic acid, food interaction with, 113
Ethmoidal sinuses, 225; *see also* Paranasal sinuses
Ethnic and cultural considerations, 27-38
  in acquired immunodeficiency syndrome, 179
  for anus, rectum, and prostate, 564, 574
  assessment and, 28-29
  for auditory system, 251, 258, 265
  for breast, 427
  cultural diversity in, 27
  cultural sensitivity in, 27
  in dental care, 229
  for eye and visual system, 301
  factual information in, 28, 30-37
  for female reproductive system, 517, 520
  for gastrointestinal system, 470, 471, 474
  for head and neck, 190, 191, 195, 200, 202, 207
  for heart and peripheral vessels, 384, 385, 390, 394, 398
  for interview, 42

Ethnic and cultural considerations—*cont'd*
 language barrier in, 27
 for lymph nodes, 174, 177
 of major cultural groups, 30-37
 for male genitalia, 549
 for musculoskeletal system, 625
 for neurologic system, 675, 677, 678
 in oral cavity cancer, 243
 in pregnancy, 496
 for respiratory system, 326, 346, 351, 352
 for skin, hair, and nails, 145
 stereotyping in, 28
 for teeth variations, 237
Evaluation in nursing process, 1, 2
Evaluation of Family Functioning Scale, 24
Eversion, 585
Exaggerated pectoriloquy, 342
Examination, physical; *see* Physical assessment
Excoriation, 130
Exercise
 health promotion and, 635
 pelvic muscle, 527
Exophthalmos, 192, 288, 304
Exotropia, 286, 303
Expert Committee on Clinical Guidelines for Over-
 weight in Adolescent Preventive Services, 110
Expiration, muscles of, 317
Exposure to respiratory irritants, 325-326
Expressive dysphasia, 651
Extension, 585
 joint, goniometer for measuring, 69
External ear; *see* Ear, external
External ear canal; *see* Auditory canal, external
External genitalia, female
 anatomy and physiology of, 481-482
 examination of, 498-501
External otitis, 249, 250
External rotation, 585
Extraocular muscles, 277, 278, 653
 in child, 297
 common problems or conditions of, 308
 of infant, 280, 296
 inspection of, 286, 296, 297
Extremities
 cold, 374
 inspection of, 595, 597
 lower
  assessment of, 693
  coordination in, 658, 660
  supporting structures of, 590
  measurement of, 596, 597
  muscular strength, sensation, and reflexes in,
   660-664
  of newborn, 623-624
 upper
  assessment of, 608-609
  coordination in, 658
  supporting structures of, 589-590
Eye and visual system, 277-316
 of adolescent, 298
  health history and, 283
  health promotion and, 315
 age-related variations in, 296-298
 alignment of, in child, 297
 anatomy and physiology of, 277-280
 of child, 297

Eye and visual system—*cont'd*
 developmental considerations for, 280
 health history and, 283
 health promotion and, 315
 common problems or conditions of, 303-312
  in external eye, 303-307
  extraocular muscles in, 308
  internal eye in, 308-312
  nursing diagnoses and, 313-314
  peripheral visual defects in, 307
 developmental considerations for, 280
 discharge from, 282
 dry, in older adult, 280
 ethnic and cultural variations in, 301
 examination of, 66-67, 284-302, 653
  external structures in, 288-290, 302
  globe in, 288, 290-292
  internal eye in, 292-295, 302
  ophthalmoscopic, 292-295, 302
  vision in; *see* Vision
 external structures of
  anatomy and physiology of, 277
  common problems or conditions in, 303-307
  examination of, 288-290, 302
 extraocular muscles of, 277, 278, 653
  in child, 297
  common problems or conditions of, 308
  in infant, 280, 296
  inspection of, 286, 296, 297
 globe of, 277-279, 288, 294
  inspection of, 290-292
 health history and, 281-283
 health promotion for, 315
 of infant, 296
  developmental considerations for, 280
  health history and, 282
 internal structures of
  anatomy and physiology of, 277-279, 294
  common problems or conditions of,
   308-312
  examination of, 288, 290-295, 302
  in older adult, 298
 movement of, 277, 278, 653
  in child, 297
  common problems or conditions of, 308
  in infant, 280, 296
  inspection of, 286, 296, 297
 nutrition and, 98
 of older adult, 298
  developmental considerations for, 280
  health history and, 283
  health promotion and, 315
 ophthalmoscopic examination of, 292-295, 302
 pain in, 281
 in pregnancy, 299
  developmental considerations for, 280
 prosthetic eye in, 299
 racial variation in, 288, 290, 294
 redness of, 282
 in review of systems, 45-46
  documentation of, 49
  of infant and child, 50
  of newborn, 49
  in pregnant woman, 55
 situational variations in, 299-300
 swelling of, 282

Eye and visual system—*cont'd*
 vision and; *see* Vision
 watering of, 282
Eyebrows, 196, 277
 in infant, 296
 inspection of, 288
 in older adult, 298
Eyelashes, 277
 in infant, 296
 inspection of, 288
Eyelids, 277
 eversion of upper, 290
 in infant, 296
 inspection of, 288
 in older adult, 298

F

Face
 bony structures of, 196
 movement and sensation of, 653-654, 655
 racial variation of, 590
FACES; *see* Family Adaptability and Cohesion
 Evaluation Scales
Facial hair, 133
 increased growth of, 157
Facial nerve, 642, 643, 644
 edema of brainstem and, 291
 eye and, 277
 teeth alignment and, 228
 tests for, 654, 655
Facilitation in data collection interview, 41
Fahrenheit temperature conversion, 76
Failure-to-thrive, 108
Fallopian tubes, 483
Fallot tetralogy, 393
Falls in older adults, 594
Falx cerebri, 637, 638
Family
 assessment of, 20
 development of, 20
 developmental tasks of, 20
 ethnic and cultural influences on, 29, 36-37
 functions of, 20
 health history of, 44
  documentation of, 57
  of infant and child, 50
  of newborn, 49
  in older adult, 53
  of pregnant woman, 55
 nonnuclear or nontraditional, 20
 psychosocial status of, 51
 single-parent, 20
Family Adaptability and Cohesion Evaluation
 Scales, 24
Family Environment assessment instrument, 24
Family Inventory of Life Events and Changes, 24
FAS; *see* Fetal alcohol syndrome
Fat
 distribution of, 82
 in food pyramid, 102
 in health eating guidelines, 97
Fathering Assessment Tool, 21
Fatigue
 cardiac output and, 365
 as nursing diagnosis

Fatigue—*cont'd*
  as nursing diagnosis—*cont'd*
    in depression, 680
    in thyroid dysfunction, 211
Fat-soluble vitamins, recommended dietary allowances for, 100
Fear, as nursing diagnosis
  in breast lumps, 433
  in cough, 355
  in female reproductive system disorders, 526
Fecal incontinence, 564
Feeding reflexes in infant, 671
Feet
  assessment of, 616-617, 627
  of newborn, 623-624
Female condom, 528
Female reproductive system, 481-529
  of adolescent, 511
    developmental considerations for, 486, 487
    health history and, 494-495
  age-related variations in, 510-512
  anatomy and physiology of, 481-485, 486
  bony pelvis in, 483, 486
  of child, 510-511
    developmental considerations for, 486
    health history and, 493-494
  common problems and conditions of, 518-524
    cervix in, 518
    nursing diagnosis in, 525-526
    ovaries in, 520
    sample documentation of, 525-526
    sexually transmitted disease in, 522-524
    uterus in, 518-520
    vulva and vagina in, 520-521
  developmental considerations for, 486-488
  ethnic and cultural variations in, 517, 520
  examination of, 497-517
    bimanual examination for, 506-509
    external genitalia, 498-501
    rectovaginal examination in, 509-510
    speculum examination for, 501-506
  external genitalia in
    anatomy and physiology of, 481-482
    examination of, 498-501, 693-694
  health history and, 489-496
  surgery in, 492
  health promotion for, 527-528
  hysterectomy and, 516
  of infant, 510
    developmental considerations for, 486
    health history and, 493
  internal genitalia in
    anatomy and physiology of, 482-483
    bimanual examination for, 506-509, 693
    rectovaginal examination of, 509-510
    speculum examination for, 501-506, 693
  in menopause, health history and, 491
  menstrual cycle in, 483, 484, 485
  of older woman, 512
    developmental considerations for, 486-488
    health history and, 491, 495-496
  of preadolescent
    developmental considerations for, 486, 487
    health history and, 494
  in pregnancy, 512-516
    developmental considerations for, 486-488

Female reproductive system—*cont'd*
  in pregnancy—*cont'd*
    health history and, 492-493, 496
    racial variation in, 498
    situational variations in, 512-517
Femoral arteries, bruits and, 451
Femoral pulse, 372
Femur, racial variation of, 590
FES assessment instrument; *see* Family Environment assessment instrument
Fetal alcohol syndrome, 207, 496
Fetal assessment, 55
  heart in, 87, 384, 470, 471
  position and, 468-469, 515
Fetal development of male genitalia, 534
Fetal head position, 515
Fetal heart rate, 87, 384, 470
Fetal heart tones, 471
Fetal lie, 469
Fetal position, palpation of, 468-469
Fetal presentation, 469
Fetoscopy, 87
Fiber in diet, 563
Fibrinolysin, prostate gland and, 559
Fibroadenoma of breast, 429
Fibrocystic disease of breast, 404, 405, 429
Fibroids of uterus, 519
Fibrous joints, 583-584
FILE; *see* Family Inventory of Life Events and Changes
Filipino health practices, 34, 35
Financial status, documentation of, 58
Fine motor function, examination of, 660
Finger
  assessment of, 610, 611
  clubbing of, 134
  coordination in, 659
  deformities of, 624
  range of motion of, 612, 613
Fingernails; *see* Nails
Finger-rubbing test, 259
First heart sound, 381
Fish in food pyramid, 102
Fissures, 130
  palpebral, 277
    racial variation in, 288
  rectal, 563, 575
Flat warts, 126
Flexion, 585
  joint, goniometer for measuring, 69
Flexion contractures of hip, 621
Floaters, 281
Floating mass in abdomen, 465, 471
Floppy infant syndrome, 594
Fluid, body
  transilluminator for differentiation of, 70
  universal precautions for, 71
Fluid intelligence, 8
Fluid volume deficit, risk for, 181
Fluorescein dye with Wood's lamp, 70
FOC; *see* Head, circumference of
FOC-to-MAC ratio, 106-107
Focused health assessment, 40
Folate; *see* Folic acid
Folic acid
  deficiency of, 98, 99
  recommended dietary allowances of, 101

Folk remedies, alternative, 27, 34-35
Folliculitis, 156
Fontanels, 188
  sunken, 193
  on vaginal examination, 516
Food and drug interactions in older adult, 112, 113
Food and Nutrition Board, National Academy of Sciences Recommended Dietary Allowances, revised 1989, 100-101
Food intolerance, 444
Food poisoning, 479
Food pyramid, 97, 102
Food records, 93
Food-frequency questionnaire, 93
Foot, supporting structures of, 590
Foreign body
  in ear, 269, 275
  in nose, 245
Formula-feeding, stools and, 565
Fortune telling, 35
Fovea centralis, 295
Fractures, 629
  assessment for, 597
Freckles, 122, 123
Fremitus, 335
Friction rub, pleural, 334, 335, 341
Frio, 34
Frontal bones, 185
Frontal sinuses, 225; *see also* Paranasal sinuses
  transillumination of, 226
Fruits in food pyramid, 102
Fundus
  of eye, 294
  uterine
    height of, 468
    palpation of, 467, 470
Fungal infection
  of female reproductive system, 522
  of skin, hair, and nails, 151, 158
  Wood's lamp for detecting, 70
Funnel chest, 331, 332
Furosemide
  food interaction with, 113
  as ototoxic drug, 250
Furuncle, 153
Fusiform aneurysm, 395

G

Gag reflex, 656
Gait, 595
  in child, 624, 672
  Parkinson's disease and, 678
  in pregnancy, 625
Galactorrhea, 431
Galactose in neonate and infant, 107
Gallbladder, 439, 440; *see also* Gastrointestinal system
  common problems or conditions of, 474-475
  examination of, 458
  palpation of, 458
  in pregnancy, 441
Ganglia, basal, 643
  Parkinson's disease and, 678
Gardnerella vaginalis, 505, 524
Gas bubbles, 75
Gas exchange, impaired, in cough, 355

Gastritis, 456-457
Gastroenteritis, 456-457, 562
Gastroesophageal reflux, 445, 456-457, 472
Gastrointestinal system, 437-480
  of adolescent, 446
  age-related variations in, 466-467
  anatomy and physiology of, 437-440
  of child, 466
    health history and, 445
  common problems or conditions of, 472-476
    nursing diagnoses and sample documentation
      for, 477-478
  developmental considerations for, 440-441
  ethnic and cultural variations in, 470, 471, 474
  examination of, 448-471
    abdomen in, 450-452, 454-458, 461-465, 471;
      see also Abdomen
    abdominal floating mass in, 465, 471
    abdominal fluid in, 462-463, 471
    abdominal pain in, 463-464, 471
    abdominal reflexes in, 461
    gallbladder in, 458
    guidelines for, 448-449
    inguinal nodes in, 460
    kidneys in, 459, 461-462, 471
    liver in, 452-453, 458
    spleen in, 454, 459
  health history and, 442-447
  health promotion for, 479
  of infant, 466
    health history and, 445
    problems or conditions and, 476
  nutrition and, 99; see also Nutrition
  of older adult, 467
    developmental considerations for, 441
    health history and, 446-447
  in pregnancy, 101-103, 467-471
    developmental considerations for, 440-441
    problems or conditions and, 476
  racial variation in, 470
  in review of systems, 46
    of adolescent, 52
    documentation of, 57
    of newborn, 49
    in pregnant woman, 55
Gay men, 538
  male genitalia examination in, 549
Gaze, cardinal fields of, 286
Gender, blood pressure and, 81
General health status; see Health status, general
General physical assessment, 82, 83; see also
  Physical assessment
Genital herpes
  eye infection of newborn and, 282
  in female, 522
  in male, 552
Genital self-examination
  by female, 527
  by male, 557
Genital warts
  in female, 522, 524
  in male, 552
Genitalia
  female external
    anatomy and physiology of, 481-482
    examination of, 498-501, 693-694

Genitalia—cont'd
  female internal
    anatomy and physiology of, 482-483
    bimanual examination for, 506-509, 693
    speculum examination for, 501-506, 693
  male, 531-558; see also Male genitalia
  in review of systems, 47
    of adolescent, 52
    documentation of, 57
    of infant and child
    of newborn, 49
    in pregnant woman, 56
Genogram, 45
Gentamicin, ototoxicity of, 250
Genu valgum, 614
Genu varum, 614
Geriatric Scale of Recent Life Events, 23
German measles, 150
Gestation
  multiple, 104; see also Pregnancy
  period of, racial variations in, 470
Gingival cysts in infant, 234
Glandular tissue, nutrition and, 99
Glans penis, 531
Glasgow Coma Scale, 667, 668
Glaucoma, 282, 312
Glomerulonephritis, 476
Glossitis, 98
Glossopharyngeal nerve, 642, 643, 644
  tests for, 656
Gloves for universal blood and body fluid precau-
  tions, 71
Glucose, blood
  in neonate and infant, 107
  nutritional status and, 96
  in pregnancy, 101
Gluteal folds, uneven, 624
Goiter, 198
Golfer's elbow, 609
Goniometer, 69, 599
Gonorrhea, 523
  collection of cultures for, 505
  eye infection of newborn and, 282
  health history and, 492
  signs and symptoms of, 524
Goodenough-Harris Drawing Test, 22
Gout, 616, 628
Gower's sign, 672
Gowns for universal blood and body fluid precau-
  tions, 71
Grain products in food pyramid, 102
Graphesthesia, 661, 662
Graves' disease, 192, 208
Graves' speculum, 70
Great vessels, 359
  heart and; see Heart
Grid light of ophthalmoscope, 67
Grip strength, 612
Groin
  lymph nodes in, 168, 169, 170
    examination of, 175
  pain in, 536
Grooming, mental status and, 665
Growth and development
  altered
    high risk for, in child with ear disorders, 273

Growth and development—cont'd
  altered—cont'd
    potential for, in male genitalia problems, 555
  growth curves for, 88-91
  of infant, 9, 10-11
  of preschooler, 12, 16
  of school-age child, 13
  of toddler, 12
Grunting in infant, 343
Guillain-Barré syndrome, 679
Gums
  common problems or conditions of, 240
  inspection of, 229-230
  nutrition and, 98
Gynecomastia, 403, 406, 432, 522

H

Habits
  of infant and child, 51
  personal; see Personal habits
Haemophilus influenzae type b conjugate vaccine,
  162-163
Haemophilus vaginalis, 505
Hair, 115-164
  age-related variations in, 136-142
    health history and, 120-121
  anatomy and physiology of, 115-116
  cells in, 116
  common problems or conditions of, 156-157
    nursing diagnoses and sample documentation
      for, 159-160
  developmental considerations for, 116-117
  ethnic and cultural variations in, 145
  examination of, 132-133
  health history and, 119
    age-related variations in, 120-121
  health promotion and, 161
  loss of, 132
  nutrition and, 98
    of preschool and school-age child, 109
  racial variation in, 133
  situational variations in, 142-145
  terminal, 116
Hairy tongue, 241
Haitian health practices, 37
Hallux valgus, 616
Halos, 281
Hammer, percussion or reflex, 68
Hammer toes, 616
Hamstring muscles, 614
Hand
  assessment of, 610, 611, 626-627
    in integrated examination, 686-687
  racial variation of, 590
  supporting structures of, 590
Handle of otoscope, 67
Handwashing in universal blood and body fluid
  precautions, 71
Hard palate, 232
HBV; see Hepatitis B virus vaccine
Head, 185-212
  of adolescent, 201
    developmental considerations for, 188
    health history and, 194
  age-related variations in, 200-202
  anatomy and physiology of, 185, 186, 187

Head—*cont'd*
  arteries of, 637, 640
  of child, 201
    health history and, 193
  circumference of
    of child, 86, 87, 200
    of newborn and infant, 83, 86, 87, 106-107, 200
  common problems or conditions of, 203-207
    nursing diagnoses and sample documentation for, 210-211
  developmental considerations for, 188
  ethnic and cultural variations of, 190, 191, 195, 200, 202
  examination of, 195-196, 203
    in integrated examination, 687-689
  health history and, 189-194
  health promotion for, 212
  of infant, 200-201
    developmental considerations for, 188
    health history and, 193
  injury to, 190-191, 678
    adolescent risk for, 194
    childhood risk for, 193
  lymph nodes in, 166, 167, 168
    examination of, 167, 172-173
  of older adult, 202
    developmental considerations for, 188
    health history and, 194
  of otoscope, 67
  in pregnancy, 202
    developmental considerations for, 188
  racial variation of, 196
  in review of systems, 45
    documentation of, 57
  rhythmic movements of, 196
  situational variations in, 202
  of stethoscope, 61
Headache, 189-190
  in adolescent, 194
  in health history, 648
  in infection, 193
  in older adult, 194
Head-to-toe examination and documentation, 685-700
  model integrated physical assessment in, 685-695
  pediatric, 695-697
  special considerations in, 685
  write-up of, 697-699
Health
  environmental; *see* Environmental health
  personal beliefs about, 28
Health assessment
  comprehensive, 39-40
  developmental; *see* Developmental assessment
  ethnic and cultural considerations in, 28-29; *see also* Ethnic and cultural considerations
  focused, 40
  interview in; *see* Interview for health history
  physical assessment in; *see* Physical assessment
  purposes of, 2
    location and, 2-3
  reasons for learning skills of, 1-5
  recording data collected in, 3
  types of data in, 2
Health beliefs, ethnic and cultural influences on, 28, 34-35

Health care providers, alternative, 27
Health care utilization, ethnic and cultural influences on, 30-31
Health history
  age-related variations in, 48-55
  biographic data in, 43
  data collection for
    extent of, 39-40
    scope of, 43-48
    techniques for, 41-42
  documentation of, 56
  environmental health in, 48
  family, 44
    documentation of, 57
  past, 43-44, 45
    documentation of, 57
    of infant and child, 50
    of newborn, 48-49
    in older adult, 53
    of pregnant woman, 44, 55-56
  pregnancy and, 44, 55-56, 490-491, 496
  present health status in, 43
  psychosocial status in, 47-48
  reason for seeking care in, 43
  review of systems in, 44-47
  situational variations in, 55-56
  symptom analysis in, 44
Health maintenance, altered, as nursing diagnosis
  in breast lumps, 433
  in cardiovascular risks, 396
  in epigastric pain, 478
Health practices, ethnic and cultural influences on, 34-35
Health status
  ethnic and cultural influences on, 32-33
  general, 45
    documentation of, 57
    ethnic and cultural influences on, 32-33
    of infant and child, 50
    of newborn, 49
  present, 43, 45
    documentation of, 56
    of infant and child, 50
    of newborn, 48
    in older adult, 53
    of pregnant woman, 55
Health-seeking behavior as nursing diagnosis
  in child with lazy eye, 313
  in infant check-ups, 210
  in lymphatic system disorders, 182
Hearing
  anatomy and physiology of, 247-248
  evaluation of
    audiometer for, 68
    tuning fork for, 67
  examination of, 259-261
    in child, 263
    in impaired hearing, 265
    neurologic system and, 655
    routine, 274
  health history and, 250-251
  loss of, 271
    in child, 253
    conductive or sensorineural, 248, 260, 271, 655
    health history and, 250-251
    in infant, 252

Hearing—*cont'd*
  loss of—*cont'd*
    measurement of, 265
    in older adult, 248, 250, 253, 264
Hearing aids, 251
Heart, 359-399; *see also* Cardiovascular system
  age-related variations in, 382-383
  anatomy and physiology of, 359-361, 362
  blood flow through, 359-360, 361
  borders of, 379
  of child, 382-383
    health history and, 367
  common problems or conditions of, 386-393
    nursing diagnoses and sample documentation for, 396-397
  congenital defects of, 382, 391-393
    health history and, 366, 367
  developmental considerations for, 362
  electric conduction of, 360, 361
  ethnic and cultural variations in, 384, 385, 390, 394, 398
  examination of, 377-379, 385
    auscultation in, 379-381
    peripheral vessels and, 368-377
  health history and, 363-367
  health promotion and, 398
  of infant, 382
    health history and, 366-367
  muscle of, 359, 360
  of newborn, 382
    health history and, 366-367
  of older adult, 383
    health history and, 367
  in pregnancy, 384
    health history and, 367
  situational variations in, 384
Heart disease, valvular, 389
Heart failure, 390
  congestive, 364, 365, 390
    in infant, 367
  right-sided, jugular vein pulsations in, 375, 376
Heart murmurs, 377, 378, 386-389
  in infant, 382
  in older adult, 383
Heart rate
  fetal, 384
  normal, 78
  in pregnancy, 87
Heart sounds, 379-381
  abnormal, 387
  in infant, 382
Heartburn in pregnancy, 103
Heave, 377
Heberden's nodes, 610, 611
Height, 82, 84-85, 94
  of adolescent, 87
  of child, 86, 87-91
  energy intake per centimeter of, 109
  in height and weight tables, 94
    for older adult, 111
  skinfold thickness and, 84-85
  of newborn and infant, 83
  of older adult, 87, 111
Helix, 247

Hemangiomas, 127, 137
Hematocrit
   in neonate and infant, 107
   nutritional status and, 96
   in pregnancy, 100
   in toddler, 108
Hemianopia, bilateral, 307
Hemiplegia, 143-144
Hemoglobin
   in neonate and infant, 107
   nutritional status and, 96
   in pregnancy, 100
   in toddler, 108
Hemoptysis, 364
Hemorrhoids, 563-564, 568, 575
   internal, 559
   in pregnancy, 362, 561, 566
Hemothorax, 353
Hepatitis, 443, 452
   viral, 474
Hepatitis B virus vaccine, 162-163
Hepatobiliary system, common problems or conditions of, 474-475
Hepatomegaly, 453
   nutrition and, 99
Hernia
   hiatal, 472
   male, 550-551
      assessment of, 546
   neural, 630
Heroin, eye signs and, 300
Herpendem skin calipers, 69
Herpes simplex virus
   I, 148, 239
   II, 522
   cold sores and, 148, 239
   health history and, 492
   sexually transmitted diseases and, 522
      eye infection of newborn and, 282
      signs and symptoms of, 524
Herpes varicella, 149
Herpes zoster, 149
Hertz, 68
Hex, 34
Hiatal hernia, 472
Hib; see Haemophilus influenzae type b conjugate vaccine
High risk; see also Risks
   for altered growth and development in child with ear disorders, 273
   for infection in male genitalia disorders, 556
   for injury in cerebrovascular accident, 556
Hinge joints, 584
Hip
   assessment of, 614, 615, 627
      in integrated examination, 693
   congenital dislocation of, 630
      tests for, 623, 624
   flexion contractures of, 621
   range of motion of, 614, 615
   supporting structures of, 590
Hip clicks with abduction, 624
Hirschberg test, 286-287
Hirsutism, 133, 157
His, bundle of, 360
Hispanic/Mexican culture, 30-36

History
   health; see Health history
   obstetric, 44
HIV encephalopathy, 677
Hives, history of, 118
Hoarseness, 221
   in thyroid tumor, 192
Holosystolic murmur, 389
Home environmental exposure to respiratory irritants, 326
Hopelessness as nursing diagnosis, 680
Hordeolum, 288, 305
Hormones
   in older adults, 117
   in replacement therapy, 491
      breast cancer and, 408
Horner's syndrome, 310
Hospitalizations in health history, 44
Housekeeping ability, assessment of, 54
Houston valves, 559
Human immunodeficiency virus, safe sex and, 528
Humerus, racial variation of, 590
Hydramnios, 476
Hydrocele, 553
   in infant, 547
Hydrocephalus, 204
Hymen, 482
   remnants of, 499
Hypercholesterolemia, 363, 398; see also Cholesterol
Hyperemesis gravidarum, 104
Hyperkeratosis, 98, 155
Hyperpigmentation of breast, 411
Hyperplasia, sebaceous, 41, 140
Hyperpnea, 80, 332, 333
Hyperresonance, 74, 336
Hypersensitivity of abdominal skin, 454, 455
Hypertelorism, 296
Hypertension, 394
   cardiovascular disease risks and, 398
   headache in, 190
   nursing diagnoses and documentation for, 396
   pulmonary, 378
Hypertensive retinopathy, 312
Hyperthyroidism, 192, 208
   apical pulsations in, 377
Hypertrophy
   of nail, 135
   of nodule, 127
   prostatic, benign, 576
   scar, 129
Hyperventilation, 332, 333
   central neurogenic, 80
Hypervitaminosis A, 104
Hypodermis, 116
Hypoglossal nerve, 642, 643, 644
   tests for, 656
   tongue movement and, 231
Hypospadias, 544
Hypotelorism, 296
Hypotension, orthostatic, 369
Hypothermia as nursing diagnosis in thyroid dysfunction, 211
Hypothyroidism, 192, 209
   congenital, 212
   headache in, 190
Hypotonia of muscle, 594

Hypoventilation, 332, 333
Hysterectomy, 516
Hz; see Hertz

I

Icterus, 443
Ileostomy, 573-574
Iliac arteries, bruits and, 451
Iliac crests, assessment of, 603
Iliopsoas muscle test, 464
Ilium, 483, 486
Illness
   chronic, in health history, 44
   patterns of, ethnic and cultural influences on, 32-33
   personal beliefs about, 28, 34-35
Immune deficiency, 179
Immunizations, 161, 162, 479
   history of, 44
   recommended schedule for, 161
Immunoglobulins, 165
   pregnancy and, 170
Immunosuppressed clients, lymph node examination in, 177
Impaired gas exchange as nursing diagnosis in cough, 355
Impaired physical mobility as nursing diagnosis
   in cerebrovascular accident, 681
   in osteoarthritis, 634
   in wrist disorders, 633
Impaired skin integrity as nursing diagnosis, 160
   risk for, 159
Imperforate anus, 564
Impetigo, 152
Implementation in nursing process, 1, 2
Impotence, 537
Incarceration of hernia, 550
Incontinence, fecal, 564
Indirect inguinal hernia, 550
Individual, role of, ethnic and cultural influences on, 29
Indocin; see Indomethacin
Indomethacin
   food interaction with, 113
   as ototoxic drug, 250
Ineffective breathing pattern in asthma, 354
Ineffective coping in asthma, 354
Infant
   behavioral development of, 9, 10-11
   circumference measurements in, 83-84, 86, 87, 106-107, 200
   delivery of, preparing for, 515-516
   development of, expected at various months, 10-11
   developmental assessment of, 9-11
   developmental tasks of, 9, 19-11
   external genitalia examination for, 510
   frequency of measurements in, 106
   head-to-toe examination and documentation for, 695-697
   health history of, 49-52
   length of, 83, 106
   nutrition and, 106-108
   physical assessment of, 83-86
   physical growth of, 9, 10-11
   presenting part of, 515, 516
   reflexes in, 670-671
   stool characteristics of, 565

Infant—*cont'd*
  vital signs of, 78, 79, 84-85
  weight of, 83, 106
Infarction, myocardial, 390
  pain in, 191
Infection
  axillary lymphatic drainage and, 416
  headache in, 193
  of kidneys, back pain in, 444
  lymph nodes enlargement in, 172
  monilial, 241
  risk for, as nursing diagnoses
    in foreign body in nose, 245
    in male genitalia disorders, 556
  sinus, 219
  stiff neck in, 193
  thyroid gland tenderness in, 199
  viral hepatitis in, 474
Infestations of skin, 155
Inflammation
  of Bartholin glands, 520
  lymphatic system in, 180
Inframammary ridge, 419
Ingrown toenail, 158
  prevention of, 161
Inguinal area
  inspection of
    in female, 498
    in integrated assessment, 695
    in male, 546
  lymph nodes in, 168, 169, 170
    examination of, 175
  male, 534, 546
  hernia and, 550-551
Inguinal ligament, 437
Inguinal nodes, 459
  examination of, 460
Inhalants, health promotion and, 356
Injury
  during delivery, 594
  to ear, 249
  head, 190-191, 678
    adolescent risk for, 194
    childhood risk for, 193
  in health history, 44
  high risk for, in cerebrovascular accident, 556
  lumbar disk, test for, 622
  to musculoskeletal system, 629
    prevention of, 635
  to spinal cord, 677
Inner canthus, 277
Inner ear, 247
Inspection in physical assessment, 73; *see also* individual organ system
Inspiration, muscles of, 317
Instruments for inspection, 73
Integrated physical assessment, model, 685-695
Integumentary system, 45
  in review of systems
    of infant and child, 50
    in pregnant woman, 55
    sample documentation of, 57
Intelligence, adult, 8
Intensity of sound, 76
Intercostal spaces, 381

Internal genitalia
  female; *see also* Female reproductive system
    anatomy and physiology of, 482-483
    bimanual examination for, 506-509
    rectovaginal examination in, 509-510
    speculum examination for, 501-506
  male, 531-534; *see also* Male genitalia
Internal hemorrhoids, 559, 568, 575
Internal rotation, 585
Interphalangeal joints, 610, 611
Interpretation in data collection interview, 41
Interruptions in data collection interview, 42
Interspinous diameter of pelvis, 513, 514
Intertuberous diameter of pelvis, 515
Interview for health history, 39-59; *see also* Health history
  age-related variations in, 48-55
  awkward moments in, 42-43
  communicating with client in, 40-43
  data collection for
    extent of, 39-40
    scope of, 43-48
    techniques for, 41-42
  documentation of, 56
  purpose of, 39
  questions in, 40-41
  setting for, 39
  situational variations in, 55-56
Intestinal obstruction, pain in, 456-457
Intoxication
  alcohol, 478
    ethnic and cultural influences on, 33
  drug, eye in, 299-300; *see also* Drugs, abuse of
Intracranial pressure, increased, 653
Intraductal papilloma of breast, 430
Intrauterine devices, 528
Intrinsic and Extrinsic Rewards Satisfaction Scale, 23
Intussusception, 476
Inversion, 585
Involution, lactation and, 403
Iodine
  deficiency of, 99
  in diet, 212
  recommended dietary allowances of, 101
Iridectomy, 310
Iridocyclitis, 309
Iridodialysis, 310
Iris, 277-278
  inspection of, 292
Iritis, 309
Iron
  deficiency of, 98, 99
  in infant formula, 445
  in older adult, 112
  in pregnancy, 103
  recommended dietary allowances of, 101
  stool color and, 566
Iron deficiency anemia
  in adolescent, 110
  in pregnancy, 100
  in toddler, 108
Irritable bowel disease, 562
  pain in, 456-457
Irritants
  contact, 146
  respiratory, exposure to, 325-326

Ischium, 483, 486
Ishihara's test, 297
Isthmus of thyroid, 185, 187
Itching
  of ear, 250
  history of, 118
  rectal, 563-564

J

Jaeger near vision chart, 66, 284
Japanese health practices, 34, 35, 37
Jaundice, 119, 123, 124, 443
  physiologic, 136
Jaw, bony structures of, 196
Jejunum, 438
Job Descriptive Index, 23
Jock itch, 542
Joint, 583-585
  clicking of, 593
  flexion or extension of, goniometer for measuring, 69
  inspection of, 595
  movement of, 585-586, 589, 590
  pain in, 592-593
  position sense of, 660-661
  range of motion of, 585-586, 589, 590
Joint capsule, 586
Judgments, value, in data collection interview, 42
Jugular veins, 637, 640
  pressure in, 375-376, 383
  pulsations of, 375-376, 383

K

Kaposi's sarcoma, 153
  in mouth, 243
Kegel exercises, 527
Keith-Wagner-Barker system of retinopathy classification, 312
Keloid, 129
Keratomalacia, 98
Keratoses, seborrheic, 41, 140
Kernig's sign, 667, 668
Ketones, pregnancy and, 101
Kidneys, 439-440
  examination of, 459, 461-462, 471
  infection of, back pain in, 444
  palpation of, 459
Kiesselbach area, 224
Kinesthetic sensation, 660-661
Knee
  assessment of, 614-616, 627
  fluid on, 619
  locking of, 621
  range of motion of, 616
  supporting structures of, 590
Knee-chest position, 77
Knock knee, 614
Knowledge deficit as nursing diagnosis
  in cardiovascular risks, 396
  in female reproductive system disorders, 525
  in infant check-ups, 210
  in male genitalia problems, 555, 556
  in nasal foreign body, 245
KOH testing; *see* Potassium hydroxide testing
Koilonychia, 135
Koplik's spots, 230, 243

Korotkoff sounds, 80-81, 82
Kussmaul respirations, 80, 332, 333
Kyphosis, 330, 603

L

Labia, 481-482
  inspection of, 498-499
Lacrimal apparatus
  in infant, 296
  in older adult, 298
Lacrimal glands, 277
Lacrimal puncta, inspection of, 289
Lacrimation, excessive, 282, 289
Lactation
  breast in, 425-426
    developmental considerations for, 403
    health history and, 409
    nipple of, 409, 425-426
  health promotion and, 435
  not associated with childbirth, 431
  nutrition in
    assessment of, 105-106
    high-risk conditions for, 104
Lactiferous duct, 401, 402
  clogged, 425
Lamps, Wood's, 70
Lang skin calipers, 69
Language
  of preschooler, 16
  primary, 29
Language barriers, 27
Language behavior, 7
Lanugo, 117, 138
Large for gestational age, 106
Large intestine, 438; see also Gastrointestinal
  system
Lasix; see Furosemide
Last examinations in health history, 44
Lateral recumbent position, 77
Laxatives, 563
  food interaction with, 113
Lead exposure, 651
Lead poisoning, 479
Left bundle branch block, 381
Left ventricular hypertrophy, 390
  apical pulsations in, 377
Leg
  cramps or pain in, 366
  dependent edema of, 365
  lymph nodes in, 169, 170
  muscles of, 587
  racial variation of, 590
  supporting structures of, 590
Legal aspects of documentation, 3
Legal blindness, 284
Legumes in food pyramid, 102
Length of newborn and infant, 83, 106
Lens of eye, 279
  accommodation and, 280; see also Accommodation
Lens selector dial, 66
Lentigines, senile, 41, 140
Leopold maneuvers, 470
Lesbians, 492
LeSègue's test, 622
Leukoedema, 230

Leukonychia punctata, 157
Leukoplakia, 232, 242
  of external female genitalia, 498
Levine's sign, 363
LGA; see Large for gestational age
Lice, 139, 156
  pubic, 542
Lichen planus, 135
Lichenification, 129
Life expectancy, ethnic and cultural influences on,
  32-33
Lift, 377
Ligaments, 586-587, 590
Light
  for ophthalmoscope, 66
  penlight, 69
  testing sensation for, 286-287, 653-654
    pupillary abnormalities and, 309
  Wood's, 70
Light touch sensation, examination of, 660-661
Lightening, 486
Lighting for inspection, 73
Limbic system, 643
Limitations of self-care behaviors, 593-594
Limited range of motion of neck, 197
Linea alba, 437
Linea nigra, 142
  in pregnant abdomen, 467
Lip
  cleft, 240
  common problems or conditions of, 239-243
    documentation for, 244-245
    nursing diagnoses for, 244-245
  health promotion and, 244-245
  inspection of, 227, 228
  nutrition and, 98
  racial variation in, 227
  squamous cell carcinoma of, 240
  ulceration of, 228
Lipoproteins in pregnancy, 101
Listening, active, 41
Lithotomy position, 77, 497-498
Liver, 438-439, 440; see also Gastrointestinal
  system
  common problems or conditions of, 474-475
  examination of, 452-453, 458
    in infant and child, 466
    in older adult, 441
    palpation of, 458
Liver spots, 41, 140
Lobar emphysema, 350
Lochia, 488
Lollipop Test, 21
Long bones, racial variation of, 590
Lordosis, 603
  in child, 624
  in pregnancy, 591, 625
Loss of consciousness in head injury, 191
Louis, angle of, 320
Lower abdominal pain, 489
Lower airway, 317
Lower extremities
  coordination in, 658, 660
  examination of, in integrated assessment, 693
  supporting structures of, 590
Lumbar disk injury, test for, 622

Lumbar spine
  assessment of, 603, 604, 626
  range of motion of, 603, 604
Lumps in breast, 404, 405, 429
Lung, 317-357; see also Respiratory system
  cancer of, 352
  lobes of, 317
  obstructive disease of, 345, 349
  percussion of, 74, 75, 336, 337
  transfer of gases in, 317
Lymph, 165, 166
Lymph nodes, 165-169; see also Lymphatic system
  of neck, 185
    enlargement of, 192
  palpation of, 74
  regional, 166-169
Lymph tissue, sites of, 165
Lymphadenitis, acute, 180
Lymphangitis, acute, 180
Lymphatic system, 165-183; see also Lymph nodes
  age-related variations in, 176
  anatomy and physiology of, 165-170
  breast and, 166-169, 401
  common problems or conditions in, 179-180
    nursing diagnosis for, 181-182
    sample documentation of, 181-182
  developmental considerations for, 170
  ethnic and cultural variations in, 177
  examination of, 172-178
  fluid circulation in, 165, 166
  in health history, 171
  health promotion for, 183
  situational variations in, 177
Lymphedema, 179
Lymphocytes, 165
Lymphogranuloma venereum, 552

M

MAC; see Mid-arm circumference
Macrocephaly, 195, 205
Macroglossia in infant, 234
Macula, 279
  inspection of, 295
Macule, 126
Magnesium, recommended dietary allowances of, 101
Male genitalia, 531-558
  of adolescent, 548
    developmental considerations for, 534, 535
    health history and, 540-541
  age-related variations in, 547-548
  anatomy and physiology of, 531-534
    external, 531, 532, 533
    inguinal area, 534
    internal, 531-534
  of child, 547-548
    developmental considerations for, 534
    health history and, 539-540
  common problems or conditions of, 550-554
    nursing diagnoses in, 555-556
    sample documentation of, 555-556
  developmental considerations for, 534, 535
  ethnic and cultural variations in, 549
  examination of, 542-549
    in integrated assessment, 693
  external
    anatomy and physiology of, 531, 532, 533

Male genitalia—cont'd
  health history and, 536-541
  health promotion and, 557
  of infant, 547
    developmental considerations for, 534
    health history and, 539
  inguinal area and, 534
  internal, 531-534
  of older adult, 548
    developmental considerations for, 534
    health history and, 541
  of preadolescent, developmental considerations
    for, 534, 535
  racial variation in, 531, 542
  situational variations in, 548-549
Male reproductive system, genitalia of, 531-558;
  see also Male genitalia
Male sexual dysfunction, 537-538
Malignant neoplasms; see also Carcinoma
  lymphatic system and, 172, 179
  melanoma in, 154
    early signs of, 161
Malnourishment, 98-99
  in toddler, 108
Malnutrition, 183
Malocclusion, 228-229
  in older adult, 236
Mammary bud, 402
Mammary glands, 401; see also Breast
Mammography, 435
Manubriosternal junction, 320
Marijuana, eye signs and, 300
Masks for universal blood and body fluid precau-
  tions, 71
Mass
  in abdomen, floating, examination of, 465, 471
  breast
    characteristics in, 418
    differentiation in, 431
    palpation of, 417
    subareolar, in adolescent male, 424
  neck, 192
  rectal, 579
Mastectomy, 427
  radical, 177
Mastitis, 431
Mastoiditis, 255
Mate selection, 18
Maternal mortality, ethnic and cultural influences
  on, 32-33
Maxillary sinuses, 225; see also Paranasal sinuses
  transillumination of, 226
McMurray test, 620
Measles, 150
  German, 150
  Koplik's spots in, 243
Measles, mumps, and rubella viruses vaccine,
  162-163
Measurement, ruler or tape measure for, 69
Meat in food pyramid, 102
Mechanical barrier contraceptives, 528
Meckel diverticulum, 476
Meconium ileus, 476
Meconium stool, 561
Medial canthus, 277
Medications; see Drugs

Meibomian cyst, 288
Meibomian gland, 277
Melanoma, malignant, 154
  early signs of, 161
Membrane, tympanic; see Tympanic membrane
Memory, mental status and, 667
Menarche
  breasts and, 402
  health history and, 407, 494
Meniere's disease, 190, 248, 250, 271
  nausea and vomiting in, 443
Meninges, 637, 638
  irritation of, 667
Meningitis, 677
  symptoms in, 193
Meningocele, 630
Meniscus, 586
  torn or damaged, 620
Menopause, 403, 488
  health history and, 491
Menstrual cycle, 483, 484, 485
  health history and, 489
Menstruation in adolescent, 110
Mental confusion, nutrition and, 99
Mental status
  disorders of, 677, 680
  examination for, 665-667
Mercury
  in sphygmomanometer, 63, 79
  in thermometer, 61, 62, 76
Metacarpophalangeal joints, 610, 611
Metasystematic operations, 8
Metatarsus adductus, 631
Metatarsus varus, 624, 631
Metropolitan height and weight tables, 94
Mexican culture, 30-36
Microaneurysm of retinal fundus, 294
Microcephaly, 195, 205
Microcirculation, 166
Mid-arm circumference
  in neonate and infant, 106
  in toddler, 108
Midaxillary line, 322
Midclavicular lines, 320
Midclavicular liver span, 452-453
Middle adulthood
  assessment tools for, 19
  developmental assessment in, 18, 19
  developmental tasks in, 19
Middle ear, 247, 248
  common problems or conditions of, 270-271
Midplane of pelvis, 513
Midspinal line, 322
Midsternal line, 320
Migraine headache, 189-190, 203
Milia, 137, 138
Milk in food pyramid, 102
Milk duct, 401, 402
  clogged, 425
Milk line from embryonic ridge, 415
Milroy disease, 179
Mineral oil, 113
Minerals
  pregnancy and, 103
  recommended dietary allowances for, 101
Mini-mental state test, 665, 667

Miosis, 292, 309
Mitral valve, heart sounds and, 379, 380, 388-389
Mixed eating disorders, pregnancy and, 104
MMR; see Measles, mumps, and rubella viruses
  vaccine
Mobility
  assessment of, 54
  health history and, 649
  impaired physical, as nursing diagnosis
    in cerebrovascular accident, 681
    in osteoarthritis, 634
    in wrist disorders, 633
  in older adults, 594
  of skin, 132
Model integrated physical assessment, 685-695
Modes of Adaptation Patterns Scale, 23
Molar, congenitally absent, 215, 228
Molding, 200
Moles, 126
  changes in, 119, 123
Molluscum contagiosum, 523
Mongolian spots, 136
Monilial infection, 241, 522
  in male, 542
Mononucleosis, Epstein-Barr, 180
Mons pubis, inspection of, 498
Montgomery glands, 401, 402
Montgomery tubercles, 413
Morgagni columns, 559
Morning sickness, 440
  in pregnancy, 101
Moro reflex, 670
Motor activity in infant, 669
Motor cortex topography, 641
Motor development, 7
  of infant, expected at various months, 10-11
  racial variations in, 651
Motor fibers of spinal nerves, 644
Motor function
  in child, testing for, 672, 673-674
  fine, examination of, 660
Motor vehicle crashes, 191
Mouth
  age-related variations in, 234-236
    health history and, 220-221
  anatomy and physiology of, 215, 216
  in child, 235-236
  common problems or conditions of, 239-243
    nursing diagnoses and sample documentation
      for, 244-245
  developmental considerations for, 217-218
  ethnic and cultural variations in, 237
  examination of, 227-233, 238, 656
  health history and, 220-221
    age-related variations in, 220-221
  health promotion and, 244-245
  in infant, 234-235
  Kaposi's sarcoma in, 243
  lesions in, 220
  nutrition and, 98
  in older adult, 218, 236
  pain in, 220
  in pregnancy, 218, 237
  in review of systems, 46
    of infant and child, 51
    of newborn, 49

Mouth—*cont'd*
in review of systems—*cont'd*
in pregnant woman, 55
situational variations in, 237
Movement; *see also* Mobility
eye; *see* Eye and visual system
facial, examination of, 653-654, 655
Mucosa
buccal, 230
common problems or conditions of, 241-243
nutrition and, 98
Mucus, respiratory system, variations in, 323-324
Multiple gestation, 104
Multiple sclerosis, 677
health history and, 649
Mumps, vaccine for, 162-163
Murmurs, heart, 377, 378, 386-389
in infant, 382
in older adult, 383
Murphy's sign, 458
Muscles; *see also* Musculoskeletal system
of abdomen, 437-438
atrophy of, 595
dystrophy of, 631
inspection of, 595-599
pain in, 592
percussion of, 75
sprain of, 629
strain of, 629
strength of, 597, 598, 599
wasting of, 99
weakness and deformity of, 593, 597, 598, 599
Muscular dystrophy, 631
Musculoskeletal system, 583-636; *see also*
Muscles
of adolescent, 624
health history and, 594
age-related variations in, 623-625
anatomy and physiology of, 583-590
of child, 624
health history and, 594
developmental considerations for, 591
ethnic and cultural variations of, 625
examination of, 595-627
ankles in, 616-617
arms in, 608-609
cervical spine in, 601
elbows in, 608-609
feet in, 616-617
fingers in, 610-612, 613
hand in, 610-612, 613
hips in, 614, 615
in integrated assessment, 695
knees in, 614-616
neck in, 601-602
routine, 595-599
shoulder and shoulder girdle in, 605-606, 607
special tests for, 618-622
spine in, 601, 603-605
temporomandibular joint and jaw in, 600
wrist in, 610, 611, 613
health history and, 592-594
of infant, 623-624
health history and, 594
injuries to, 629
nutrition and, 98-99

Musculoskeletal system—*cont'd*
of older adult, 625
health history and, 594
in pregnancy, 625
racial variation of, 583, 590, 617
in review of systems, 47
documentation of, 57
of infant and child, 49
of newborn, 49
in pregnant woman, 56
situational variations of, 625
Myasthenia gravis, 593, 679
health history and, 649
Mydriasis, 292, 309
Myelomeningocele, 630
Myers-Briggs Type Indicator, 23
Myocardial infarction, 390
pain in, 191
Myocardium, 359, 360
Myomas of uterus, 519
Myopathy, 593
Myopia, 284
Myringotomy tube, 271
Myxedema, 208

N

Nabothian cyst, 518
Nails, 115-164
age-related variations in, 136-142
health history and, 120-121
anatomy and physiology of, 115-116
arterial pulse assessment and, 374
cells in, 116
clubbing of, 134, 374
common problems or conditions of, 157-158
nursing diagnoses and sample documentation
for, 159-160
developmental considerations for, 116-117
ethnic and cultural variations in, 145
examination of, 134-135
health history and, 120
age-related variations in, 120-121
health promotion and, 161
in heart and peripheral vascular examination, 374
nutrition and, 98
racial variation in, 116, 134
situational variations in, 142-145
structures of, 116
NANDA diagnoses, 4-5
Nasal air flow, obstruction of, 219
Nasal cavity
bones of, 213
inspection of, 223-224, 225
Nasal discharge, 219, 223
Nasal flaring in infant, 343
Nasal foreign body
health promotion and, 245
nursing diagnoses in, 245
Nasal polyps, 224, 239
Nasal septum, deviated, 224
Nasal speculum, 67, 223-224, 225
Nasal turbinates, 224
Nasolabial folds, 196
Nasopharynx in review of systems, 46
documentation of, 57
of newborn, 49

National Academy of Science, pregnancy recommendations of, 104
National Child Assessment Form, 21
National Cholesterol Education Program Guidelines, 97
for preschool and school-age child, 109
National Standard for Health Statistics growth grids, 88-91, 109
Nausea and vomiting
history of, 443
in pregnancy, 103, 440
NCEP; *see* National Cholesterol Education Program Guidelines
NCHS; *see* National Standard for Health Statistics growth grids
Near vision chart, 66
Nearsightedness, 284
Neck, 185-212
of adolescent, 201
developmental considerations for, 188
health history and, 194
age-related variations in, 200-202
anatomy and physiology of, 185, 186, 187
arteries of, 637, 640
of child, 201
health history and, 193
common problems or conditions of, 207-209
nursing diagnoses and sample documentation
for, 210-211
developmental considerations for, 188
ethnic and cultural variations of, 190, 191, 200, 202
examination of, 196-199, 203, 601-602
in integrated examination, 687-689
health history and, 191-194
health promotion for, 212
of infant, 200-201
developmental considerations for, 188
health history and, 193
limited motion of, 191
lymph nodes in, 166, 167, 168
examination of, 167, 172-173
mass in, 192
movement of, 657
muscle strength of, 657
muscle symmetry in, 196-197
of older adult, 202
developmental considerations for, 188
health history and, 194
pain in, 191
in older adult, 194
in pregnancy, 202
developmental considerations for, 188
racial variation of, 196
range of motion of, 197, 601
in review of systems, 46
documentation of, 57
situational variations in, 202
supporting structures of, 589
in tonic neck reflex, 670
wry, 207
Need Satisfaction Questionnaire, 23
Needles in universal blood and body fluid precautions, 71
Neomycin, ototoxicity of, 250
Neonate; *see* Newborn

Neoplasms
  malignant
    lymphatic system and, 172, 179
    melanoma in, 154
      early signs of, 161
  of skin, 153-154
Nerve compression, pain in, 592
Nerve root irritation, 622
Nervous system; see Neurologic system
Neural herniation, 630
Neural tube defects, 104
Neuralgia, trigeminal, 600, 654
Neuritis, sciatic, 622
Neurogenic hyperventilation, central, 80
Neurologic soft signs, 672, 673-674
Neurologic system, 637-683
  age-related variations in, 669-674
  anatomy and physiology of, 637-646, 647
    autonomic nervous system, 644, 646
    central nervous system, 637-644, 645
    peripheral nervous system, 644, 645, 647
  central nervous system in; see Central nervous
    system
  of child, 672, 673-674
    developmental considerations for, 647
    disorders and, 677
    health history and, 650-651
  common problems or conditions of, 677-679
    nursing diagnoses and sample documentation
      for, 680-681
  developmental considerations for, 647
  ethnic and cultural variations in, 675, 677, 678
  examination of, 652-675
    abdominal superficial reflexes in, 647, 665
    balance in, 657-658
    Brudzinski's sign in, 667, 668
    cerebellar function in, 657-660
    coordination in, 658-660
    extremity muscular strength, sensation, and re-
      flexes in, 660-664
    facial movement and sensation in, 653-654, 655
    Glasgow Coma Scale in, 667, 668
    hearing in, 655
    in integrated assessment, 694-695
    Kernig's sign in, 667, 668
    mental status in, 665-667
    mouth and tongue in, 656
    neck movement and muscle strength in, 657
    shoulder movement and muscle strength in, 657
    smell in, 652
    speech in, 652
    taste in, 656
    vision in, 653
  health history and, 648-651
  health promotion for, 682
  of infant, 107-108
    developmental considerations for, 647
    examination of, 669, 670-671
    health history and, 650
  mental status in
    disorders of, 677, 680
    examination for, 665-667
  in newborn, 107-108, 669, 670-671
  nutrition and, 99
  of older adult
    developmental considerations for, 647

Neurologic system—cont'd
  of older adult—cont'd
    health history and, 650-651
    peripheral nervous system in
      anatomy and physiology of, 644, 645, 647
      disorders of, 677
    in pregnancy, 675
      developmental considerations for, 647
    racial variation in, 651
    in review of systems, 47
    situational variations in, 675
    of special needs client, health history
      and, 651
Neurologic vibratory evaluation, 67
Neuropathy, 593
Nevi, pigmented
  changes in, 119, 123
  inspection of, 125
Newborn
  apnea in, 327
  chest circumference of, 83-84, 86, 87, 106
  external genitalia examination for, 510
  head circumference of, 83, 86, 87, 106, 200
  head-to-toe examination and documentation for,
    695-697
  health history of, 48-49
  length of, 83, 106
  male genitalia in, 534
  nutrition of, 106-108
  physical assessment of, 83-86
  respirations in, 343
  vital signs of, 78, 84-85
  weight of, 83, 106
Niacin
  deficiency of, 98
  recommended dietary allowances of, 101
Nicotine effects, 363
Night blindness, 281
Nipple, 320
  changes in, 405
  discharge from, 414, 420
    cytology of, 414
  inspection of, 413-414
  in lactation, 409, 425-426
  supernumerary, 414, 415, 417
  variations in, 412-413
Nitrofurantoin, ototoxicity of, 250
Nitrogen balance in neonate and infant, 107
Nits, 139, 156
Nocturia, 364
Node, 127
  Bouchard's, 610, 611
  Heberden's, 610, 611
  inguinal, 460
  rectal, 579
  sinoatrial and atrioventricular, 359, 360
Nodule, 127; see also Node
Noise
  hearing loss from, 250
  levels of, 274
  protection from, 274
Noncompliance as nursing diagnosis
  in asthma, 354
  in gout, 272
  in male genitalia disorders, 556
Normocephalic skull, 195

Nose
  age-related variations in, 234-236
    health history and, 220-221
  anatomy and physiology of, 213-215
  in child, 235
  common problems or conditions of, 239
    nursing diagnoses and sample documentation
      for, 244-245
  developmental considerations for, 217-218
  discharge from, 219, 223
  ethnic and cultural variations in, 237
  examination of, 223-226, 238
  foreign body in, 245
  health history and, 219-220
    age-related variations in, 220-221
  health promotion and, 244-245
  in infant, 234
  nasal speculum for, 67, 223-224, 225
  in older adult, 218, 236
  in pregnancy, 218, 237
  racial variation in, 234
  in review of systems, 46
    documentation of, 57
    of newborn, 49
    in pregnant woman, 55
  situational variations in, 237
  smell and, 652
Nose sprays, 246
Nosebleed, 220
Notch, suprasternal, 320
Nursing diagnoses for problems or conditions
  of auditory system, 272-273
  of breast, 433-434
  documentation of, 699
  of female reproductive system, 525-526
  of hair, 159-160
  of head and neck, 210-211
  of lip, 244-245
  of lymphatic system, 181-182
  of mouth, 244-245
  of nail, 159-160
  of nose, 244-245
  of oropharynx, 244-245
  of paranasal sinuses, 244-245
  of respiratory system, 354-355
  of skin, 159-160
  of skin, hair, or nails, 159-160
  of teeth, 244-245
Nursing process, 1
Nutrition, 93-114; see also Eating
  in adolescent, 110-111
  in adults, 93-97
  altered
    less than body requirements, in temporo-
      mandibular joint dysfunction, 244
    more than body requirements
      in child, 477
      in male breast enlargement, 434
      in obesity in older adult, 314
  body mass index in, 94, 95, 96
  documentation of, 49
  food pyramid in, 97, 102
  health promotion and, 479
  of infant and child, 50
  infection risk and, 183
  iodine and, 212

Nutrition—*cont'd*
malnourishment in, 98-99
Metropolitan height and weight tables in, 94
in neonates and infants, 106-108
in older adult, 111-113, 446-447
in postpartum and lactating women, 105-106
in pregnant women, 97-105
in preschooler, 109-110
questionnaire for, 105
Recommended Dietary Allowances in, 97, 100-101
supplements in, 103
in toddler, 108-109
Nutrition During Pregnancy and Lactation: an Implementation Guide, 104
Nutrition During Pregnancy: Part II, Nutrient Supplements, 103
Nuts in food pyramid, 102
Nystagmus, 286
in child, 297
drug intoxication and, 300

O

Obesity, 93
in adolescent, 110
cardiovascular system and, 363, 398
in child, 477
Objective data, 2
Obstetric conjugate, 513, 514
Obstetric history, 44, 490-491
documentation of, 57
Obstruction
bile duct, 458
intestinal, pain in, 456-457
of nasal air flow, 219
Obstructive lung disease, 345, 349
Obturator muscle test, 464
Occipital bones, 185
Occult blood in stool, 571
Occupational environmental exposure to respiratory irritants, 326
Ocular problems, 282; *see also* Eye and visual system
Ocular tissue, nutrition and, 98
Oculomotor nerve, 642, 643, 644, 653
damage to, 309, 310
eye anatomy and, 277-278, 279, 280
eye movement and, 286
pupils of eye and, 292
Odor of breath, 227
Oily skin, history of, 118
Old lady in alternative health practices, 34
Older adult
assessment tools for, 19
developmental assessment of, 19
developmental tasks of, 19
external genitalia examination for, 512
health history of, 52-55
nutrition and, 111-113
vital signs of, 87
weight and height of, 87
Olecranon process, 608, 609
Olfactory nerve, 223, 642, 644, 652
Open-ended questions, 41
Ophthalmoscope, 66-67
Ophthalmoscopic examination, 292-295, 302

Optic disk, 279
inspection of, 292-293
Optic nerve, 642, 644
destruction of, 309
in eye anatomy and physiology, 277, 279, 280
pupils of eye and, 292
Optic tracts, 280
OPV; *see* Oral poliovirus vaccine
Oral cavity
in nutritional assessment, 97
of preschool and school-age child, 109
in older adult, 112
Oral contraceptives; *see* Contraceptives
Oral poliovirus vaccine, 162-163
Oral temperature, 76
Organ of Corti, 248
Organic brain syndrome
in older adult, 651
orientation in, 667
Oropharynx
age-related variations in, 234-236
health history and, 220-221
anatomy and physiology of, 215, 217
in child, 235-236
common problems or conditions of, 239-243
nursing diagnoses and sample documentation for, 244-245
developmental considerations for, 217-218
ethnic and cultural variations in, 237
examination of, 227-233, 238
health history and, 220-221
health promotion and, 244-245
in infant, 234-235
in older adult, 236
in pregnancy, 218
racial variation in, 230, 232
in review of systems, 46
documentation of, 57
of infant and child, 51
of newborn, 49
situational variations in, 237
Orthopnea, 364
Orthostatic hypotension, 369
Ossification of sutures, 188
Osteoarthritis, 610, 611, 632, 634
Osteoma of external auditory meatus, 269
Osteomyelitis, 628
Osteoporosis, 632
racial variations in incidence of, 625
risk factors for, 634
Otitis externa, 247, 249, 250, 256, 269
Otitis media, 249
bacterial, 270
in child, 252, 253
hearing loss from, 253
secretory, 270
serous, 258, 270
Otoscope, 67, 256
Ototoxic drugs, 250
Outcome identification in nursing process, 1, 2
Outer canthus in child, 297
Outer ear, 247
Ovaries, 483
cancer of, 520
Papanicolaou smear and, 491, 504-505

Ovaries—*cont'd*
common problems and conditions of, 520
palpation of, 509
Overload Index, 22
Ovulation, 484, 485
Oximetry, pulse, 64
Oxygen transfer in respiratory system, 317
Oxygenation, general, 332

P

Pace of Life Index, 22
Pacific Islander culture, 31-37
Paget's disease of breast, 405, 414, 430
Pain
abdominal; *see* Abdominal pain
back, 614
blood pressure and, 81
in breast, 404
chest, 325, 363-364
ear
in child, 253
health history and, 249-250
nursing diagnosis for, 273
epigastric, 478
in eye, 281
leg, 366
male genitalia and, 536
in mouth, 220
musculoskeletal, 592-593
neck, 191
in older adult, 194
neurologic, health history and, 650
as nursing diagnosis
in earache, 273
in lymphatic system disorders, 181
in rectal bleeding, 578
in temporomandibular joint dysfunction, 244
in wrist disorders, 633
pelvic, 489
rectal, 563
sinus, 219
superficial sensation of, examination of, 660-661
in wrist, 633
Pain medications, health history and, 650
Palate
hard, 232
soft, movement of, 656
Pallor, 123, 124, 332
of extremities, 374
nutrition and, 99
Palmar erythema, 362
Palmar grasp reflex, 670
Palmaris longus muscle, 612
Palpation
bimanual technique for, 74
light or deep, 73-74
in physical assessment, 73-74
Palpebral conjunctiva, 277
inspection of, 289-290
Palpebral fissures, 196, 277
racial variation in, 288
Palpebral slant of eye, upper, 296, 301, 307
Pancreas, 439, 440; *see also* Gastrointestinal system
common problems or conditions of, 475
Pancreatitis, 475
pain in, 442, 456-457

Pap smear; *see* Papanicolaou smear
Papanicolaou smear, 491
   collection of, 504-505
Papilledema, 292
Papilloma of breast, intraductal, 430
Papule, 126
Paradoxic splitting of heart sound, 381
Paradoxical pulse, 369, 370
Paralysis
   male genitalia examination in, 548
   of shoulder and upper arm muscles, 624
Paranasal sinuses
   age-related variations in, 234-236
      health history and, 220-221
   anatomy and physiology of, 213-215
   in child, 218, 235
   common problems or conditions of, documenta-
      tion for, 244-245
   congestion or pain in, 219
   developmental considerations for, 217-218
   ethnic and cultural variations in, 237
   examination of, 223-226, 238
   health history and, 219-221
   health promotion and, 244-245
   in infant, 217
   in older adult, 236
   in review of systems, 46
      documentation of, 57
      of newborn, 49
   situational variations in, 237
   transillumination of, 226
Paraphimosis, 544, 551
Paraplegia, 143-144
Parasympathetic nervous system, 644, 646
Paravertebral muscles, 605
Parenting Satisfaction Scale, 24
Parkinson's disease, 206, 649, 678
Paronychia, 135
Paroxysmal nocturnal dyspnea, 324, 364
Pars flaccida, 247
Pars tensa, 247
Partial hysterectomy, 516
Past health history, 43-44, 45
   documentation of, 57
   of infant and child, 50
   of newborn, 48-49
   in older adult, 53
   of pregnant woman, 55
Patch, 126
   Peyer's, 165, 170
   salmon, 136, 137
Patellar reflex, testing for, 662-664
Patent ductus arteriosus, 391
Paternalistic data collection interview, 42
Patrick test, 614, 615
Patterns of elimination, altered; *see* Elimination,
   altered
Pay Satisfaction Scale, 23
PCP, eye signs and, 300
PDA; *see* Patent ductus arteriosus
PDQ; *see* Prescreening Developmental Questionnaire
Peas in food pyramid, 102
Peau d'orange appearance, 412
Pectus carinatum, 331
Pectus excavatum, 331, 332
Pedal pulse, 373

Pederson speculum, 70
Pediatric head-to-toe examination, 695-697
Pediatric vaginal speculum, 70
Pediculosis, 156
Pelvis
   abscess in, 464
   biischial diameter of, 515
   bones of, 585
      female, 483, 486
   diameters of, 513-515
   examination of, in integrated assessment, 693
   floor of, 482
   inflammatory disease of, 507
   inlet of, 513
   midplane of, 513
   muscles of, 588
      exercises for, 527
   pain in, 489
   in pregnancy, 513-515
   racial variation of, 590
Penis
   anatomy and physiology of, 531, 532
   carcinoma of, 551
   common problems of, 551
   discharge from, 537
   examination of, 543-544
   lesions of, 537
   maturity development and, 535
Penlight, 69
Peptic ulcer, 472
   nausea and vomiting in, 443
   pain in, 456-457
Perceptual alteration as nursing diagnosis, 313, 314
Percussion
   direct or indirect, 74
   lung tones in, 74, 75, 336, 337
   in physical assessment, 74
   technique for chest, 336, 337
Percussion hammer, 68
Perfusion, 79
   altered peripheral tissue, in arterial insufficiency,
      397; *see also* Peripheral vessels
   respiratory, 317
Perianal area, 567
   examination of, in pregnancy, 576
Pericardial effusion, 379
Pericarditis, 391
Pericardium, 359, 360
Perineum
   inspection of, 499
   palpation of, 501
Peripheral atherosclerosis, 394
Peripheral cyanosis, 375, 376
Peripheral edema, 375, 376
Peripheral nervous system; *see also* Cranial nerves
   anatomy and physiology of, 644, 645, 647
   disorders of, 677
Peripheral vessels, 359-399; *see also* Cardiovascular system
   age-related variations in, 382-383
   anatomy and physiology of, 359-361, 362
   of child, 382-383
      health history and, 367
   common problems or conditions of, 393-395
      nursing diagnoses and sample documentation
         for, 396-397

Peripheral vessels—*cont'd*
   developmental considerations for, 362
   elasticity of, 362
   ethnic and cultural variations in, 384, 385, 390,
      394, 398
   examination of, 368-385
      arterial, 368-374
      auscultation in, 379-381
      blood pressure in, 368-369
      heart and, 377-379, 385
      pulses in, 369-373
      skin, hair, and nails in, 374
      venous, 375-377
   health history and, 363-367
   health promotion and, 398
   of infant, 382
      health history and, 366-367
   of newborn, 382
      health history and, 366-367
   of older adult, 383
      health history and, 367
   in pregnancy, 384
      health history and, 367
   racial variation in, 361, 385
   situational variations in, 384
Peripheral vision, 653
   defects of, 307
   testing for, 285, 307, 653
Peristalsis
   bowel sounds and, 451
   visible, 450
Peritoneum, 437-438
   irritation of, 454, 463
Peroneus tertius muscle, 617
Personal Assessment of Intimacy Relationships, 23
Personal beliefs
   about health and illness, 28
   stereotyping and, 28
Personal exposure to respiratory irritants, 325-326
Personal habits
   blood pressure and, 81
   circulatory system and, 363
   gastrointestinal system disorders and, 445
Personal protection
   equipment for patient care and, 71
   for sexually active male, 557
Personal questions to interviewer, 42
Personality development, theories of, 7-8
Petechiae, 98, 124, 125
Peyer's patches, 165, 170
Phalen's sign, 618
Pharyngitis, streptococcal, 180
Pharynx
   inspection of, 233
   in pregnancy, 218
   streptococcal infection of, 180
Phenothiazines, galactorrhea and, 431
Phenylketonuria, 107
Phimosis, 543
Phosphorus, recommended dietary allowances
   of, 101
Photoreceptor cells, 279
Physical assessment, 73-92; *see also* Health as-
   sessment; individual organ or system
   age-related variations in, 83-87, 88-91
   auscultation in, 74-76

Physical assessment—*cont'd*
  clinical guidelines for, 686-695
  equipment for, 61-72, 686; *see also*
   Equipment
  fetal, in pregnant woman, 55
  general, 82, 83
  head-to-toe, 685-700
    infant, 695-697
    model integrated, 685-695
    special considerations in, 685
    write-up of, 697-699
  of height, 82
  for infant, 695-697
  inspection in, 73
  model integrated, 685-695
  nutrition and, 96-97, 98-99; *see also*
   Nutrition
  palpation in, 73-74
  percussion in, 74
  positioning for, 76, 77
  in pregnancy, 87, 101-104
  previous, 44
  situational variations in, 87
  skinfold thickness in, 69, 82, 83-85, 94
  special considerations in, 685
  vital signs in, 76-82
  of weight, 82, 83, 84, 94
  write-up of, 697-699
Physical examination; *see* Physical assessment
Physical growth
  of infant, 9, 10-11
  of preschooler, 12, 16
  of school-age child, 13
  of toddler, 12
Physical mobility; *see* Mobility
Physiologic cup, 293
Physiologic jaundice, 136
Piaget's theory of personality development, 7-8
Pica, 104, 445
PID; *see* Pelvis, inflammatory disease of
Pigeon chest, 331
Pigeon toe, 624
Pigmentation of skin; *see* Skin pigmentation
Pigmented nevi
  changes in, 119, 123
  inspection of, 125
Pilonidal cyst or sinus, 567, 575
Pitch of sound, 76
Pitting
  edematous, 376
  of nail, 135
Pityriasis rosea, 148
Pivot joints, 584
PKU; *see* Phenylketonuria
Planning in nursing process, 1, 2
Plantar reflex
  in infant grasp, 670
  testing for, 662-664
Plaque, 98, 126
Pleural effusion, 352
Pleural friction rub, 334, 335, 341
PMS; *see* Premenstrual syndrome
Pneumatic attachment for otoscope, 67
Pneumococcal pneumonia, 351
Pneumonia with lobar consolidation, 351
Pneumothorax, 353, 379

Poisoning
  food, 479
  lead, 479
Polycythemia, 382
Polydactyly, 624
Polyhydramnios, 476
Polyps
  in ear, 269
  nasal, 224, 239
  rectal, 575
Popliteal artery, 369
Popliteal edema, 616
Popliteal pulse, 78, 373
Portage Guide to Early Education, 21
Port-wine stain, 137
Position
  for examination, 76, 77
    of female reproductive system, 497-498
  joint, sense of, 660-661
Posterior chamber of eye, 277
Posterior tibial pulse, 373
Postmenopausal bleeding, 495
Postpartum and lactating women, nutrition and, 105-106
Postural hypotension, 369
Posture
  inspection of, 596
  Parkinson's disease and, 678
Potassium hydroxide testing for vaginal or cervical
  specimens, 505
Potential for altered growth and development in
  male genitalia problems, 555
Pouch in ileostomy or colostomy, 573
Poultry in food pyramid, 102
Poupart's ligament, 437-438, 534
Prealbumin
  in neonate and infant, 107
  nutritional status and, 95-96
Preauricular nodes, 172
Precordium, palpation of, 377-378
Preeclampsia, 104
Pregnancy
  of adolescent
    ethnic and cultural influences on, 32-33
    high-risk nutritional conditions during, 104
  alcohol in, 103
  anemia in, 100
  anthropometrics in, 100
  anus in, 561, 565-566, 573
  auditory system in, 264
    developmental considerations for, 248
  biochemical tests in, 100-101
  blood glucose in, 101
  blood pressure in, 87, 362, 384
  breast in, 101, 402, 408, 425
    developmental considerations for, 402
    health history and, 408
  Centers for Disease Control and Prevention rec-
    ommendations for, 104
  cervix during, 486, 488
  constipation in, 103, 561, 566
  developmental considerations for, 486-488
  ectopic, 456-457
  edema in, 362
  estrogens during, 486
  ethnic and cultural considerations for, 496
    teenager and, 32-33

Pregnancy—*cont'd*
  eye and visual system in, 299
    developmental considerations for, 280
  gait in, 625
  gallbladder in, 441
  gastrointestinal system in, 101-103, 467-471
    developmental considerations for, 440-441
    problems or conditions and, 476
  head and neck in, 188, 202
  health history and, 44, 55-56, 490-491, 496
  heart and peripheral vessels in, 367, 384
  heart rate in, 87
  hematocrit in, 100
  hemoglobin in, 100
  hemorrhoids in, 362, 561, 566
  history of previous, 44
  immunoglobulins in, 170
  iron and, 100, 103
  lordosis in, 591, 625
  morning sickness in, 101
  mouth in, 218, 237
  musculoskeletal system in, 625
  National Academy of Science recommendations
    for, 104
  nausea and vomiting in, 103, 440
  neurologic system in, 675
    developmental considerations for, 647
  nose and pharynx in, 218, 237
  nutrition in, 97-105
    high-risk conditions for, 104
  oropharynx in, 218
  pelvis in, 513-515
  perianal examination in, 576
  physical assessment in, 87, 101-104
  progesterone in, 440, 486
    respiratory system and, 322
  pulse in, 87
  Recommended Dietary Allowances in, 103-104
  rectum in, 573
    developmental considerations for, 561
    health history and, 565-566
  reproductive system changes in, 512-516
  respirations in, 87
  respiratory system in, 322
    examination of, 345
  serum albumin in, 100-101
  skin in, 117
  smoking in, 103
  spiders of breast in, 425
  supplements in, 103
  tidal volume in, 322
  uterus during, 486, 488
  vagina during, 488
  varicosities in, 142, 362
  vital signs in, 87
  vitamin A in, 104
  vomiting in, 440
  weight in, 87, 97
Premenstrual syndrome, 489, 518
  health promotion and, 527
Prenatal history, hearing loss and, 252
Prepuce, 531
Presbycusis, 248, 250
Presbyopia, 280, 284
Preschooler, 12, 16
  assessment tools for, 12
  behavioral development of, 12, 16

Preschooler—*cont'd*
  developmental tasks of, 16
  normal heart rates of, 78
  normal respiratory rates of, 79
  nutrition in, 109-110
  physical growth of, 12, 16
Prescreening Developmental Questionnaire, 21
Present health status, 43, 45
  documentation of, 56
  of infant and child, 50
  of newborn, 48
  in older adult, 53
  of pregnant woman, 55
Presentation of fetus, 469
Presenting part of infant, 515, 516
Pressure
  blood; *see* Blood pressure
  pulse, 79, 368
Pressure areas, bony prominences vulnerable to, '143, 144
Prevention of injury, 635
Priapism, 536
Primary skin lesions, 126-128
Problem list
  documentation of, 699
  subjective, documentation of, 58
Professional terminology in data collection interview, 42
Progesterone, 483
  fluid retention and, 365
  in pregnancy, 440, 486
    respiratory system and, 322
Prolactin, galactorrhea and, 431
Prolapse
  of rectum, 576
  of uterus, 501, 519
Prominences, bony, vulnerable to pressure, 143, 144
Pronation, 585
Prone position, 77
Prostate gland, 559-581
  age-related variations in, 572
  anatomy and physiology of, 534, 559, 561
  benign hypertrophy of, 576
  cancer of, 577
    health promotion in, 580
  common problems or conditions of, 576-577
    nursing diagnoses and sample documentation for, 578-579
  developmental considerations for, 561
  enlargement of, classification of, 571
  ethnic and cultural variations in, 564, 574
  examination of, 569, 570-571
  health history and, 564, 566
  health promotion and, 580
  of older adult, 572
    developmental considerations for, 561
    health history and, 566
Prostatitis, 537, 576
Prosthesis for eye, 299
Protection from noise, 274
Protein
  deficiency of, 98, 99
  in neonate and infant, 107
  recommended dietary allowances of, 100
  retinol binding, 107
Pruritus; *see* Itching

Pseudoaneurysm, 395
Psoriasis, 147
Psychosocial status, 47-48
  of adolescent, 53
  documentation of, 58
  of infant and child, 51
  of newborn, 49
  of older adult, 53-55
  of pregnant woman, 56
Pterygium, 289, 305
Ptosis, 288, 305
Puberty, 402, 486
  health history and, 406, 494
Pubescence, 486
Pubic hair, 133
  development of, 486, 487
  increased growth of, 157
  inspection of, 498
  male, 542
    maturity development and, 535
Pubic lice, 542
Pubis, 483, 486
Pudendum, 481
Pulmonary arteries, 359, 361
Pulmonary hypertension, 378
Pulmonic valves, 359
  heart sounds and, 379, 380
    abnormal, 388-389
  stenosis of, 378, 388-389
Pulse, 78, 369-373
  abnormalities in, 370
  amplitude of, 78, 369
  contour of, 78
  of newborn and infant, 85
  in pregnancy, 87
  venous, 375-377, 383
Pulse oximetry, 64
Pulse pressure, 79, 368
Pulsus alternans, 369, 370
Pulsus bisferiens, 370
Pulsus paradoxus, 369, 370
Pupil of eye, 277
  abnormalities of, 308-310
  constriction of, 309, 653
  dilation of, 309
    drugs and, 281
  drug intoxication and, 300
  in infant, 296
  inspection of, 292
Purification, 34
Purkinje fibers, 360
Purpura, 125
Pustule, 128
Pyelonephritis, 459, 476
  in male, 536
Pyloric sphincter, 438
Pyloric stenosis, 476
Pyorrhea, advanced, 240
Pyramid, food, 102
Pyridoxine, deficiency of, 98

Q

Quadriceps muscles, 614
Quadriplegia, 143-144
Questions
  about sensitive issues, 41

Questions—*cont'd*
  interview, 40-41
    why, 42
  personal, to interviewer, 42
  in questionnaire for nutritional assessment, 105
Quinine, ototoxicity of, 250

R

Racial variations
  in auditory system, 257
  in blood pressure, 81, 369, 385, 394
  in breast, 415, 417
  in eye and visual system, 288, 290, 294
  in female reproductive system, 498
  in gastrointestinal system, 470
  in gestational period, 470
  in hair, 133
  in head, 196
  in lips, 227
  in lungs and respiratory system, 320, 327
  in male genitalia, 531, 542
  in musculoskeletal system, 583, 590, 617
  in nails, 116, 134
  in neurologic system, 651
  in nose, 234
  in oropharynx, 230, 232
  in osteoporosis incidence, 625
  in peripheral vessels, 361, 385
  in skeleton, 625
  in skin pigmentation, 124
    aging and, 140
    in newborn, 136
    in older adult, 140
    pressure areas and, 143
  in sweat glands, 116
  in teeth, 215, 217, 221
Radial pulse, 78, 372
Radical mastectomy, 177
Range of motion, 585-586, 589, 590
  of ankle, 617
  assessment of, 597, 598, 599
  of elbow, 609
  of fingers, 612, 613
  of hips, 614, 615
  of jaw, 600
  of knee, 616
  of neck, 197, 601
  of shoulder, 606, 607
  of spine, 604
  of trunk, 603
  of wrist, 612, 613
Rape prevention guidelines, 527
Rash, 124
  diaper, 493, 539
  history of, 118
The Rating-Ranking Scale of Child Behavior, 22
Raynaud's phenomenon or disease, 395
Reason for seeking care, 43
  documentation of, 56
  in infant and child health history, 50
  in newborn health history, 48
  in older adult, 53
  of pregnant woman, 55
Rebound tenderness in abdomen, 463
Recommended Dietary Allowances, 97, 100-101
  in postpartum and lactating women, 106

Recommended Dietary Allowances—*cont'd*
  in pregnancy, 103-104
Recommended immunization schedule, 161
Record, food, 93
Recording of data collected in health assessment, 3;
  see also Documentation
Recreation, safe, 682
Rectal temperature, 76
Rectal wall, palpation of, 510
Rectocele, 501, 521
Rectovaginal examination, 509-510
Rectum, 438, 559-581; *see also* Gastrointestinal
  system
  of adolescent, 572
  age-related variations in, 572
  anatomy and physiology of, 559, 560, 561
  bleeding from, 563
    nursing diagnosis and documentation in, 578
  cancer of, 575
    health promotion in, 580
    risk factors for, 562
  of child, 572
    developmental considerations for, 561
    health history and, 565
  common problems or conditions of, 575-576
    nursing diagnoses and sample documentation
      for, 578-579
  developmental considerations for, 561
  ethnic and cultural variations in, 574
  examination of, 567-569, 570
    in integrated assessment, 693-694
    stool specimen in, 571
  fissures of, 563, 575
  health history and, 562-566
  health promotion and, 580
  of infant, 572
    developmental considerations for, 561
    health history and, 564-565
  itching, burning, and stinging of, 563-564
  in male, health history and, 566
  masses of, 579
  of older adult, 572
    developmental considerations for, 561
    health history and, 566
  pain in, 563
  polyps of, 575
  in pregnancy, 573
    developmental considerations for, 561
    health history and, 565-566
  prolapse of, 576
  situational variations in, 573-574
Rectus abdominis muscle, 437
Recumbent position, dorsal or lateral, 77
Red reflex, 292, 293
  in infant, 296
Red-free filter, 66
Reflection in data collection interview, 41
Reflex
  corneal, 286-287
    drug intoxication and, 300
    in older adult, 280
  cremasteric, 665
  deep tendon; *see* Deep tendon reflexes
  gag, 656
  in infant, 670-671
  in older adult, 674

Reflex—*cont'd*
  red, 292, 293
    in infant, 296
  superficial, 644, 647
    abdominal, neurologic examination of, 647, 665
Reflex arc, 644, 645, 647
Reflex hammer, 68
Reflux, gastroesophageal, 445, 456-457, 472
Regurgitation
  aortic or pulmonic valve, 378, 388-389
  gastrointestinal, in infant, 445
Relationships, family; *see* Family
Religious influences, 29
Renal arteries, bruits and, 451
Renal calculi, 476
Renal failure, acute or chronic, 476
Reproductive system
  female, 481-529; *see also* Female reproductive
    system
  male, 531-558; *see also* Male genitalia
Resonance, vocal, 340-342
Respirations, 79, 80; *see also* Breathing
  depth of, in child, 344
  of newborn and infant, 85
  normal, 79, 80
  patterns of, 80
  in pregnancy, 87
Respiratory compromise or distress, 330
Respiratory depth, 79, 80
Respiratory effort, 332-333
Respiratory excursion, 336-338
Respiratory irritants, exposure to, 325-326
Respiratory rates, 79, 80
Respiratory system, 317-357
  of adolescent, 344
    health history and, 327-328
  age-related variations in, 343-345
  anatomy and physiology of, 317-322
    external, 317-322
    internal, 317, 318, 319
  breathing problems in, 323-325
  of child, 322
    examination of, 344
    health history and, 327-328
    respiratory rates and, 343
  common problems and conditions of, 348-353
    nursing diagnoses and sample documentation
      for, 354-355
  developmental considerations for, 322
  ethnic and cultural considerations for, 326, 346,
    351, 352
  examination of, 330-342, 347
    anterior and posterior chest, 333-342
    breath sounds in, 338-340, 341
    chest wall configuration in, 330-332
    general presentation in, 330
    oxygenation in, 332
    percussion tones over lungs in, 336, 337
    respiratory effort in, 332-333
  in health history, 323-329
    of child and adolescent, 327-328
    of infants, 326-327
    of older adult, 328-329
  health promotion and, 356
  of infant, 322
    examination of, 343

Respiratory system—*cont'd*
  of infant—*cont'd*
    health history and, 326-327
    respiratory rates and, 343
  of older adult, 322
    examination of, 344-346
    health history and, 328-329
  in pregnancy, 322
    examination of, 345
  racial variation in, 320, 327
  in review of systems, 46
    documentation of, 57
    of infant and child
    of newborn, 49
    in pregnant woman, 55
  situational variations in, 345-346
  topographic markers of, 320-322
Restatement in data collection interview, 41
Retina, 279
  disorders of, 311, 312
  inspection of, 294
Retinal arteries, 293
Retinal veins, 293
Retinol binding protein, 107
Retinopathy
  diabetic, 311
  hypertensive, 312
Retractions
  chest wall, 377
  supraclavicular, in infant, 343
Retroflexed or retroverted uterus, 508
Reverse splitting of heart sound, 381
Review of systems, 44-47
  of adolescent, 52
  documentation of, 57
  of infant and child, 50-52
  of newborn, 49
  of pregnant woman, 55-56
Rheumatic heart disease, 366, 367
Rheumatoid arthritis, 592, 608, 609, 610, 629
Rhinitis, 224
Rhonchi, 341
Rib cage, 317-320
Riboflavin
  deficiency of, 98
  recommended dietary allowances of, 100
Right ventricular hypertrophy, 390
Rigidity, abdominal, 454
Ringing in ears, 250
Ringworm, 151
Rinne test, 260, 655
Risks
  for breast cancer, 406
  for cardiovascular disease, 398
  for colorectal cancer, 562
  documentation of, 699
  for fluid volume deficit in lymphatic system dis-
    orders, 181
  for impaired skin integrity, 159
  for infection, 183
    in male genitalia disorders, 556
    in nasal foreign body, 245
  for injury in cerebrovascular accident, 556
  for osteoporosis, 634
Rituals, 29
Rods, 279

Romberg test, 261, 657
Rooting reflex, 671
Root-work and Root doctor, 34
ROS; *see* Review of systems
Rosenbaum near vision chart, 66, 284, 285
Rotation, external or internal, 585
Rubella, 150
  congenital, 366
  vaccine for, 162-163
Rubeola, 150
Ruler, 69
Rupture
  of appendix, 464
  of tympanic membrane, 249, 255, 257

S

SA node; *see* Sinoatrial nodes
Saccular aneurysm, 395
Sacrococcygeal area, 567
Safe sex, 528
Safe travel or recreation, 682
Safety in sports, 594
Sagittal suture, 188
  visible on vaginal examination before delivery, 516
Saliva in universal blood and body fluid precautions, 71
Salivary glands, 215, 216
  in infant, 217
Salivation in child, 235
Salmon patch, 136, 137
Sandor Clinical Assessment–Geriatric, 23
Sarcomas, Kaposi's, 153
  in mouth, 243
Saturated fat in healthy eating guidelines, 97, 100
Scabies, 130, 139, 155, 156
SCAG; *see* Sandor Clinical Assessment–Geriatric
Scale, 129
Scaling skin, 98
Scalp hair in newborn, 138
Scapular line, 322
Scar, 124, 129
Scarlet fever, 152
Schlemm's canal, 278
School experiences of child, 51
School-age child, 13-17
  assessment tools for, 13
  behavioral development of, 13
  developmental tasks of, 17
  experiences of, 51
  normal heart rates of, 78
  normal respiratory rates of, 79
  physical growth of, 13
Sciatic neuritis, 622
Sclera, 277
  in infant, 296
  inspection of, 290
  in older adult, 298
Scoliosis, 330, 603, 632
Screening
  for breast problems or conditions, 435
  for eye disorders, 315
  for hearing acuity, 67, 68
  for hearing impairment, 274
  of neurologic soft signs, 672, 673-674
Scrotum
  anatomy and physiology of, 531, 533

Scrotum—*cont'd*
  common problems or conditions of, 553-554
  examination of, 545-546
    in integrated assessment, 695
    in infant, 547
    maturity development and, 535
Scurvy, 99
Sebaceous cyst, 128, 268
Sebaceous glands, 116
  breast and, 401
Sebaceous hyperplasia, 41, 140
Seborrheic dermatitis, 146
  in newborn, 138
Seborrheic keratoses, 41, 140
Second heart sound, 381
Secondary skin lesions, 129-131
Secretory otitis media, 270
Sedatives, sexual function and, 538, 541
Seizures, 677
  in health history, 648-649
  in infant, 650
Selenium, recommended dietary allowances of, 101
Self-awareness, cultural sensitivity and, 27
Self-care
  assessment of, 54
  deficit or limitations in, 593-594
Self-esteem disturbance as nursing diagnoses
  in depression, 680
  in obesity, 477
Self-examination
  of breast, 421
  of genitalia
    by female, 527
    by male, 557
Self-image, disturbance of; *see* Body image disturbance
Semilunar valves, 359
Seminal vesicles, 534
Seminiferous tubules, 531
Senile lentigines, 41, 140
Senile tremor, 651
Sensation
  altered
    health history and, 649
    as nursing diagnosis, 313, 314
  examination of, 660-664
    facial, 653-654, 655
    pediatric, 672, 673-674
Sensitive issues, questions about, 41
Sensitivity, cultural, 27
Sensorineural hearing loss, 248, 260, 271, 655
Sensory fibers of spinal nerves, 644
Sensory function in child, testing for, 672, 673-674; *see also* Sensation
Sensory/perceptual alteration as nursing diagnosis, 313, 314
Septal defects, atrial or ventricular, 392
Serous otitis media, 258, 270
Serum albumin
  in neonate and infant, 107
  nutritional status and, 95
  in older adult, 112
  in pregnancy, 100-101
Serum glucose; *see* Blood glucose
Serum prealbumin
  in neonate and infant, 107

Serum prealbumin—*cont'd*
  nutritional status and, 95-96
Serum transferrin, 107
Setting for health history interview, 39
Sexual abuse, health history and, 540
Sexual activity
  health history and, 495
  in older adult, 495-496
  personal protection for male, 557
Sexual dysfunction, male, 537-538
Sexuality
  health history and, 492
  male, 538
Sexually transmitted diseases, 522-524
  eye infection of newborn and, 282
  health history and, 492
  in male, 552-553
  safe sex and, 528
  signs and symptoms of, 524
SGA; *see* Small for gestational age
SGSS; *see* Stokes/Gordon Stress Scale
Shingles, 149
Shinto, 35
Shortness of breath, 324-325, 364
Shoulder
  assessment of, 603, 605, 626
    in integrated examination, 687
  movement of, 657
  muscle strength of, 657
  range of motion of, 606, 607
  supporting structures of, 589
Sibilant rhonchi or wheezes, 341
Sighing, 333
Signs, 2
  Brudzinski's, 667, 668
  bulge, 619
  Gower's, 672
  Kernig's, 667, 668
  Phalen's, 618
  Tinel's, 618
Silences in interview, 42
Sims' position, 77
Single-parent families, 20
Single-use thermometer strips, disposable, 61, 62
Sinoatrial nodes, 359, 360
Sinuses
  paranasal; *see* Paranasal sinuses
  pilonidal, 567, 575
Sitting positions for examination, 77
Situational variations, health history and, 55-56
Skeletal muscles, 583, 586, 587, 588
Skeleton, 583, 584, 585; *see also* Musculoskeletal system
  appendicular, 589-590
  axial, 589
  chest, deformities of, 330
  inspection of, 595
  lesions of, nutrition and, 99
  racial variations in, 625
Skene glands and duct, 482
  inspection of, 499-500
Skin, 115-164
  age-related variations in, 131, 136-142
    health history and, 120-121
  altered integrity of, in arterial insufficiency, 397
  anatomy and physiology of, 115-116

Skin—*cont'd*
arterial pulse assessment and, 374
cancer of
prevention of, 161
risk assessment for, 119
color of, 122-125
changes in, 119; *see also* Cyanosis
venous pressure and, 376
common problems or conditions of, 146-155
nursing diagnoses and sample documentation
for, 159-160
developmental considerations for, 116-117
dry, 131
history of, 118
edema and cyanosis and, 375, 376
elasticity of, 117
ethnic and cultural variations in, 145
examination of, 122-132
health history and, 118-119
age-related variations in, 120-121
health promotion and, 161
recommended immunization schedule for,
161-162
in heart and peripheral vascular
examination, 374
lesions of
characteristics of, to be noted during examination, 131
primary, 126-128
secondary, 129-131
venous pressure and, 376
mobility of, 132
in nutritional assessment, 97, 98
of preschool and school-age child, 109
oily, history of, 118
pigmentation of; *see* Skin pigmentation
situational variations in, 142-145
structures of, 115
turgor of, 132
in child, 1139
in newborn, 138
in older adult, 142
vascular abnormalities of, 125
in child, 138-139
in newborn, 136
wrinkling of, 117
Skin calipers, 69, 82, 83-85, 94
Skin pigmentation, 122-124
racial variation in, 124
in newborn, 136
in older adult, 140
pressure areas and, 143
Skin protection
altered health maintenance for, 160
promotion of, 161
Skin tags, 41, 140
Skinfold thickness, 69, 82, 83-85, 94
in neonate and infant, 106
in preschool and school-age child, 109
Skull
inspection of, 195
of newborn and infant, 83, 86, 87, 591
racial variation of, 590
supporting structures of, 589
Slit light of ophthalmoscope, 67
Small for gestational age, 106

Small intestine, 438; *see also* Gastrointestinal system
in older adult, 441
Smears, vaginal, collection of, 504-505
Smell, sense of, 223, 642, 644, 652
Smokeless tobacco, 356
Smoking, 325-326
cardiovascular disease risks and, 398
documentation of, 58
ethnic and cultural influences on, 32
health promotion and, 326, 356
in pregnancy, 103
risks of, 246, 326
vasoconstriction and, 363
Snacking in adolescent, 110
Snellen visual acuity chart, 65, 284
Soaps, lactating breast and, 409
Social Readjustment Rating Scale, 22
Social Rewards Satisfaction, 23
Social-adaptive behavior, 7
Soft palate, movement of, 656
Somesthetic cortex topography, 641
Sonorous rhonchi or wheezes, 341
Sore throat, 220
Sound
bone-conducted, 655
characteristics of, 76
quality of, 76
Sound waves, 67, 68
Special needs client, health history and, 651; *see
also* Neurologic system
Speculum
nasal, 67, 223-224, 225
vaginal, 70
in examination, 501-506
Speech, examination of, 652
Spermatocele, 554
Spermatogenesis, 531
Spermicides, vaginal, 528
Sphenoidal sinuses, 225; *see also* Paranasal sinuśes
Sphincters
cardiac, 438
pyloric, 438
stenosis of, 476
rectal, 559
Sphygmomanometer, 63, 79
Spiders, 125, 137, 138, 142, 362
breast, in pregnancy, 425
Spina bifida, 630
Spinal accessory nerve, 642, 643, 644
head turning and, 197
tests for, 657
Spinal cord, 643-644, 645
injury to, 677
Spinal nerves, 644, 645
Spinal processes of vertebrae, 605
Spine
assessment of, 603, 604, 626
range of motion of, 604
supporting structures of, 589
Spiritualist, 34
Spleen, 169-170, 439, 440; *see also* Gastrointestinal system
examination of, 454, 459
palpation of, 459
Splenomegaly, 454
Spooning of nails, 135

Sports, safety in, 594
Sprain, muscle, 629
Sputum, variations in, 323-324
Squamocolumnar junction, 483
Squamous cell carcinoma
of lips, 240
of skin, 154
Staphylococcal infection of skin, hair, and nails,
151-153, 156
Stasis dermatitis, 129, 147
Stasis ulcer, 130, 365, 366
Stations of infant's presenting part, 515, 516
STDs; *see* Sexually transmitted diseases
Stenson's duct, 230
Step in place reflex, 671
Stepfamilies, 20
Stereognosis, examination of, 661, 662
Stereotyping, 28
Sternal retractions in infant, 343
Sternocleidomastoid muscle, 185, 187
assessment of, 602
Sternum, 320
Steroids, gynecomastia and, 432
Stethoscope, 61-62, 74-75
Doppler ultrasonic, 64, 87
Stiff neck, 191, 193
in infection, 193
in older adult, 194
Stinging, rectal, 563-564
Stocking anesthesia, 374
Stokes/Gordon Stress Scale, 23
Stoma, colostomy, 573-574
Stomach, 438, 439; *see also* Abdomen
percussion of, 74, 75
Stomatitis, angular, 98
Stool
blood in, 563, 571
diet of infant and, 565
examination of, 571
in ileostomy or colostomy, 573
incontinence of, 564
jaundice and, 443
meconium, 561
variations in, 563, 571
Storkbite, 136, 137
Strabismus, 297, 308
Straight leg raising test, 622
Strain, muscle, 629
in older adults, 594
Strangulation of hernia, 550
Strawberry angioma, 125, 137
Streptococcal infection
in pharyngitis, 180
of skin, hair, and nails, 151-153
Streptomycin, ototoxicity of, 250
Stress
cardiovascular system and, 363
health promotion for, 398
coping ability for, in child, 52
Stress incontinence, 501
Striae, 122
in pregnant abdomen, 142, 467
Stridor in infant, 343
Stroke; *see* Cerebrovascular accident
Sty, 288, 305
Subjective data, 2

Subjective problem list, documentation of, 58
Sucking reflex, 671
Summary in data collection interview, 41
Sun exposure and protection, 161
Superficial reflexes, 644, 647
    abdominal, neurologic examination of, 647, 665
Superficial tactile sensation, 660-661
Supernumerary nipples, 414, 415, 417
Supination, 585
Supine position, 77
Supplements
    indications for, 103
    in pregnancy, 103
Supraclavicular lymph nodes, 173
Supraclavicular retractions in infant, 343
Suprasternal notch, 197, 320
Surgery in health history, 44
    documentation of, 57
    female reproductive system, 492
Sutures
    ossification of, 188
    sagittal, 188
        visible on vaginal examination before
        delivery, 516
Swallowing difficulty, 220, 444
    health history and, 649
Swan neck deformity, 610
Sweat glands, 116, 117
Sweets in food pyramid, 102
Swimmer's ear, 250, 269
Sympathetic nervous system, 644, 646
Symptoms, 2
    analysis of, 43, 44
Syncope, 365
Syndactyly, 624
Synovial joints, 584, 586, 589
Synovitis of knee, 616
Syphilis
    in female, 523
        health history and, 492
        signs and symptoms of, 524
    in male, 552
Syringes in universal blood and body fluid precau-
    tions, 71
Systematic operations, 8
Systemic systolic blood pressure, 79
Systems review, 44-47
    of adolescent, 52
    documentation of, 57
    of infant and child, 50-52
    of newborn, 49
    in pregnant woman, 55-56
Systole
    blood pressure and, 79, 81, 368-369
    heart and, 359-360, 361
Systolic heart murmurs, 377, 378, 386-389

T

T_3, 192
T_4
    in neonate and infant, 107
    in thyroid dysfunction, 192
T lymphocytes, 165, 169
Tachycardia, 369
    nutrition and, 99
Tachypnea, 80, 332, 333

Tactile fremitus, 335
Tactile sensation, superficial, 660-661
Tail of Spence, 401, 402
Talipes equinovarus, 624, 631
Talking too much in data collection interview, 42
Tape measure, 69
Tarsals, racial variation of, 590
Taste, examination of, 656
Taste buds, 215
Td; see Tetanus and diphtheria toxoid
Tears
    excessive, 282, 289
    lacrimal gland formation of, 277
Teenage pregnancy
    ethnic and cultural influences on, 32-33
    high-risk nutritional conditions during, 104
Teeth, 215, 216
    age-related variations in, 234-236
        health history and, 220-221
    in child, 218
        examination of, 235
        health history and, 222
    common problems or conditions of, 240
        nursing diagnoses and sample documentation
        for, 244-245
    deciduous, 217
    developmental considerations for, 217-218
    ethnic and cultural considerations for, 237
    examination of, 227-233, 238
    health history and, 221
        age-related variations in, 220-221
    health promotion and, 244-245
    inspection of, 228-229
    malocclusion of, 228
    in older adult, 218
        health history and, 222
    permanent, dentition of, 216
    racial variation in, 215, 217, 221
    situational variations in, 237
Telangiectasia, 125, 128, 137, 142, 362
Temperature, 76
    in child, 86-87
    conversion of Fahrenheit and Centigrade, 76
    of newborn and infant, 84-85
    of skin, 131
    thermometers for measurement of, 61, 62, 76
Temporal bones, 185
Temporal headache, 203
Temporal pulse, 371
Temporalis muscle, 600
Temporomandibular joint, 227
    assessment of, 600, 626
    dysfunction of, 600, 628
        nursing diagnosis in, 244
Tenderness
    in breast, 404
    in muscles, 595
Tendon, 586-587, 590
Tendon reflexes, deep; see Deep tendon reflexes
Tennis elbow, 609
Tension headache, 189, 203
Tentorium cerebelli, 637, 638
Terminal hairs, 116
Terminology in data collection interview, 42
Testes
    anatomy and physiology of, 531

Testes—cont'd
    common problems or conditions of, 553-554
    examination of, 545-546
    fetal development of, 534
    pain in, 536
    torsion of, 553
Tetanus and diphtheria toxoids, 162-163
Tetralogy of Fallot, 393
Thelarche, 402, 486
Theories of development, 7-8
Thermometers, 61, 62, 76
    disposable, single-use thermometer strips as, 61, 62
Thiamine, deficiency of, 98, 100
Thiazides, food interaction with, 113
Thigh, supporting structures of, 590
Thiouracil, breast milk and, 409
Third molar, agenesis of, 215
Thomas test, 621
Thoracic cage, 317-320
Thoracic expansion, 334
Thoracic spine
    assessment of, 603, 604, 626
    range of motion of, 604
Thorax, percussion of, 74, 75; see also Chest
Thought content disruptions, 667
Thought processes, slowed, 651
Threshold, 68
Thrill, 377, 378
Throat, sore, 220
Thrombophlebitis, 394
    contraceptives and, 365
Thrombosis, 394
    of corpora cavernosa, 536
Thrush, 241
Thymus, 169
Thyroid gland, 185, 192
    cancer of, 212
    enlargement of, nutrition and, 99
    examination of, 198-199
    nodules of, 198, 199
TIA; see Transient ischemic attack
Tibial pulse, posterior, 373
Tidal volume, pregnancy and, 322
Tinea corporis, 151
Tinea cruris, 542
Tinea pedis, 151
Tinea unguium, 158
Tinel's sign, 618
Tinnitus, 271; see also Meniere's disease
Tissue characteristics, transilluminator for differ-
    entiation of, 70
Tissue perfusion, altered peripheral, in arterial in-
    sufficiency, 397
Tobacco, 325-326
    in pregnancy, 103
    smokeless, 356
    vasoconstriction and, 363
Toddler, 12, 13
    behavioral development of, 12
    developmental tasks of, 9, 24
    eating habits of, 445
    normal heart rates of, 78
    normal respiratory rates of, 79
    nutrition of, 108-109
    physical growth of, 12
Toe, deformities of, 616, 624

Toenail, ingrown, 158
  prevention of, 161
Toilet-training, 493, 565
  in male, 539
Tongue
  anatomy and physiology of, 215
  in child, 236
  common problems or conditions of, 241
  examination of, 656
  inspection of, 231
  nutrition and, 98
  in older adult, 218
  palpation of, 231-232
Tonic neck reflex, 670
Tonic pupil, 310
Tonsils, 170
  in child, 236
  inspection of, 233
Tophi, 268
Torsion, testicular, 553
Torticollis, 207
Torus palatinus, 232
Total cholesterol
  nutritional status and, 96
  in older adult, 112
Total hysterectomy, 516
Trabecular meshwork, 278
Trachea, 317, 319
  deviation of, 330, 333
Traction-inflammatory headache, 203
Tranquilizers, sexual function and, 538, 541
Transferrin, 107
Transient ischemic attack, 649
Transillumination
  of sinuses, 226
  of skull in infant, 200-201
Transilluminator, 70
Transverse diameter of pelvis, 513, 514, 515
Trapezius muscle, 602
  strength of, 605, 606
Trauma; see Injury
Travel
  environmental exposure to respiratory irritants
    and, 326
  safe, 682
Tremor
  Parkinson's; see Parkinson's disease
  senile, 651
Trendelenburg test, 377
Triamterene, food interaction with, 113
Triangles of neck, 185, 187
Triceps reflex, 662-664
Trichomonas vaginalis, 505
Trichomoniasis, 523
  signs and symptoms of, 524
Tricuspid valve, heart sounds and, 379, 380, 388-389
Tricyclic antidepressants, 431
Trigeminal nerve, 600, 642, 643, 644
  edema of brainstem and, 291
  eye and, 277
  neuralgia in, 600, 654
  tests for, 653-654, 655
Triglycerides, nutritional status and, 96
Trochlear nerve, 642, 643, 644, 653
  eye movement and, 277, 286

Trunk
  bones of, 585
  muscles of, 588
  range of motion of, 603
TSH
  in neonate and infant, 107
  in thyroid dysfunction, 192
Tubercle
  darwinian, 254, 267
  Montgomery, 413
Tuberculosis, 351
Tubing of stethoscope, 61
Tumor, 127
Tuning fork, 67, 259, 260
Turgor of skin, 132
  in child, 139
  in newborn, 138
  in older adult, 142
  venous pressure and, 376
24-hour recall of foods eaten, 93
Two-point discrimination, 661, 662
Tympanic membrane, 247, 248
  color variations in, 258
  common problems or conditions of, 270-271
  examination of, 255-259
    in child, 263
    in infant, 262
  landmarks of, 257
  mobility variations in, 259
  normal, 258
  ruptured, 249, 255, 257
  in temperature measurement, 61, 62, 76
Tympanotomy, 271
Tympany, 74, 452, 454, 462

U

Ulcer, 130
  aphthous, 241
  corneal, 306
  of lips, 228
  peptic, 472
    nausea and vomiting in, 443
  venous stasis, 130, 365, 366
Ulcerative colitis, 473, 563
Ultrasonic stethoscope, Doppler, 64, 87
Umbilicus
  displacement of, 450
  in infant, 466
  palpation of, 458
Undernutrition in toddler, 108
Underweight, 93
Unemployment, 30-31
Universal blood and body fluid precautions, 71
Upper airway, 317
Upper extremities; see Extremities, upper
Urea nitrogen in neonate and infant, 107
Ureters, 440
Urethra, 531, 532
Urethral meatus
  inspection of, 499
  in male, 544
Urethritis, 537
Urinalysis in neonate and infant, 107
Urinary bladder, 440
  in infant and child, 466

Urinary difficulties, 444
  nursing diagnosis and sample documentation
    in, 579
Urinary incontinence
  female examination and, 500
  stress, 500
Urinary system, 439
  common problems or conditions of, 476
    nursing diagnosis and sample documentation
      in, 579
  in review of systems, 46-47
    of adolescent, 52
    documentation of, 57
    of infant and child
    of newborn, 49
    in pregnant woman, 56
Urination, changes in
  in female, 490
  in male, 536-537, 564
Urine
  color of, 443, 444
  jaundice and, 443
USDA food pyramid, 97, 102
Uterine adnexa, palpation of, 509, 510
Uterine cervix; see Cervix
Uterine fundus
  height of, 468
  palpation of, 467, 470
Uterine tubes, 483
Uterus, 483
  anteflexed, 508
  anteverted, 507
  bimanual examination for, 506-510
  common problems and conditions of, 518-520
  fibroids of, 519
  fundal height of, 513
  at midposition, 508
  during pregnancy, 486, 488
  prolapse of, 501, 519
  retroflexed, 508
  retroverted, 508
Uvea, 277
Uveitis, 309
Uvula, 232

V

Vagina, 482
  bimanual examination for, 507
  common problems and conditions of, 520-521
  discharge from, 490
    in child, 493
    inspection of, 504
  dryness and itching of, in older woman, 495
  inspection of, 499-500
  introitus of, 499
  during pregnancy, 488
  smear from, 504-505
  speculum for, 70, 501-506
  spermicides for use in, 528
  tissue examination of, 70
  wall inspection of, 506
Vaginitis
  monilial, 522
  signs and symptoms of, 524
Vagus nerve, 642, 643, 644
  tests for, 656
Value judgments in data collection interview, 42

Valves of Houston, 559
Valvular heart disease, 389
Varicocele, 554
Varicosities in pregnancy, 142, 362
Vas deferens
  anatomy and physiology of, 531-534
  examination of, 546
Vascular abnormalities of skin, 125
  in child, 138-139
  in newborn, 136
Vascular bruit; *see* Bruits
Vascular headaches, 203
Vascular spiders, 125, 128, 137, 142, 362
  of breast in pregnancy, 425
Vasculitis, headache in, 190
Vegans, pregnant, 104
Vegetables in food pyramid, 102
Vegetarians, pregnant, 104
Veins, 361, 362
Venereal warts, 522
  health history and, 492
  signs and symptoms of, 524
Venous hum, 383, 452
Venous peripheral vascular examination, 375-377
Venous pressure, jugular, 375-377, 383
Venous stasis ulcers, 130, 365, 366
Venous thrombophlebitis, 394
  contraceptives and, 365
Venous thrombosis, 394, 536
Ventilation, 79, 80
  respiratory, 317
Ventral roots of spinal nerves, 644
Ventricular hypertrophy
  left, 390
    apical pulsations in, 377
  right, 390
Ventricular septal defects, 392
Vernix caseosa, 116, 117
Verruca, 126
Vertebra prominens, 322
Vertebrae
  cervical, 185
    assessment of, 601, 626
  racial variation of, 590
  spinal column, spinal cord, and spinal nerves exiting, 643
  spinal processes of, 605
Vertebral arteries, 637, 640
Vertigo, 251
  in health history, 648
Vesicles, 127
Vesicular breath sounds, 338-340
Vestibular function
  loss of, 271
  testing of, 261
Vestibulocochlear nerve, 642, 643, 644
Vibration sensation, 67, 660-661
Vietnamese health practices, 35, 37
VII; *see* Vocational Interest Inventory
Viral hepatitis, 474
Viral infection
  of lips, 239
  of liver, 474
  of skin, hair, and nails, 148-150
Virginal speculum, 70
Viscera, percussion of, 74, 75
Vision, 279-280; *see also* Eye and visual system
  decreased or absent, 299

Vision—*cont'd*
  difficulty with, 281
  examination of, 284-287, 302
  peripheral defects of, 307
  visual acuity assessment in, 284-287, 302, 653
    in child, 297
    "E" chart for, 65, 284, 297
    health promotion and, 315
    near vision chart for, 66
    of newborn and infant, 280, 296
    in older adult, 298
    peripheral visual defects in, 285, 307
    screening and, 315
    Snellen chart for, 65, 284
Vital capacity in older adult, 322
Vital signs, 76-82
  blood pressure in, 79-81, 82
  of child, 86-87
  in integrated physical examination, 686
  of newborn and infant, 78, 84-85
  of older adult, 87
  in pregnancy, 87
  pulse in, 78
  respiration in, 79, 80
  temperature in, 76
Vitamins
  A
    deficiency of, 98
    in pregnancy, 104
  B
    deficiency of, 98, 99
    recommended dietary allowances of, 100-101
  C
    deficiency of, 98, 99
    recommended dietary allowances of, 100
  D
    deficiency of, 98
    recommended dietary allowances of, 100
  deficiency of, 98-99
    in older adult, 112
  E, 100
  fat-soluble, 100
  K
    deficiency of, 98
    recommended dietary allowances of, 100
  recommended dietary allowances of, 100-101
  stool color and, 566
  water-soluble, 100-101
Vitiligo, 119, 122, 126
Vitreous humor, hemorrhage in, 292
Vocal fremitus, 335
Vocal sounds or vocal resonance, 340-342
Vocational Interest Inventory, 22
Voice change, 221
  assessment of, 652
Vomiting
  history of, 443
  in pregnancy, 440
Voodoo, 34
VSD; *see* Ventricular septal defects
Vulva, 481
  common problems and conditions of, 520-521
  self-examination of, 527

W

Warts, 126
  venereal, 522
    health history and, 492

Warts—*cont'd*
  venereal—*cont'd*
    signs and symptoms of, 524
Washington Guide to Promoting Development in the Young Child, 22
Wasting of muscles, 99
Water-hammer pulse, 370
Water-soluble vitamins, recommended dietary allowances for, 100-101
Weakness, muscular, 593, 597, 598, 599
Weber test, 260, 655
Weight, 82, 83, 84-85, 94
  of adolescent, 86
  blood pressure and, 81
  changes in, history of, 444
  of child, 86, 87-91
  health promotion and, 635
  of newborn and infant, 83, 106
  of older adult, 87, 111-112
  in postpartum and lactating women, 105
  in pregnancy, 87, 97
  variation in desirable, 93-94
Weight-for-stature index in preschool and school-age child, 109
Wet mount, vaginal or cervical, 505
Wheal, 127
Wheezes
  sibilant, 341
  sonorous, 341
Whispered pectoriloquy, 342
Whispered voice test, 259, 655
Whiteheads, 139
Why questions in data collection interview, 42
WIC; *see* Women, Infant and Children program
Willis, circle of, 637, 640
Witchcraft, 34
Witch's milk, 423
Women, Infant and Children program, 104
Wood's lamp, 70
Wrist
  assessment of, 610, 611, 626-627
    in integrated examination, 687
  pain in, 633
  range of motion of, 612, 613
  supporting structures of, 590
Write-ups; *see* Documentation
Wry neck, 207

X

Xerosis, 98

Y

Yeast infection, 522, 524
Yin and yang, 35
Yogurt in food pyramid, 102
Young adult
  assessment tools in, 18
  developmental assessment in, 18, 19
  developmental tasks of, 19

Z

Zinc, recommended dietary allowances of, 101